Professional Issues in Speech-Language Pathology and Audiology

THIRD EDITION

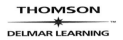

THOMSON

DELMAR LEARNING

Professional Issues in Speech-Language Pathology and Audiology

By Rosemary Lubinski and Lee Ann C. Golper

Vice President, Health Care Business Unit:
William Brottmiller

Director of Learning Solutions:
Matthew Kane

Acquisitions Editor:
Sherry Dickinson

Product Manager:
Molly Belmont

Editorial Assistant:
Angela Doolin

Marketing Director:
Jennifer McAvey

Marketing Manager:
Christopher Manion

Content Project Manager:
Katie Wachtl

Library of Congress Cataloging-in-Publication Data

Professional issues in speech-language pathology and audiology / edited by Rosemary Lubinski, Lee Ann C. Golper, Carol M. Frattali.—3rd ed.
   p. ; cm.
   Includes bibliographical references and index.
   ISBN 1-4180-1548-2 (alk. paper)
   1. Speech therapy—Practice. 2. Audiology—Practice. I. Lubinski, Rosemary. II. Golper, Lee Ann C., 1948- III. Frattali, Carol.
   [DNLM: 1. Speech-Language Pathology. 2. Audiology. 3. Professional Practice. WM 475 P9635 2007]
   RC428.5.P755 2007
   616.85'5—dc22   2006013090

ISBN: 1-4180-1548-2
ISBN-13: 978-1-4180-1548-0

NOTICE TO THE READER

✳

Professional Issues in Speech-Language Pathology and Audiology

THIRD EDITION

Edited By

ROSEMARY LUBINSKI, ED.D., CCC-SLP
University at Buffalo, SUNY

LEE ANN C. GOLPER, PH.D.
Vanderbilt University

CAROL M. FRATTALI, PH.D., BC-NCD
Formerly, National Institutes of Health

THOMSON
✳ ™
DELMAR LEARNING

Australia • Brazil • Canada • Mexico • Singapore • Spain
United Kingdom • United States

To the Memory of Carol Frattali

Carol Frattali wanted us to be the very best professionals that we can be. Rosemary and Lee Ann now continue the tradition, and Carol remains its guiding spirit.

In the end, we are the memories others have of us and the stories they still tell about us. Our Carol stories and our Carol memories are all beautiful.

Audrey Holland, Ph.D.

Contents

3   Professional Organizations 74

SECTION IV   Providing Quality Care 409

19 Policies and Procedures 411

Foreword

On professional issues in speech-language pathology—*Professional Issues in Speech-Language Pathology and Audiology* is a remarkable compilation of the most essential and useful information a practitioner needs to navigate the daily challenges encountered in the delivery of speech-language pathology services. Regardless of the setting (education, private practice, early intervention or health care), in which the services are rendered, this book provides information, strategies and techniques the reader will find useful. There are chapters packed with specifics helpful in certain work settings as well as chapters with information that applies to all settings, such as competencies, ethics, evidence-based practice, professional liability, and professional autonomy. Clinicians will find themselves frequently reaching for this book when they have a 'professional' question.

Faculty will find the text essential when teaching professional issues courses as they help prepare students to begin their careers. Some of the chapters can also be integrated into clinical courses. Armed with the information they'll learn from this text, graduates will find themselves well prepared to enter the work force and will find that they'll refer to this text over and over whenever they meet a new professional challenge.

Nancy B. Swigert, M.A., CCC/SLP
Past President of ASHA

On professional issues in audiology—The ancestors of the professions were very insightful in establishing the basic principles on which the discipline is founded, and identifying the challenges we would face with the growth of the professions. The chapter detailing the history and milestones in the development of the professions should be a must read for students. As the decades have passed, audiology has evolved from an almost purely "service" profession to one of greater entrepreneurial emphasis, covering a scope of practice, that has expanded markedly as technology and the science of the profession has enhanced our understanding of the vestibular, auditory and neurological systems. The practical, professional, social and regulatory information provides practitioners, faculty and students valuable perspectives, better preparing them to utilize their critical thinking-reasoning skills by making more informed, evidence-based decisions affecting the lives of patients and students. The authors have done an outstanding job of addressing the challenges of practicing in an environment where professional autonomy is emerging, new interdisciplinary alliances are being formed, funding streams are limited, evidence-based practice is a requirement, and the knowledge base has demanded a doctoral degree be the minimum standard for independent practice in audiology. The text offers a realistic look at the professional issues surrounding audiology and the resultant practice of the profession. At its best, providing diagnostic information and treatment that was unimaginable a few decades ago, and, at its worst, fragmented and fraught with challenges as to where, and how it fits in the health care and educational systems of today.

The wealth of information contained in the text helps everyone from seasoned professionals to students understand the historical value of issues, and offers a perspective on the complexities of implementing the provision of highest quality services, and strategies for teaching it to others. Each chapter demonstrates how practitioners and students can pose problems of practical importance, and search efficiently and effectively for solutions using the most current relevant evidence as a guide.

This is a "must have" text for practicing professionals, faculty and students by recognized experts in each of the professional issues addressed. It is an extraordinary compilation of information organized into a logical, understandable text that effectively describes the internal and external, professional, social and regulatory influences that affect the science of the profession, education of audiologists, and practice of audiology: e.g., who we are, how we got here, and why we do what we do.

Lawrence W. Higdon, M.S., CCC-A
Past President of ASHA

Preface

The 3rd edition of *Professional Issues in Speech-Language Pathology and Audiology,* like the earlier versions, is intended as a primary text and resource for faculty, students, and practicing clinicians seeking a comprehensive review of contemporary issues in communication sciences and disorders. This book is aimed at helping entry-level and practicing clinicians better understand the critical challenges facing the professions of audiology and speech-language pathology today. We have again brought together subject matter experts across a wide array of topics with the goal of providing within a single text a range and depth of treatment of contemporary subjects of relevance to audiology and speech-language pathology that cannot be found elsewhere. Several chapters are dense with terminology, facts, resource lists, websites, and reference documents. This information should serve as a desk reference for audiologists and speech-language pathologists in clinical practice and academic settings.

ORGANIZATION OF THE TEXT

The twenty eight chapters in this text are organized within five sections: Overview of the Profession, Employment Issues, Expanding Clinical Populations and Settings, Providing Quality Care, and Evidence Based Practice. Each chapter in the book begins with a description of the scope of the subject matter to be addressed and ends with a summary of the key points covered. Some chapters also include case studies and illustrative vignettes, which are intended to provide a real life context for the subjects discussed. Section I, Overview of the Professions, includes chapters that have global application to the discipline of communication sciences and disorders. The intent of this section is to examine how we organize ourselves professionally, the competencies we need to do our jobs, the ethical and legal issues we face, the clinical specializations we might move into, and the international scope of the discipline. In Chapter 1, Lubinski and Golper introduce professional issues such as access to services, maintaining currency, and successful "survival skills" in our profession, discussions that will be taken up again elsewhere in the book. They also provide a thumbnail look and chronology of some of the history of audiology and speech-pathology to provide a context for a number of contemporary issues. Chapter 2 contains information of critical importance both to the developing and seasoned clinician: establishing competencies and credentials. Battle provides us with a comprehensive review of education, certification, and licensure requirements and practices in the professions. Hale and Bess highlight the history, purposes, structures, and operations of our major professional associations in Chapter 3. In Chapter 4, Miller focuses our attention on professional ethics that is followed by a new chapter on a critically important topic by Horner, professional liability, Chapter 5. Tying up this section is Chapter 6 by Worrall and Hickson discussing audiology and speech-language pathology outside of the U.S. and international alliances.

Section II, Employment Issues, moves to the general topic of work settings and employment. Slater starts us thinking about some of the global work force issues facing the professions in Chapter 7. Lubinski advises clinicians about how to prepare for employment in Chapter 8, including how to transition from one employment setting to another. In Chapter 9, Brown and Handlesman discuss the importance of achieving professional autonomy as well as collaboration between professionals. And, this section ends with a discussion of the topic of support personnel within the discipline by Paul and Sparks, Chapter 10.

In Section III, Expanding Clinical Populations and Professional Settings, we take a look at specific populations and service settings in our professions. This section begins with an overview of special populations in Chapter 11 by Lubinski and Masters. Next we provide a series of chapters covering an array of policy and regulatory issues of particular significance to the profession, beginning with White's chapter on health care legislation, regulation, and financing, Chapter 12 and service delivery in health care settings by Cornett, Chapter 13. We

then turn to early intervention and education settings, with Chapter 14, on educational policy by Eger; Chapter 15 on service delivery in educational settings by Staskowski and Nelson; and Chapter 16 by Koury on service delivery with very young children in early intervention programs. Wolf then provides us with a glimpse at the world and issues faced in private practice service delivery settings in Chapter 17. This section ends with how to promote access to audiology and speech-language pathology services across service settings, Chapter 18 by Hallowell and Henri.

In Section IV, Providing Quality Care, we begin by considering Rao's guidance on establishing and implementing policies and procedures as guideposts for quality, Chapter 19. Next Kummer's chapter, Chapter 20, emphasizes the importance of leadership in defining and achieving quality goals and outcomes. Topics specifically related to quality improvement programs within service settings include a chapter on infection control and prevention, by Lubinski, Chapter 21; and identifying and preventing abuse within our client populations across the age span, Chapter 22, also by Lubinski. Next, Kayser, Chapter 23, discusses the elements that are necessary to achieve and maintain quality services within culturally and linguistically diverse clinical populations. The key to maintaining quality service rests with developing and maintaining competencies in clinical staff; thus, McCrae and Golper review the supervisory processes in both clinical training programs and in the work place, Chapter 24. In Chapter 25, Torrens gives us a comprehensive review of the variety of ways in which technology can enhance service delivery and improve efficiencies and the quality of services provided. Finally, this section ends with the interpersonal and attitudinal side of quality—how to reduce stress and deal with conflict in the workplace by Lubinski, Chapter 26.

In the last section, Section V, we end the text with an emphasis on maintaining our scientific bases and Evidence-Based Practice. In Chapter 27, Kent provides an analysis of the current status and future of our science, and in Chapter 28 Golper and Brown provide a review and tutorial on applying some of the tools of evidence-based practice to evaluate, guide, and enhance clinical service delivery. We are pleased to be able to bring such an expert panel of contributors to a discussion of these issues of vital interest to audiologists and speech-language pathologists.

In this 3rd Edition, Lee Ann C. Golper agreed to serve as co-editor as a labor of love in tribute to the memory of her dear friend and colleague, Carol M. Frattali. Lubinski and Frattali had co-edited the first two editions of this text, published in 1994 and 2001, setting a standard of excellence that we hope has been maintained in this edition. No one could ever fill the many spaces left empty by Carol Frattali's untimely passing. This text is dedicated to her memory.

NEW TO THIS EDITION

New to the 3rd edition is Table A guiding the reader to the content of the chapters that is tied to the Council for Clinical Certification (CFCC) standards for the Certificate of Clinical Competence (CCC) in both audiology and speech-language pathology. Review of this table will help faculty and students access information relevant to these standards. The matrix contains a list of chapters across one axis and a listing of the standards down the other. Table A is found right before Section I of the book (pg. xlii).

Many of the chapters feature useful appendices. The appendices are comprised of frequently referred to documents, forms, and guidelines.

Another important feature in this edition is the "Critical Thinking" section at the end of each chapter. In the earlier editions this section was referred to as "Discussion Questions." In this edition, the contributors are taking the discussion questions one step further by asking the reader "what do you think?" We are asked to consider critically what we have just read; to judge the validity, biases, or incongruities of the information or opinions contained in the chapter; and to apply the information to address real world dilemmas and problems. We are asked to consider the pros and cons in various solutions. The goal is to spark classroom discussions that might yield divergent opinions and points of view. As is so often the case in our professional lives, when we reflect on complex issues and consider all of the sides of a problem there may be no single right answer or a simple solution.

This text also includes new subjects that were requested by consumers and reviewers of previous editions, with discussion of a variety of new topics, such as our historical roots, professional liability, technology, leadership, and supervision in the workplace as well as in clinical education, evidence-based practices, and other topics.

About the Authors

Rosemary Lubinski received her B.S. from Bloomsburg University (PA) and her M.A. and Ed.D. from Columbia University. She is Professor of Speech-Language Pathology in the Department of Communicative Disorders and Sciences at the University of Buffalo where she has spent her entire academic career. Dr. Lubinski has worked as a university professor and clinical supervisor as well as a clinician in the schools, a hospital outpatient rehabilitation center, a nursing home, and home health care. Her primary interests are in the communication problems of the elderly and those with dementia, aphasia, and traumatic brain injury. She is a frequent presenter at national and international conferences and the author of numerous articles and chapters as well as the texts *Dementia and Communication, Communication Technologies for the Elderly: Vision, Hearing and Speech,* and now the third edition of this text. A Fellow of ASHA, Dr. Lubinski's current research is funded by the Alzheimer's Society of Canada. She is active in ASHA's Special Interest 15 Gerontology.

Lee Ann C. Golper completed her B.A. at Indiana University, M.S. at Portland State University, and Ph.D. at University of Oregon. Her principal interests are in medical speech-language pathology, neurologic communication disorders, and health services administration. She is the author the text *Sourcebook for Medical Speech Pathology,* now in its second edition and the coeditor of *Business Matters: A Guide of Speech-Language Pathologists,* a publication of the American Speech-Language-Hearing Association. She and Robert T. Wertz are the co-editors of the Clinical Competence Series, Thomson Delmar Learning. She is Board Certified in Neurogenic Communication Disorders (BC-NCD) in Adults by the Academy of Neurologic Communication Disorders and Sciences. She has been a faculty member in neurology and otolaryngology departments within medical center training programs and in communication sciences and disorders graduate programs since 1978. She worked for several years as a staff speech pathologist in the Department of Veterans Affairs Medical Centers in Portland, OR, and Louisville, KY, and for the past 13 years has been an administrator of multidisciplinary health services programs within university medical centers. She is currently an associate professor and Director of the Speech-Language Pathology Division in the Department of

Hearing and Speech Sciences, School of Medicine, Vanderbilt University. Dr. Golper is a Fellow of the American Speech-Language-Hearing Association, a Fellow of the American Academy of Otolaryngology-Head and Neck Surgery, and a Scientific Fellow of the American Heart Association-American Stroke Association.

Carol M. Frattali received her B.S. in Speech-Language Pathology and Audiology at Ithaca College, her M.A. in Speech-Language Pathology at the San Francisco State University, and her Ph.D. in Speech-Language Pathology at the University of Pittsburgh. Her clinical and research interests were in the areas of the neurocognitive bases of language and its disorders, with an emphasis in discourse processing, social discourse production, and neuro-linguistic approaches to assessment and treatment in aphasia. Her extensive publications include a textbook focused on outcomes assessment methods, *Measuring Outcomes in Speech-Language Pathology.* She held Board Certified in Neurologic Communication Disorders in Adults (BCNCD-A) from the Academy of Neurologic Communication Disorders and Sciences (ANCDS) and was a Fellow in the American Speech-Language Hearing Association (ASHA). Dr. Frattali was the Research Coordinator, in Speech and Language Pathology at the National Institutes of Health Clinical Center and an Adjunct Professor in the Department of Hearing and Speech Sciences, at the University of Maryland at College Park, and a Research Professor at the George Washington University, Department of Speech and Hearing Sciences.

Acknowledgments

Dolores Battle would like to acknowledge the help given by Charles Diggs, Director of State and Consumer Advocacy, American Speech-Language Hearing Association.

Lee Ann C. Golper and Rosemary Lubinski offer their sincere thanks to Sue Hale for her review and assistance with the Council for Clinical Certification Standards reference guide provided within the front section of this text. They also wish to acknowledge the commentary and expertise provided by Judith Felson Duchan in her review of the historical information and chronology included in Chapter 1.

Ann Kummer would like to acknowledge Cincinnati Children's Hospital Medical center where she has been extremely fortunate to spend her career. She says, "Much of what I know about leadership and communication comes from working in an environment where there is strong leadership and positive communication at all levels. Cincinnati Children's is an organization that not only models this, but also encourages and recognizes these skills in all employees."

Diane Paul and Susan Sparks gratefully acknowledge the assistance of Vic S. Gladstone, Ph.D., CCC-A (Chief Staff Officer for Audiology, American Speech-Language-Hearing Association Rockville, MD) and Nancy K. Madison, MA, CCC-A (Madison Audiology Consulting Services, Cheney, Washington) in the preparation of her chapter. The authors also want to acknowledge Tobi Frymark, Tracy Schooling, and Beverly Wang (National Center for Evidence-Based Practice in Communication Disorders, Rockville, MD) for assisting with the systematic literature search.

John Torrens would like to acknowledge his wife, Deanna Torrens, for her support and InterActive Therapy Group for providing the professional environment to pursue a variety of professional interests.

Linda Worrall and Louise Hickson wish to acknowledge the research assistance provided by Joanne Castner.

Finally, the editors want to express their appreciation for the comments, corrections, and suggestions made by the reviewers of earlier versions of this edition; several of those suggestions have been incorporated into the final text.

—Rosemary Lubinski, Ed.D.
—Lee Ann C. Golper, Ph.D.

Contributors

Dolores E. Battle, Ph.D.
Professor Speech-Language Pathology and
    Senior Advisor to President For Equity
    and Campus Diversity
Buffalo State College
Buffalo, New York

Fred H. Bess, Ph.D.
Professor of Audiology
Chair of Hearing and Speech Sciences
    Department
Vanderbilt Bill Wilkerson Center
Vanderbilt University
Nashville, Tennessee

Karen E. Brown, Ph.D.
Vanderbilt Bill Wilkerson Center
Vanderbilt University
Nashville, Tennessee

Janet Brown, M.A.
Director, Health Care Services in Speech-
    Language Pathology
American Speech-Language-Hearing Association
Rockville, Maryland

Becky Sutherland Cornett, Ph.D.
Associate Compliance Director
The Ohio State University Medical Center
Columbus, Ohio

Diane L. Eger, Ph.D.
Diacomm Consulting, Inc.
Moon Township, Pennsylvania

Lee Ann C. Golper, Ph.D.
Associate Professor and Administrative Director
    of Clinical Programs in Speech-Language
    Pathology
Department of Hearing and Speech Sciences
Vanderbilt Bill Wilkerson Center
Vanderbilt University
Nashville, Tennessee

Sue T. Hale, M.C.D.
Assistant Professor
Director of Clinical Education
Department of Hearing and Speech Sciences
Vanderbilt Bill Wilkerson Center
Vanderbilt University
Nashville, Tennessee

Brooke Hallowell, Ph.D.
Director and Associate Professor
School of Hearing, Speech and Language
    Sciences
Ohio University
Athens, Ohio

Jaynee Handelsman, Ph.D.
Assistant Director Vestibular Testing Center
Department of Otolaryngology
University of Michigan Health System
Ann Arbor, Michigan

Bernard P. Henri, Ph.D.
Executive Director
Cleveland Hearing and Speech Center
Cleveland, Ohio

Louise Hickson, Ph.D.
Associate Professor in Audiology and Deputy
    Head of School
Communication Disability in Ageing Research
    Centre
School of Health and Rehabilitation Sciences
The University of Queensland
Brisbane, Australia

Jennifer Horner, Ph.D., J.D.
Associate Professor, and Program Director,
    Communication Sciences and Disorders
Chair, Department of Rehabilitation Sciences
Medical University of South Carolina
College of Health Professions
Charleston, South Carolina

Hortencia Kayser, Ph.D.
Professor
Department of Communication Sciences
    & Disorders
Saint Louis University
St. Louis, Missouri

Raymond D. Kent, Ph.D.
Professor
Department of Communicative Disorders
University of Wisconsin-Madison
Madison, Wisconsin

Laurie Nash Koury, M.A.
Private Practitioner
Research Specialist
Department of Communication Disorders
    and Sciences
University at Buffalo
Buffalo, New York

Ann W. Kummer, Ph.D.
Senior Director, Division of Speech-Language
    Pathology
Cincinnati Children's Hospital Medical Center
    and Professor of Clinical Pediatrics
University of Cincinnati Medical Center
Cincinnati, Ohio

Rosemary Lubinski, Ed.D.
Professor
Department of Communicative Disorders
    and Sciences
University of Buffalo, SUNY
Buffalo, New York

M. Gay Masters, Ph.D.
Assistant Professor
Department of Surgery
University of Louisville
Louisville, Kentucky

Elizabeth S. McCrea, Ph.D.
Clinical Professor
Department of Speech and Hearing Sciences
Indiana University
Bloomington, Indiana

Thomas D. Miller, Ph.D., J.D.
Professor
Department of Communication Sciences
    and Disorders
Nazareth College of Rochester
Rochester, New York

Nicola Nelson, Ph.D.
Charles Van Riper Professor
Department of Speech-Language Pathology
    and Audiology
Director Ph.D. in Interdisciplinary Health Studies
College of Health and Human Services
Western Michigan University
Kalamazoo, Michigan

Diane R. Paul, Ph.D.
Director, Clinical Issues in Speech-Language
    Pathology
American Speech-Language-Hearing Association
Rockville, Maryland

Paul R. Rao, Ph.D.
Vice President, Clinical Services, Quality
    Improvement, and Corporate Compliance
Privacy Liaison
National Rehabilitation Hospital
Washington, DC
Visiting Professor, University of Maryland
College Park, Maryland

Sarah Slater, M.S.
Director, Survey Research
American Speech-Language-Hearing
    Association
Rockville, Maryland

Susan E. Sparks, M.A.
Speech-Language Pathology Assistant Program
Shoreline Community College
Seattle, Washington

Maureen Staskowski, Ph.D.
Consultant for Speech and Language Impaired
Macomb Intermediate School District
Clinton Township, Michigan

John Torrens, Ph.D.
Interactive Therapy Group
Jamesville, NY

Steven C. White, Ph.D.
Director, Health Care Economics and Advocacy
American Speech-Language-Hearing Association
Rockville, Maryland

Kenneth E. Wolf, Ph.D.
Professor of Otolaryngology
Associate Dean for Educational Affairs
Charles R. Drew University of Medicine
    and Science
Los Angeles, California

Linda Worrall, Ph.D.
Professor
Communication Disability in Ageing Research
    Centre
School of Health and Rehabilitation Sciences
The University of Queensland
Brisbane, Australia

T A B L E A Matrix of Chapter Content Relevant to the Council for Clinical Certification Standards for the Certificates of Clinical Competence

	Ch 1	Ch 2	Ch 3	Ch 4	Ch 5	Ch 6	Ch 7	Ch 8	Ch 9	Ch 10	Ch 11	Ch 12
Audiology Standards												
IV-B1. Professional Codes of Ethics		X	X	X	X	X			X	X		
IV-B2- Patient Characteristics											X	
IV-B12 Infection/universal precautions												
IV-B15 Research	X											
IV-B17 Health Care/Education										X		X
IV-B18 Cultural Diversity	X					X	X				X	
IV-B19 Supervision										X		
IV-B20 Laws, reg, etc		X		X	X			X		X		X
Speech-Language Standards												
IV-C Prevention/Identification												
C1 Interact with others	X											
C3 Identify at risk for hearing							X				X	
IV-D Evaluation												
D1 Interact with others	X											
C2 Evaluation information												X
D15 Maintain Records				X	X							
D16 Communicates Results	X			X	X				X			
IV-E Treatment												
E1 Interact with others	X											
E5 Culturally sensitive	X										X	
E6 Collaborate with others	X										X	
E12 Assess efficacy	X											
E14 Serve as advocate	X								X		X	
E16 Maintain records				X	X							
E17 Communicate results	X											
III-E Knowledge of Ethical Conduct		X	X	X	X							
III-F Research	X											
III-G Contemporary Prof Issues	X	X	X	X	X	X	X	X	X	X	X	X
III-H Credentialing		X	X									X

Ch 13	Ch 14	Ch 15	Ch 16	Ch 17	Ch 18	Ch 19	Ch 20	Ch 21	Ch 22	Ch 23	Ch 24	Ch 25	Ch 26	Ch 27	Ch 28
				X											
			X		X					X					
								X							
														X	X
X	X	X	X	X	X	X		X							
			X							X					
							X				X				
X	X	X	X	X	X	X	X	X	X						
									X						
		X	X		X		X						X		
			X							X					
		X	X		X		X						X		
X	X	X	X												X
						X	X								
X		X	X				X								
		X	X		X		X						X		
			X							X					
X	X	X	X		X										
															X
X	X	X	X		X	X									
X		X				X	X								
								X							
								X							
														X	X
X	X	X	X	X	X	X	X	X	X	X	X	X	X	X	X
X	X	X													

Overview of the Professions

1

Professional Issues: From Roots to Reality

ROSEMARY LUBINSKI, EDD
LEE ANN C. GOLPER, PHD

SCOPE OF CHAPTER

Most of us were attracted to the professions of speech-language pathology and audiology because of our genuine desire to help individuals communicate better. A certain noble motivation pervades our professional identity. We assess and diagnose communication and swallowing disorders; select appropriate technologies; provide management to correct or improve hearing, speech, language, voice, and swallowing; counsel clients and their significant others; ensure individuals with hearing, speech, language, and swallowing impairments are able to achieve their maximal functional capability; participate in prevention programs; educate others about hearing, speech, language, voice, and swallowing; and conduct basic and applied research to advance the scientific bases of our professions.

Students in communicative disorders are particularly eager to learn how to begin assessing and treating clients. Efficacious, effective, and cost-effective evaluation and treatment services are at the core of much of what we do. Practicing professionals are always seeking better assessment and intervention techniques and technologies to serve clients. For communication disorders professions to remain viable in today's society, they must balance their ideals with the realism that is imposed by clients, caregivers, payers, and policy makers. Our commitment to improving communication skills and opportunities across the age span must be constantly infused with new ideas and technologies to address the societal and economic forces that challenge and enhance our efforts.

Today's professionals need to be equally knowledgeable and skilled in the most current and evidence-based assessment and intervention techniques *and* with societal trends, policy making, and challenges to ethical practice. In addition, your own interpersonal skills must enhance the services you provide. You must be able to articulate convincingly the value of your service. Thomas Friedman in his book *The World is Flat* (2005) talks about the changes to all professions through globalization and technology. He says that to survive in today's work world, we must not get mired in the past; rather we must embrace change and ". . . create value through leadership, relationships, and creativity" (p. 14). Our value will emanate from a professional culture that is based in science, leadership, interpersonal skills, and vision.

In the past two editions of *Professional Issues in Speech-Language Pathology and Audiology,* we asked readers to think broadly about the factors that influence our daily practice. Certainly the changes in health care and education have headed the list, as have expanding scopes of practice. (See the Appendix at the end of this chapter for the most current Scopes of Practice in Audiology and Speech-Language Pathology). While these issues remain dynamic and important, let us also consider some other themes that influence how we think about our profession and those we serve.

It is about 80 years since the first individuals met to form a professional organization concerned with communication sciences and disorders. The early pioneers in the professions are gone, but their legacies are still evident, and we need to maintain a historical record of the roots of our professions. Few students today know the names or contributions of the founding women and men in our professions. Thus, we begin this chapter with a brief history of the professions to provide today's practitioners with some conception of their heritage.

A second topic we introduce in this chapter is *access*. Access is a theme that underlies so much of what we do. How do clients access our services and what factors influence that access? How do our ser-

vices help our clients access the educational, medical, employment, and social opportunities they need? What types of technologies provide communication access for our clients? How do legal considerations and economic issues affect access to audiology and speech-language pathology services? How does the community provide access to opportunities that enhance communication? Our work should be one of helping clients have "access-ability."

A third philosophical topic we would like you to consider is *currency*. Those of us who entered the professions a decade or more ago appreciate that the skills and knowledge needed to provide state-of-the art service have expanded exponentially. We serve a more diverse group of clients who have more challenging needs. The demands from today's educational and health care marketplace require that each of us can provide technologically sophisticated, evidence-based procedures that result in functional outcomes. The dollars to support our services are limited, and coverage is typically determined by groups and individuals outside the professions. Further, requirements for continuing education from national organizations and state licensure agencies dictate that clinicians maintain their clinical currency. Clinical mastery can only be accomplished through actively seeking continuing education and professional development.

The final topic we discuss is *success skills* in the workplace. As undergraduate and graduate students, you invest your time in learning the scientific knowledge and clinical skills that will make you a professional audiologist or speech-language pathologist. What you will soon learn as you enter the professional arena is that you must acquire numerous other thinking and interpersonal skills to work efficiently and effectively as a member of a team in any workplace.

These topics evoke numerous practice-related issues that eventually must lead to new strategies if our professions are to provide the highest quality and most efficient service. Although presented individually, these themes of history, accessibility, currency, and workplace success skills have important implications for how we learn to be communication disorders specialists and how we practice. This chapter challenges new and mature clinicians to consider their vision of themselves as professionals: Do you consider yourself to be a reactive or proactive clinician? Would you say your professional roots are shallow or deep and branching? Are your clinical approaches aligned with the values of today's society? Do you use science and technology as the basis of your work? Do you respect the uniqueness of individual clients? Today's professional needs to demonstrate a new intelligence that emerges from this type of continued critical evaluation of how we approach our values and our work.

HISTORY OF THE PROFESSIONS

Human beings undoubtedly have been fascinated by normal and disordered communication since the time we first discovered the capacity to use our speech and hearing to communicate. That fascination and a shared passion to improve the lives of individuals with hearing and speech disorders brought groups of people together in the early part of the past century to lay the cornerstones of the discipline of communication sciences and disorders and pave the way for the professions of audiology and speech-language pathology. This section offers a brief look at a few of the events and influences that were a part of that history.

What Is a Profession?

To appreciate the multilayered history of audiology and speech-language pathology, let's consider some of the features of a "profession." A profession is made up of a *body of people* with specialized *knowledge* who are engaged in similar endeavors or a *shared occupation* with recognized *standards* for *education* and *technical skills* and *credentials*. These people follow a consensual code of *conduct* and *ethics*. Our profession defines us. When we say we belong to a particular profession or we have a particular occupation, we are expressing who we are. Our profession tells others something about our interests, employment, education, skills and knowledge, credentials, socioeconomic status, and

standards of behavior; consequently, it is important that we carefully consider and define the practices that are a part of our profession—our scope of practice. The scopes of practice for audiologists and speech-language pathologists have been thoughtfully framed in the policy documents within the American Speech-Language-Hearing Association's Scope of Practice in Audiology (ASHA, 2004c) and Scope of Practice in Speech-Language Pathology (ASHA, 2001). See the Appendix after this chapter for copies of the Scopes of Practice.

A profession has multiple dimensions and layers, as does its history. Thus, to understand the origins of our occupational titles, or the principles and practices that are the basis of our profession today, we would need to understand who the founding mothers and fathers were, how science and technologies have changed practices, how standards have affected our education, how professional organizations originated and evolved, and how other factors, such as world events and economic factors, have shaped our practices. We cannot begin to address more than a few aspects of this history in just a few pages here. At best we can highlight selected parts of the evolutionary development of our history and its influences in a cursory manner and take at quick look at a superficial chronology. The reader is encouraged to refer to more comprehensive historical reviews elsewhere, listed in the references and resources sections, where the details have been far better elaborated. We should emphasize, though, that history helps us to put contemporary issues into context; thus, a historical context is a part of the discussions of specific topics in several other chapters in this text.

Roots

Publications going back to antiquity contain references to speech, hearing, and the science of sound (Hunt, 1978). Some of the earliest textbooks in medicine dating back to the 1600s described the structures of the ear and vocal mechanism and proposed theories of audition and phonation (Fabricus, 1600). Most historians, however, point to the work and writings coming out of Europe in the early to mid-1800s as a period when the basic ideas and concepts that led to the formation of our professions really began to take shape (O'Neill, 1987). We can appreciate the importance of the 1800s as a formative period for the professions of audiology and speech-language pathology by considering how often contemporary literature related to hearing, deafness, stuttering, aphasia, and child development begins with citations of seminal work published by 19th-century authors. It was during that time that the early roots of our professions emerged from the work of theorists and practitioners across several disciplines, mainly in medicine, psychology, linguistics, phonetics, acoustics, elocution, and education.

Within this formative era one finds common roots for the professions of audiology and speech-language pathology. Although we conventionally think of these two professional areas of practice as having a distinct history, they did not spring up from different parts of the world, at different points in time, with different parent disciplines, or from practitioners or investigators who had different interests—nor did God create the first audiologist out of the rib of a speech-language pathologist. The two fields share a common, interrelated parentage.

In his review, O'Neill (1987) discusses the early history of audiology and speech-language pathology and notes overlapping and converging interests in speech, language, and hearing by medical practitioners in continental Europe and both physicians and elocutionists in Great Britain in the mid-1800s. O'Neill describes how interest in developing remediation approaches to improve the speech of deaf speakers in Scotland and England ultimately sparked the development of the profession of *speech correction*. While interest in habilitation of deaf speakers was growing in Britain and Europe, clinical diagnostic tests of hearing using tuning forks were being introduced (the Rinne and Weber tests) and the use of electrically powered audiometers was being investigated. Among European physicians, there was growing interest in diseases of the ear (otology). Notably, two such physicians, Urbanschitsch and Bezold, had a particular interest in speech and auditory training for the deaf (see Silverman's translation, Urbanschitsch, 1982). Bezold's method focused

on units of speech while Urbanschitsch emphasized individual speech sounds (O'Neill, 1987). O'Neill notes that these two physicians, referred to as the "fathers of audiology," were principally known for their interests in techniques aimed at improving speech production in the deaf and aural habilitation for individuals with hearing loss. Bezold and Urbanschitsch can be viewed as early pioneers in aural habilitation as well as rehabilitative audiology.

Let's consider another example of the common origins of audiology and speech-language pathology by looking at the legacies of Alexander Graham Bell. Working with his father (both were elocutionists) in Edinburgh, Scotland, in 1860, the Bells developed and applied a formal system of speech rehabilitation for the deaf, termed "Visible Speech." A. G. Bell went on to conduct experiments based on the idea of transmitting speech signals through electric energy and ultimately invented one of the first telephones (historians suggest the original inventor of the telephone was in fact not Bell, but rather an Italian-American named Meucci or, possibly, a German inventor). The photophone (in which sound is transferred by light) and wax recorders for sound recording (leading to the invention of the Gramaphone at Bell Laboratory) were also invented by Bell. Bell worked on one of the earliest versions of the audiometer at roughly the same time he developed a school of vocal physiology in Boston. Motivated by his experiences with deafness in his own family, he investigated the causes of deafness, including its inheritability. Later, during World War II as part of war-related research, scientists in the laboratory named for him, Bell Laboratory, invented the sound spectrograph (Bruce, 1973; Duchan, 2005; Eber, 1982), a technology that has been integral to the fields of hearing and speech sciences.

Many of principles, procedures, and technologies that are fundamental to the professions of speech-language pathology and audiology, as well as speech science and hearing science, can be traced to the legacies of Bell and his colleagues. He was interested in speech physiology, aural habilitation, hearing assessment, signal transmission, amplification, acoustics, and genetics. Bell, Thomas Gallaudet, and others contributed to the origins of the field of deaf education as well as audiology and the subspecialties of rehabilitative audiology and aural habilitation in speech-language pathology. Additionally, Bell was among the first to explore the genetics of hearing loss. Bell was clearly a creative thinker and interested in all sides of the problem in his approach to deafness, speech, and communication, and his work illustrates the common origins and interests of audiology and speech-language pathology.

What's in a Name?

Audiologist The first graduate degree in audiology in the United States was granted in 1946 at Northwestern University. This first program was headed by Dr. Raymond Carhart within the Department of Speech Communication (theater, rhetoric, drama), where the Speech Disorders program was already housed (see the chronology later in this chapter). Dr. Carhart is sometimes credited with having been the first to use the word *audiology,* but Northwestern University's archives credit Stanley Nowak, a hearing-aid distributor, as the individual who coined the term in 1939 (see Northwestern University Archives reference in the Resources section). Dr. Carhart noted the University of Illinois had the distinction of making the first academic faculty appointment in audiology, but Northwestern was the first to establish a school in that discipline. It is conceivable that the term *audiology* was in common usage at least by the early part of the 1940s. The first Doctor of Philosophy (PhD) degree in audiology was conferred in 1948 at Northwestern, and soon afterward PhDs in that field were conferred at other universities across the country where speech pathology programs were already housed. After the initial granting of graduate degrees in audiology, the occupational title *audiologist* came to be the preferred occupational designation, as it is today (see the definition of an audiologist in the Appendix).

Speech-Language Pathologist The history of the occupational title *speech-language pathologist* is less straightforward. One way to trace the evolution of the title *speech correctionist* to *speech-language pathologist* is by looking at how these terms were treated

within our professional societies and graduate programs. The term *speech correctionist* had been around for nearly a century before the first interest groups in speech correction began to organize themselves into formal societies. Physicians, elocutionists, educators, and others had been referring to their remediation practices for speech disorders as speech *correction*. In the early 1900s, groups with special interests in speech correction were formed within the National Education Association (NEA), a society mainly made up of individuals who were working in school settings, and slightly later within the National Association of Teachers of Speech (NATS), a professional society for individuals with interests in rhetoric, theater, and public speaking. These special interest groups eventually became formal societies. In 1918, the National Society for the Study and Correction of Speech Disorders (NSSCSD) was formed out of a special interest group in the NEA. The NSSCSD was headed by Walter Babcock Swift, a faculty member of Cleveland's Western Reserve University. The charter members, like the members of its parent organization, the NEA were principally working in school settings.

In 1925, the American Academy of Speech Correction (AASC) was (unofficially) chartered out of a special interest group within the National Association of Teachers of Speech (NATS). The NATS still exists today but has also undergone several name changes; it is now the National Communication Association. The initial members of the AASC were academics, psychologists, physicians, administrators, and individuals interested in speech communication, speech correction, and the study of speech disorders. This gave the AASC a somewhat different—more academic, multidisciplinary, and medical—orientation than that of Swift's school-allied organization.

The individual most instrumental in establishing the AASC is Carl Seashore of the University of Iowa. We will look more specifically at the legacies of the University of Iowa speech program, its leaders, and alumni later in this section. Dr. Seashore earned the first PhD in psychology from Yale in 1895. He went on to teach at the University of Iowa and was eventually appointed the dean of the graduate school where he founded the Department of Speech Disorders and appointed Lee Edward Travis as the first director. Dr. Travis had just earned his PhD in the Psychology Department at Iowa with emphasis in speech pathology in 1924. In 1925, Dr. Seashore organized a conference to bring together individuals from various disciplines with interests in speech disorders, its causes, symptoms, and treatment. A handful of individuals attending that Iowa conference convened at Lee Edward Travis' home to discuss forming a separate society; one of those individuals was Robert West. In his historical review of the origins of ASHA, Malone (1999) quotes West's description of how the decision to form a new society was made: "the Association began as an informal and impromptu meeting in Lee Travis' dining room in Iowa City. . . . The determination was expressed to call together a rump session of those interested in speech correction at the convention of the NATS" (p. 5). Thus, the American Academy of Speech Correction was formed. Chartered unofficially in 1925, the AASC had a small and selective membership made up of physicians (a psychiatrist and two otolaryngologists), psychologists, professors of English and speech, phoneticians, and speech correctionists, including those who were the first individuals to obtain doctor of philosophy degrees with emphasis in speech disorders: Sara Stinchfield (Hawke), who received her doctorate from University of Wisconsin in 1921; Lee Edward Travis, who received his doctorate from University of Iowa in 1924; and Robert West (the AASC's first president), who received his doctorate from University of Wisconsin in 1927 (Neidecker & Blosser, 1993; Duchan, 2004). Both Stinchfield and West were the first doctoral graduates of the University of Wisconsin's graduate program in speech disorders. Established in 1914, the University of Wisconsin's graduate program in speech disorders was the first such program in this country.

AASC eventually evolved to become ASHA. AASC was the more academic and medically allied organization, and it had a more exclusive membership than Swift's society, the NSSCSD (Duchan, 2004). The bylaws of the AASC, for example, allowed five new members to be added per year, and membership was limited to individuals who had graduate degrees (MD, PhD, DDS, or master's degrees), demonstrated scholarship (research and publications), and interest in speech correction and disorders. The founders of the AASC were motivated by a desire to establish standards and ethics and to initiate collaboration between disciplines with shared interests in speech disorders. The first activities of the AASC charter members were to draft a Code of Ethics and practice standards and to establish the AASC's authority to define the scope of practice. Due to his leadership role in the AASC and in establishing standards, West has been referred to as the "founding father" of the field of speech-language pathology (Duchan, 2004). West's interests spanned a variety of topics, including stuttering, voice, phonetics, and aphasia, but the work he is best known for is the text *The Rehabilitation of Speech: A Textbook of Diagnostic and Corrective Procedures,* written in 1937 with coauthors Kennedy and Carr, and a later edition, in 1947, with Kennedy, Carr, and Backus. As the AASC evolved, it later became the American Speech Correction Association (ASCA), then the American Speech and Hearing Association (ASHA), and ultimately, the American Speech-Language-Hearing Association (same acronym).

As we trace the development of the profession and its societies, there seems to have been a number of factors that contributed to shifting references to the occupational title away from *speech correctionist* to the more medically oriented *speech pathologist*. A move toward dropping the term *correctionist* was evident early in the development of the profession. The constitution of the AASC contained reference to a requirement for fellowship to include "knowledge of speech and its disorders" rather than knowledge of speech *correction* as stated in an earlier version. In 1934, when the AASC was renamed the American Speech Correction Association and officially separated itself from the general speech or speech communication members NATS, the revised constitution of the ASCA required its Fellow members to have "knowledge of speech *pathology*"—an official nod to the term *pathology* to refer to the work of the profession. By the early 1930s the reference to speech pathology was in common usage; consider Lee Edward Travis's popular handbook entitled *Speech Pathology* published in 1931. An additional influence came with the United States' involvement in World War II, which resulted in bringing speech and hearing clinicians into Veterans Administration hospitals to treat combat related communication impairments (e.g., aphasia, traumatic brain injury, hearing loss). The occupational title *speech pathologist* seems better aligned with this practice setting. It is evident that by the mid-1940s the reference to correctionist had virtually lost favor, and clinicians used the occupational titles of speech pathologist, speech clinician, or speech therapist. Other occupational titles, such as *communicologist,* and the occupational title commonly found in European countries, *logopedist,* have been suggested in the United States and rejected (Malone, 1999).

In 1976 the term *language* began to be added to the professional title in an effort to acknowledge language and speech as distinctive constructs and areas of concern and practice. In 1976, the Legislative Council of ASHA (LC 10-76) endorsed the use of *speech-language pathologist,* and in 1978, ASHA officially changed the name of the association to the American Speech-Language-Hearing Association (LC 22-78). Despite, or perhaps as a result of all of the name debates, and addition of more hyphens and more syllables, confusion continues among the general public and within the profession itself as to the preferred occupational title. The general public refers to us as *speech therapists,* and within the profession we sometimes revert to *speech pathologist,* as it is less of a mouthful. *Speech and Language Therapist* (SLT) is the standard occupational title in the United Kingdom, but ASHA's leadership has consistently cautioned against its use with the arguments: (1) *therapy* is only part of the scope of practice of speech-language pathology, and (2) *therapy* implies services that are physician-prescribed, an implication that works against the Association's efforts to achieve and maintain autonomy. Despite the Association's objections, however, references to "speech therapy" and "speech therapist" are frequently encountered in job descriptions, public policies, federal statutes, insurance policies, and other references to the profession. We continue to be challenged to increase the public's awareness and to discipline ourselves to use the preferred professional title, speech-language pathologist (SLP).

University of Iowa and Lee Edward Travis

We cannot consider the history of our profession without taking special note of the formative and pioneering role played by the University of Iowa and its graduates. We have mentioned earlier the role Carl Seashore and Lee Edward Travis played in chartering one of the first professional societies in the United States. Seashore and Travis were two of the most important and influential individuals in the history of our profession. When Seashore was the head of the Department of Psychology at University of Iowa, he brought together a faculty from medicine, psychology, and speech correction to form a program in speech correction headed by Travis. Travis completed his PhD in Psychology with emphasis in speech disorders in 1924, and subsequently Seashore invited him to serve as Director of the Psychology Clinic and Professor of Psychology and Speech at Iowa. Travis is known for his research in the cerebral dominance theory of stuttering and was among the first to use electrophysiological measurements of brain functions. Under Travis's leadership, the Iowa program adopted a philosophy that stressed the importance of understanding normal processes before we can understand abnormal processes. The Iowa program also promoted the principle that treatment should be referenced by research. In Chapter 2 of this text, Battle points out that the standard curriculum and course work in communication sciences and disorders requires that normal processes are studied before the course work in communication disorders. That perspective can be traced to the Iowa program, and it remains the cornerstone of the curriculum in communication sciences and disorders today. It would seem, however, that we have been less mindful of Travis's admonition to reference research in designing our treatment. Had we followed that principle more closely, our professions might be better situated to respond to the current demand for evidence-based practices (see Chapter 28).

In addition to establishing one of the first programs for the study of communication disorders in this country, the University of Iowa and the department heads for that program have been among the giants in our profession, starting with Travis and including Wendell Johnson, James Curtis, Kenneth Moll, and Hughlett Morris. The University of Iowa also has graduated some of our profession's premiere leaders and legends: Charles Van Riper, Grant Fairbanks, Max David (Mack) Steer, Herbert Koepp-Baker, and Charles Strother, to mention just a few of the alumni. Many of the Iowa alumni went on to establish and direct speech and hearing programs at other universities throughout the country, bringing the traditions and values laid down by Travis to subsequent generations of clinicians, educators, and scientists in communication sciences and disorders. Those of us who completed graduate programs in the United States are arguably less than "six degrees of separation" from Travis and the University of Iowa.

Stuttering and Autonomy

Stuttering deserves special discussion when considering our history. Stuttering was an early and prominent interest to scientists and practitioners who were concerned about protecting the public from charlatans providing "cures" for stuttering. These concerns motivated the formation of the AASC and its emphasis on standards and a Code of Ethics. Therapy for and causal theories about "stuttering and stammering" have a particularly long, and somewhat notorious, history, and stuttering has remained one of the speech disorders receiving the greatest attention in our literature. O'Neill (1987) points out during the 1800s, there were a number of theories regarding the causes and treatment of stuttering. An especially large number of textbooks were published on this topic, both in the United States and Great Britain; for example a text on the causes and treatment of stuttering and stammering (Hunt, 1870) was in its seventh edition in 1870. Consider also that the Boston Stammerers' Institute was established in 1867. Treatment theories ranged from surgical mutations of the tongue to a range of highly touted "curative methods" (Duchan, 2001;

O'Neill, 1987; Wollock & Perelló, 1989). Within the various practitioner circles with interest in stuttering in the late 1800s, the question of who should rightfully be treating this condition emerged. Rockey (1980) observes that the debate in Britain at that time over who should treat stutterers—speech correctionists or physicians—ultimately contributed to establishing our professional autonomy by identifying speech correction as a field of practice separate from a subspecialty of medicine.

Speech-Language Pathology and Audiology in the United States

A number of published historical reviews focus on the fields of speech-language pathology and audiology. Even though we said earlier that the 1800s were foundational to the profession, Wollock and Perrelló (1989) claim the French historian Jean Itard published a paper containing a historical, era-by-era review of the study of speech disorders—in 1817! Wollock's 1997 text, *The Noblest Animate Motion: Speech, Physiology and Medicine in Pre-Cartesian Linguistic Thought,* traces the theory of speech-language pathology from the 5th century BC through the 17th century AD. Wollock and Perrelló (1989), at the invitation of the International Association of Logopedics and Phoniatrics, presented a comprehensive bibliography listing several hundred published articles and texts, each containing some mention of the history of speech, language, and hearing remediation in the world's literature. This bibliography is retrievable at Mankato State University's Web site. An extensive world literature related to hearing, speech, and language goes far beyond the British and European writings of the 1800s that are typically referred to as relevant to developments in the United States.

Readers interested in finding out more about the history of the professions should explore the references and Web sites at the end of this chapter. Looking specifically at the development of audiology and speech-language pathology in the United States, O'Neill's 1987 chapter in Herbert Oyer's text provides an excellent review. Another comprehensive, era-by-era review is found on a Web site by Duchan (2001). Duchan (2002) also authored a summary article appearing in the *ASHA Leader,* an extensive bibiliography related to the history of audiology and speech-language pathology in America, and a related article on the topic (2004) of professional identity, "Professional Identity: Then and Now."

A brief narrative on "The History of Audiology" can be found on the ASHA Web site. Another good source of historical review is Levitt's (2003) *ASHA Leader* article on "Audiology and Communications Technology: A Symbiotic Relationship." In his review, Levitt illustrates how technologic advancements in amplification instrumentation and hearing assessment have correspondingly advanced the scope of practice in audiology.

Professional Associations and ASHA

We have already discussed the evolution of the early societies that evolved to the American Speech-Language-Hearing Association. Commentary on the first 50 years of ASHA can be found in Paden (1975) and Spahr (1987). Spahr, the Executive Director of ASHA for many years, outlines the history of the ASHA national office. More recently, Malone (1999) provides a highly entertaining collection of oral interviews on the history of ASHA's first 75 years. These include commentaries and candid interviews with leaders within the Association membership and the national office. For more about the development of ASHA and the American Academy of Audiology (AAA), see Chapter 3, Professional Associations.

Chronology

With the caveat that we have not verified the dates or accuracy of the review articles or citations from the original compilers, we will select just a few random tidbits of history out of the references cited previously to create a summary chronology. Additional sources are added, where noted, along with the authors' own reminiscence of events. Let's look at a chronology of some of the layers of our profession's history, with primary emphasis on events in the United States and mainly in the formative decades, up to the 1990s:

- 1800s—Physicians, grammarians, and elocutionists sharing interests in speech correction, deafness, stuttering, voice, aphasia, and aural habilitation, beginning mainly in Europe and Great Britain and later in the United States, collectively laid the cornerstones of the principles, practices, and science of audiology and speech-language pathology.

- 1882—The first textbook on speech disorders was published in Philadelphia, authored by a physician who practiced in Britain, Samuel Otway Lewis Potter, titled *Speech and Its Defects: Considered Physiologically, Pathologically, Historically, and Remedially.*

- 1899–1901—Although the first U.S. patent was filed in 1862, the first commercially available hearing aid was manufactured at the turn of the century. These were large component devices with carbon dust microphones, costing about $400.

- Early 1900s—Individuals who identify themselves as *speech correctionists* formed a special interest group within larger organizations, including the National Education Association (NEA) and the National Association of Teachers of Speech (NATS).

- 1910—The first text on *Experimental Phonetics,* authored by Rousselot, was published.

- 1914—University of Wisconsin established a graduate program and clinic in speech disorders.

- 1916 through early 1920s—Speech clinics in privately funded and university-based centers began to be established across the country.

- 1918—Walter Babcock Swift organized the speech correctionists' special interest group (mentioned previously) in the NEA and chartered the National Society for the Study and Correction of Speech Disorders.

- 1921—Sara Stinchfield (Hawke) received her PhD in speech disorders from the University of Wisconsin.

- 1924—Lee Edward Travis received his PhD in Psychology, with emphasis in speech disorders, from the University of Iowa.

- 1925—The American Academy of Speech Correction (AASC) was formed out of an interest group within the NATS.

- 1920s—The first audiometers were commercially available.

- 1927—The AASC became the American Society for the Study of Disorders of Speech (ASSDS).

- 1927—The Council of Physical Therapy in the American Medical Association, in conjunction with the American Standards Association, established standards for audiometers.

- 1927—Robert West was awarded a PhD in speech pathology from the University of Wisconsin.

- 1928—Sara Stinchfield published a text entitled *The Psychology of Speech*.

- 1928—Travis becomes the Director of the Psychology Clinic and Professor of Psychology and Speech at the University of Iowa.

- 1929—A group of 40 scientists and engineers at the A. G. Bell Laboratory in New York City formed The Acoustical Society of America (ASA) and published the first quarterly *Journal of the Acoustical Society of America* (JASA) that same year.

- Early 1930s—Wearable multipart hearing aids became commercially available.

- 1931—Lee Edward Travis published the first edition of his book *Speech Pathology;* later editions of this classic text come to be referred to as "The Travis Handbook."

- 1934—ASSDS became the American Speech Correction Association (ASCA).

- 1935—A Code of Ethics was written for the ASCA.

- 1936—The *Journal of Speech Disorders* was first published.

- 1937—Samuel Orton wrote the book *Reading, Writing and Speech Problems in Children*.

- 1939—Mildred McGinnis wrote her master's thesis on the aphasia in children, with

- treatment techniques influenced by Orton. Charles Van Riper published the first edition of *Speech Correction: Principles and Methods.*

- Late 1930s, early 1940s—Influential European academicians immigrated to the United States, including: neuropsychiatrist Karl Goldstein, whose ideas influenced neurologists in this country, such as Norman Geschwind; otolaryngologist Emil Froeschels, who proposed voice therapy techniques and motor speech treatment procedures that are still applied; and psychologist Heinz Werner, who applied Goldstein's theories to the study of normal language development.

- 1940s—Battery-powered, vacuum-tube hearing aids were manufactured in the United States.

- 1943—Mildred Berry and Jon Eisenson published their text *The Defective in Speech,* emphasizing motoric and linguistic factors in speech and including references to speech disorders in the hearing impaired, deaf, and developmentally delayed child.

- Early and mid-1940s—Soldiers returned from battle in World War II, putting high numbers of veterans with neurologic injuries and hearing losses into VA hospitals, requiring the Veterans Administration (now the United States Department of Veterans Affairs) to bring "speech correctionists" and audiologists into VA hospitals to work with these veterans, including notable researchers such as Jon Eisensen and Joseph Wepman. Battlefield injuries created a high demand for audiologists to provide hearing testing and rehabilitation for combat related hearing-impaired veterans. Since that time, the VA has been a leader in providing research and development of diagnostic methods, prosthetic aids, and rehabilitation to better the lives of adults with hearing, speech, and language disorders.

- Mid-1940s—A. G. Bell Laboratory researchers developed the sound spectrograph as part of their war-related research projects.

- 1946—Raymond Carhart offered the first course in audiology in the School of

Communication at Northwestern University (NU), which already housed a program in speech pathology.

- 1947—The ASCA became the American Speech and Hearing Association (ASHA), formally recognizing the increasingly important role of audiology and hearing science in the profession of communication sciences and disorders and in the Association. Consistent with the name change, that same year the *Journal of Speech Disorders* was renamed to the more inclusive *Journal of Speech and Hearing Disorders.*

- Around 1949 and 1950—Federal funding through the Children's Bureau and Maternal and Child Health and Services for Crippled Children became available, enhancing access to services for communicatively impaired children and providing traineeships in audiology and speech-language pathology.

- 1951—Vanderbilt University formed the Division of Audiology and Speech, under the authority of John B. Youmans, Dean of the School of Medicine (McConnell, 1978).

- 1952—Standards for clinical certification by ASHA were established with the basic certificate requiring 30 hours of course work, 275 hours of practicum, and one year of professional practice; no graduate degree or national examination were yet required.

- 1951—*Speech Therapy with Children* by Ollie Backus and Jane Beasley's was published.

- Through the 1950s—Joseph Wepman, Jon Eisensen, and Hildred Schuell provided their unique theoretical bases and taxonomies for the diagnosis and treatment of aphasia, thus establishing the specialty of clinical aphasiology within speech-language pathology.

- 1953—Pocket model hearing aids became available.

- 1957—Helmur Mykelbust's *Auditory Disorders in Children* and Mildred Templin's *Certain Language Skills in Children* were published.

- 1958—The *Journal of Speech and Hearing Research* was launched, after considerable debate within the ASHA leadership about the need for an additional journal.

- Late 1950s and early 1960s—Noam Chomsky, an MIT (Massachusettes Institute of Technology) linguist, proposed a theory of transformational (generative) grammar as the basis for language development. Other linguists such as Jean Berko-Gleason, Ursula Bellugi, and Roger Brown provided evidence for the regularity and generative nature of language development in children, further establishing the importance of psycholinguistic theories in language development and language disorders.

- 1957—Small transistor hearing aids were available, followed by over-the-ear aids.

- 1959—The American Boards of Examiners in Speech Pathology and Audiology was formed.

- 1964–65—The Academy of Rehabilitative Audiology was formed.

- 1965—ASHA established accreditation standards for graduate programs in audiology and speech-language pathology and required a master's degree as a standard for membership in the Association.

- 1965—The standards for the Certificate of Clinical Competence (CCC) were implemented, whereby audiologists and speech pathologists would be required to hold a master's degree or equivalent from a graduate program with a standard clinical and academic curriculum of 60 (equivalent) semester hours of credit, 275 hours of clinical practicum, 9 months of supervised full-time experience, a letter from the candidate's academic program director, and a passing score in a national examination before they were eligible for this credential.

- Early 1970s—In-the-canal hearing aids became available.

- 1973—Clinical practicum clock hours requirement for the CCC was increased to 300.

- Mid 1970s—Federal funding for coverage of clinical services under Medicare included speech therapy, which encouraged large numbers of speech-language pathologists to join occupational and physical therapists in service delivery within health care settings (hospitals, rehabilitation centers, home health, and nursing homes).

- Mid 1970s—Speech and language management was influenced by new theories about "pragmatics," emphasizing function over the form of language in communication and leading clinicians to focus treatment within the context of the social purposes and functions of communication in everyday life.

- 1977—American Academy of Dispensing Audiologists was formed.

- 1978—American Speech and Hearing Association became the American Speech-Language-Hearing Association.

- 1979—ASHA's proscription against selling hearing aids by audiologists for profit was rescinded.

- Early 1980s—Diagnosis Related Groups (DRGs) for Medicare coverage for hospital-related services is introduced, effectively reducing the lengths of stay in hospitals and curtailing hospital staffing for speech-language pathology and occupational therapy and physical therapy services. This change diminished the extent of services provided to inpatients and shifted the services to nursing homes, rehabilitation centers, and hospital-based outpatient programs.

- 1987—ASHA's Legislative Council recognized the growing number of developing specialties within its membership and approved the formation of Special Interest Divisions.

- 1988—Under the leadership of James Jerger of Baylor College of Medicine, audiologists formed the American Academy of Audiology.

- 1989—ASHA recognized audiology and speech-language pathology as two distinct professions within the discipline of communication sciences and disorders.

- 1993—ASHA required a master's or doctoral degree (no longer accepting "equivalency") in speech-language pathology and audiology for the Certificate of Clinical Competency, as well as 75 hours of course work, including basic sciences, 375 hours of observation and practicum, with 250 hours of those required at the graduate level, and a 36-week Clinical Fellowship with periodic evaluations.

- 1994—ASHA initiated a program to confer Specialty Recognition status for ASHA members who demonstrate exceptional knowledge and mastery level skills in clinical specialties.

- 1997—New requirements were adopted for the CCC in audiology with at least 75 hours of post-baccalaureate study, 12 months of full-time, supervised experience, and a doctoral degree. The first two requirements become effective January 1, 2007, and the doctoral degree requirement (clinical doctorate, or Doctor of Audiology) takes effect in 2012.

- From the mid to late 1990s—Changes and regulations related to federal funding under Medicare coverage for nursing home, home health, and rehabilitation (with other payers following suit) continued to define the nature of services provided by speech-language pathologists in health service settings.

- Today and beyond—Amazing advancements in science and technologies include augmentative and alternative communication technologies, multiple channel cochlear implants, and functional MRI. Among the growing populations who require highly specialized clinical management are individuals with balance disorders, frail elders, children with autism spectrum disorders, and individuals surviving catastrophic injuries and illnesses who have chronic cognitive-communicative disorders. Meanwhile, the educational curriculum expands, the cry for greater autonomy of the professions continues, and the public increasingly demands the application of the best scientific knowledge to service delivery.

Observations on Our History

The preceding historical review and thumbnail chronology are intended to be illustrative and not comprehensive. Although we have mentioned some of the legacies of a few founding fathers and mothers, many important events and individuals have not been mentioned. The reader is encouraged to go to the references provided to flesh out better this fascinating history. Several of these reviews are easily retrievable through the World Wide Web (Duchan, 2001, 2002, 2004, 2005; Levitt, 2003; O'Neill, 1987; Wollock & Pelleró, 1989). This brief review allows us to make some observations about our profession: The principles, practices, and science of hearing, speech, and language can be traced back through two centuries. Multiple disciplines contributed to the earliest foundations of communication sciences and disorders. The professions of audiology and speech-language pathology share common roots. The principles and values of our founding fathers and mothers are still evident. Professionals continuously redefine themselves, and professional organizations and societies constantly change. New societies are sometimes formed out of interest groups within an existing organization. Clinical practices are also constantly changed and advanced by new discoveries in science and technology. Economic factors, world events, and societal attitudes have shaped the scope of practices and the growth and development of our profession. Creative and passionate clinicians, educators, administrators, and scientists have inspired, challenged, and sustained us throughout the history of our professions.

ACCESS

From a look at our roots, we now turn to modern-day reality and consider how we can make our clinical services accessible to those who need them. Access to clinical services in audiology and speech-language pathology involves at least five factors: demographics, outcome measurement, funding, technology, and community inclusion.

Demographics

Our clients and their families as well as their insurers, educators, and caregivers must know what services we provide and how these services are of value to them. We know that disabilities affect at least 22 percent of all Americans (Centers for Disease Control, 2001). Disabilities that impair sensory, physical, and mental abilities disproportionately affect young children under 5 years of age (12.3 percent) and the oldest over age 65 (36.4 percent) (U.S. Census Bureau, 2000). Estimates also indicate that at least one in six Americans has a communication disability (ASHA, 2004a).

The percentage of minorities is increasing in the general population, particularly among Hispanic, Asian, and Native Americans. Unfortunately, the data on the prevalence and incidence of disabilities among these populations are limited, but indications reveal that these groups are at high risk for disability. In addition, they are also vulnerable to poverty, unemployment, and poor health status (National Council on Disability, 1993). For example, African Americans, nearly a quarter of whom have income below the poverty rate, are twice as likely as their Caucasian counterparts to have a stroke (National Institute on Deafness and Other Communication Disorders, 2004; U.S. Census Bureau, 2005).

The Agency for Healthcare Research and Quality (2000) indicates that minority residents of nursing homes are less likely to have sensory aids such as glasses and hearing aids. Caesar and Williams (2002) posit that minorities, in comparison with whites, have poorer access to medical care and what they do receive is of lower quality. They also hypothesize that the causes of racial differences in health care delivery are multifaceted. For example, disparities may be related to overt or unintentional discrimination on the part of health care workers and their settings, the unequal distribution of medical resources, and lack of patient awareness of medical procedures. Limited language skills in English may also be a barrier for some minorities and those with linguistic differences.

Little demographic research has been done in recent years by our professions to identify how many individuals in each of these groups have communication, hearing, and/or swallowing problems. Indeed, a conference devoted to epidemiology of communication disorders recently convened by the National Institute on Deafness and Other Communication Disorders (2005) stated that "modern epidemiology, which encompasses analytical studies, clinical trials, outcomes research, and health services delivery, has received scant attention in the field of hearing research." The institute also recognized the need for studies of communication across the life span and among minority groups. The current lack of information means it is difficult to provide data to support the argument that communication disorders are common and have a significant impact on individuals and society.

There is some recognition by the federal government, evident in IDEA legislation, that early identification of disabilities and intervention with young children are critical. There is less recognition by the government that the critical needs of elders who have a communication problem may require more than a limited amount of speech therapy. Medicare pays for only limited hearing evaluations and does not cover hearing aids for elders. Third party payers similarly assume that only a minimal amount of therapy is appropriate for all clients—a "one small size fits all" view.

As communication disorders professionals, we each have an obligation to educate the broad social and political community regarding the nature of communication, hearing, and swallowing problems, their effects, and the benefits of intervention. We cannot assume that others will raise our standard. We also need to document any disparities in service delivery to various populations, including minorities and those who reside in rural or less accessible areas.

Outcome Measurement

Accessibility to communication disorders services will be enhanced if we can illustrate convincingly the personal, economic, educational, vocational, and social value of communication intervention. We are responsible for demonstrating that what we do has positive, functional, and lasting outcomes for clients and their caregivers. It is insufficient to say that

clients improve a certain number of percentage points on a communication test. Everyone wants to know what observable difference our intervention makes in the daily life of the client and significant others. New types of valid, reliable, and quick-to-administer outcome measures must be developed, including those that focus on function in daily environments, changes in educational and vocational performance, changes in the psychosocial well-being of clients, and changes in the health and emotional status of the significant others. Most importantly, we need to design studies that will document the cost effectiveness of communication intervention. We need to think more broadly as to how our intervention affects our clients. For example, do those clients who improve their communication or swallowing need fewer hours of skilled nursing care per week in a care facility? Do the family members of those with dementia who participate in communication counseling report less stress when communicating? Do they increase their communication interaction? Can we provide long-term follow-up on the effects of preschool intervention on educational achievement and high school graduation rate? Such studies are labor intensive and require multiple sites, intensive and lengthy data collection, and long-term analysis. They will provide, however, a richer and more varied spectrum of outcome data.

Funding

Remember this simple rule: People pay for what they deem valuable. Communication disorders specialists cannot assume that clients and payers know the value of our services to child development, educational progress, employment opportunities, participation in health care, or personal fulfillment. Nor can we assume that services provided at no charge are valued. It has become the rule rather than the exception that our services will be paid for by a third party, such as an insurer or a school district, rather than the client/patient or family. Funding for services from government programs and insurers is generally limited, and the affected individuals assume that if the school or insurer does not cover the service, then it must not be of value. Thus, while some are financially unable to pay for our services, others are unwilling to make a personal investment once covered services are discontinued. As a result, we suspect that many clients from young children through the elderly are underserved; they simply do not receive enough therapy to make a meaningful or lasting difference.

In many cases, however, we lack the evidence to know what "enough" therapy is. Thus, it is difficult to provide sufficient proof that intervention is effective. Are we as communication disorders specialists satisfied when our clients are dismissed due to funding limitations? What responsibility do we have to find new funding sources or innovative and cost-effective ways to deliver services? How can we provide long-term services for those with complex or progressively degenerative problems?

Audiologists and speech-language pathologists must come to their positions knowledgeable about financing clinical services. You need to know business practices as well as clinical practices. Specifically, even as a new professional, you must know the nature of a variety of reimbursement systems, how your services are covered by them, and what you can do to maximize the resources the client brings. You must also be aware of changes in legislation that affect the financial coverage for your services. You should be prepared to advocate for legislation that will fairly reimburse our services. You cannot depend on someone else to do this. Remember that every vote, letter, and phone call is meaningful in influencing legislation and funding.

Technology

Technology has improved access to communication partners and opportunities for those with hearing and communication difficulties. Under the broad rubrics of "techno-health," these devices and systems affect all aspects of our diagnostic and service delivery as well as our own educational opportunities. Rapid advances in technology serve those with hearing, communication, cognitive, and swallowing disorders. The variety of individual types of technologies is discussed in Chapter 25, but let's consider some examples that demonstrate their vast potential. An increasing number of today's consumers are technology literate and expect some type of technology to be available to assist them with their communication difficulties. Clients are increasingly more likely to put their faith in devices over the hard work of behavioral therapy.

Programmable advanced digital hearing aids now provide improved sound clarity, reduced circuit noise, faster processing, and improved ability to listen in noise. Cochlear implants have been surgically implanted in more than 13,000 individuals, including 10,000 children, to help provide a sense of sound for the profoundly deaf and severely hard of hearing (National Institute of Deafness and Communication Disorders, 2002). A variety of environmental assistive listening devices make hearing easier in community settings. A wide variety of high- to low-technology augmentative speech devices make graphic communication and even speech possible for those with severe speech unintelligibility. These devices have become more portable, adaptable, intelligent, and user friendly. For those with memory and attention disabilities, portable computer systems and smart environments have been developed to assist with cuing and planning. Environmental technologies provide safer and more communication-friendly environments for those with vision, hearing, and cognitive disorders.

Technology has also become essential in assessment and therapy. For example, technologies are available to provide objective data about respiration, phonation, resonation, and articulation before and after therapy. Tele-audiology employs the use of a desktop or palm computer and an Internet connection to provide a real-time assessment of hearing (Givens & Elangovan, 2003). Therapy for fluency disorders, aphasia, and cognitive disorders may employ computers or other technology-assisted intervention.

Technology has been particularly useful in the delivery of clinical services to those in rural and remote environments. Known as *telehealth* or *telepractice,* technology is used to provide assessment and individual therapy for a variety of disorders as well as information and counseling to clients and their families. Audiologists are using telepractice for screenings, hearing aid programming and counseling, aural rehabilitation, and other audiometric testing such as auditory brainstem response and otoacoustic emissions. Similarly, speech-language pathologists use telepractice for assessment and intervention across all disorders in school and home settings. All of these provide improved access to communication services for those in distant and rural areas.

ASHA has recently published several position statements on telepractice for speech-language pathologists and audiologists (ASHA, 2005a, b). Importantly, these professional position papers all include the following admonition: "The use of telepractice does not remove any existing responsibilities in delivering services, including adherence to the Code of Ethics, Scope of Practice, state and federal laws (e.g. licensure, HIPAA, etc.), and ASHA policy documents on professional practices."

Technology provides clinicians with quicker access to patient records and faster documentation. Most third party payers, including Medicare, now require electronic billing. Thus, with the submission of these data, large databases are being created that allow payers to look at practice patterns and to set benchmarks for practice (e.g., the typical number of treatment visits for a given condition in setting A compared to setting B). Technology also offers a variety of educational opportunities. Simple examples include the use of video-recorded conferences and demonstrations. Others may attend live audio or video conferences using their own technology at home or office. The decreasing cost and widespread availability of sophisticated technology allows clinicians 24/7 access to information. Numerous colleges and universities offer practicing audiologists opportunities to upgrade their education to the doctoral level through technology-enhanced programs. The use of distance education is becoming a component of some graduate programs in speech-language pathology and audiology. The Internet facilitates clinical discussions and access to a wide variety of scientific and related information. Today's clinicians must be highly familiar and comfortable with the remote delivery of services and use it to

their own advantage to pursue continuing education and discussion with other practitioners nationally and internationally. See Chapter 25 on technology in this text for a more in-depth discussion of this topic.

Community Inclusion

It is insufficient to provide state-of-the-art intervention and the latest technology and to prove that communication services have functional and lasting value if there is not a home and broader social community that provides communication opportunities where these skills may be realized. As communication disorders specialists, many of us assume that "fixing" the communication problem means that the client will axiomatically have access to a variety of meaningful communication opportunities. Many of our pediatric clients return to environments bereft of cognitive and communicative stimulation and opportunities. Elders may return to settings where they are physically and socially isolated from people and activities of choice. Some clients have few opportunities in their community to demonstrate new or improving communication skills learned in therapy. What is learned in therapy needs environmental support to be functional and meaningful.

Accessibility to communication opportunities means that the individual can easily get to people and activities that enhance cognitive, communicative, and emotional well-being. This accessibility is enhanced when the physical environment is user friendly for those with motoric, sensory, communicative, and cognitive limitations. Further, family and others must realize their social obligation to be active and skilled communication partners for those with communication problems. Thus, communication disorders specialists have a responsibility to work directly with family, teachers, and other caregivers to help them understand the concept of a positive physical and social communication environment and to develop skills that will augment and solidify therapeutic improvements in that environment.

Examples of this intervention principle in action include the work of Lubinski (e.g., 1994) on creating a positive communication environment for adults with aphasia and dementia and the work done in England by Byng and Pound on living healthy with aphasia. Innovatively, Byng and Pound helped establish an Aphasia Day to educate the community about aphasia and created community-based conversation groups for stroke survivors and their families. Such intervention empowers clients and their significant others to use improving skills and cultivate even better ways to communicate in the community.

CURRENCY

A major issue facing both professions is how to prepare professionals to meet the ever-expanding scopes of practice with more diverse and complicated clients in a climate of fiscal restraint. Practicing clinicians soon realize they must be able to work collaboratively with other professionals and articulate convincingly clients' needs and progress through outcome data. It is no longer good enough to "do your best," but your best must be observable, measurable, and cost effective to the consumer and payer. Even beginning clinicians need to have good business sense so they can offer the best possible services at reasonable cost. Clinicians in every setting find that their knowledge base must be updated regularly to meet these challenges.

The first challenge for preparation begins at the preprofessional level. At present, audiology has decided to require, by 2012, the doctorate as its entry level degree. Beginning audiologists will need to meet the academic and clinical requirements of either PhD or AuD degrees to meet ASHA certification requirements. These doctoral-level entry practitioners will enter with an increased academic and clinical preparation. Three- to 5-year doctoral programs will give audiologists in training more time to study hearing science, hearing disorders, assessment and rehabilitation, business, and other areas in greater depth and vastly increase the number of preprofessional practicum hours in several settings. What is unknown is whether the marketplace will

be prepared to financially compensate this level of practitioner.

Some also propose that more professional doctoral programs emerge for speech-language pathologists. Lubinski (2003) revisits the need for doctoral professionals in medical settings. Typical 2-year master's level training programs cannot offer the breadth and depth of education and practicum necessary to provide sophisticated clinical services to those with complicated diagnostics and intervention for neurogenic and medically related disorders across the age span. Others argue that this level of expertise can be gained on the job and through continuing education and that the marketplace will not reward adequately the increased level of education.

In contrast, there is a move within speech-language pathology to develop a paraprofessional level of practitioner, variously called *speech therapy aides, assistants, paraprofessionals,* or *support personnel.* This move is seen as helping to meet workforce shortages and to free master's- and doctoral-level practitioners to conduct skilled diagnostic and intervention services as well as to reduce the costs of service. There is disagreement as to the ultimate impact of this level of practitioner on the availability of jobs, the quality of services offered, and the need for supervision.

A second challenge is the need to upgrade the professional knowledge base of practicing speech-language pathologists and audiologists once they have entered the workforce, regardless of degree held. Many states have mandated continuing education as a requirement for maintaining licensure or certification. As of January 1, 2003, ASHA has required that audiologists obtain 30 hours of continuing education per 3-year period (ASHA, 2003). Similarly, speech-language pathologists began this requirement on January 1, 2005. Continuing education can be acquired through a variety of venues (ASHA, 2004b).

How to access meaningful, state-of-the-art, and economical continuing education is a real issue for many professionals. Some settings have begun to offer regular in-house continuing education programs specifically tailored to their professionals' populations and needs. They may use their own master clinicians as presenters or invite outside specialists. Attendance at local, state, and national conferences is another way to access this education. Participation in audio or video conferences, journal reading programs, and taking traditional college coursework are other continuing education mechanisms. Further, those offering continuing education need to be aware of the knowledge level and clinical needs of their audience. Too many professionals question the clinical utility of some presentations. They want information that they can apply immediately to service delivery. Again, the Internet increasingly offers continuing education and opportunities for discussion among clinicians about professional issues, new technologies, and challenging cases.

Colleges and universities have a special obligation to find innovative ways to offer continuing education to their communities. Such offerings help maintain the currency of their own supervisors and local clinicians who frequently serve as externship supervisors. Busy clinicians are more likely to take short intensive courses that can be accomplished in a day or a long weekend than semesters of course work with 1st year graduate students. Establishing consortia of colleges to offer nontraditional continuing education to their local communities is both efficient and effective in enhancing clinical currency in their communities.

Clinicians who participate in continuing education, particularly those who focus their education and practice in a specific area, may want specialty recognition or certification. Such acknowledgment may be personally, professionally, and financially rewarding. ASHA, AAA, and the Academy of Neurologic Communication Disorders and Sciences (ANCDS) are examples of three groups that provide specialty recognition or board certification for expertise in one or more areas of professional practice.

The issue of currency cannot be discussed without attention to the insufficient number of research doctorates in our professions. The current and projected lack of doctoral-level professionals will have a dramatic impact on the availability and quality of training programs, the production of basic and applied research in our disciplines, and the availability of continuing education programs. Strategies need to be formulated to encourage qualified individuals to consider academia and research as professional goals. Possible suggestions include identification and encouragement of highly qualified students at the undergraduate level, development of special tracks for such students so they can simultaneously attain their clinical and research goals, and development of innovative programs to attract working professionals back to school. Academic programs and professional settings might partner to identify and support professionals who may be qualified and want to pursue an advanced graduate degree. Once graduated, these doctorates might split their time between academia and clinic. Many working professionals would return for doctoral programs if adequate fellowships or other forms of work study options were available. While graduate programs desire full-time doctoral students as a means of training researchers, the increasing need for doctoral-level academics and researchers may necessitate new programming options.

Clinical currency is critical if our professional work is to be valued and sought after. Without doubt, the practitioner who is most current will provide the best quality service and command the best salary. Hopefully, our practitioners will assume a philosophy that lifelong learning emanates from an inner drive for self-improvement.

POSITIVE WORKPLACE SKILLS

When discussing plans for the third edition of this book with colleagues, one repeated theme was the need to emphasize "professional attitude" in the workplace. Professionals in both audiology and speech-language pathology recognize that clinical skills must be matched with positive workplace skills. In 2000, an ASHA briefing paper for academicians, practitioners, employers, and students was prepared entitled "Responding to the Changing Needs of Speech-Language Pathology and Audiology Students in the 21st Century." Nine workplace skills were identified as critical to successful employment:

- Planning and priority setting
- Organizing and time management

- Managing diversity
- Team building
- Interpersonal savvy and peer relationships
- Organizational agility
- Conflict management
- Problem solving, perspective, and creativity
- Dealing with paradox and learning on the fly

Review of these skills places them into two broad categories: (1) executive skills that help us to plan, implement, and evaluate what we do and make appropriate accommodations and (2) positive interpersonal communication and leadership skills. You will be more successful in your practice across settings if you have an efficient and organized work plan. Others must perceive that you are competent and confident in what you do. You will be expected to keep to a schedule, find ways to maximize billable time, and submit accurate reports on time. Remember that "time is money." The successful clinician seamlessly blends skill, sensitivity, efficiency, and effectiveness.

Critical to your workplace success are your abilities to communicate effectively in oral presentations and written reports. Your speech and writing represent you as a professional to your department or program, your profession, and most of all to your clients. You need to be able to make a data-based, logical, and concise argument that your client needs service and will benefit from your intervention. Further, your communication skills build bridges to colleagues, clients, and their families. You will need these individuals to implement and reinforce your interventions. Every workplace involves teamwork, and your ability to work collaboratively is essential to your success. Your work will be more productive if others reinforce the strategies and interventions you provide. It is insufficient to be technically competent as a clinician unless you also demonstrate consistent and positive workplace skills. See Chapter 8, Preparing for Employment; Chapter 9, Professional Autonomy and Collaboration; Chapter 26, on stress and conflict; and Chapter 29, Leadership and Communication Skills for further related discussion.

SUMMARY

This chapter discussed four general topics that influence what we do and how we do it as speech-language pathologists and audiologists. First, we have briefly visited our historical roots to understand how our professions have originated and evolved. Ours are relatively young professions that emerged as hybrids from a variety of disciplines. Understanding where we have come from should help us see issues that have persisted throughout our history and to predict the trajectory of our future.

Second, we discussed the fact that our services must be accessible to those who need them. Accessibility is influenced by the demographics of our clientele, funding availability, the use of technology, outcome measures, and community inclusion. Our clients present with diverse backgrounds, needs, and resources that require sensitive and innovative provision of services. Keep in mind that our goal is to help the client to have more communication "access-ability."

Next we discussed the importance of maintaining our clinical currency. Professionals must maintain a commitment to lifelong learning and the use of evidence-based practice to be viable in today's health care and educational marketplaces. As our scopes of practice evolve, so must our knowledge base.

Finally, we discussed the executive, communication, and leadership skills that are essential to implementing all of the clinical skills and knowledge you have into the workplace. A professional is a hybrid of clinical knowledge and skills, cultural and societal intelligence, and social competence.

Given this armament of skills and knowledge, we will be ready for challenges from third party payers, educational and health care policy makers, some colleagues, and even clients and families.

As we proceed, let us do so with a sense of achievement for what we have firmly accomplished in our more than 80 year history as professions and with a positive attitude toward what we plan to achieve in our clinical and research efforts in this new century.

CRITICAL THINKING

1. What factors influenced your decision to enter the profession of audiology or speech-language pathology?

2. How do you think the changes in demographic statistics will affect academia, research, the scopes of practice, and job availability in audiology and speech-language pathology in the next 5, 10, or 20 years?

3. What will professional historians in communication disorders say about professional practice in the first quarter of the 21st century?

4. Select two or three names from this list and research their biographies: Hallowell Davis, Richard Silverman, Bryng Bryngelson, Stanley Ainsworth, Geog Von Bekesy, Kenneth O. Johnson, Robert L. Milisen, Richard Schieflebusch, James Jerger, Louis M. DiCarlo, Frederick L. Darley, Mildred Berry, Ira Ventry, Herold Lillywhite, Mildred Templin, Rolland Van Hattum, Frank Kleffner, and Marion Downs. What did these individuals do to earn the Honors of the Association from the American Speech-Language-Hearing Association? What were their major accomplishments and contributions to the professions of audiology and speech-language pathology? Did any of those contributions affect you in some way?

5. What factors do you feel influence the accessibility of our services to clients from birth through old age?

6. How do you think technology will affect the delivery of our services in the next 10 years?

7. Why is continuing education so critical to our professions? How do you plan to maintain your clinical currency? What factors will influence your ability to implement this plan?

8. What are some innovative ways universities can offer both continuing education and opportunities for doctoral study? What would induce you to access these programs?

9. What executive and interpersonal skills do you feel are most important for you to develop and why? How would you rate your ability to communicate with colleagues, clients, and families? How might you acquire and refine the people skills you need to succeed as a professional?

REFERENCES

Agency for Healthcare Research and Quality. (2000). *Addressing racial and ethnic disparities in health care.* Available at http://www.ahrq.gov

American Speech-Language-Hearing Association. (2000). Responding to the changing needs of speech-language pathology and audiology students in the 21st century. Available at http://www.asha.org

American Speech-Language-Hearing Association. (2003). New audiology standards. Available at http://www.asha.org

American Speech-Language-Hearing Association. (2004a). Incidence and prevalence of speech, voice, and language disorders in adults in the United States. Available at http://www.asha.org

American Speech-Language-Hearing Association. (2004b). Maintenance of certification in speech-language pathology. Available at http://www.asha.org

American Speech-Language-Hearing Association. (2005a). Audiologists providing clinical services via telepractice (position statement). *ASHA Supplement, 25.*

American Speech-Language-Hearing Association. (2005b). Speech-language pathologists providing clinical services via telepractice (position statement). *ASHA Supplement, 25.*

American Speech-Language-Hearing Association. (2005c). *The history of audiology.* Available at http://www.asha.org

Bruce, E. V. (1973). *Alexander Graham Bell: The conquest of silence.* Boston: Little, Brown.

Caesar, L., & Williams, D. (2002). Socioculture and the delivery of health care: Who gets what and why. *The ASHA Leader.* Available at http://www.asha.org

Duchan, J. (2001). Getting here: The first hundred years of speech pathology in America. Available at http://www.acsu.buffalo.edu/~duchan/history.html

Duchan, J. (2002). The history of speech-language pathology and audiology in America. Available at http://www.asha.org

Duchan, J. (2004). Professional history: Then and now. Available at http://www.speechpathology.com

Duchan, J. (2005). The phonetically-based speech therapy methods of Alexander Graham Bell. *Journal of Speech-Language Pathology and Audiology, 29,* 70–72.

Eber, D. (1982). *Genius at work: Images of Alexander Graham Bell.* New York: Viking Press.

Fabricus, H. (1600). *De vision, voce, et auditu.* Venice: F. Bolzetta.

Friedman, T. (2005). *The world is flat: A brief history of the twenty-first century.* New York: Farrar, Straus and Giroux.

Givens, G., & Elangovan, S. (2003). Internet application to tele-audiology—"Nothin' but Net." *American Journal of Audiology, 12,* 59–65.

Hunt, F. V. (1978). *Origins in acoustics: The science of sound from antiquity to the age of Newton.* New Haven, CT: Yale University Press.

Hunt, J. (1870). Stammering and stuttering: Their nature and treatment (7th ed.). London: Longmans, Green.

Itard, J. (1989). Mémoire sur le bégaiement. In J. Wollock & J. Perrelló (Eds.). A bibliography of writings on the history of logopedics, phoniatrics, communication disorders and allied subjects. Presented at the Conference of the International Association of Logopedics and Phoniatrics, Prague, 1989. Available at http://www.mnsu.edu (original work published in 1817).

Levitt, H. (2003). Audiology and communications technology: A symbiotic relationship. *The ASHA Leader, 8* (11), 4–5, 17. Available at http://www.asha.org

Lubinski, R. (2003). Revisiting the professional doctorate in speech-language pathology. *Journal of Medical Speech-Language Pathology,* 11.

Malone, R. (1999). *The first 75 years: An oral history of the American Speech-Language-Hearing Association.* Washington, DC: American Speech-Language-Hearing Association.

McConnell, F. (1978). *The Bill Wilkerson Hearing and Speech Center.* Nashville: The Bill Wilkerson Center.

National Council on Disability. (1993). Meeting the unique needs of minorities with disability. Available at http://www.ncd.gov/newsroom/publications/1993/minority.htm#6

National Institute of Deafness and Other Communication Disorders. (2002). *Cochlear implants.* Available at www.niacd.nih.gov/health/hearing/coch.asp

National Institute of Deafness and Other Communication Disorders. (2004). Communication disorders and stroke in African-American and other cultural groups: Multidisciplinary perspectives and research needs. Available at http://www.nidcd.nih.gov/health/misc/comm.asp

National Institute of Deafness and Other Communication Disorders. (2005). NIDCD workshop on epidemiology of communication disorders. Available at http://www.nidcd.nih.gov/funding/programs/ep/episummary.asp

Neidecker, E., & Blosser, J. (1993). *School programs in speech language: Organization and management.* Englewood Cliffs, NJ: Prentice Hall.

Northwestern University Archives. Records of the Department of Audiology. Available at http://www.library.northwestern.edu/archives

O'Neill, J. (1987). The development of speech-language pathology and audiology in the United States. In H. J. Oyer (Ed.), *Administration of programs in speech-language pathology.* Boston: Allyn and Bacon. Available at http://www.mnsu.edu

Paden, E. (1975). ASHA in retrospect: Fiftieth anniversary reflections. *Journal of the American Speech and Hearing Association, 17*(7), 439; (8), 499; (9), 571–572; (10), pp. 727–728; (11), 795.

Potter, S. O. L. (1882). *Speech and its defects.* Philadelphia: P. Blakiston Son.

Rockey, D. (1980). *Speech disorder in the nineteenth century.* London: Croom Helm.

Spahr, F. T. (1987). History of the national office: *Asha, 29*(3), 10.

Urbanschitsch, T. (1982). *Auditory training for deaf mutism and acquired deafness* (S. Richard Silverman, Trans.). Washington, DC: Alexander Graham Bell Association for the Deaf.

U.S. Census Bureau. (2000). Disability status of the civilian noninstitutionalized population by sex and selected characteristics for the United States and Puerto Rico: 2000 (PHC-T-32). Available at http:www.census.gov/population/www/cen2000/phc-t32.html

U.S. Census Bureau. (2005). Historical poverty tables. Available at http://www.census.gov

Wollock, J. (1997). *The noblest animate motion: Speech, physiology and medicine in pre-Cartesian linguistic thought.* Philadelphia: John Benjamins.

Wollock, J., & Perrelló, J. (1989). A bibliography of writings on the history of logopedics, phoniatrics, communication disorders and allied subjects. Presented at the Conference of the International Association of Logopedics and Phoniatrics, Prague. Available at: http://www.mnsu.edu

RESOURCES

ASHA Web site for History of Audiology: http://www.asha.org

Judith Felson Duchan Web site: http://www.acsu.buffalo.edu

Mankato State University's Web site: http:// www.mnsu.edu

Northwestern University Archives: http://www.library.northwestern.edu/archives

APPENDIX 1–A

Scope of Practice in Audiology

AD HOC COMMITTEE ON SCOPE OF PRACTICE IN AUDIOLOGY

This scope of practice in audiology statement is an official policy of the American Speech-Language-Hearing Association (ASHA). The document was developed by the Coordinating Committee for the ASHA vice president for professional practices in audiology and approved in 2003 by the Legislative Council (11-03). Members of the coordinating committee include Donna Fisher Smiley (chair), Michael Bergen, and Jean-Pierre Gagné with Vic S. Gladstone and Tina R. Mullins (ex officios). Susan Brannen, ASHA vice president for professional practices in audiology (2001-2003), served as monitoring vice president. This statement supersedes the Scope of Practice in Audiology statement (LC 08-95), (ASHA, 1996).

Reference this material as: American Speech-Language-Hearing Association. (2004). Scope of practice in audiology. *ASHA Supplement 24*, in press.

Index terms: ASHA reference products, AUD education and qualifications, AUD practice settings, AUD roles and activities, audiology, practice scope and patterns, World Health Organization (WHO) framework.

Documents type: practice guidelines and policies

STATEMENT OF PURPOSE

The purpose of this document is to define the scope of practice in audiology in order to (a) describe the services offered by qualified audiologists as primary

SOURCE: American Speech-Language-Hearing Association. (2001). *Scope of Practice in Audiology.* Available from http://www.asha.org/about/publications/reference-library/Reprinted with permission.

service providers, case managers, and/or members of multidisciplinary and interdisciplinary teams; (b) serve as a reference for health care, education, and other professionals, and for consumers, members of the general public, and policy makers concerned with legislation, regulation, licensure, and third party reimbursement; and (c) inform members of ASHA, certificate holders, and students of the activities for which certification in audiology is required in accordance with the ASHA Code of Ethics.

Audiologists provide comprehensive diagnostic and treatment/rehabilitative services for auditory, vestibular, and related impairments. These services are provided to individuals across the entire age span from birth through adulthood; to individuals from diverse language, ethnic, cultural, and socioeconomic backgrounds; and to individuals who have multiple disabilities. This position statement is not intended to be exhaustive; however, the activities described reflect current practice within the profession. Practice activities related to emerging clinical, technological, and scientific developments are not precluded from consideration as part of the scope of practice of an audiologist. Such innovations and advances will result in the periodic revision and updating of this document. It is also recognized that specialty areas identified within the scope of practice will vary among the individual providers. ASHA also recognizes that credentialed professionals in related fields may have knowledge, skills, and experience that could be applied to some areas within the scope of audiology practice. Defining the scope of practice of audiologists is not meant to exclude other appropriately credentialed postgraduate professionals from rendering services in common practice areas.

Audiologists serve diverse populations. The patient/client population includes persons of different race, age, gender, religion, national origin, and sexual orientation. Audiologists' caseloads include individuals from diverse ethnic, cultural, or linguistic backgrounds, and persons with disabilities. Although audiologists are prohibited from discriminating in the provision of professional services based on these factors, in some cases such factors may be relevant to the development of an appropriate treatment plan. These factors may be considered in treatment plans

only when firmly grounded in scientific and professional knowledge.

This scope of practice does not supersede existing state licensure laws or affect the interpretation or implementation of such laws. It may serve, however, as a model for the development or modification of licensure laws.

The schema in Figure 1A–1 depicts the relationship of the scope of practice to ASHA's policy documents that address current and emerging audiology practice areas; that is, preferred practice patterns, guidelines, and position statements. ASHA members and ASHA-certified professionals are bound by the ASHA Code of Ethics to provide services that are consistent with the scope of their competence, education, and experience (ASHA, 2003). There are other existing legislative and regulatory bodies that govern the practice of audiology.

FRAMEWORK FOR PRACTICE

The practice of audiology includes both the prevention of and assessment of auditory, vestibular, and related impairments as well as the habilitation/rehabilitation and maintenance of persons with these impairments. The overall goal of the provision of audiology services should be to optimize and enhance the ability of an individual to hear, as well as to communicate in his/her everyday or natural environment. In addition, audiologists provide comprehensive services to individuals with normal hearing who interact with persons with a hearing impairment. The overall goal of audiologic services is to improve the quality of life for all of these individuals.

The World Health Organization (WHO) has developed a multipurpose health classification system known as the International Classification of Functioning, Disability, and Health (ICF) (WHO, 2001). The purpose of this classification system is to provide a standard language and framework for the description of functioning and health. The ICF framework is useful in describing the role of audiologists in the prevention, assessment, and habilitation/rehabilitation of auditory, vestibular, and other related impairments and restrictions or limitations of functioning.

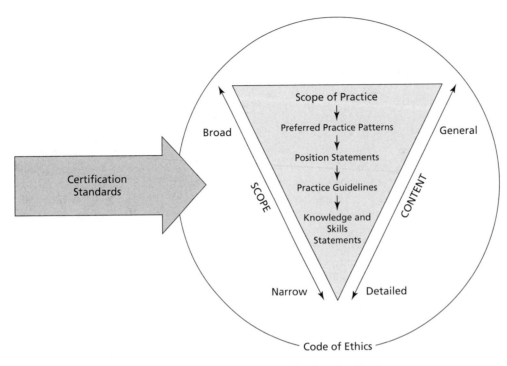

Certification Standards

Scope of Practice
↓
Preferred Practice Patterns
↓
Position Statements
↓
Practice Guidelines
↓
Knowledge and Skills Statements

Broad

General

Narrow

Detailed

SCOPE

CONTENT

Code of Ethics

F I G U R E   1A–1 Conceptual Framework of ASHA Standards and Policy Statements

The ICF is organized into two parts. The first part deals with Functioning and Disability while the second part deals with Contextual Factors. Each part has two components. The components of Functioning and Disability are:

- **Body Functions and Structures:** Body Functions are the physiological functions of body systems and Body Structures are the anatomical parts of the body and their components. Impairments are limitations or variations in Body Function or Structure such as a deviation or loss. An example of a Body Function that might be evaluated by an audiologist would be hearing sensitivity. The use of typanometry to access the mobility of the tympanic membrane is an example of a Body Structure that might be evaluated by an audiologist.

- **Activity/Participation:** In the ICF, Activity and Participation are realized as one list.

Activity refers to the execution of a task or action by an individual. Participation is the involvement in a life situation. Activity limitations are difficulties an individual may experience while executing a given activity. Participation restrictions are difficulties that may limit an individual's involvement in life situations. The Activity/Participation construct thus represents the effects that hearing, vestibular, and related impairments could have on the life of an individual. These effects could include the ability to hold conversations, participate in sports, attend religious services, understand a teacher in a classroom, and walk up and down stairs.

The components of Contextual Factors are:

- **Environmental Factors:** Environmental Factors make up the physical, social, and attitudinal environment in which people live and conduct their lives. Examples of

Environmental Factors, as they relate to audiology, include the acoustical properties of a given space and any type of hearing assistive technology.

- **Personal Factors:** Personal Factors are the internal influences on an individual's functioning and disability and are not a part of the health condition. These factors may include but are not limited to age, gender, social background, and profession.

Functioning and Disability are interactive and evolutionary processes. Figure 1A–2 on the following page illustrates the interaction of the various components of the ICF. Each component of the ICF can be expressed on a continuum of function. On one end of the continuum is intact functioning. At the opposite end of the continuum is completely compromised functioning. Contextual Factors (Environmental and Personal Factors) may interact with any of the components of functioning and disability. Environmental and Personal Factors may act as facilitators or barriers to functioning.

The scope of practice in audiology encompasses all of the components of the ICF. During the assessment phase, audiologists perform tests of Body Function and Structure. Examples of these types of tests include otoscopic examination, pure-tone audiometry, tympanometry, otoacoustic emissions measurements, and speech audiometry. Activity/Participation limitations and restrictions are sometimes addressed by audiologists through case history, interview, questionnaire, and counseling. For example, a question such as "Do you have trouble understanding while on the telephone?" or "Can you describe the difficulties you experience when you participate in a conversation with someone who is not familiar to you?" would be considered an assessment of Activity/Participation limitation or restriction. Questionnaires that require clients to report the magnitude of difficulty that they experience in certain specified settings can sometimes be used to measure aspects of Activity/Participation. For example: "Because of my hearing problems, I have difficulty conversing with others in a restaurant." In addition, Environmental and Personal Factors also need to be taken into consideration by audiologists as they treat individuals with auditory, vestibular, and other related impairments. In the above question regarding conversation in a restaurant, if the factor of "noise" (i.e., a noisy restaurant) is added to the question, this represents an Environmental Factor. Examples of Personal Factors might include a person's background or culture that influences his or her reaction to the use of a hearing aid or cochlear implant. The use of the ICF framework (WHO, 2001) may help audiologists broaden their perspective concerning their role in evaluating a client's needs or when designing and providing comprehensive services to their clients. Overall, audiologists work to improve quality of life by reducing impairments of body functions and structures, Activity limitations/Participation restrictions and Environmental barriers of the individuals they serve.

DEFINITION OF AN AUDIOLOGIST

Audiologists are professionals engaged in autonomous practice to promote healthy hearing, communication competency, and quality of life for persons of all ages through the prevention, identification, assessment, and rehabilitation of hearing, auditory function, balance, and other related systems. They facilitate prevention through the fitting of hearing protective devices, education programs for industry and the public, hearing screening/conservation programs, and research. The audiologist is the professional responsible for the identification of impairments and dysfunction of the auditory, balance, and other related systems. Their unique education and training provides them with the skills to assess and diagnose dysfunction in hearing, auditory function, balance, and related disorders. The delivery of audiologic (re)habilitation services includes not only the selecting, fitting, and dispensing of hearing aids and other hearing assistive devices, but also the assessment and follow-up services for persons with cochlear implants. The audiologist providing audiologic (re)habilitation does so through a

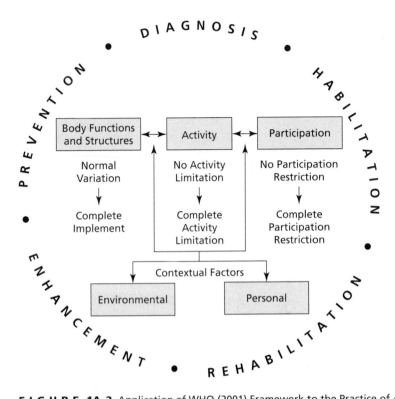

FIGURE 1A–2 Application of WHO (2001) Framework to the Practice of Audiology

comprehensive program of therapeutic services, devices, counseling, and other management strategies. Functional diagnosis of vestibular disorders and management of balance rehabilitation is another aspect of the professional responsibilities of the audiologist. Audiologists engage in research pertinent to all of these domains.

Audiologists currently hold a master's or doctoral degree in audiology from a program accredited by the Council on Academic Accreditation in Audiology and Speech-Language Pathology (CAA) of the American Speech-Language-Hearing Association. ASHA-certified audiologists complete a supervised postgraduate professional experience or a similar supervised professional experience during the completion of the doctoral degree as described in the ASHA certification standards. Beginning January 1, 2012, all applicants for the Certificate of Clinical Competence in Audiology must have a doctoral

degree from a CAA-accredited university program. Demonstration of continued professional development is mandated for the maintenance of the Certificate of Clinical Competence in Audiology. Where required, audiologists are licensed or registered by the state in which they practice.

PROFESSIONAL ROLES AND ACTIVITIES

Audiologists serve a diverse population and may function in one or more of a variety of activities. The practice of audiology includes:

A. Prevention

1. Promotion of hearing wellness, as well as the prevention of hearing loss and protection of hearing function by designing,

implementing, and coordinating occupational, school, and community hearing conservation and identification programs;

2. Participation in noise measurements of the acoustic environment to improve accessibility and to promote hearing wellness.

B. Identification
1. Activities that identify dysfunction in hearing, balance, and other auditory-related systems;
2. Supervision, implementation, and follow-up of newborn and school hearing screening programs;
3. Screening for speech, orofacial myofunctional disorders, language, cognitive communication disorders, and/or preferred communication modalities that may affect education, health, development or communication and may result in recommendations for rescreening or comprehensive speech-language pathology assessment or in referral for other examinations or services;
4. Identification of populations and individuals with or at risk for hearing loss and other auditory dysfunction, balance impairments, tinnitus, and associated communication impairments as well as of those with normal hearing;
5. In collaboration with speech-language pathologists, identification of populations and individuals at risk for developing speech-language impairments.

C. Assessment
1. The conduct and interpretation of behavioral, electroacoustic, and/or electrophysiologic methods to assess hearing, auditory function, balance, and related systems;
2. Measurement and interpretation of sensory and motor evoked potentials, electromyography, and other electrodiagnostic tests for purposes of neurophysiologic intraoperative monitoring and cranial nerve assessment;
3. Evaluation and management of children and adults with auditory-related processing disorders;

4. Performance of otoscopy for appropriate audiological management or to provide a basis for medical referral;
5. Cerumen management to prevent obstruction of the external ear canal and of amplification devices;
6. Preparation of a report including interpreting data, summarizing findings, generating recommendations and developing an audiologic treatment/management plan;
7. Referrals to other professions, agencies, and/or consumer organizations.

D. Rehabilitation
1. As part of the comprehensive audiologic (re)habilitation program, evaluates, selects, fits and dispenses hearing assistive technology devices to include hearing aids;
2. Assessment of candidacy of persons with hearing loss for cochlear implants and provision of fitting, mapping, and audiologic rehabilitation to optimize device use;
3. Development of a culturally appropriate, audiologic rehabilitative management plan including, when appropriate:
   a. Recommendations for fitting and dispensing, and educating the consumer and family/caregivers in the use of and adjustment to sensory aids, hearing assistive devices, alerting systems, and captioning devices;
   b. Availability of counseling relating to psycho social aspects of hearing loss, and other auditory dysfunction, and processes to enhance communication competence;
   c. Skills training and consultation concerning environmental modifications to facilitate development of receptive and expressive communication;
   d. Evaluation and modification of the audiologic management plan.
4. Provision of comprehensive audiologic rehabilitation services, including management procedures for speech and language habilitation and/or rehabilitation for

persons with hearing loss or other auditory dysfunction, including but not exclusive to speechreading, auditory training, communication strategies, manual communication and counseling for psychosocial adjustment for persons with hearing loss or other auditory dysfunction and their families/caregivers;

5. Consultation and provision of vestibular and balance rehabilitation therapy to persons with vestibular and balance impairments;

6. Assessment and non-medical management of tinnitus using biofeedback, behavioral management, masking, hearing aids, education, and counseling;

7. Provision of training for professionals of related and/or allied services when needed;

8. Participation in the development of an Individual Education Program (IEP) for school-age children or an Individual Family Service Plan (IFSP) for children from birth to 36 months old;

9. Provision of in-service programs for school personnel, and advising school districts in planning educational programs and accessibility for students with hearing loss and other auditory dysfunction;

10. Measurement of noise levels and provision of recommendations for environmental modifications in order to reduce the noise level;

11. Management of the selection, purchase, installation, and evaluation of large-area amplification systems.

E. Advocacy/Consultation

1. Advocacy for communication needs of all individuals that may include advocating for the rights/funding of services for those with hearing loss, auditory, or vestibular disorders;

2. Advocacy for issues (i.e., acoustic accessibility) that affect the rights of individuals with normal hearing;

3. Consultation with professionals of related and/or allied services when needed;

4. Consultation in development of an Individual Education Program (IEP) for school-age children or an Individual Family Service Plan (IFSP) for children from birth to 36 months old;

5. Consultation to educators as members of interdisciplinary teams about communication management, educational implications of hearing loss and other auditory dysfunction, educational programming, classroom acoustics, and large-area amplification systems for children with hearing loss and other auditory dysfunction;

6. Consultation about accessibility for persons with hearing loss and other auditory dysfunction in public and private buildings, programs, and services;

7. Consultation to individuals, public and private agencies, and governmental bodies, or as an expert witness regarding legal interpretations of audiology findings, effects of hearing loss and other auditory dysfunction, balance system impairments, and relevant noise-related considerations;

8. Case management and service as a liaison for the consumer, family, and agencies in order to monitor audiologic status and management and to make recommendations about educational and vocational programming;

9. Consultation to industry on the development of products and instrumentation related to the measurement and management of auditory or balance function.

F. Education/Research/Administration

1. Education, supervision, and administration for audiology graduate and other professional education programs;

2. Measurement of functional outcomes, consumer satisfaction, efficacy, effectiveness, and efficiency of practices and

programs to maintain and improve the quality of audiologic services;

3. Design and conduct of basic and applied audiologic research to increase the knowledge base, to develop new methods and programs, and to determine the efficacy, effectiveness, and efficiency of assessment and treatment paradigms; disseminate research findings to other professionals and to the public;

4. Participation in the development of professional and technical standards;

5. Participation in quality improvement programs;

6. Program administration and supervision of professionals as well as support personnel.

PRACTICE SETTINGS

Audiologists provide services in private practice; medical settings such as hospitals and physicians' offices; community and university hearing and speech centers; managed care systems; industry; the military; various state agencies; home health, subacute rehabilitation, long-term care, and intermediate-care facilities; and school systems. Audiologists provide academic education to students and practitioners in universities, to medical and surgical students and residents, and to other related professionals. Such education pertains to the identification, functional diagnosis/assessment, and non-medical treatment/management of auditory, vestibular, balance, and related impairments.

REFERENCES

American Speech-Language-Hearing Association. (1996, Spring). Scope of practice in audiology. *Asha, 38* (Suppl. 16), 12–15.

American Speech-Language-Hearing Association. (2003). Code of ethics (revised). *ASHA Supplement, 23,* 13–15.

World Health Organization (WHO). (2001). *ICF: International classification of functioning, disability and health.* Geneva: Author.

RESOURCES

General

American Speech-Language-Hearing Association. (1979, March). Severely hearing handicapped. *Asha, 21.*

American Speech-Language-Hearing Association. (1985, June). Clinical supervision in speech-language pathology and audiology. *Asha, 27,* 57–60.

American Speech-Language-Hearing Association. (1986, May). Autonomy of speech-language pathology and audiology. *Asha, 28,* 53–57.

American Speech-Language-Hearing Association. (1987, June). Calibration of speech signals delivered via earphones. *Asha, 29,* 44–48.

American Speech-Language-Hearing Association. (1988). *Mental retardation and developmental disabili-ties curriculum guide for speech-language pathologists and audiologists.* Rockville, MD: Author.

American Speech-Language-Hearing Association. (1989, March). Bilingual speech-language pathologists and audiologists: Definition. *Asha, 31,* 93.

American Speech-Language-Hearing Association. (1989, June/July). AIDS/HIV: Implications for speech-language pathologists and audiologists. *Asha, 31,* 33–38.

American Speech-Language-Hearing Association. (1990). The role of speech-language pathologists and audiologists in service delivery for persons with mental retardation and developmental disabilities in community settings. *Asha, 32* (Suppl. 2), 5–6.

American Speech-Language-Hearing Association. (1990, April). Major issues affecting delivery of services in hospital settings: Recommendations and strategies. *Asha, 32,* 67–70.

American Speech-Language-Hearing Association. (1991). Sound field measurement tutorial. *Asha, 33* (Suppl. 3), 25–37.

American Speech-Language-Hearing Association. (1992). 1992 U.S. Department of Labor definition of speech-language pathologists and audiologists. *Asha, 4,* 563–565.

American Speech-Language-Hearing Association. (1992). Sedation and topical anesthetics in audiology and speech-language pathology. *Asha, 34* (March, Suppl. 7), 41–42.

American Speech-Language-Hearing Association. (1993). National health policy: Back to the future (technical report). *Asha, 35,* (Suppl. 10), 2–10.

American Speech-Language-Hearing Association. (1993). Position statement on national health policy. *Asha, 35* (Suppl. 10), 1.

American Speech-Language-Hearing Association. (1993). Professional performance appraisal by individuals outside the professions of speech-language pathology and audiology. *Asha, 35,* (Suppl. 10), 11–13.

American Speech-Language-Hearing Association. (1994, January). The protection of rights of people receiving audiology or speech-language pathology services. *Asha, 36,* 60–63.

American Speech-Language-Hearing Association. (1994, March). Guidelines for the audiologic management of individuals receiving cochleotoxic drug therapy. *Asha, 36* (Suppl. 12), 11–19.

American Speech-Language-Hearing Association. (1995, March). Guidelines for education in audiology practice management. *Asha, 37* (Suppl. 14), 20.

American Speech-Language-Hearing Association. (1997). *Preferred practice patterns for the profession of audiology.* Rockville, MD: Author.

American Speech-Language-Hearing Association. (1997, Spring). Position statement: Multiskilled personnel. *Asha, 39* (Suppl. 17), 13.

American Speech-Language-Hearing Association. (1998). Position statement and guidelines on support personnel in audiology. *Asha, 40* (Suppl. 18), 19–21.

American Speech-Language-Hearing Association. (2001). *Scope of practice in speech-language pathology.* Rockville, MD: Author.

American Speech-Language-Hearing Association. (2002). *Certification and membership handbook: Audiology.* Rockville, MD: Author.

American Speech-Language-Hearing Association. (2003). Code of ethics (revised). *ASHA Supplement 23,* 13–15.

Joint Audiology Committee on Clinical Practice. (1999). *Clinical practice statements and algorithms.* Rockville, MD: American Speech-Language-Hearing Association.

Joint Committee of the American Speech-Language-Hearing Association (ASHA) and the Council on Education of the Deaf (CED). (1998). Hearing loss: Terminology and classification: Position statement and technical report. *Asha, 40* (Suppl. 18), 22.

Paul-Brown, Diane. (1994, May). Clinical record keeping in audiology and speech pathology. *Asha, 36,* 40–43.

AMPLIFICATION

American Speech-Language-Hearing Association. (1991). Amplification as a remediation technique for children with normal peripheral hearing. *Asha, 33* (Suppl. 3), 22–24.

American Speech-Language-Hearing Association. (1998). Guidelines for hearing aid fitting for adults. *American Journal of Audiology, 7*(1), 5–13.

American Speech-Language-Hearing Association. (2000). Guidelines for graduate education in amplification. *ASHA Supplement, 20,* 22–27.

American Speech-Language-Hearing Association. (2002). Guidelines for fitting and monitoring FM systems. *ASHA Desk Reference,* vol. 2, 151–172.

American Speech-Language Hearing Association. (2004). Technical report: Cochlear implants. *ASHA Supplement, 24,* in press.

AUDIOLOGIC REHABILITATION

American Speech-Language-Hearing Association. (1981, April). On the definition of hearing handicap. *Asha, 23,* 293–297.

American Speech-Language-Hearing Association. (1984, May). Definition of and competencies for aural rehabilitation. *Asha, 26,* 37–41.

American Speech-Language-Hearing Association. (1990). Aural rehabilitation: An annotated bibliography. *Asha, 32* (Suppl. 1), 1–12.

American Speech-Language-Hearing Association. (1992, March). Electrical stimulation for cochlear implant selection and rehabilitation. *Asha, 34* (Suppl. 7), 13–16.

American Speech-Language-Hearing Association. (2001). *ARBIB: Audiologic rehabilitation—basic information bibliography.* Rockville, MD: Author.

American Speech-Language-Hearing Association. (2001). *Knowledge and skills required for the practice of audiologic/aural rehabilitation.* Rockville, MD: Author.

AUDIOLOGIC SCREENING

American Speech-Language-Hearing Association. (1988, November). Telephone hearing screening. *Asha, 30,* 53.

American Speech-Language-Hearing Association. (1994, June/July). Audiologic screening (Executive summary). *Asha, 36,* 53–54.

American Speech-Language-Hearing Association Audiologic Assessment Panel 1996. (1997). *Guidelines for audiologic screening.* Rockville, MD: Author.

(CENTRAL) AUDITORY PROCESSING DISORDERS

American Speech-Language-Hearing Association. (1979, December). The role of the speech-language pathologist and audiologist in learning disabilities. *Asha, 21,* 1015.

American Speech-Language-Hearing Association. (1990). Audiological assessment of central auditory processing: An annotated bibliography. *Asha, 32* (Suppl. 1), 13–30.

American Speech-Language-Hearing Association. (1996, July). Central auditory processing: Current status of research and implications for clinical practice. *American Journal of Audiology, 5*(2), 41–54.

BUSINESS PRACTICES

American Speech-Language-Hearing Association. (1987, March). Private practice. *Asha, 29,* 35.

American Speech-Language-Hearing Association. (1991). Business, marketing, ethics, and professionalism in audiology: An updated annotated bibliography (1986–1989). *Asha, 33* (Suppl. 3), 39–45.

American Speech-Language-Hearing Association. (1991). Considerations for establishing a private practice in audiology and/or speech-language pathology. *Asha, 33* (Suppl. 3), 10–21.

American Speech-Language-Hearing Association. (1991). Report on private practice. *Asha, 33* (Suppl. 6), 1–4.

American Speech-Language-Hearing Association. (1994). Professional liability and risk management for the audiology and special-language pathology professions. *Asha, 36* (March, Suppl. 12), 25–38.

DIAGNOSTIC PROCEDURES

American Speech-Language-Hearing Association. (1978). Guidelines for manual pure-tone threshold audiometry. *Asha, 20,* 297–301.

American Speech-Language-Hearing Association. (1988, March). Guidelines for determining threshold level for speech. *Asha,* 85–89.

American Speech-Language-Hearing Association. (1988, November). Tutorial: Tympanometry. *Journal of Speech and Hearing Disorders, 53,* 354–377.

American Speech-Language-Hearing Association. (1990). Guidelines for audiometric symbols. *Asha, 32* (Suppl. 2), 25–30.

American Speech-Language-Hearing Association. (1991). Acoustic-immittance measures: A bibliography. *Asha, 33* (Suppl. 4), 1–44.

American Speech-Language-Hearing Association. (1992, March). External auditory canal examination and cerumen management. *Asha, 34* (Suppl. 7), 22–24.

EDUCATIONAL AUDIOLOGY

American Speech-Language-Hearing Association. (1991). Utilization of Medicaid and other third party funds for covered services in the schools. *Asha, 33* (Suppl. 5), 51–59.

American Speech-Language-Hearing Association. (1995, March). Acoustics in educational settings: Position statement and guidelines. *Asha, 37* (Suppl. 14), 15–19.

American Speech-Language-Hearing Association. (1997). Trends and issues in school reform and their effects on speech-language pathologists, audiologists, and students with communication disorders. *ASHA Desk Reference,* Vol. 4, 317–326.

American Speech-Language-Hearing Association. (1997, Spring). Position statement: Roles of audiologists and speech-language-pathologists working with persons with attention deficit hyperactivity disorder: Position statement and technical report. *Asha, 39* (Suppl. 17), 14.

American Speech-Language-Hearing Association. (2002). *Guidelines for audiology service provision in and for schools.* Rockville, MD: Author.

American Speech-Language-Hearing Association. (2002). Appropriate school facilities for students with speech-language-hearing disorders: Technical report. *ASHA Supplement 23,* 83–86.

ELECTROPHYSIOLOGICAL ASSESSMENT

American Speech-Language-Hearing Association. (1987). *Short latency auditory evoked potentials.* Rockville, MD: Author.

American Speech-Language-Hearing Association. (1992, March). Neurophysiologic intraoperative monitoring. *Asha, 34* (Suppl. 7), 34–36.

American Speech-Language-Hearing Association. (2003). Guidelines for competencies in auditory evoked potential measurement and clinical applications. *ASHA Supplement 23,* 35–40.

GERIATRIC AUDIOLOGY

American Speech-Language-Hearing Association. (1988, March). Provision of audiology and speech-language pathology services to older persons in nursing homes. *Asha,* 772–774.

American Speech-Language-Hearing Association. (1988, March). The roles of speech-language pathologists and audiologists in working with older persons. *Asha, 30,* 80–84.

American Speech-Language-Hearing Association. (1997, Spring). Guidelines for audiology

service delivery in nursing homes. *Asha, 39* (Suppl. 17), 15–29.

OCCUPATIONAL AUDIOLOGY

American Speech-Language-Hearing Association. (1996, Spring). Guidelines on the audiologist's role in occupational and environmental hearing conservation. *Asha, 38* (Suppl. 16), 34–41.

American Speech-Language-Hearing Association. (1997, Spring). Issues: Occupational and environmental hearing conservation. *Asha, 39* (Suppl. 17), 30–34.

American Speech-Language-Hearing Association (2004). The audiologist's role in occupational

hearing conservation and hearing loss prevention programs. *ASHA Supplement 24.* In press. —what type of document is this? Different from the following reference?

American Speech-Language-Hearing Association (2004). The audiologist's role in occupational hearing conservation and hearing loss prevention programs: Technical report. *ASHA Supplement 24,* in press.

PEDIATRIC AUDIOLOGY

American Speech-Language-Hearing Association. (1991). Guidelines for the audiological assessment of children from birth through 36 months of age. *Asha, 33* (Suppl. 5), 37–43.

American Speech-Language-Hearing Association. (1991). The use of FM amplification instruments for infants and preschool children with hearing impairment. *Asha, 33* (Suppl. 5), 1–2.

American Speech-Language-Hearing Association. (1994, August). Service provision under the Indi-

viduals with Disabilities Education Act-Part H, as amended (IDEA-Part H) to children who are deaf and hard of hearing—ages birth to 36 months. *Asha, 36,* 117–121.

Joint Committee on Infant Hearing. (2000). JCIH year 2000 position statement: Principles and guidelines for early hearing detection and intervention programs. *American Journal of Audiology, 9,* 9–29.

VESTIBULAR

American Speech-Language-Hearing Association. (1992, March). Balance system assessment. *Asha, 34* (Suppl. 7), 9–12.

American Speech-Language-Hearing Association. (1999, March). Role of audiologists in vestibular

and balance rehabilitation: Position statement, guidelines, and technical report. *Asha, 41* (Suppl. 19), 13–22.

APPENDIX 1–B

Scope of Practice in

Speech-Language Pathology

AD HOC COMMITTEE ON SCOPE OF PRACTICE IN SPEECH-LANGUAGE PATHOLOGY

This document was approved by the ASHA Legislative Council in April 2001 (LC 7-01). Members of the 000 Ad Hoc Committee on Scope of Practice in Speech-Language Pathology who developed this document are Nicholas Bankson (chair), Allan Diefendorf, Roberta Elman, Susan Forsythe, Elizabeth Gavett, Alex Johnson (vice president for professional practices in speech-language pathology who serves as Executive Board liaison), Lori Lombard, Ninevah Murray, Arlene Pietranton (ex officio), and Carmen Vega-Barachowitz.

STATEMENT OF PURPOSE

The purpose of this document is to define the scope of practice in speech-language pathology in order to:

1. Delineate areas of speech-language pathology professional practice provided by members of the American Speech-Language-Hearing Association (ASHA) and clinical certification holders in accordance with the ASHA Code of Ethics;

2. Educate health care, education, and other professionals, consumers, payers, regulators, and members of the general public about profes-

sional services offered by speech-language pathologists as qualified providers;

3. Assist ASHA members and certificate holders in the provision of high quality and evidence-based services to individuals across the life span who present with communication, swallowing, or other upper aerodigestive concerns[1];

4. Provide guidance for education programs in speech-language pathology curriculum.

The scope of practice defined here and the areas specifically set forth describe the breadth of professional practice offered within the profession. Levels of education, experience, skill, and proficiency with respect to the activities identified within this scope of practice vary among individual providers; a speech-language pathologist does not typically practice in all areas of the field. As the ASHA Code of Ethics specifies, individuals may only practice in areas in which they are competent based on their education, training, and experience. However, speech-language pathologists may expand

Reference this material as: American Speech-Language-Hearing Association. (2001). *Scope of practice in speech-language pathology.* Rockville, MD: Author.

Index terms: ASHA reference products, practice scope and patterns. SLP education and qualifications, SLP practice settings, SLP roles and activities, speech-language pathology, World Health Organization (WHO) framework

Document type: Practice guidelines and policies

SOURCE: American Speech-Language-Hearing Association. (2001). *Scope of Practice in Speech-Language Pathology.* Available from http://www.asha.org/about/publications/reference-library/Reprinted with permission.
[1]Aeromechanical events related to communication, respiration, and swallowing (e.g., speaking valve selection, respiratory retraining for paradoxical vocal fold motion, stomal stenosis management, and insufflation testing after total laryngectomy).

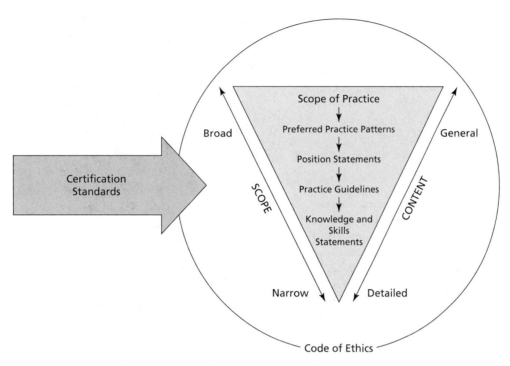

FIGURE 1B–1 Conceptual Framework of ASHA Standards and Policy Statements

their current level of expertise. Certain situations may necessitate that speech-language pathologists pursue additional education or training to expand their personal scope of practice.

This scope of practice statement does not supersede existing state licensure laws or affect the interpretation or implementation of such laws. It may serve, however, as a model for the development or modification of licensure laws.

The schema in Figure 1B-1 (see above) depicts the relationship of the scope of practice to practice policy documents, certification standards, and the ASHA Code of Ethics. As indicated, individuals must fulfill the speech-language pathology certification standards in order to enter the practice of the profession. Practice policy documents (i.e., preferred practice patterns, position statements, guidelines, and knowledge and skills statements) address current and emerging speech-language pathology practice areas. These documents build on the knowledge, skills, and experiences required by the certification standards.

The ASHA Code of Ethics sets forth the fundamental principles and rules considered essential to the preservation of the highest standards of integrity and ethical conduct to which members of the profession of speech-language pathology are bound.

Speech-language pathology is a dynamic and continuously developing profession; listing specific areas within this scope of practice does not exclude emerging areas of practice. Although not specifically identified in this document, in certain instances speech-language pathologists may be called on to perform services (e.g., "multiskilling" in a health care setting, collaborative service delivery in schools) for the well-being of the individual(s) they are serving. In such instances it is both ethically and legally incumbent upon professionals to determine that they have the knowledge and skills necessary to conduct such tasks. Finally, it should be indicated that factors such as changes in service delivery systems, increasing numbers of people needing services, projected United States population growth of cultural and linguistic minority groups, and technological and scientific advances mandate that a scope of practice statement for the profession of speech-language pathology be dynamic in nature. For these reasons, this document will undergo periodic review and possible revision.

FRAMEWORK FOR PRACTICE

The domain of speech-language pathology includes human communication behaviors and disorders as well as swallowing or other upper aerodigestive functions and disorders. The overall objective of speech-language pathology services is to optimize individuals' ability to communicate and/or swallow in natural environments, and thus improve their quality of life. This objective is best achieved through the provision of integrated services in meaningful life contexts. The World Health Organization (WHO) is in the process of finalizing a multipurpose health classification system identified as the International Classification of Functioning, Disability and Health (ICIDH-2)* that offers clinical service providers an internationally recognized conceptual framework and common language for discussing and describing human functioning and disability (WHO, 2000). This framework can be used to describe the role of speech-language pathologists in enhancing quality of life by optimizing human communication behavior, swallowing, or other upper aerodigestive functions regardless of setting. The ICIDH-2 [ICF] framework has two parts. The first is termed Functioning and Disability; the second refers to Contextual Factors. Functioning and Disability includes the following two components:

- **Body Functions and Structures:** Body Functions refers to the physiological or psychological functions of body systems; Body Structures refers to the anatomic parts of the body and their components.
- **Activity/Participation:** Activity refers to the performance of a task or action of a given

individual; Participation refers to an individual's involvement in a life situation. Both Activity and Participation components are modified with Capacity and Performance qualifiers. The Capacity qualifier describes an individual's ability to execute a task or an action in a standardized or uniform environment. The Performance qualifier describes what an individual does in the current environment or actual context in which s/he lives.

Figure 1B–2 illustrates the components of the framework as applied to the practice of speech-language pathology. Each component can be expressed as a continuum of function. One end of the continuum indicates intact or neutral functioning; the other indicates completely compromised function or disability (e.g., impairment, activity limitation [formerly referred to as *disability* (WHO, 1980)], or participation restriction [formerly referred to as *handicap* (WHO, 1980)]). For example, the component of Body Functions and Structures has a continuum that ranges from normal variation to complete impairment; Activity ranges from no activity limitation to complete activity limitation; and Participation ranges from no participation restriction to complete participation restriction.

The second part of the ICIDH-2 [ICF] framework refers to Contextual Factors. Contextual Factors may interact with Body Functions and Structures, Activity, or Participation as facilitators or barriers to functioning. Contextual Factors include the following two components:

- **Environmental Factors:** defined as the physical, social, and attitudinal environment in which people live.
- **Personal Factors:** include such features of an individual as age, race, gender, educational background, and lifestyle. Although not formally classified in the ICIDH-2 [ICF], Personal Factors are acknowledged to be contributors to intervention outcomes.

The scope of practice in speech-language pathology encompasses all components and factors

---

*Editor's note: In 2001 the original acronym, ICIDH-2, was changed to ICF.

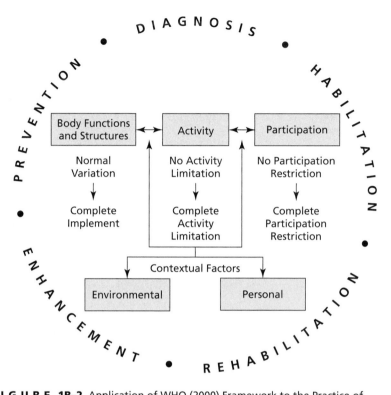

FIGURE 1B–2 Application of WHO (2000) Framework to the Practice of Speech-Language Pathology

identified in the WHO framework. That is, speech-language pathologists work to improve quality of life by reducing impairments of body functions and structures, activity limitations, participation restrictions, and environmental barriers of the individuals they serve. They serve individuals with known disease processes (e.g., aphasia, cleft palate) as well as those with activity limitations or participation restrictions (e.g., individuals needing classroom support services or special educational placement), including when such limitations or restrictions occur in the absence of known disease processes or impairments (e.g., individuals with differences in dialect). The role of speech-language pathologists includes prevention of communication, swallowing, or other upper aerodigestive disorders as well as diagnosis, habilitation, rehabilitation, and enhancement of these functions.

EDUCATION AND QUALIFICATIONS

Speech-language pathologists must hold a graduate degree, the Certificate of Clinical Competence (CCC-SLP) of the American Speech-Language-Hearing Association (ASHA), and where applicable, other required credentials (e.g., state licensure, teaching certification).

As primary care providers for communication, swallowing, or other upper aerodigestive disorders, speech-language pathologists are autonomous professionals; that is, their services need not be prescribed or supervised by individuals in other professions. However, in many cases individuals are best served when speech-language pathologists work collaboratively with other professionals.

SCOPE OF PRACTICE

The practice of speech-language pathology includes prevention, diagnosis, habilitation, and rehabilitation of communication, swallowing, or other upper aerodigestive disorders; elective modification of communication behaviors; and enhancement of communication. This includes services that address the dimensions of body structure and function, activity, and/or participation as proposed by the World Health Organization model (WHO, 2000). The practice of speech-language pathology involves:

1. Providing prevention, screening, consultation, assessment and diagnosis, treatment, intervention, management, counseling, and follow-up services for disorders of:

   - speech (i.e., articulation, fluency, resonance, and voice including aeromechanical components of respiration);

   - language (i.e., phonology, morphology, syntax, semantics, and pragmatic/social aspects of communication) including comprehension and expression in oral, written, graphic, and manual modalities; language processing; preliteracy and language-based literacy skills, including phonological awareness;

   - swallowing or other upper aerodigestive functions such as infant feeding and aeromechanical events (evaluation of esophageal function is for the purpose of referral to medical professionals);

   - cognitive aspects of communication (e.g., attention, memory, problem solving, executive functions);

   - sensory awareness related to communication, swallowing, or other upper aerodigestive functions.

2. Establishing augmentative and alternative communication techniques and strategies including developing, selecting, and prescribing of such systems and devices (e.g., speech generating devices);

3. Providing services to individuals with hearing loss and their families/caregivers (e.g., auditory training; speechreading; speech and language intervention secondary to hearing loss; visual inspection and listening checks of amplification devices for the purpose of troubleshooting, including verification of appropriate battery voltage);

4. Screening hearing of individuals who can participate in conventional pure-tone air conduction methods, as well as screening for middle ear pathology through screening tympanometry for the purpose of referral of individuals for further evaluation and management;

5. Using instrumentation (e.g., videofluoroscopy, EMG, nasendoscopy, stroboscopy, computer technology) to observe, collect data, and measure parameters of communication and swallowing or other upper aerodigestive functions in accordance with the principles of evidence-based practice;

6. Selecting, fitting, and establishing effective use of prosthetic/adaptive devices for communication, swallowing, or other upper aerodigestive functions (e.g., tracheoesophageal prostheses, speaking valves, electrolarynges). This does not include sensory devices used by individuals with hearing loss or other auditory perceptual deficits;

7. Collaborating in the assessment of central auditory processing disorders and providing intervention where there is evidence of speech, language, and/or other cognitive-communication disorders;

8. Educating and counseling individuals, families, co-workers, educators, and other persons in the community regarding acceptance, adaptation, and decision making about communication, swallowing, or other upper aerodigestive concerns;

9. Advocating for individuals through community awareness, education, and training programs to promote and facilitate access to full

participation in communication, including the elimination of societal barriers.

10. Collaborating with and providing referrals and information to audiologists, educators, and health professionals as individual needs dictate;

11. Addressing behaviors (e.g., perseverative or disruptive actions) and environments (e.g., seating, positioning for swallowing safety or attention, communication opportunities) that affect communication, swallowing, or other upper aerodigestive functions;

12. Providing services to modify or enhance communication performance (e.g., accent modification, transgendered voice, care and improvement of the professional voice, personal/ professional communication effectiveness);

13. Recognizing the need to provide and appropriately accommodate diagnostic and treatment services to individuals from diverse cultural backgrounds and adjust treatment and assessment services accordingly.

PROFESSIONAL ROLES AND ACTIVITIES

Speech-language pathologists serve individuals, families, groups, and the general public through a broad range of professional activities. They:

- Identify, define, and diagnose disorders of human communication and swallowing and assist in localization and diagnosis of diseases and conditions;

- Provide direct services using a variety of service delivery models to treat and/or address communication, swallowing, or other upper aerodigestive concerns;

- Conduct research related to communication sciences and disorders, swallowing, or other upper aerodigestive functions;

- Educate, supervise, and mentor future speech-language pathologists;

- Serve as case managers and service delivery coordinators;

- Administer and manage clinical and academic programs;

- Educate and provide in-service training to families, caregivers, and other professionals;

- Participate in outcomes measurement activities and use data to guide clinical decision making and determine the effectiveness of services provided in accordance with the principles of evidence-based practice;

- Train, supervise, and manage speech-language pathology assistants and other support personnel.

- Promote healthy lifestyle practices for the prevention of communication, hearing, swallowing, or other upper aerodigestive disorders;

- Foster public awareness of speech, language, hearing, swallowing, and other upper aerodigestive disorders and their treatment;

- Advocate at the local, state, and national levels for access to and funding for services to address communication, hearing, swallowing, and other upper aerodigestive disorders;

- Serve as expert witnesses;

- Collaborate with audiologists in identifying neonates and infants at risk for hearing loss;

- Recognize the special needs of culturally diverse populations by providing services that are free of potential biases, including selection and/or adaptation of materials to ensure ethnic and linguistic sensitivity;

- Provide services using tele-electronic diagnostic measures and treatment methodologies (including remote applications);

PRACTICE SETTINGS

Speech-language pathologists provide services in a wide variety of settings, which may include but are not exclusive to:

- Public and private schools
- Health care settings (e.g., hospitals, medical rehabilitation facilities, long-term care

facilities, home health agencies, community clinics, behavioral/mental health facilities)
- Private practice settings
- Universities and university clinics
- Individuals' homes
- Group homes and sheltered workshops

- Neonatal intensive care units, early intervention settings, preschools, and daycare centers
- Community and state agencies and institutions
- Correctional institutions
- Research facilities
- Corporate and industrial settings

REFERENCE AND RESOURCE LIST

General

American Speech-Language-Hearing Association. (1986, May). The autonomy of speech-language pathology and audiology. *Asha, 28,* 53–57.

American Speech-Language-Hearing Association. (1992). Sedation and topical anesthetics in audiology and speech-language pathology. *Asha, 34* (Suppl. 7), 41–42.

American Speech-Language-Hearing Association. (1993). Definition of communication disorders and variations. *Asha, 35* (Suppl. 10), 40–41.

American Speech-Language-Hearing Association. (1993). Guidelines for caseload size and speech-language pathology service delivery in the school. *Asha, 35* (Suppl.10), 33–39.

American Speech-Language-Hearing Association. (1994). *Admission/discharge criteria in speech-language pathology.* Unpublished report. Rockville, MD: Author.

American Speech-Language-Hearing Association. (1994). Code of ethics. *Asha, 36* (Suppl. 13), 1–2. *under revision*

American Speech-Language-Hearing Association. (1996). Inclusive practices for children and youths with communication disorders. *Asha, 38* (Suppl. 16), 35–44.

American Speech-Language-Hearing Association. (1996). Scope of practice in audiology. *Asha, 38* (Suppl. 16), 12–15.

American Speech-Language-Hearing Association. (1997). Position statement and technical report: Multiskilled personnel. *Asha, 39* (Suppl. 17), 13.

American Speech-Language-Hearing Association. (1997). *Preferred practice patterns for the profession of speechlanguage pathology.* Rockville, MD: Author.

American Speech-Language-Hearing Association. (1999). *Guidelines for the roles and responsibilities of the school-based speech-language pathologist.* Rockville, MD: Author.

American Speech-Language-Hearing Association. (2000). *IDEA and your caseload: A template for eligibility and dismissal criteria for students ages 3 to 21.* Rockville, MD: Author.

Council on Professional Standards in Speech-Language Pathology and Audiology. (2000). *Speech-language pathology certification standards.* Rockville, MD: Author.

World Health Organization. (2000). *International classification of functioning, disability and health: Prefinal draft.* Geneva, Switzerland: Author.

Augmentative and Alternative Communication

American Speech-Language-Hearing Association. (1989). Competencies for speech-language pathologists providing services in augmentative communication. *Asha, 31*(3), 107–110.

American Speech-Language-Hearing Association. (1991). Augmentative and alternative communication. *Asha, 33* (Suppl. 5), 8.

American Speech-Language-Hearing Association. (1991). Report: Augmentative and alternative communication. *Asha, 33* (Suppl. 5), 9–12.

American Speech-Language-Hearing Association. (1998). Maximizing the provision of appropriate technology services and devices for students in schools. *Asha, 40* (Suppl. 18), 33–42.

National Joint Committee for the Communicative Needs of Persons with Severe Disabilities. (1992). Guidelines for meeting the communication needs of persons with severe disabilities. *Asha, 34* (Suppl. 7), 1–8.

Cognitive Aspects of Communication

American Speech-Language-Hearing Association. (1982). Serving the communicatively handicapped mentally retarded individual. *Asha, 24*(8), 547–553.

American Speech-Language-Hearing Association. (1987). The role of speech-language pathologists in the habilitation and rehabilitation of cognitively impaired individuals. *Asha, 29*(6), 53–55.

American Speech-Language-Hearing Association. (1988). Mental retardation and developmental disabilities curriculum guide for speech-language pathologists and audiologists. *ASHA Desk Reference*, vol. 4, 185–189.

American Speech-Language-Hearing Association. (1988). The role of speech-language pathologists in the identification, diagnosis, and treatment of individuals with cognitive-communicative impairments. *Asha, 30*(3), 79.

American Speech-Language-Hearing Association. (1990). Interdisciplinary approaches to brain damage. *Asha, 32* (Suppl. 2), 3.

American Speech-Language-Hearing Association. (1990). The role of speech-language pathologists and audiologists in service delivery for persons with mental retardation and developmental disabilities in community settings. *Asha, 32* (Suppl. 2), 5–6.

American Speech-Language-Hearing Association. (1991). Guidelines for speech-language pathologists serving persons with language, socio-communicative and/or cognitive-communicative impairments. *Asha, 33* (Suppl.5), 21–28.

American Speech-Language-Hearing Association. (1995). Guidelines for the structure and function of an interdisciplinary team for persons with brain injury. *Asha, 37* (Suppl. 14), 23.

Deaf and Hard of Hearing

American Speech-Language-Hearing Association. (1984). Competencies for aural rehabilitation. *Asha, 26* (5), 37–41.

American Speech-Language-Hearing Association. (1990). Aural rehabilitation: an annotated bibliography. *Asha, 32* (Suppl. 1), 1–12.

American Speech-Language-Hearing Association. (1994, August). Service provision under the Individuals with Disabilities Education Act–Part H, as Amended (IDEA–Part H) to children who are deaf and hard of hearing ages birth to 36 months. *Asha, 36*, 117–121.

Hearing Screening

American National Standards Institute. (1996). *Specifications for audiometers* (ANSI S3.6.-1996). New York: Acoustical Society of America.

American National Standards Institute. (1991). *Maximum permissible ambient noise levels for audiometric test rooms* (ANSI S3.1-1991). New York: Acoustical Society of America.

American Speech-Language-Hearing Association. (1994). Clinical practice by certificate holders in the profession in which they are not certified. *Asha, 36*(13), 11–12.

American Speech-Language-Hearing Association. (1997). *Guidelines for audiologic screening*. Rockville, MD: Author.

Joint Committee on Infant Hearing. (2000). Year 2000 position statement: Principles and guidelines for early hearing detection and intervention programs. *American Journal of Audiology, 9*, 9–29.

Language and Literacy

American Speech-Language-Hearing Association. (1982). Definition of language. *Asha, 24* (6), 44.

American Speech-Language-Hearing Association. (1982). Position statement on language learning disorders. *Asha, 24* (11), 937–944.

American Speech-Language-Hearing Association. (1989). Issues in determining eligibility for language intervention. *Asha, 31 (3)*, 113–118.

American Speech-Language-Hearing Association. (1991). A model for collaborative service delivery for students with language-learning disorders in the public schools. *Asha, 33* (Suppl. 5), 44–50.

American Speech-Language-Hearing Association. (1991). Guidelines for speech-language pathologists serving persons with language, socio-communicative and/or cognitive-communicative impairments. *Asha, 33* (Suppl. 5), 21–28.

American Speech-Language-Hearing Association Task Force on Central Auditory Processing Consensus Development. (1995). *Central auditory processing: Current status of research and implications for clinical practice.* Rockville, MD: ASHA.

American Speech-Language-Hearing Association. (2000). *Guidelines on the roles and responsibilities of speechlanguage pathologists with respect to reading and writing in children and adolescents.* Rockville, MD: Author.

American Speech-Language-Hearing Association. (2000). *Position statement on the roles and responsibilities of speechlanguage pathologists with respect to reading and writing in children and adolescents.* Rockville, MD: Author.

American Speech-Language-Hearing Association. (2000). *Technical report on the roles and responsibilities of speechlanguage pathologists with respect to reading and writing in children and adolescents.* Rockville, MD: Author.

National Joint Committee on Learning Disabilities. (1989). Communication-based services for infants, toddlers, and their families. *ASHA Desk Reference,* vol. 3, 159–163.

Multicultural Issues

American Speech-Language-Hearing Association. (1983). Social dialects (and implications). *Asha, 25*(9), 23–27.

American Speech-Language-Hearing Association. (1985). Clinical management of communicatively handicapped minority language populations. Asha, 27(6), 29–32.

American Speech-Language-Hearing Association. (1989). Bilingual speech-language pathologists and audiologists. *Asha, 31,* 93.

American Speech-Language-Hearing Association. (1998). Provision of English-as-a-second-language instruction by speech-language pathologists in school settings: Position statement and technical report. *Asha, 40* (Suppl. 18), 24–27.

Prevention

American Speech-Language-Hearing Association. (1982). Prevention of speech, language, hearing problems. *Asha, 24,* 425, 431.

American Speech-Language-Hearing Association. (1988, March). Prevention of communication disorders. *Asha, 30,* 90.

American Speech-Language-Hearing Association. (1991). The prevention of communication disorders tutorial. *Asha, 33* (Suppl. 6), 15–41.

Research

American Speech-Language-Hearing Association. (1992). Ethics in research and professional practice. *Asha, 34* (Suppl. 9), 11–12.

Speech: Articulation, Fluency, Voice, Resonance

American Speech-Language-Hearing Association. (1992). Position statement and guidelines for evaluation and treatment for tracheoesophageal fistulization/puncture. *Asha, 34* (Suppl. 7), 17–21.

American Speech-Language-Hearing Association. (1992). Position statement and guidelines for vocal tract visualization and imaging. *Asha, 34* (Suppl. 7), 31–40.

American Speech-Language-Hearing Association. (1993). Position statement and guidelines for oral and oropharyngeal prostheses. *Asha, 35* (Suppl. 10), 14–16.

American Speech-Language-Hearing Association. (1993). Position statement and guidelines on the use of voice prostheses in tracheotomized persons with or without ventilatory dependence. *Asha, 35* (Suppl. 10), 17–20.

American Speech-Language-Hearing Association. (1993). The role of the speech-language pathologist and teacher of voice in the remediation of singers with voice disorders. *Asha, 35*(1), 63.

American Speech-Language-Hearing Association. (1995, March). Guidelines for practice in stuttering treatment. *Asha, 37* (Suppl. 14), 26–35.

American Speech-Language-Hearing Association. (1998). Roles of otolaryngologists and speech-language pathologists in the performance and interpretation of strobovideolaryngoscopy. *Asha, 40* (Suppl. 18), 32.

ASHA Special Interest Division 3: Voice and Voice Disorders. (1997). *Training guidelines for laryngeal videoendoscopy/stroboscopy*. Unpublished report. Rockville: MD. Author.

Supervision

American Speech-Language-Hearing Association. (1985). Clinical supervision in speech-language pathology and audiology. *Asha, 28*(6), 57–60.

American Speech-Language-Hearing Association. (1989). Preparation models for the supervisory process in speech-language pathology and audiology. *Asha, 32*(3), 97–106.

American Speech-Language-Hearing Association. (1992). Supervision of student clinicians. *Asha, 34* (Suppl. 9), 8.

American Speech-Language-Hearing Association. (1992). Clinical fellowship supervisor's responsibilities. *Asha, 34* (Suppl. 9), 16–17.

American Speech-Language-Hearing Association. (1996, Spring). Guidelines for the training, credentialing, use, and supervision of speech-language pathology assistants. *Asha, 38* (Suppl. 16), 21–34.

American Speech-Language-Hearing Association. (in preparation). Knowledge and skills for supervision of speech-language pathology assistants.

Swallowing/Upper Aerodigestive Function

American Speech-Language-Hearing Association. (1987). Ad hoc committee on dysphagia report. *Asha, 29*(4), 57–58.

American Speech-Language-Hearing Association. (1989). Report: Ad hoc committee on labial-lingual posturing function. *Asha, 31*(11), 92–94.

American Speech-Language-Hearing Association. (1990). Knowledge and skills needed by speech-language pathologists providing services to dysphagic patients/clients. *Asha, 32* (Suppl. 2), 7–12.

American Speech-Language-Hearing Association. (1991). The role of the speech-language pathologist in assessment and management of oral myofunctional disorders. *Asha, 33* (Suppl. 5), 7.

American Speech-Language-Hearing Association. (1992). Position statement and guidelines for instrumental diagnostic procedures for swallowing, *Asha, 34* (Suppl. 7), 25–33.

American Speech-Language-Hearing Association. (1993). Orofacial myofunctional disorders: knowledge and skills. *Asha, 35* (Suppl. 10), 21–23.

American Speech-Language-Hearing Association. (2000). Clinical indicators for instrumental assessment of dysphagia (guidelines): Executive summary. *ASHA Suppl. 20,* 18–9.

American Speech-Language-Hearing Association. (2000). Roles of the speech-language pathologist and otolaryngologist in the performance and interpretation of endoscopic examination of swallowing (position statement). *ASHA Suppl. 20,* 17.

ASHA Special Interest Division 13: Swallowing and Swallowing Disorders (Dysphagia). (1997). Graduate curriculum on swallowing and swallowing disorders (adult and pediatric dysphagia). *ASHA Desk Reference,* vol. 3, 248a–248n.

Establishing Professional Competencies Through Education, Certification, and Licensure

DOLORES E. BATTLE, PHD

SCOPE OF CHAPTER

Speech-language pathologists and audiologists must have the professional skills and knowledge to ensure their services are of high quality and do no harm to the consumer. Preparation for careers in speech-language pathology and audiology typically begins at the undergraduate level and continues through the graduate degree and beyond. Education continues through the professional career to maintain competence and currency in the area of practice.

On completion of a graduate degree in communication sciences and disorders, speech-language pathologists and audiologists can practice their professions. Speech-language pathologists and audiologists are also eligible to obtain the Certificate of Clinical Competence (CCC), the credential that identifies them as meeting the national standards for entry into their profession as established by ASHA's Council for Clinical Certification (CFCC). They will also be eligible for a license to practice in their state, if applicable, and teacher certification/licensure. Some audiologists may seek board certification from AAA's American Board of Audiology. Integration of education and credentialing for practice of the professions is necessary to ensure that services are delivered by qualified personnel according to the highest ethical standards of the professions. This chapter provides an overview of the standards for professional education, certification, and licensure necessary for entry into the professions of speech-language pathology and audiology.

PROFESSIONAL EDUCATION

An academic degree is an award conferred on an individual by a college or university signifying the completion of a course of study or attainments in research or within a profession (Knowles, 1977). Traditionally, in English-speaking countries, there are four stages in higher education represented by associate's, bachelor's, master's, and doctoral degrees. Accreditation is the means by which educational institutions assure the public that the degrees offered meet standards of a quality education as validated by external accrediting agencies. The validity of academic accreditation programs in the United States is assured by standards set by the Secretary of Education and the Council on Higher Education Accreditation (CHEA). CHEA accredits graduate educational accreditation programs that provide entry-level professional education. Most colleges and universities in the United States are accredited by one of six regional accrediting agencies that oversee the general quality of the educational programs and services the academic institutions offer. The regional associations are identified by the region of the country in which the college or university is located such as the Middle States Association, New England Association of Schools and Colleges, or the Southern Association of Colleges and Schools.

In addition to regional accreditation for colleges and universities, academic institutions seek specialty accreditation to assure consumers and students that they are offering a quality educational program that meets the standards of a profession. For example, the National Council for Accreditation of Teacher Education (NCATE) accredits teacher education programs. Council on Academic Accreditation (CAA) accredits speech-language pathology and audiology programs. The Accreditation Commission for Audiology Education (ACAE) of AAA has developed accreditation standards for education of Doctor of Audiology training programs and is seeking CHEA recognition for this accreditation program.

Accreditation is intended to protect the interests of students, benefit the public, and improve the quality of teaching, learning, research, and professional practice (ASHA, 2005). Accreditation offers assurance that an academic program meets nationally established standards in five areas: (1) administrative structure and governance, (2) faculty and instructional staff, (3) curriculum, including both academic and clinical education, (4) students, and (5) program resources. Inherent in the values associated with accreditation is the belief that all professionals who provide services to the public have an obligation to ensure, as far as possible, that the services they provide are of high professional quality. One way of meeting this obligation is to establish minimum standards of educational quality for new professionals and to identify publicly those programs that meet or exceed these standards.

To obtain accreditation by the CAA, academic programs in speech-language pathology and audiology must demonstrate that they have engaged in extensive self-study to evaluate the quality of the program, including an assessment of the outcomes of the program and how the educational unit uses the study's outcomes to improve its quality. The program must submit a detailed report that addresses each of the standards. It must also have an on-site visit by a team of specially trained peers who verify the information and supportive materials submitted with the application.

Accreditation from CAA may be granted for a maximum of 8 years; however, annual reports provide an ongoing assessment of program quality. If a program fails to meet or maintain the standards for accreditation, the program may be placed on probation or the accreditation may be withdrawn.

A newly established educational program in the process of obtaining accreditation is called a *program in candidacy*. To obtain candidacy status, the educational program must submit a detailed report indicating how it will meet all standards for accreditation within a 5-year period. The program may also have a site visit by the CAA to assure that reasonable progress is being made toward meeting all standards for full accreditation during the five-year candidacy period. Students enrolled in the program in candidacy are considered to be in an accredited program when they apply for clinical certification.

According to the standards for the Certificates of Clinical Competence (CCC) of the ASHA, all graduate education and practicum must be initiated and completed in a program that is accredited by the CAA or is in an approved candidacy status. Current information on the accreditation status of a program can be obtained at ASHA's Web site. (See the Resources section at the end of this chapter for further information and Web site addresses.)

Undergraduate Preprofessional Education

More than 280 colleges and universities provide undergraduate or preprofessional education in communication sciences and disorders in the United States. Approximately 75 percent of the programs also provide graduate education. Undergraduate education in communication sciences and disorders is considered preprofessional education in that bachelor's level graduates do not qualify for certification by ASHA or state licensure. Its purpose is to provide students with a foundation in education or the liberal arts and sciences, some exposure to the discipline of communication sciences, and an introduction to communication disorders.

There is no accreditation process for undergraduate programs in communication sciences and disorders. The CAA accredits only clinical graduate programs that prepare students for independent practice of the professions. The ASHA Ad Hoc Committee on Undergraduate Education has developed a set of advisements for undergraduate programs (ASHA, 1990) delineating the expectations of a quality undergraduate program. The advisements are centered on three primary features: program administration, faculty, and curriculum and clinical competencies. They give direction so that programs are administered well and include regular evaluation of effectiveness. The advisements also suggest that the faculty be of sufficient size and competence to teach the courses for which they have responsibility. The advisements encourage programs to develop a curriculum that will provide for the development of critical skills and knowledge consistent with a traditional liberal arts education and preparation for graduate professional education.

Admission to the Undergraduate Program Applicants to undergraduate programs in communication sciences and disorders are usually required to provide evidence of a strong college preparatory high school program that includes laboratory sciences; computational mathematics, including algebra, trigonometry, and precalculus; and some exposure to a language other than English. Many programs require a satisfactory performance on the Scholastic Aptitude Test (SAT), the American College Testing Program (ACT), or a similar standardized test used to predict success in college. In addition, programs often prefer students who have had some experience in human services such as working with young children, adults, or persons with disabilities through volunteer work or employment. In some institutions, students apply for admission to the communication disorders undergraduate program at admission to the college or during their first year. In others, admission is not permitted until the sophomore or junior year. Students who are admitted to the program are usually expected to have a grade point average (GPA) of at least 2.5 (on a 4-point scale). Many programs require that students have completed some of the basic science course work or other specific course work before admission to the program. Prospective students are urged to check with the program in which they plan to enroll for specific admission requirements.

Undergraduate Curriculum Students completing undergraduate study in communication sciences and disorders must usually demonstrate skill in the following areas: oral and written communication, computer and technological literacy, and computational skills and scientific reasoning; the ability to think and critically solve problems; an understanding of cultural and linguistic diversity; an understanding of typical and atypical human development across the life span; and the ability to analyze, synthesize, and apply information (ASHA, 1990). Although the CCC is not awarded until the applicant has a graduate degree, knowledge of the principles of biological sciences, physical sciences, mathematics, and social/behavioral sciences can be completed in the undergraduate program as part of a broad liberal arts and sciences background.

Although the specific coursework in an undergraduate program is defined by the degree-granting institution, undergraduate coursework in the discipline usually provides the student with knowledge of the basic human communication and swallowing processes, including their biological, neurological, acoustic, psychological, developmental and linguistic, and cultural bases. The program may include courses such as anatomy and physiology of the speech and hearing mechanism, articulatory and acoustic phonetics and/or linguistics, physics of sound or speech acoustics, development of speech and language, instrumentation or technology in communication science, the neural basis of communication, hearing sciences, and introduction to the nature and prevention of communication disorders. More clinically focused coursework is also typically included, such as the nature of hearing and hearing disorders, aural rehabilitation, language and phonological disorders, clinical methods, and observation. In addition, many programs require coursework in statistics.

Because they are preprofessional in nature, many programs do not provide undergraduate students with practicum experience other than 25 hours of supervised observation. Programs that offer supervised clinical practice may limit the experience to the senior year. Some may offer a student teaching experience at the undergraduate level.

Transition to Graduate School Undergraduate students who wish to pursue graduate education in communication sciences and disorders usually prepare for the transition early in their senior year. Most graduate programs require the Graduate Record Examination (GRE) for admission; thus, students should prepare to take the examination early in their senior year. Letters of recommendation from faculty who can attest to their ability to succeed in graduate school and a personal statement or letter of intent are also frequently required. Because graduate programs vary, students should also work with their advisor to identify the graduate schools that will serve their individual needs. Special attention should be paid to application deadlines for admission and for financial aid. Information about

accredited graduate programs can be found on the ASHA Web site. The Council of Academic Programs in Communication Sciences and Disorders (CAPCSD) also provides information about graduate programs in the discipline. Again, see the Resources section for Web addresses.

Graduate Education

A graduate degree is the minimal degree required for the practice of speech-language pathology and audiology by both state licensure and professional certification. A master's degree is required for clinical certification in speech-language pathology. In 2012, the required degree for clinical certification in audiology will be the doctoral degree (e.g. Doctor of Philosophy (PhD) or Doctor of Audiology (AuD) degree).

The first graduate degrees in the discipline were awarded in the 1920s. Today, approximately 250 academic institutions offer accredited programs in speech-language pathology, audiology, or both in the United States (ASHA, 2005). The major objective of graduate education in the professions is to prepare students for independent practice of the professions. Academic programs also prepare students for careers in speech and hearing science or for advancement to doctoral programs; however, only those programs that prepare students for entry into the professions are accredited by the CAA.

Admission to the Graduate Program Admission to graduate programs in communication sciences and disorders requires a strong undergraduate record in liberal arts and sciences in addition to preprofessional course work in the basic sciences and communications sciences. The preprofessional course work is usually completed as part of an undergraduate program in communication sciences and disorders. Students who have a bachelor's degree but have not completed a preprofessional curriculum in communication sciences and disorders usually complete 18 to 30 semester hours of preprofessional course work to qualify for acceptance into the graduate program. This requirement varies across programs. Some programs allow the preprofessional course work to be taken after admission to the graduate program. Because these students are matriculated into the graduate program, financial aid may be available. Other programs expect all preprofessional course work to be completed before admission to the graduate program. These students are usually nonmatriculated and may be classified as nondegree, make-up, premajor, conditional, or "qualifier" students. Financial aid is usually not available to nonmatriculated graduate students.

Although requirements for admission to graduate study in communication sciences and disorders vary, programs usually require applicants to submit the following: (1) scores on the verbal reasoning, quantitative reasoning, and/or analytical writing sections of the Graduate Record Examination (GRE) or the Millers Analogies Test (MAT); (2) official transcripts indicating successful completion of the bachelor's degree and required course work; (3) three letters of recommendation from persons knowledgeable about the student's ability to be successful in graduate study; and (4) a written personal statement expressing the applicant's interest in the chosen career or other topic chosen by the program. A personal interview is usually optional but is highly recommended. International students may be required to present additional documentation and scores from the Test of English as a Foreign Language (TOEFL) or the SPEAK oral proficiency test. Applicants must be sure to know the dates when tests are given and the time required to have scores reported to the institution.

Graduate Curriculum According to the standards for academic accreditation in speech-language pathology or audiology, the curriculum of graduate programs must be sufficient to permit students to meet recognized national standards for entry into the practice of the profession (ASHA, 2005). Academic programs that meet this standard may be accredited by the CAA. The CAA currently accredits 249 programs that offer a master's degree in speech-language pathology or that are in candidacy, 55 master's degree programs in audiology, and 59 clinical doctoral programs in audiology, including one doctoral consortium program. The CAA will not accredit master's degree programs in audiology after 2007 because of the changes in certification standards that will be in effect in 2012.

The curricula of individual graduate programs often reflect the interests and strengths of the individual members of the program faculty but must also meet the standards established by the CAA. All CAA-accredited programs provide course work and clinical practicum for those who are seeking the ASHA CCC as well as state licensure and teacher certification for those who require or desire these additional credentials. Some programs offer coursework in speech and hearing science that does not lead to clinical certification.

Graduate programs for speech-language pathology and audiology have different curricula as these professions are distinctly separate. Preparation in both professions has the following similar features for completion: (1) academic coursework, (2) clinical practicum, and (3) a culminating activity such as a comprehensive examination, research project, externship, or thesis.

Speech-Language Pathology Curriculum The graduate curriculum for speech-language pathology usually requires a minimum of 75 semester credit hours, including 36 at the graduate-level culminating in a master's, doctoral, or other recognized postbaccalaureate degree. Graduate course work and graduate clinical practicum must be initiated and completed in a program accredited by the CAA in speech-language pathology. The course of study must be of sufficient breadth and depth to achieve specified knowledge and skills outcomes to cover the scope of practice of the profession. The curriculum also includes a practicum experience that encompasses the current scope of practice with children and adults resulting in a minimum of 400 hours of supervised practice. Three hundred seventy-five hours must be with direct patient contact, and 25 hours may focus on clinical observation. A 36-week clinical fellowship (CF) that establishes collaboration between the clinical fellow and a mentor follows the completion of the degree. A maintenance of certification requirement went into effect on January 1, 2005, to assure continued competence for the practice of the profession.

The academic course work in speech-language pathology typically builds on the foundation of normal basis of communication established in the preprofessional program and leads to completion of the academic and clinical practicum requirements for the CCC. Most programs require five semesters (including at least one summer) beyond the bachelor's degree. The curriculum should lead to the development of the knowledge base in the professional discipline and application of that knowledge to the assessment and treatment associated with the scope of practice. Curricula often include advanced course work in basic human communication sciences and swallowing processes, including their biological, neurological, acoustic, psychological, developmental and linguistic, and cultural bases. The curriculum must also provide knowledge of the nature of speech, language, hearing, and communication disorders and differences and swallowing disorders, including the etiologies, characteristics, and anatomical/physiological, acoustic, psychological, developmental, linguistic, and cultural correlates. The academic programs usually also provide course work in specific clinical disorders, conditions, or concerns, such as aphasia, dysphagia, motor speech disorders, articulation disorders, fluency disorders, voice and resonance disorders, craniofacial anomalies and associated communication disorders, cognitive and language disorders, augmentative and alternative communication, hearing disorders, and aural rehabilitation. Course work also usually includes instruction related to professional issues, cultural and linguistic diversity, research principles, and ethics. (See the ASHA Web site for the certification handbooks that outline the Council for Clinical Certification [CFCC] standards and provide a complete description of course work and other requirements for certification.)

According to the current standards for accreditation, the program must be able to provide students with all clinical education necessary to fulfill the ASHA Standards for the CCC in the area(s) in which accreditation is sought (ASHA, 2005). These CCC standards are established by the CFCC. Although the exact nature of the clinical practica varies with the educational program, most provide extensive supervised practice in an on-campus clinic prior to required supervised experience in hospital, educational, rehabilitation center, and outpatient clinic settings.

Audiology Curriculum Beginning in 2012, persons seeking clinical certification in audiology by the ASHA must have a doctoral degree. Many academic programs are now offering the clinical doctorate instead of the master's degree. The clinical degree designator may be the AuD or ScD. Most programs accept students into the doctoral program without their first completing a master's degree; others offer a post-master's degree program for students who already have a masters' degree, and a few offer opportunities for both. Postbaccalaureate degree accredited programs are for individuals who hold an undergraduate degree. They usually require 4 years of full-time study, including a residency year that allows them to be eligible for ASHA certification upon program completion. Postmaster's degree programs are for students who have completed a master's degree prior to entry into the doctoral program. The length of time of enrollment varies depending on the student's prior academic and clinical preparation.

Students in audiology graduate programs typically have completed course work in basic and communication sciences in a communication sciences and disorders undergraduate program. Audiology graduate students usually complete additional course work in basic communication sciences related to audiology and hearing, such as anatomy and physiology of the hearing mechanism, hearing science, and electrophysiology at the graduate level. Effective 2007, graduate students in audiology are required to complete a minimum of 75 semester credit hours of postbaccalaureate study that culminates in a master's, doctoral, or otherwise recognized graduate academic degree. A doctoral degree will be required for persons who apply for ASHA certification after December 31, 2011. The course of study must include a minimum of 12 months of full-time equivalent supervised clinical practicum in sufficient depth and breadth to achieve the requisite knowledge and skills to provide a high level of professional care in audiology prior to awarding the degree.

The professional course work related to audiology includes courses such as amplification, diseases and disorders of the hearing mechanism, pharmacology, tinnitus, vestibular functioning and balance, counseling, central auditory testing and processing, evaluation and fitting of hearing aids and other assistive listening devices, hearing conservation, calibration, real ear measurements, pediatric audiology, cochlear implants, and specific diagnostic testing such as auditory brainstem response and evoked oto-acoustic emissions. In addition, programs include course work in ethical standards, research principles, and current regulations affecting the profession. The practicum experience is equivalent to a minimum of 12 months of full-time supervised experience. The clinical practicum for programs in audiology must meet the requirements specified for the CCC, if the program is accredited by CAA.

Culminating Activity The graduate degree usually requires a culminating activity designed to demonstrate that the student has acquired an appropriate knowledge base in the discipline and can use that knowledge in an integrated manner to address problems in the discipline or the profession. The culminating activity is usually undertaken toward the end of the graduate program and is the final step toward completion of the degree. The specific options vary with the institution and/or the program. They usually consist of one or more of the following: a comprehensive examination, a capstone or research project, an externship, or a thesis.

Comprehensive Examination Comprehensive examinations are designed to allow the student to demonstrate the ability to synthesize knowledge gained during the academic program and to apply that knowledge to solve clinical or theoretical problems. They may be oral, written, or a combination of both. Comprehensive examinations may be questions or problems developed by the faculty that are related to the curriculum and clinical experiences of the program. These examinations are one way to measure program outcomes. Some programs do not require in-house comprehensive examinations but choose to use data about performance of program

graduates on the Praxis II Examination in Speech-Language Pathology or Audiology to inform the program regarding achievement of knowledge outcomes. Summary data from program graduates are provided to programs on an annual basis by the test administrator (Educational Testing Service) for such use, and summative results are grouped according to content areas. However, the Praxis II examinations as measures of individual performance may not be required or used by accredited programs as a comprehensive examination.

The Master's or Capstone Project A master's or capstone project is an independent project developed by the student with the guidance of a faculty member. Master's projects are usually case studies, research projects of a limited scale, literature reviews to answer a specific question or to review a particular topic area, or a similar activity that requires the student to integrate knowledge obtained in the course of study. Some programs specify that the project be presented before the faculty or student peers. The project report is usually retained in the department.

Thesis A thesis is an original research study examining hypotheses or clinical questions following a prescribed method of inquiry. The thesis is developed with the guidance of a faculty member in consultation with a committee of faculty scholars. The product is a written document encompassing the literature reviewed to develop the statement of the problem and hypotheses, the method and procedures used in the study, the results, and an analysis and discussion of the results, including the significance or application of the findings to the discipline. The student is required to "defend" the thesis to a thesis committee or present the study to faculty members and student peers. The thesis document must be prepared in a prescribed format and is usually bound, submitted to the graduate school for approval, and retained in the library of the institution. Students who intend to pursue doctoral education are strongly encouraged to complete a thesis as their culminating activity to prepare for doctoral research and study.

Doctoral Education

The doctoral degree is the highest degree granted by educational institutions (Knowles, 1977). The University of Paris awarded the first doctorates in religion in 1150. The Doctor of Philosophy (PhD) was first conferred in Paris in the mid-13th century. The doctoral degree, as granted in the United States and several other nations, is a relatively modern development. Until well into the 19th century, the bachelor's degree was the highest degree awarded in the United States. German institutions, famed for their development of scientific method, began to attract American students to study for the doctoral degree. The German doctorate became so prestigious that steps were taken to create similar programs in the United States. As the history in Chapter 1 described, the first American doctoral degree in speech-language pathology was awarded to Sara M. Stinchfield (Hawke) at the University of Wisconsin in 1921 (Neidecker & Blosser, 1993). Presently, several hundred institutions in the United States award the doctoral degree, including 61 in speech-language pathology and audiology.

Doctoral education is more than an extension of the master's degree program. A doctoral degree requires demonstrated achievement in three broad areas: (1) mastery of the essential theory and knowledge in the field in which the degree is awarded, (2) completion of pertinent research or scholarship relevant to the field, and (3) a dissertation or scholarly work that is an original contribution to the knowledge base in the particular field (Council of Graduate Schools in the United States, 1990). Potential doctoral students choose the program because of the opportunity to study with a particular professor or to study within a specialty at a particular institution.

Two types of doctoral degrees are awarded in the United States—honorary degrees and earned degrees. Earned degrees may be research degrees or professional degrees.

Honrary Doctoral Degrees Universities grant honorary degrees known as *honoris causa ad gradum* to recognize outstanding professional attainment or public service. Honorary degrees require no academic work. Persons holding the honorary doctorate do not use the title of "doctor."

Earned Doctoral Degrees Earned degrees require significant academic work in a discipline. Doctoral degrees represent a significant advancement in the discipline with a specialization in a specific area of research and scholarship or clinical practice. Three types of earned doctoral degrees awarded in the United States—the research doctorate, the professional doctorate, and the clinical doctorate, which is a combination of the research and professional doctorate.

The Research Doctorate The research doctorate is a mark of highest academic achievement in a particular field (Council of Graduate Schools in the United States, 1990). The research doctorate prepares students for academic or research careers. There may or may not be a clinical component. Research doctorates usually involve study within the discipline as well as interdisciplinary areas to prepare the student for specialization and contributions to the knowledge base of the discipline through original research. A modern reflection of the German roots and the scientific method, the research doctorate is awarded to recognize creative scholarship and original research that makes a contribution to the knowledge base of a particular field. The research doctorate requires course work, oral and written examinations, and a dissertation representing original research or a publication of an original work deemed to be a substantial contribution to knowledge by a group of scholars in the field of study. A PhD degree is usually awarded at the completion of a research doctoral program regardless of the field of study. In audiology, hearing science, speech-language pathology, and speech-language science, persons holding the PhD or other research doctorates usually are employed by colleges or universities, but many seek employment in hospitals or other service-delivery settings where research and clinical teaching are a part of the facility or institution's mission.

The Clinical Doctorate The clinical doctorate refers to specialized preparation for those who wish to do clinical or applied research and/or become direct service providers to the public or to other professions. Preparation in applied or clinical research and the completion of a research project related to a clinical problem are usually required for the completion of a clinical doctorate. Persons holding the clinical doctorate often seek employment in university or college clinics, teaching hospitals, and rehabilitation or other health care programs. Some also enter private practice.

The Professional Doctorate While research and clinical doctorates place emphasis on research, professional doctorates place emphasis on clinical practice. The professional doctorate is defined as "the highest university award given in a particular field in recognition of completion of academic preparation for professional practice" (Council of Graduate Schools in the United States, 1990, p. 1). Professional doctorates vary in their requirements, although most require vocationally or professionally oriented course work, proven expertise in the field, examinations and, in some cases, research. The major objective of the professional doctorate is to produce professionals who are competent to provide a wide array of services associated with independent professional practice.

The most frequently awarded professional doctorate in the United States is the Doctor of Education (EdD), first awarded at Harvard University in 1920. Another commonly awarded professional doctorate is the Doctor of Social Work (DSW). The Doctor of Medicine (MD) and Doctor of Dental Science (DDS) occupy a middle ground between the research and professional doctorates. They are referred to as first professional doctoral degrees. Other examples of professional doctorates include, for example, the Doctor of Juris prudence (JD), the Doctor of Chiropractics (DC), Doctor of Osteopathy (DO), Doctor of Pharmacy (PharmD), Doctor of Veterinary Medicine (DVM), Doctor of Physical Therapy (DPT), and Doctor of Optometry (OD). Persons who hold a first professional degree may also seek a research degree. For example, a medical researcher who does research may hold both the MD and the PhD.

Doctor of Audiology New in the area of professional doctorates is the Doctor of Audiology (AuD). The most common degrees granted by programs offering doctoral degrees in audiology are now the AuD and the ScD (Doctor of Science). The clinical doctorate in audiology is a graduate professional degree earned by those audiologists who are competent to perform a wide variety of diagnostic, remedial, and other services associated with the independent practice of audiology.

The clinical doctorate in audiology places major emphasis on clinical education, with a major component of the program being clinical practice in a variety of settings and with a variety of clients whose hearing disorders require a high degree of expertise for appropriate evaluation and treatment. Some programs also require clinical research as a component of the degree program.

Although only in existence since the early 1990s, the number of academic programs that offer the entry-level clinical doctorate degree in audiology continues to grow. There are currently 59 clinical doctorate programs in the United States. ASHA has identified the doctoral degree, with AuD as the preferred title, for entry into the practice of the profession of audiology. The doctoral degree will be required for clinical ASHA certification in Audiology as of January 1, 2012. It is currently required for Board Certification in Audiology by the American Board of Audiology of AAA. Four states—Ohio, Indiana, New Mexico, and Oklahoma—currently require the doctoral degree for state license in audiology. Persons holding the clinical doctorate often are employed in hospitals, rehabilitation facilities, private practice, or industry.

Doctoral Curriculum Research doctoral programs in speech-language pathology, audiology, and speech-language or hearing sciences typically require 3 or 4 years of study beyond the master's degree or 4 to 6 years beyond the bachelor's degree without an intervening master's degree. There are no set times for gaining the research doctorate; however, some universities set a maximum time of 6 to 7 years to prevent students from extending their work indefinitely. Clinical doctoral programs typically require 3 to 4 years beyond the bachelor's degree.

Academic Course Work in Doctoral Programs

The curriculum of a doctoral program is individualized, with the flexibility to allow doctoral candidates to prepare as scholars and/or practitioners in their area of choice. The curriculum, however, must ensure that graduates are familiar with the scientific and professional knowledge base of their particular area of study. Course work may include courses in related disciplines such as linguistics, neuroscience, or pharmacology in addition to specific advanced course work within the discipline. If the program is a research doctorate, there must be sufficient curriculum to provide a firm basis in the development and analysis of research and laboratory sciences, including research design, methods of scientific inquiry, and statistics. For the clinical doctorate, there must be a sufficient knowledge base and analytical skills to develop and analyze the results of clinical inquiry.

For the professional doctorate, such as the AuD, there must be a sufficient knowledge base to assure the development of expertise necessary for the development of clinical skills that are robust both in depth and breadth of clinical practice. In addition, the students must be able to interpret pertinent research and apply it to clinical practice. To ensure that the chosen program of study is strong and consistent with the university standards for awarding the degree, all doctoral students must file a plan of study with the university early in their program.

Preliminary and Qualifying Examinations

Most doctoral programs require that preliminary examinations be taken early in the degree program to assess the student's knowledge of the field so that an appropriate plan of study can be designed. At or near the end of the formal course work portion of the program, doctoral students take qualifying examinations to verify the student has the necessary foundation in the discipline on which to develop individual research or advanced clinical practice. The examinations usually require that the candidate integrate knowledge from various areas of the discipline.

Upon completion of the qualifying examination, the student is admitted to candidacy and is referred to as a doctoral *candidate*. Universities vary in the nature and timing of such activities and have publications outlining requirements, sequence of study, and time lines.

Residency Most doctoral programs recognize that, in order to develop the intensity of involvement in the doctoral study, at least one year of the doctoral program must be completed on a full-time basis. The year of full-time study is called the *residency period*. It allows the student the opportunity to engage fully in interaction with faculty and other students in scholarly and clinical pursuits. Interaction with scholars and practitioners is essential to develop the problem-solving, research, and critical thinking skills necessary for completion of the degree.

Dissertation or Culminating Activity All doctoral programs require the completion of a culminating activity to achieve the degree. This is typically called a *dissertation*, an independent research or capstone project, or an advanced clinical study, depending on the type of degree to be earned. The culminating activity is usually begun after the completion of the academic curriculum and the comprehensive examination. It may be initiated during the year of residency. Doctoral candidates usually develop an original hypothesis or clinical problem and design a study or project to test the hypothesis or solve the problem using methods of scientific inquiry. The culminating activity is directed by a primary faculty advisor, or major professor, assisted by a doctoral program committee of scholars, researchers, or practitioners. The requirements for membership on the doctoral program committee and the dissertation committee vary by institution, but most programs require the majority of members of the committee to be members of the graduate faculty of the institution.

After completion of the research project in the research doctoral program, the doctoral candidate writes the dissertation that describes the basis of the research or problem, methodology, results, and conclusions. The dissertation also includes a discussion of the implications of the findings for future research, or for the profession and clinical practice (Blake, 1995). Because the dissertation or culminating activity is intended to make an important and unique contribution to the field of knowledge, the dissertation is usually evaluated by at least one person outside of the university who has agreed to serve this purpose. This is usually a recognized scholar with expertise in the field of inquiry. Acting as an objective reviewer, the external evaluator attests to the rigor used in the study and the value of the contribution to the field of knowledge.

Doctoral programs usually require that the candidate defend the dissertation or capstone before a body of scholars, researchers, and practitioners, as appropriate to the project. The oral defense allows the doctoral candidate to demonstrate mastery of the knowledge and skills required for the degree to assure the degree was earned according to the standards established by the granting university.

Postdoctoral Study

Postdoctoral study, usually referred to as "post doc," is highly specialized study taken by an individual after the completion of a research doctoral degree. It usually consists of 1 to 3 years of advanced study in a specialized area of research or clinical study in collaboration with a known scholar or expert in a particular field. Government grants, foundations such as the American Speech-Language-Hearing Foundation (ASHF), and private agencies in a particular area of demonstrated need often fund postdoctoral study. Postdoctoral fellows focus on refining research and grant-writing skills, making connections in research circles, and building a list of publications as a prelude to obtaining faculty or research positions.

Distance Education

Distance education is instruction that occurs when the instructor and student are separated by distance, time, or both. Distance education programs are used by persons who are unable to attend a typical university program because they are not geographically close to the university, or are not able to attend the college courses at the time when they are offered.

Distance education is not new. In the 19th century, education could be obtained by mail order correspondence courses. As technology improved, education became available to students in remote geographical areas through audio recordings, videotapes, telephone, and telecourses. Advances in technology and the need for new models of education that function with changes in lifestyle have made distance education available for continuing education, specific academic course work, and some academic degrees. Nearly all academic programs use some form of distance education to enhance instruction. Online programs, such as Blackboard (Blackboard, 1997), Angel (2005), and other forms of electronic learning management systems, enable instructors to use the Internet to enhance instruction and student interaction outside of the classroom through virtual learning environments.

About three dozen academic programs that provide some academic courses and/or degrees through distance education in speech-language pathology or audiology. Most of the programs offer graduate course work; however, one program offers courses for students with bachelor's degrees in other disciplines who are completing course work for admission to graduate programs (Boswell, 2005). Distance education programs are often designed to assist persons who are unable to attend classes on site or are unable to relocate to obtain a master's degree on site. Distance education programs use Web-based technology, interactive video conferencing with video streaming, Web conferencing, prerecorded CD-ROMs, and other technology to expose students to academic and theoretical knowledge, clinical education, exposure to virtual clients, directed readings, online discussions, and class and individual projects and examinations. Most, if not all, of the instruction is provided in synchronous or asynchronous formats. Synchronous instruction is real-time instruction through video conference or other live instruction. Asynchronous distance instruction is provided at a different time through Web-based, CD-ROM, or other instruction that is recorded and viewed at a time selected by the student.

Clinical instruction and supervision are provided in some distance education programs by live video conferencing or video recording. Students completing courses or accredited degree programs through distance education are expected to meet the same academic standards of the degree-granting institution as students attending the regular on-site program (Dudding & Purcell, 2003).

Some issues have arisen as distance education programs have grown in availability. These issues include the access to and sufficiency of faculty to respond to student questions and concerns, the security of examinations, and library availability. Those participating in such programs should discuss these issues with a representative of the distance education program prior to enrolling. See Chapter 25 on Technology for more discussion of distance education.

PROFESSIONAL LICENSURE AND CERTIFICATION

The regulation of the practices of speech-language pathology and audiology is to protect the consumer from unscrupulous or incompetent practice. Consumers place their faith in the services received from persons they believe to be experts. They may not be able to make reasoned judgments about the competence of the person providing services. Professional regulation serves to protect the consumer from harm resulting from improper diagnosis and treatment (Lynch & Hesse, 1997). It also assures the consumer that services are being provided in a manner that meets professional standards for ethical practice.

Professional regulation began in the 1850s with the licensing of physicians. Through the next century, professional licensing expanded to other professions such as dentists and attorneys. Professional regulation of persons providing speech-language pathology and audiology services began in the 1950s with teacher certification. In 1969, Florida became the first state to regulate the practice of speech-language pathology and audiology in noneducational settings. Professional regulations

establish the minimal standards necessary for entry into the general practice of a profession. The standards for the credentials are established by either governmental regulatory agencies or by professional associations. Governmental agencies issue professional licenses or certificates, such as the license in speech-language pathology or audiology or the teaching certificate. Government licenses and certificates are mandatory for professional practice in the area of the agency's jurisdiction or regulating body's. Professional associations also issue certificates such as the CCC from ASHA's Council for Clinical Certification (CFCC) or Board Certification by the American Board of Audiology of AAA. Certification from professional associations is voluntary and may exist for reasons other than consumer protection, including establishing professional standards and identity.

The State License

Licensure defines for the public the minimum qualifications necessary for entry into the practice of a profession within a given state (Flower, Ohta, Stephens, Quinn, & Orahood, 1986). In most states, the regulations for obtaining a license in speech-language pathology and audiology were developed after a model provided by the ASHA. Consequently, the requirements are similar across the states. Some states refer directly to the ASHA standards for the CCC so that the state requirements are identical to those of the CCC, including all revisions. Most states, however, identify the requirements independent of the CCC and are thus unaffected by changes in the CCC unless specific modifications are made in state laws or regulations. This distinction is important because the requirements for the CCC are changing to require a doctorate in audiology in 2012.

Licensing is the process by which a state government grants an individual the right to practice a given profession in a defined scope of practice. Licensure is based on the belief that stringent entry requirements and ongoing scrutiny by the state will protect the health, safety, and welfare of the public from unscrupulous or incompetent practice. Permission to practice the profession is granted when the applicant can demonstrate that the minimal degree of competence has been attained. Professional licenses issued by governmental agencies are usually required for practice in areas where the agency has legal jurisdiction, such as the public schools or health care agencies. The credentials issued by governmental agencies include the professional license, teacher licensure or certification, or registration.

Licensing laws containing broad provisions governing the practice of the professions are established by legislative acts. Because they are the laws of the state, licensure laws can only be changed by legislative act. Rules or regulations are established by authorized agencies to implement the provisions established in the law, such as a state Department of Education or Department of Health. Changes in the rules or regulations can be made by the authorized agency. For example, the law may state that the applicant must hold a graduate degree consisting of coursework and practice acceptable to the governing agency. The governing agency may specify in its regulations that the graduate degree must be a master's or doctoral degree in speech-language pathology, audiology, or a related field and that the graduate degree contains specific course work and practice related to the area in which the license is sought. The license may also specify that the person hold certification such as the ASHA CCC or equivalent.

As shown in Table 2–1, nearly all states regulate the professions of speech-language pathology and audiology. All 50 states regulate audiology, but the District of Columbia does not. Forty-nine states regulate audiology by licensure, and one (Colorado) regulates by registration. Forty-seven states regulate SLPs by licensure. There is no regulation in Colorado, Michigan, South Dakota, or the District of Columbia for SLPs. See Table 2–1 for further information regarding states that regulate persons who are support personnel to the professions, such as speech-language pathology or audiology assistants. The ASHA Web site provides the most current summary of licensure requirements by state.

Components of Licensure Laws Although the specific content of the licensure laws varies from state to state, each law has certain basic components:

a statement of intent, definition of the area of practice, prohibited acts, requirements, provisions for discipline, and identification of the regulatory body. The law may also have special provisions about transferability, exemptions, or other matters particular to the state.

Intent Licensure laws usually include a statement that explains the purpose of the statute. For example, the Declaration of Policy and Legislative Intent in the Alabama Licensure Law for Speech Pathologists and Audiologists (1975 amended in 1997 Section 34-28A-2) states:

> The practice of speech pathology and audiology is a privilege which is granted to qualified persons by legislative authority in the interest of public health, safety, and welfare, and, in enacting this law it is the intent of the legislature to require educational training and licensure of any persons who engage in the practice of speech-language pathology and/or audiology, to encourage better educational training programs, to prohibit the unauthorized and unqualified practice of speech pathology and/or to practice speech pathology and audiology, and to provide enforcement of the chapter and penalties for its violation.

Definition of Practice Licensure laws, also referred to as *practice acts*, usually establish a "scope of practice"—that is, they define what the person covered by the act is allowed to do in the practice of the profession. For example, The New York State Education Law Article 159 (1974) defines the practice of audiology as:

> The application of principles, methods, and procedures of measurement, testing, evaluation, consultation, counseling, instruction, and habilitation or rehabilitation related to hearing, its disorders and related communication impairments and vestibular disorders for the purpose of nonmedical diagnosis, prevention, identification, amelioration, or modification of such disorders and conditions in individuals and/or groups of individuals.

T A B L E 2–1 States Regulating Speech-Language Pathologists (SLP), Audiologists (A), and Support Personnel (SP) (as of February 2006)

(L=License   R=Registration   O= Other Regulation   C=Certification   X=None)

State	SLP	A	SP	State	SLP	A	SP
Alabama	L	L	R	Nebraska	L	L	R
Alaska	L	L	R	Nevada	L	L	O
Arkansas	L	L	R	New Hampshire	L	L*	O
California	L	L	R	New Jersey	L	L	X
Colorado	X	R	X	New Mexico	L*	L*	L
Connecticut	L*	L*	O	New York	L	L	X
Delaware	L*	L*	R	North Carolina	L	L	R
Florida	L	L	R	North Dakota	L	L	O
Georgia	L	L	R	Ohio	L*	L*	L
Hawaii	L*	L*	X	Oklahoma	L	L	R
Idaho	L	L	L	Oregon	L	L	L
Illinois	L	L	L	Pennsylvania	L	L	R
Indiana	L*	L*	R	Rhode Island	L	L	R
Iowa	L	L	R	South Carolina	L	L	L
Kansas	L*	L*	R	South Dakota	X	L*	X
Kentucky	L	L	L	Tennessee	L	L	R
Louisiana	L*	L*	L	Texas	L*	L*	L
Maine	L	L	R	Utah	L	L	R
Maryland	L	L*	L	Vermont	L	L	O
Massachusetts	L*	L*	C	Virginia	L	L	O
Michigan	X	L	O	Washington	L	L	O
Minnesota	L	L	O	Washington, DC	X	X	X
Mississippi	L	L	R	West Virginia	L	L	R
Missouri	L	L	R	Wisconsin	L	L	O
Montana	L*	L*	R	Wyoming	L	L	R

*Indicates school-based personnel are required to be licensed

Prohibited Acts Many state licensure laws prohibit the use of the professional title by persons not holding the license. This prohibition assures the public that anyone using the title has met the standards established by the law and regulatory agency. For example, the Alabama licensure law prohibits "any person who shall use in connection with his name or otherwise assume, use or advertise any title or description tending to convey the impression that he is a speech pathologist or audiologist without being licensed." According to New York State Law (1975), "anyone not authorized to use a professional title and who uses the professional title is guilty of a class A misdemeanor. In addition, anyone who knowingly aids or abets three or more persons not authorized to use a professional title or knowingly employs three or more persons not authorized to use a professional title, or who uses such title in the course of such employment, shall be guilty of a class E felony." See Chapter 5, Professional Liability, for in-depth discussion of this topic.

State Regulatory Board of Examiners Licensure laws usually establish a board of examiners or an advisory council that is appointed by the regulatory agency. The boards include licensed professionals. They usually include at least one consumer or public member to ensure that consumer needs are protected and represented in board activity. It is not unusual for boards to also include representatives from other professions as well. The boards of examiners ensure the self-regulatory function of the professions within the state. Their duties and responsibilities usually include, but are not limited to, oversight of the law and regulations, proposing policy, counsel on professional discipline, handling complaints from consumers, and processing or making recommendations on applications for licensure. The boards advise the regulatory authority concerning the specific requirements for the license to practice the profession.

Education All state laws regulating speech-language pathologists and audiologists specify the master's degree, a graduate degree, or equivalent as the minimum for receipt of the license. In some states, the area of the degree is not specified. In others, such as the Nebraska Statutes Relating to Audiology and Speech Pathology (2003), the education requirement states, "Every applicant for a license to practice audiology or speech-language pathology shall (1) present proof of a master's degree or its equivalent in audiology or speech-language pathology from an academic program approved by the Board." Other states, however, specify the academic course work directly in the law itself. The Alabama licensure law, for example, details the specific courses that provide information about and training in the management of speech, hearing, and language disorders and that provide information supplementary to these areas (Section 34-28A-21 of the Laws of Alabama).

Experience Most states require applicants for the license to have completed a minimum of 325 clock

hours at the graduate level, or 400 required supervised clock hours in speech-language pathology or audiology. A nine-month, full-time supervised clinical experience after awarding the degree is required for licensure in SLP in most states. Some states, such as Nevada, North Dakota, and Virginia, have no specific experience requirements. Because educational training programs in audiology have responded to standards changes for the CCC and for Board Certification by AAA which require a clinical doctorate degree, audiologists in many states are working with regulatory boards to move the professional experience requirement to become part of the educational requirements for licensure of audiologists. State regulatory agencies have chosen to respond to these requests in a variety of ways. Because the regulatory responses have been so varied, it is important for those wishing to practice in the area of audiology in a particular state to check on the status of applicable laws or regulations carefully to determine the requirements for eligibility for licensure.

Examination All state licensure laws require applicants to demonstrate their professional knowledge in the area of practice. The laws often do not identify or specify a particular examination, leaving such decisions to the rules and regulations; however, several states have adopted the Praxis II Examinations in Speech-Language Pathology and Audiology as the appropriate examinations for this purpose. The examination is owned by the Educational Testing Service and developed in consultation with professional speech-language pathologists and audiologists. This is the same examination required for the clinical certification in speech-language pathology by the CFCC of ASHA; however, the states must set their own passing score for satisfying the knowledge requirement based on standardizing this score in relation to the performance of the licensed individuals in the state.

Exemptions Many state licensure laws have provisions that exempt certain persons from holding the license to practice the professions. Federal employees such as those employed by the VA hospitals or military are usually exempt because the federal government has sole jurisdiction over its employees. Some states have provisions that exempt persons holding teacher licensure or certification by the state department of education from holding the professional license. However, by the personnel standards of the 2004 Individuals with Disabilities Education Act (IDEA), persons providing services to students with disabilities must hold the appropriate credential in the state as consistent with any state-approved or state-recognized certification, licensing, or other comparable requirement applicable to a specific professional discipline. Such personnel must not have had their certification or licensure requirements waived on an emergency, temporary, or provisional basis (IDEA, 2004). Although not all states are yet in compliance with the mandates of IDEA, all personnel providing services to students with disabilities are expected to have professional development so they can meet the legal requirements.

Some states also exempt persons from the license who practice professions under other state licensing laws (e.g., physicians, surgeons, students and trainees providing services under supervision of licensed professionals, and persons fulfilling postgraduate professional supervised experience requirements). Additionally, some states exempt nurses, teachers of the deaf, and persons, such as laryngectomees using alaryngeal speech, who are providing services to other persons with similar disabilities.

Continuing Education Of the states that regulate the practice of audiology or speech-language pathology or both through licensure or title registration, 41 states require a prescribed program of continuing education for renewal of the license (Table 2–2). Continuing education assures that the licensee maintains currency and continues to uphold the standards of practice acceptable to the

T A B L E 2–2 Continuing Competence Requirements by State (as of February 2006)

	#CE hours	Time (years)	ASHA CEU Preapproved	Comments
Alabama	12	1		
Alaska	none			
Arizona	8	1		
Arkansas	10	1		
California	24	2	X	
Colorado	none			
Connecticut	none			
Delaware	20	2		Minimum 14 hours focusing on clinical skills
Florida	30	2	X	18 hours clinical skills, 2 hours prevention of medical errors
Georgia	25	2		
Hawaii	none			
Idaho	NA	NA		
Illinois	20	2	X	
Indiana	36	2		Up to 6 hours of self-study permitted
Iowa	30	2		
Kansas	20	2		
Kentucky	15	1	X	May carry over up to 5 hours
Louisiana	10	1	X	At least 5 hours must be in area of licensure

(Continued)

T A B L E 2–2 (*Continued*)

	#CE hours	Time (years)	ASHA CEU Preapproved	Comments
Maine	50	2	X	May carry over unlimited number of hours
Maryland	20	2		Up to 5 hours of self-study permitted
Massachusetts	20	2	X	Minimum 10 hours in area of licensure
Michigan	NA	NA		
Minnesota	30	2	X	At least 20 hours directly related to area of licensure
Mississippi	10	1	X	Minimum 10 hours directly related to clinical practicum
Missouri	30	2	X	Minimum 20 hours from approved sponsors
Montana	40	2	X	At least 25 hours from approved sponsors
Nebraska	20	2	X	Up to 3 hours of self-study permitted
Nevada	15	1		Maximum 8 hours in practice management
New Hampshire (SLP only)	50	3	X	
New Jersey	20	2	X	Minimum 15 hours directly related to practice
New Mexico	10	1	X	May carry over up to 10 hours
New York	30	3		At least 20 hours directly related to area of licensure
North Carolina	none			
North Dakota	10	1		
Ohio	20	2	X	Minimum 10 hours related to clinical practice
Oklahoma	20	2		
Oregon	10	1	X	
Pennsylvania	20	2		
Rhode Island	20	2	X	
South Carolina	32	2	X	Minimum 8 hours in clinical practice
South Dakota	12	1		
Tennessee	10	1		
Texas	10	1		May carry over up to 20 hours
Utah	20	2		
Vermont	NA			
Virginia	30	2	X	Minimum 15 hours related to area of licensure
Washington	none			
West Virginia	10	2		
Wisconsin	20	2		
Wyoming	20	1	X	

profession. There is considerable variation in the requirement for the demonstration of continued competence across states.

The amount of continuing education is expressed in a number of Continuing Education (CE) or clock hours within a particular time period. The number of CE hours per year ranges from about 8 to 30 hours within a 1 to 3-year period. Typically states require an average of 10 hours per year. Arizona, for example, requires 8 clock hours of continuing education in 1 year, California requires 24 hours within 2 years, Montana requires 40 hours in 2 years, and both Idaho and New York require 30 hours in 3 years.

The specifics of the continuing education requirements are as varied as the amount of continuing education required. Continuing education may be permitted through independent or self-study, journal study groups, earned academic credit beyond that required for the graduate degree, preparing and providing instruction, publishing an article in a peer-reviewed publication, or learning related to clinical fellow supervision or through programs approved by ASHA, AAA, or other organizations. Some states allow pre-approved CE courses to meet the requirements; however, other states require that the CE is related to clinical practice.

ASHA maintains a fee-based Continuing Education Registry of continuing education units earned in ASHA-approved continuing education programs. The Association also offers Awards of Continuing Education (ACE) to persons who earn at least 70 hours of continuing education in a 36-month period. AAA members may also use the Academy's Continuing Education Registry to store and organize Academy-approved courses. It, too, issues CE transcripts upon request.

Professional Discipline Ongoing scrutiny of persons who hold the license is maintained by a requirement that the licensee adheres to standards of clinical and ethical practice. Licensure laws contain provisions for persons who violate the professional code of conduct. The board of examiners, the state attorney general, the local district attorney, or other bodies, depending on the specific charges and/or authorized body within a state, usually review alleged violations. In New York, for example, the Division of Professional Discipline processes the violations after consultation with members of the Board of Examiners in Speech-Language Pathology and Audiology. Procedures for discipline are usually specified in rules and regulations. The sanctions for violations of a state license may include probation, suspension or revocation of the license, and/or payment of a fine. The individual may also be referred to the attorney general for possible prosecution if a felony is alleged to have been committed.

Transferability and Reciprocity A license to practice in one state is not directly transferable to another state. There are no reciprocal agreements among the states. Persons must apply for a license in each state where they wish to practice. Several states, however, have special provisions for persons who are licensed in another state or who hold the CCC, such as waiver of the examination requirement. All states require, as a minimum, an application and the presentation of official academic transcripts to verify completion of the degree and course work requirements.

Interim Practice of Temporary Licenses Interim practice provisions allow a person to practice for a period of time before the actual license is issued or while a license is pending. The interim license must be granted prior to independent practice. Provisions for interim practice or temporary licenses vary across the states. In some states, a temporary license is issued for a period of time (e.g., 30 days) while the application is pending. In other states, a temporary license is issued to allow practice if all requirements have been met except the passing of the required examination. In these cases, it is usual for the temporary license to be in effect until the next administration of the required examination. Additionally, some states issue a temporary license to individuals who are completing the professional experience requirement with full licensure provided once the experience, typically 9 months of full-time work, is completed.

SUPPORT PERSONNEL

More personnel are sometimes needed to provide speech-language and audiology services because of increased demand, a more diverse client base, and an expanding scope of practice. Some tasks performed by speech-language pathologists and audiologists can be performed by personnel with less training than the licensed or certified professional. These support personnel are often referred to as *speech-language pathology* or *audiology assistants* or *aides*. National standards for education and training of support personnel or in regard to appropriate tasks to be performed by these individuals were not specified by a national credential when states began recognizing or licensing them. As a result, there is considerable variation in nearly all aspects of regulation of support personnel across states. Support personnel, following academic or on-the-job training, perform tasks as prescribed, directed, and supervised by a certified and/or licensed speech-language pathologist or audiologist as appropriate. Supervision may be direct or indirect. Chapter 24, Supervision, discusses this topic in more detail.

Several issues involving support personnel remain controversial in the discipline. Some professionals fear that support personnel will be used to supplant more highly qualified and paid licensed or certified professionals. Others may perceive that administrators impose support personnel on professionals who may not be prepared to supervise them. Support personnel may come with varied education and experiences in various states. The consumer and other professionals may not know how to distinguish the roles and responsibilities of both positions. See Chapter 10 on the topic of support personnel.

Support Personnel in SLP

Speech-language assistants have been permitted and regulated by many states since the 1970s. As shown in Table 2–1, 34 states currently regulate the use of support personnel; however, regulations vary considerably. Support personnel in both audiology and speech-language pathology are regulated in 20 states. Speech-language pathology support personnel are regulated in 14 states.

Of the 34 states, 10 states (Idaho, Illinois, Kentucky, Louisiana, Maryland, New Mexico, Ohio, Oregon, South Carolina, and Texas) regulate support personnel through licensure, the most stringent form of regulation. Twenty-three states regulate support personnel through registration and one through certification. Although not officially regulated, support personnel are acknowledged in five additional states. In four states (Connecticut, New Hampshire, Virginia, and Wisconsin), support personnel are not directly regulated; however, licensed speech-language pathologists or audiologists who use support personnel are required to use specific supervisory guidelines. Some states that regulate speech-language pathology, such as New York, do not permit the use of speech-language pathology support personnel.

Education Requirements The most common term for support personnel is *assistant,* with 13 states using the term. Ten states use the term *aides,* and four states use both *assistant* and *aide,* depending on the level of education. In some states both terms are used depending on the level of educational requirements and the specified level of practice.

The level of education required of support personnel varies from state to state. Some states (Montana, New Mexico, and Rhode Island) require a bachelor's degree in the area plus enrollment in a master's degree program. Six states (Arkansas, Kansas, Louisiana, Rhode Island, South Carolina, and Texas) require a bachelor's degree and some practicum. Six states (Alabama, Florida, Idaho, Indiana, Missouri, and West Virginia) require a bachelor's degree. Sixteen other states require as little as a high school diploma plus additional on-the-job training. Still other states do not specify any specific training.

As of September 2003, there were at least 27 operational associate degree programs for speech-language pathology assistants, and 73 institutions are considering and/or developing programs. Some of these programs are exploring training opportunities through distance learning and collaboration between community colleges and institutions of higher education. Ten states require continuing education for support personnel similar to the continuing education requirements for licensed speech-language pathologists or audiologists.

Because state laws differ, the tasks permitted by assistants vary from state to state. All require that support personnel work under the supervision or direction of an appropriately licensed or certified speech-language pathologist or audiologist. The level of supervision varies across the states. Some states limit the number of support personnel that a licensed professional may supervise. Others specify the amount and type of supervision that must be provided and/or the tasks support personnel are permitted to perform.

Support Personnel in Audiology

Audiology assistants are also regulated in some states. Depending on the level of training, they may perform tasks such as conducting speech-language or hearing screenings, following documented treatment plans or protocols, assisting during assessment, conducting calibration checks, and maintaining equipment. Most states do not permit assistants to interpret diagnostic test results, modify individual treatment plans, or make clinical decisions.

ASHA and Support Personnel

ASHA does not credential support personnel in speech-language pathology or audiology. However, the Association has had guidelines for the use of support personnel since 1969. In 1995, the ASHA Legislative Council approved a position paper and guidelines for the training, credentialing, and use of speech-language pathology assistants (ASHA, 2004 a, b). The ASHA guidelines call for assistants to complete a minimum of an associate's degree or equivalent course of study. According to the guidelines, support personnel, following academic training or on-the-job training, perform tasks as prescribed, directed, and supervised by an ASHA-certified speech-language pathologist or audiologist as appropriate. Supervision must be provided directly on site by an SLP or audiologist while an assigned activity is performed by support personnel or indirectly through demonstration, record review, or evaluating. Because the guidelines are national in scope, they may serve to bring about more uniformity in the terms used to identify speech-language pathology support personnel, training requirements, and supervisory responsibilities.

In 1997, ASHA approved a position paper and guidelines on support personnel in audiology (ASHA, 1998). The position paper states that support personnel may assist audiologists in delivery of services when appropriate. According to ASHA, training for audiology assistants should be competency-based and provided through a variety of formal and informal instructional methods. Support personnel should be provided with information on roles and functions by the supervising audiologist. The supervising audiologist should maintain written documentation of training activities and provide continuing opportunities for their assistants (ASHA, 1997). Supervising audiologists should assign specific tasks to the support person. The amount and type of supervision required should be based on the skills and experience of the assistant, the needs of patients/clients served, the service delivery setting, the tasks assigned, and other factors. The number of support personnel supervised by a given audiologist must be consistent with the delivery of appropriate, quality service (ASHA, 1998).

PROFESSIONAL CERTIFICATION: CERTIFICATE OF CLINICAL COMPETENCE AND BOARD CERTIFICATION

The credentials issued by professional associations such as ASHA or AAA are usually voluntary unless required by an agency where there is no governmental jurisdiction. The credential issued by ASHA is the Certificate of Clinical Competence (CCC), while AAA issues the American Board of Audiology (ABA) certification.

ASHA CERTIFICATION

ASHA developed its first standards for the practice of the professions in 1942. As the profession developed, the need for more stringent standards became necessary. In 1951, two levels of certification were awarded. Practitioners holding a bachelor's degree were awarded the Basic Certificate, and those holding a master's degree were awarded the Advanced Certificate. In 1962, ASHA adopted the master's degree as the minimum degree required for membership in the association, and consequently, new certification standards requiring the master's degree were adopted in 1965.

In 1972, the dual certification program was altered to establish the single level of certification known as the Certificate of Clinical Competence, which became the standard for entry into the practice of speech-language pathology or audiology. The CCC permits the holder to provide independent clinical services and to supervise the clinical practice of student trainees, other clinicians who do not hold certification, and support personnel.

Requirements for the Certificate of Clinical Competence

ASHA's Council for Clinical Certification (CFCC) develops the standards and is responsible for awarding the CCC in both speech-language pathology and audiology. The standards for the CCC include a required academic degree, course work in basic communication sciences and disorders, a supervised clinical practicum, a period of supervised professional practice, adherence to the ASHA Code of Ethics, and a passing score on the Praxis II Examination in Speech-Language Pathology or Audiology. The standards for the CCCs have been revised several times since their establishment to ensure that the standards are consistent with the contemporary scope of practice of the professions. They are developed following a rigorous validation study of the knowledge and skills necessary for entry into independent practice of the profession. Validation studies are conducted periodically by an independent organization to determine whether the standards continue to meet the needs of independent practice. Changes in the requirements are made, if necessary.

ASHA CCC in Speech-Language Pathology The salient features of the current standards for the CCC in Speech-Language Pathology include the following:

1. A master's, doctoral, or other recognized post-baccalaureate degree;

2. Graduate course work and graduate clinical practicum initiated and completed in a program accredited in speech-language pathology by ASHA's Council of Academic Accreditation in Audiology and Speech-Language Pathology (CAA);

3. A program of study with a minimum of 75 semester credit hours, including a minimum of 36 graduate credit hours of academic credit; that reflect a well-integrated program of study dealing with biological/physical sciences and mathematics; behavioral and/or social sciences, including normal aspects of human behavior and communication; and prevention, evaluation, and treatment of speech-language, hearing, and related disorders. Some course work must deal with issues pertaining to normal and abnormal development and behavior across the life span and to culturally diverse populations;

standards of ethical conduct, processes used in research, and the integration of research principles into evidence-based clinical practice; and contemporary professional issues;

4. A minimum of 400 clock hours of supervised clinical practicum, of which at least 375 clock hours must be direct client/patient contact and 325 of these must be obtained while the candidate was engaged in graduate study and 25 hours of supervised observation;

5. A passing score on a national examination adopted by ASHA for purposes of certification in speech-language pathology;

6. Completion of a full-time supervised speech-language pathology clinical fellowship of at least 36 weeks that establishes a collaboration between the clinical fellow and a mentor;

7. A maintenance of certification requirement that went into effect on January 1, 2005, requiring a minimum of 30 hours of professional development over a 3-year period.

Specific information on the standards for the CCC in speech-language pathology can be obtained from the ASHA Web site in the Resources section at the end of the chapter.

ASHA CCC in Audiology The scope of practice of the profession of audiology has changed rapidly in the last decade. In response to data presented by audiologists and an extensive skills validation study, the standards for the CCC in Audiology go into effect in 2007 and are fully implemented in 2012. The salient features of the 2007 Standards for the CCC in Audiology include the following:

1. The applicant must have a minimum of 75 graduate semester credit hours of postbaccalaureate study that culminates in a master's, doctoral, or other recognized academic graduate degree. The course of study must address the knowledge and skills pertinent to the field of audiology;

2. After December 31, 2011, the applicant must have a doctoral degree;

3. Graduate education in audiology must have been initiated and completed in a program accredited by the CAA;

4. The applicant must have prerequisite knowledge and skills in oral and written or other forms of communication;

5. The applicant must have prerequisite skills of life sciences, physical sciences, behavioral sciences, and mathematics;

6. The program of study must be of sufficient depth and breadth to achieve the knowledge and skills in four areas: foundations of practice, prevention and identification, evaluation, and treatment;

7. The program of study must include a practicum experience that is equivalent to a minimum of 12 months of full-time, supervised experience prior to awarding the degree;

8. The applicant must demonstrate successful achievement of the required knowledge and skills by means of both formative and summative assessments;

9. A maintenance of certification requirement took effect on January 1, 2003. Specific information on the standards for the CCC in Audiology can be obtained from ASHA's Web site.

Certification by the American Board of Audiology

The American Academy of Audiology (AAA) is a professional organization for audiologists. The AAA has established a certification program for audiologists administered by the American Board of Audiology (ABA). The purpose of the certification program is to generate and promulgate universally recognized standards in professional practice and to encourage audiologists to meet or exceed these standards. The ABA began granting certification to audiologists in January 1999. Persons seeking certification by the ABA must demonstrate evidence of initial mastery of the core elements of audiologic knowledge. To be eligible for certification, audiologists must have earned either a master's or doctoral degree in audiology from a regionally accredited college or university. Beginning in 2007, all persons eligible for the ABA certification must have earned a doctoral degree in audiology (e.g., AuD, PhD, EdD) from a regionally accredited college or university. In addition, applicants for certification must have obtained a passing score on a national examination as required by the ABA, completed 375 hours of supervised direct patient care, and completed 2,000 hours of mentored professional practice within a three-year time period after completion of academic course work. The mentor must verify the experience and make a recommendation for granting board certification. The mentor must hold a current state license or registration in audiology or hold current ABA certification (American Board of Audiology, 2005). Currently, persons who have completed the academic coursework and the 375 contact hours of patient care of the ABA certification requirements may apply for provisional board certification. When they have passed the national examination in audiology and completed the 2,000 hours of mentored experience, they may apply for full board certification.

After 2008, certified individuals must be recertified for a three-year period by completing 60 clock hours of continuing education in audiology, including at least three hours in professional ethics. These certification hours may be obtained in a wide variety of contexts, including attending approved conferences, courses, seminars, and workshops; participating in professional boards; authoring audiology articles in peer-reviewed journals, chapters, or professional books; or providing academic instruction. Effective January 1, 2008, additional requirements for the nature of continuing education activities go into effect. For more information about certification and continuing education by the ABA, see its Web site address in the Resources section of this chapter.

SPECIALTY RECOGNITION

Specialty recognition is a voluntary program that recognizes individual practitioners who have obtained advanced knowledge and experience in a given specialty area such as fluency or voice disorders. It is not a program of certification, nor is it intended to replace the ASHA's CCC or certification through AAA. It is a means for consumers, professionals, and referral and payer sources to identify practitioners who choose to meet established educational and experience criteria and who focus all or part of their practice in a particular specialty area recognized by ASHA or other professional groups. The program assumes that the majority of professionals will maintain a broad-based practice. To date, third party payers have not required that practitioners have specialty recognition for reimbursement purposes; however, some voice concern that this may be a future problem.

There are three programs of specialty recognition: the ASHA program of specialty recognition; the Academy of Neurologic Communication Disorders & Sciences (ANCDS); and the AAA specialty certification for cochlear implant audiologists. See the Web sites of these organizations for specific details.

The ASHA Program of Specialty Recognition

The minimum requirement for specialty recognition is holding the CCC. The specialty recognition program builds on a specific experience and knowledge base beyond that held by the standards established for the CCC. A petitioning group with special expertise in an area of practice (e.g., an ASHA Special Interest Division) must petition the Council for Clinical Specialty Recognition (CCSR) to sponsor a recognition program in a particular area. The petitioning group then completes a two-stage application process. At the present time, specialty recognition is available in fluency, swallowing and swallowing disorders, and child language. The requirements for specialty recognition vary for each area. For additional information on specialty recognition, contact ASHA.

Board Certification in Neurologic Communication Disorders (BC-NCD)

The Academy of Neurologic Communication Disorders (ANCDS) certification is granted for demonstrated expertise in working with adults, children, or children and adults (dual) who have neurologic communication disorders. Requirements for the certification include holding the CCC in speech-language pathology, a minimum of five years of experience with neurologic communication disorders, a passing score on an examination, and a written case summary and oral presentation before members of the board. For additional information on this certification, see the ANCDS Web address in the Resources section of this chapter.

ABA Specialization in Cochlear Implants

The ABA Board Certification with a Specialty in Cochlear Implants was developed to recognize those audiologists who have special knowledge and skill to be considered a cochlear implant specialist. In addition to holding the ABA certification, applicants must have verified experience working with cochlear implants and pass a written examination developed for this purpose. The first administration of the specialist examinations was conducted in 2005. For additional information about specialization in cochlear implants, see the Resources section at the end of this chapter.

INTERNATIONAL ISSUES

There are professional preparation programs for speech-language pathologists and audiologists in many countries around the world (Cheng, 2006). Each country has its own educational requirements and standards for professional practice. Many countries follow the general format for education and training in the United States; however, many do not. Some countries prepare students for independent practice at the bachelor's degree level, others require the master's degree, and still others have a system of required specialization. The educational requirements range from a bachelor's to a doctoral degree. Several countries also require certification and licenses for practice. While the requirements are generally similar, they differ in the required course work and the amount and type of supervised clinical practicum, experience, and examinations.

In some countries education in speech-language pathology is taken simultaneously with education in a second profession, such as audiology/hearing science, education, psychology, or generalist rehabilitation (International Association of Phoniatrica et Logopaedica, 1999). The content of the educational programs is usually course work in speech and language science, behavioral science, and biomedical sciences. In addition, there are guidelines for supervised clinical practicum, a practical examination, and recommended preparation in culturally and linguistically appropriate assessment and intervention. English language instruction may be necessary as much of the literature in the discipline is in English. For information on educational programs around the world, see the Web address for the International Association of Logopedics and Phoniatrics. See Chapter 6 for more in-depth discussion of international alliances.

International Guidelines for Education in Speech-Language Pathology

The International Association of Logopedics and Phoniatrics (IALP) has developed guidelines for Initial Education in Logopedics (1998). The guidelines recognize a variety of social, cultural, and educational influences that need to be considered in establishing education programs for the practice of speech-language pathology. Because of significant differences in the availability of educational programs in countries around the world, the IALP has also developed Guiding Principles for Training Support Workers in Communication Disabilities in Underserved Areas (1999). The guidelines are intended for those countries that have limited resources to begin a university-level program.

ASHA Certification: International Issues

The standards for clinical certification by ASHA require that graduate education be initiated and completed in an educational program accredited by the CAA. Because of its accreditation from the U.S. Department of Education and the Council for Higher Education Accreditation (CHEA), the CAA can only accredit programs in the United States. Persons who receive their professional education in other countries are only eligible for the CCC if they are currently certified by a certification agency having a reciprocal agreement with ASHA.

ASHA has a mutual recognition agreement with the Canadian Association of Speech-Language Pathology and Audiology (CASLPA). In recognition of increased trade and mobility between the United States and Canada, ASHA and CASLPA have endorsed each other's certification program in the professions of speech-language pathology and audiology as providing a substantially equivalent determination of the individual's qualifications to engage in independent clinical practice.

The Bologna Agreement in Europe

In recognition of the need for mobility between speech-language pathologists practicing in countries in the European Union, a recent agreement was made to standardize the standards for clinical practice among countries in the European Union. The Bologna Agreement (2005) aims to increase the alignment of higher education systems across Europe. A Directive of the European Parliament and the Council on the Recognition of Professional Qualifications was adopted in June 2005. The directive aims for mutual recognition of qualifications to practice the professions among the European countries. The Bologna Process aims to establish a European Higher Education Area by 2010. By 2005, 40 countries had agreed to harmonize their systems of higher education to facilitate professional recognition so that degrees and professional standards are comparable. The common framework for the standards is for an undergraduate bachelor's degree with at least three years of study, followed by a postgraduate master level with one or two years of study. Discussion continues about whether the professional qualification should be at the bachelor's, master's, or doctoral level.

Mutual Recognition Agreement Among English-Speaking Countries

The credentials in several English-speaking countries, while similar to those of ASHA, are not considered essentially equivalent. A quadrilateral agreement exists between ASHA, CASLPA, the Royal College of Speech and Language Therapists (RCSLT) in the United Kingdom, and the Speech Pathology Association of Australia Limited. This quadrilateral agreement recognizes common standards in academic and clinical practice and streamlines the recognition process for speech-language pathologists credentialed by the associations who seek accreditation of another association in the agreement. Speech Pathology New Zealand and Ireland have expressed an interest in being included in the agreement. The program does not extend to audiologists. Specific information on the credentialing of persons educated in foreign countries can be obtained from ASHA.

International Terminology

Discussions on the mutual recognition of credentials brought an awareness of the need to have an understanding of professional terminology used in the various English-speaking countries. The International Group on Terminology (IGOT) with representatives from 10 professional associations, including the International Association of Logopedics and Phoniatrics, has begun discussions to identify common terminology used in the professions.

CODE OF ETHICS

The preservation of the highest standards of integrity and ethical principles is vital to the responsible discharge of obligations in the professions of speech-language pathology and audiology. Speech-language pathologists and audiologists who hold the ASHA CCC must abide by the Code of Ethics (ASHA, 2003) to assure the public they hold paramount the welfare of the persons they serve professionally, achieve and maintain the highest level of professional competence, and honor their responsibility to the public and to the professions. The Board of Ethics, which consists of members of the profession as well as consumers, reviews violations of the code. Violations of the code may result in probation or revocation of the CCC. In addition, persons who are certified by the American Board of Audiologists must abide by the code of ethics of the American Academy of Audiology. See Chapter 4, Professional Ethics, and Chapter 5, Professional Liability, for further discussion of this topic.

SUMMARY

Communication is a complex human behavior. The study of communication sciences and disorders and the practice of the professions of speech-language pathology and audiology are changing to meet the challenges of advancing knowledge of the complexities of speech, language, swallowing, and hearing impairments. The standards for practice must be current to assure the public will not be harmed by improper evaluation or treatment. The assessment and treatment of communication disorders and the investigation of the nature of speech, language, swallowing, and hearing requires a highly skilled professional. The practice of speech-language pathology requires a graduate degree with assurance of continuing competence. The practice of audiology soon will require a doctoral degree as a minimum standard for entry into the profession's practice. The public must also be assured that professionals follow standards of clinical and ethical practice. This assurance is met by regulation through professional certification and/or professional licensure. By adherence to codes of professional conduct and ethical standards, the public can be assured that services provided by competent speech-language pathologists and audiologists who are worthy of their trust.

CRITICAL THINKING

1. Review the licensure law for speech-language pathologists and audiologists in your state or that of a neighboring state. Do the requirements differ from the requirements for the ASHA CCC?

2. What harm could result from the delivery of speech-language pathology or audiology services by an unlicensed or noncertified person?

3. What will be the impact of the required doctoral degree for the ASHA CCC in audiology on the profession of audiology?

4. How will the requirement for the doctoral degree in audiology affect master's degree programs in audiology? How do you think the public and third party payers will perceive the doctorate in audiology?

5. Should the certification standards for speech-language pathology be changed to require a doctoral degree? What would be the advantages and disadvantages of such a requirement?

6. What are the advantages and disadvantages of professional standards for support personnel?

7. Why is continuing education a critical component to the education of speech-language pathologists and audiologists? How do you intend to meet the continuing education requirements of state licensure and professional certification?

8. What issues related to certification and licensing are related to professional practice in other countries?

9. What are the advantages and disadvantages of having two major audiology professional organizations (ASHA and AAA)?

REFERENCES

Alabama Licensure Law for Speech Pathologists and Audiologists, Acts of 1975. 34–28A-2 (revised September 3, 2005).

American Board of Audiology. (2005). *Application handbook.* Reston, VA: Author.

American Speech-Language-Hearing Association. (1990). *Report of the Ad-Hoc Committee on Undergraduate Education.* Rockville, MD: Author.

American Speech-Language-Hearing Association. (1998). Position statement and guidelines on support personnel in audiology. *Asha, 40* (Spring Supplement 18), 19–21.

American Speech-Language-Hearing Association. (2003). Code of Ethics (revised). *Asha Supplement, 23,* 13–15.

American Speech-Language-Hearing Association. (2004a). Guidelines for credentialing, use and supervision of speech-language pathology assistants. Available at http://www.asha.org

American Speech-Language Hearing Association (2004b). Training, use and supervision of support personnel in speech-language pathology. Available at http://www.asha.org

American Speech-Language-Hearing Association. (2005). Background information for the standards and implementation for the certificate of clinical competence in audiology. Available at http://www.asha.org

Angel Learning. (2005). Indianapolis, IN: Thomson Higher Education.

Blackboard Academic Suite. (2005). Washington, DC: Blackboard.

Blake, D. (1995). *The dictionary of educational terms.* Brookfield, VT: Ashgate Publishing.

Bologna Agreement. (2005). CQ3 Chapter 2 International Context. Available at http://www.rcslt.org/resources/CQ3_Chapter_2.pdf

Boswell, S. (2005, May 24). Opening doors for future clinicians: Distance learning at Longwood targets students from other disciplines. *The ASHA Leader, 10,* 2 & 24.

Cheng, L. (Ed.). (2006). *Education of speech language pathologists around the world. Folia Phoniatrica et Logopaedica, 58,* 1.

Council of Graduate Schools in the United States. (1990). *The doctor of philosophy degree.* Washington, DC: Author.

Council on Academic Accreditation in Audiology and Speech-Language Pathology. (2004). Standards for accreditation of graduate education in educational programs in audiology and speech-language pathology. Available at http://www.asha.org

Dudding, C. C., & Purcell-Robertson, R. M. (2003, June 10). Beyond the technology: How to navigate distance education. *The ASHA Leader, 8,* 6–7, 16.

Flower, R. M., Ohta, D., Stephens, M., & Orahood, R. (1986). Perspectives on licensure. *Asha, 28,* 19–23.

Individuals with Disabilities Education Improvement Act, Public Law 108–446 (2004).

International Association of Logopedics and Phoniatrics. (1998). Guidelines for the initial education in logopedics. *Folia Phoniatrica et Logopaedica, 50,* 230–234.

International Association of Phoniatrica et Logopaedica (1999). Guiding principles of training of support workers in communication disabilities in underserved areas. *Folia Phoniatrica et Logopaedica, 51,* 239–242.

Knowles, A. (Ed.). (1977). Degrees, diplomas, and certificates. *International encyclopedia of higher education, 4* (pp. 1230–1241). San Francisco: Jossey-Bass.

Lynch, C., & Hesse, J. (1997). Characteristics of state licensure laws. Rockville, MD: American Speech-Language-Hearing Association, State & Consumer Advocacy.

Nebraska Statutes for Practice of Audiology and Speech Pathology. §71-1, 190 (p. 4). Lincoln, NE: (2003). Department of Health and Human Services Regulations and Licensure Credentialing Division.

Neidecker, E., & Blosser, J. (1993). *School programs in speech language: Organization and management.* Englewood Cliffs, NJ: Prentice Hall.

New York State Education Law Article 159. (1974). Speech-language pathologists and audiologists '8203, 1974, c.1055; '8202 amended L. 1983, c.43.'1.

RESOURCES

American Academy of Audiology
   11730 Plaza America Drive, Suite 300
   Reston, VA 20190
   Phone: 800-AAA-2336, 703-790-8466
   Fax: 703-790-8631
   Web site: http://www.audiology.org/

American Academy of Neurologic Communication
   Disorders
   P.O. Box 26532
   Minneapolis, MN 55426
   Phone: 952-920-0484
   Fax: 952-920-6098
   Web site: www.ancds.org

American Speech-Language-Hearing Association
   10801 Rockville Pike, Rockville, MD 20852
   Phone: 301-897-5700
   Web site: http://www.asha.org.

Online Guide to Graduate Education: For information
   on graduate programs, including the Online
   Guide to Graduate Education in Speech-Language
   Pathology and Audiology, consult http://www.asha
   .org/gradguide/

le Comité Permanent de Liaison des Orthophonistes et
   Logopédes de L'Union Européenne: For information on European standards, contact CPLOL at
   http://www.cplol.org

The Council of Academic Programs in Communication
   Sciences and Disorders (CAPCSD)
   Web site: http://www.capcsd.org

International Association of Logopedics and Phoniatrics
   Web site: http//www.ialp.info

FINANCIAL AID
AND SCHOLARSHIPS

Information on scholarships available from ASHA
   can be obtained from the American Speech-
   Language-Hearing Foundation, 10801 Rockville
   Pike, Rockville, MD 20852.

Information on federal scholarships and assistantships
   through federally funded grants and contracts can
   be obtained through individual colleges and universities or the U.S. Department of Education,
   Office of Special Education and Rehabilitative
   Services, Division of Personnel Preparation,
   Washington, DC 20202.

Sertoma International Communication Disorders
   Scholarships of $1,000 each to cover tuition,
   books, and supplies are available from the
   Sertoma Foundation, 1912 E. Meyer Boulevard,
   Kansas City, MO 64132.

Specific information on financial assistance, including
   privately funded scholarships for graduate study
   in communication sciences and disorders, is available from the financial aid office at the college or
   university you wish to attend.

3

Professional Organizations

SUE T. HALE, MCD, AND
FRED H. BESS, PHD

SCOPE OF CHAPTER

This chapter introduces students to opportunities for affiliating with professional organizations. The benefits of membership are highlighted, but the more important objective is to help students discover the service, leadership, and learning opportunities these organizations present. Scenarios in the opening section set the stage for what associations can do for their members. A brief review of the construct of professional organizations is provided. The American Speech-Language-Hearing Association (ASHA) and the American Academy of Audiology (AAA) are highlighted as the two primary organizations for our professions. Related professional organizations, state associations, and student organizations are also described.

PRACTICAL DILEMMAS
AND AFFILIATION

Consider the following:

- The only speech-language pathologist working in a rural school district has concerns about the size of the caseload the school district requires to be served. Unlike the predecessor in this position, this clinician serves a number of children who exhibit multiple and severe handicaps. How does the speech-language pathologist demonstrate that the current caseload/workload with fewer children is equivalent in effort to that of the previous clinician who saw greater numbers of children with less severe disorders?

- An audiologist is approached by a hearing aid manufacturer who offers an all-expense-paid educational opportunity regarding a new product line the manufacturer sells. The conference will take place for 2 hours a day during a 5-day stay at an exclusive ski resort. The company representative also encourages the audiologist to invite a family member or spouse to come along. How should the audiologist respond?

- A speech-language pathologist in a medical setting is assigned to provide intervention for patients who require systems for alternative/augmentative communication, an area of practice with which the clinician has had little experience or education. How can the clinician locate relevant educational events and materials to assist in developing the necessary skills and knowledge to provide services in this area?

- An audiologist wants to communicate with other audiologists who are researching hearing aid products and cochlear implants. Where can the audiologist locate colleagues with similar interests?

- A speech-language pathologist is concerned that the arbitrary cap on reimbursement for services provided to hospital outpatients will soon be reinstated if legislation is not passed to eliminate the therapy cap. How can the speech-language pathologist maximize the value of advocacy efforts for legislation of this nature?

In each instance, affiliation with a professional association and taking advantage of the member benefits of that association will assist the professionals facing these practical dilemmas. Professional associations available to speech-language pathologists and audiologists support members in dealing with all of the instances listed previously: clarifying caseload versus workload issues to employers, handling ethical dilemmas in the workplace, accessing continuing education opportunities, affiliating with other professionals who have similar interests, and participating in grassroots and coordinated advocacy efforts. These are just a few of the benefits available to speech-language pathologists and audiologists who are members of professional associations.

Students in training who affiliate with organizations targeted to their interests and needs gain firsthand knowledge of the structure and benefits of these associations prior to entering the workforce. Student organizations provide opportunities for leadership development and volunteer service as well as educational materials and scholarly and professional publications. These organizations facilitate students as they transition to the workplace in regard to standards and credentialing, ethics, and networking. Two organizations available to students in communication sciences and disorders are the National Student Speech-Language-Hearing Association (NSSLHA), which is affiliated with ASHA, and the National Association of Future Doctors of Audiology (NAFDA), which is affiliated with AAA. These organizations will be described in more detail later in the chapter.

HOW DO PROFESSIONAL
ASSOCIATIONS WORK?

Professional associations offer an array of services and benefits to members as well as providing support and advocating on behalf of consumers served by those members. Professional associations have a targeted scope of activity, typically related to a particular discipline. Individuals who wish to affiliate with the association often have to meet requirements that relate to degrees held and other educational and professional qualifications.

Professional associations have a number of common characteristics. These organizations often take responsibility for providing members with educational programs and materials, scientific and professional publications, targeted legislative advocacy activities, standards and scopes of practice, marketing resources, and public information. An important characteristic of most professional organizations is a requirement that members agree to abide by a Code of Ethics, a set of standards for professional conduct that delineate responsibilities of the members to consumers, colleagues, and the profession. Professional associations are usually non-profit organizations governed by a board of directors and operated with publicly accessible bylaws. The bylaws, which contain the organization's mission and goals, also describe the governance structure and how the work of the association is conducted. Most professional organizations operate with a combination of volunteer leaders, who often assume positions on the board of directors or other policy-making groups, and paid staff members who engage in day-to-day operations and support member services.

Professional organizations derive a large portion of the operating budget from member dues, but additional fiscal resources are often generated by conventions and continuing education activities, publications and product sales, affiliations with commercial entities (affinity credit cards, professional and casualty insurers, convention exhibitors), corporate sponsors, and investments. These sources of income support the member benefits and consumer advocacy goals of the organization.

ASHA and AAA are two national organizations with members from the professions of speech-language pathology and audiology. ASHA has members from both professions, while AAA has members from the profession of audiology.

ASHA: A NATIONAL PROFESSIONAL ORGANIZATION FOR SPEECH-LANGUAGE PATHOLOGISTS AND AUDIOLOGISTS

The American Speech-Language-Hearing Association is the largest and oldest scientific and professional organization representing the professions of speech-language pathology and audiology. ASHA began with a meeting in May 1925 in the home of Lee Edward Travis. There were fewer than 25 individuals at that first meeting, and they came together because they all held an interest in speech and its disorders. It was more than a decade before the number of members reached 60, and the organization began publishing its first scholarly journal. In 1947, the organization embraced the profession of audiology and was named the American Speech and Hearing Association. The association established national standards for graduate training program accreditation and credentialing of service providers in the 1960s. In 1978, the organization changed its name once again to reflect the component of language in its research and clinical pursuits and became the American Speech-Language-Hearing Association. Throughout its history, the association has been characterized by enormous growth in membership and a corresponding need for greater staff support. In 1981 the association moved to its current headquarters in Rockville, Maryland, but the need for more space resulted in a 2004 decision to expand the size of the national office. The association will soon break ground on a 150,000-square-foot facility, also in Rockville, which is expected to open in late 2007 (Uffen, 2005).

Purpose

Bylaws address the purposes of an association. The purposes of ASHA, as stated in its bylaws (ASHA, 2004), are:

(1) To encourage basic scientific study of the processes of individual human communication

with special reference to speech, language, and hearing;

(2) To promote appropriate academic and clinical preparation of individuals entering the discipline of human communication sciences and disorders and promote the maintenance of current knowledge and skills of those within the discipline;

(3) To promote investigation and prevention of disorders of human communication;

(4) To foster improvement of clinical services and procedures concerning such disorders;

(5) To stimulate exchange of information among persons and organizations thus engaged and to disseminate such information;

(6) To advocate the rights and interests of persons with communication disorders; and

(7) To promote the individual and collective professional interests of the members of the Association. (p. 2) (article II, 2.1).

The ASHA bylaws address many other issues and serve to provide information about all aspects of the operation and mission of the association, including governance, standards, the Code of Ethics, publications, and other key organizational components.

Membership

ASHA currently has more than 120,000 certified members, noncertified members, international affiliates, and nonmember certificate holders who are audiologists, speech-language pathologists, and speech, language, or hearing scientists. At the end of 2005, ASHA affiliates included more than 106,000 speech-language pathologists and more than 12,000 audiologists. Just less than 1,300 individuals were certified in both speech-language pathology and audiology (ASHA, 2006). At the end of 2005, 93.7 percent of ASHA members were female, a continuation of a trend that has seen a gradual reduction in the percentage of males in the association. Also at the end of 2005, 7.2 percent of those affiliated with the association were members of racial/ethnic minority groups,

and 18 percent of members were 55 years of age or older (ASHA, 2006). Three of these demographic factors are extremely concerning to the association.

Efforts have been initiated to recruit and retain males in the professions, but the numbers indicate that these efforts have not met with great success. The association has also worked to increase the number of professionals from racial and ethnic minorities, but the overall percentage in relation to the total membership has increased less than 1 percent since 2003. Success in the recruitment and retention of males and minority professionals is essential for a diverse workforce to be available to address the communication needs of all citizens. Finally, the large number of older members of the association suggests that retirement is on the horizon for many, particularly for the baby boomer group. Many of the professionals in this group also have PhDs and fill the ranks of academia. The shortage of younger members who hold research and teaching degrees is extremely concerning in regard to future training needs and, indeed, for the vitality of the knowledge base for the professions. ASHA is devoting large amounts of energy and resources to address the doctoral shortage.

It should be mentioned that the number of audiologists who are members of ASHA and hold the Certificate of Clinical Competence has held steady in recent years. At a time when some audiologists prefer to affiliate exclusively with AAA, whose members are only audiologists, negligible changes in the total number of audiologists affiliated with ASHA have been observed. However, the number of speech-language pathologists continues to increase annually with the result that the percentage of audiology members in relation to the total ASHA membership has declined. ASHA leaders are attempting to determine the effect on the overall percentage of members who are audiologists in relation to the move from the master's degree to the Doctor of Audiology (AuD) degree by most audiology training programs. The transition to the AuD has resulted in fewer audiology graduates during the current interim period as programs move from two-year to four-year degrees. These demographic trends will continue to engage the interest and attention of ASHA organizers for the foreseeable future.

Standards

A key component of the American Speech-Language-Hearing Association is its standards program, which addresses issues of individual credentialing as well as accreditation of academic training. ASHA has offered the Certificates of Clinical Competence (CCC) in audiology and speech-language pathology for more than 40 years. These certificates have become nationally recognized credentials by governmental and educational agencies. The CCC standards have served as the model for the state licensure requirements in many states. Additionally, ASHA supports the accreditation of graduate programs in communication sciences and disorders through the Council on Academic Accreditation (CAA), an accreditation program recognized by the Council on Higher Education Accreditation of the U.S. Department of Education. Students who wish to receive the CCC must complete the requisite academic and clinical training in a CAA-accredited graduate training program. The newest ASHA standards for graduate education and professional credentialing in both audiology and speech-language pathology emphasize the attainment of knowledge and skills to address speech, language, and hearing needs across the life span and with a variety of disorders. See Chapter 2 for in-depth discussion of ASHA accreditation and certification.

Governance

The governance structure of an association describes how policies are made, states who is responsible for certain work in the organization, and serves to guide a consumer or member in determining where to go for assistance with a certain problem or question. The governance structure of ASHA is described in detail in Article IV of the bylaws (ASHA, 2004, p. 2–7) (article IV, 4.1–4.4). A visual display of the structure is presented in Figure 3–1 (ASHA, 2005).

For ASHA, the primary work of governance in shared by the Executive Board and the Legislative Council (LC), both of whom have clearly identified duties for policy-making and fiscal responsibility. The 150 members of the Legislative Council are elected by ASHA members in each state and represent those members at two meetings each year. During those meetings, the resolutions under consideration affect policies and guidelines, budget, and member issues. The LC has two assemblies, the Audiology/Hearing Science Assembly, which considers and votes on matters specific to audiology, and the Speech-Language Pathology/Speech or Language Science Assembly, which considers issues that affect only speech-language pathology. The entire council votes on issues of general concern to the membership.

The Executive Board (EB) consists of 12 members. The President, President-Elect, Past-President, and eight Vice Presidents are elected by the membership in a mail vote. The President, Vice President for Administration and Planning, Vice President for Academic Affairs, Vice President for Research and Technology, and Vice President for Governmental and Social Policies may be audiologists or speech-language pathologists. Audiologists are represented on the EB by the Vice President for Professional Practices in Audiology and the Vice President for Quality of Service in Audiology. Similar vice presidential positions exist for speech-language pathology. The other members of EB are the Executive Director of the association, who is a nonvoting member, and the Speaker of the (Legislative) Council who is an ex officio representative elected by the LC. The EB's role is in the oversight and operation of the association and in making budgetary and programmatic recommendations to the LC. Shared governance provides for both entities to work together in addressing the principles of advocacy, autonomy, and accountability for the association (Williams, 2001, p. 26).

The National Office

In addition to the volunteer leadership of the association, a national office staff of more than 200 members works in the day-to-day operation of the association. The Executive Director works closely with Chief Staff Officers in speech-language

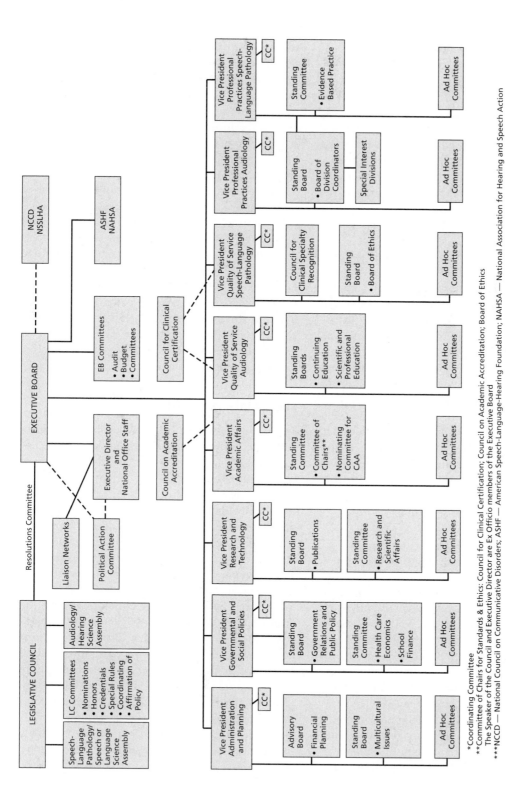

FIGURE 3–1 Association Governance Structure

*Coordinating Committee

**Committee of Chairs for Standards & Ethics: Council for Clinical Certification; Council on Academic Accreditation; Board of Ethics

The Speaker of the Council and Executive Director are Ex Officio members of the Executive Board

***NCCD — National Council on Communicative Disorders; ASHF — American Speech-Language-Hearing Foundation; NAHSA — National Association for Hearing and Speech Action

SOURCE: American Speech-Language-Hearing Association. (2005). Association Governance Structure. Rockville, MD: Author. Reprinted with permission.

79

pathology, audiology, science and research, multicultural affairs, and operations to conduct the work of the National Office. These executives, referred to as the Facilitating Team, guide the work clusters in the National Office. The work clusters include academic accreditation, certification, and ethics; audiology practice policy and consultation; speech-language pathology practices; multicultural affairs; governmental relations and public policy; governance and international affairs; professional education; marketing and sales; public relations; publishing; the Action Center; and other administrative and operational groups.

The administrators and staff in the National Office work to accomplish association purposes, develop and implement work plans to achieve association objectives, and monitor long-term operations. The National Office relates to members directly through the Action Center call line and other forms of person-to-person communication. Additionally, staff within the office maintain and update the Web portal to maximize its benefit to members, students, and consumers. (See Resources for Web addresses of associations.) Working with the volunteer leadership, the national office staff members are often the most direct link between the association and the members, and the work of the national office is essential to the association.

The Future

ASHA's future viability is dependent on many issues, many of which are tied to the ability to remain responsive and effective in a world where information must be gained and shared instantaneously and across national borders. Members will value services that meet their expectations for immediacy, accuracy, and currency. The Web portal, Web-based seminars and dialogues, and telecommunications of all types are association activities that address those expectations.

In addition, ASHA has developed a strategic plan to address concerns and issues that are considered core to the continuing mission of the association. The Strategic Plan: 2005–2007 (ASHA, 2005)

suggests a work strategy for addressing key issues for the future. These issues include the need for high-quality research to support evidence-based practice, the shortage of doctoral-level faculty to support the future of the professions, the need to constantly monitor and modify comprehensive scopes of practice, the requirement for increased knowledge and skills for the provision of culturally competent services in a diverse society, the necessity for an increased international exchange of professional knowledge and mutual international collaboration, and the need to understand and recognize cultural, linguistic, and political differences worldwide that will facilitate collaborative work with international associations (Schill & Dublinske, 2005). With the establishment of the strategic plan, ASHA moved forward with a commitment to embrace the international professional community while maintaining a commitment to the research, educational, legislative, and practice needs of its current members.

Special Interest Divisions

Special Interest Divisions were established within ASHA to promote knowledge and skills in specialized areas ASHA members may join one or more of the Divisions and have access to educational programs, research, publications, and dialogue with members with similar interests. The Divisions have their own steering committees and are financially self-supporting. This program provides the members with an opportunity to gain leadership experience and influence practice patterns within an area of specialization.

Sixteen Special Interest Divisions address the diverse areas of language learning, neurogenic disorders, voice disorders, fluency disorders, orofacial disorders, hearing research and diagnostics, aural rehabilitation, hearing conservation, hearing disorders in childhood, issues in higher education, administration and supervision, augmentative and alternative communication, swallowing and swallowing disorders, communication issues in culturally and linguistically diverse populations, gerontology, and school-based issues.

AAA: A NATIONAL PROFESSIONAL ORGANIZATION FOR AUDIOLOGISTS

The American Academy of Audiology is the world's largest professional organization of, by, and for audiologists. The impetus for AAA dates back to the 1987 ASHA convention in New Orleans when a mini-seminar was presented on "The Future of Audiology." Richard Talbott chaired the session and recruited five well-known audiologists to discuss such critical issues as future needs and potential employment of audiologists, knowledge base required to meet the future needs, level of academic training needed to achieve the knowledge base, and university faculty/supervisory personnel needs for training audiologists. One of the panel members, James Jerger, concluded his presentation by noting that it was now time for a new professional organization of, by, and for audiologists. Jerger's comments were met with an enthusiastic response. As a follow-up to the ASHA session, 32 audiology leaders met in Houston, Texas, in early 1988 at the invitation of James Jerger (Baylor College of Medicine). The purpose of the study group was to establish an independent freestanding national organization for audiologists. The group voted unanimously to develop a new organization for audiologists, to be called the American College of Audiology, and the first national office was established at Baylor College of Medicine. In addition, an ad hoc steering committee was appointed to develop bylaws. Finally, before leaving the Houston meeting, each member of the founders group contributed $20 to establish the organization's first budget.

In the few short months to follow, remarkable progress was made. The newly developed bylaws for the organization were approved, the organization was renamed the American Academy of Audiology, the Academy was incorporated under the laws of the state of Tennessee, an organizational structure was established and officers elected, dues were established, committee assignments were made, dates for the first annual meeting were determined, and a major membership drive was launched. In 1989, the first AAA convention was held at Kiawah Island, South Carolina, and the response exceeded all expectations: Close to 600 participants, including 45 "charter" exhibitors, attended the meeting and literally overflowed the conference facilities.

Since 1989, the AAA has undergone significant growth in membership and development. By 1993, the AAA reached a point in membership size and fiscal responsibilities that it became necessary to move the national office to Washington, D.C., and contract staff to assist in the organization's management. Today, the AAA national office is located in Reston, Virginia.

Purpose

According to the AAA bylaws (AAA, 2005), the Academy is a professional organization of individuals dedicated to providing quality hearing care to the public. The focus is to enhance the ability of AAA members to achieve career and practice objectives through professional development, education, research, and increased public awareness of hearing disorders and audiologic services.

Membership

AAA currently has more than 10,000 members, an impressive number given the relatively short time the organization has been in existence. Moreover, the number of new members added each year is growing substantially. The demographic breakdown of the AAA membership is similar to that of ASHA. In 2005, 71 percent of the membership of AAA was female, and 28 percent have doctoral degrees (this number will grow significantly now that the doctor of audiology degree will be required to practice in the profession). Although AAA does not have data on the number of members representing racial/ethnic minority groups, the number is small and is probably similar to that of ASHA. Finally, the number of audiologists over age 55 is 16 percent.

Both ASHA and AAA have been concerned about the inability to attract sufficient numbers of males and minorities into the profession despite the development of special recruitment initiatives.

Equally disturbing is the relatively large number of professionals who are 55 years or older, most of whom will be retiring within the next 10 years. These demographic concerns have been discussed earlier in the membership section related to ASHA.

Standards

Similar to ASHA, the AAA has developed a standards program for certifying audiologists. The program, offered by the American Board of Audiology (ABA), certifies audiologists whose knowledge base and clinical skills are consistent with professionally established standards and who continue to add to their knowledge through various forms of continuing education. The ABA is currently working toward having states and government agencies recognize ABA certification. Recently, the ABA has begun to develop specialty certifications. The first specialty certification program offered by ABA was for cochlear implant audiologists.

AAA has also begun to develop an accreditation process for universities offering AuD graduate training. Beginning in 2003, the Accreditation Commission for Audiology Education (ACAE) began developing education standards for AuD training programs. The completed standards were adopted by the ACAE Board of Directors in March 2005, following a rigorous peer review process. The standards can be found online at http://www.acaeaccred.org. In addition to ACAE, a technology company has been contracted for the development of a Web-based accreditation system. This Computerized Accreditation Program (CAP) will be an innovative online accreditation system combining high-quality standards with state-of-the art technology. The result is accreditation plus an interactive, Web-based process designed to facilitate ease in management, and provide valuable information to program directors, faculty, students and communities of interest. Some of the proposed features of the system include online participation, an interactive self-study process, the ability to retrieve national trends and analyses from a data warehouse. The ACAE and CAP programs are expected to be launched in the near future.

Governance and the National Office

The governance structure of AAA is described in Article V of the bylaws (AAA, 2005). The structure is purposely designed to be streamlined so that the leadership can respond in a timely manner to its membership as well as to topical issues on the national front that arise from time to time throughout the year. To this end, the Academy is governed by a Board of Directors composed of 12 Fellows, including the President, President-elect, Past President and 9 Members-at-Large. Each member of the board is elected by the membership at large and possesses the power to vote on issues before the board. In addition to other duties, the Board of Directors is expected to (1) grant membership to those applicants whose qualifications, in the board's judgment, meet the requirements set forth by the bylaws; (2) establish boards, committees, and task forces, as necessary, to guide and assist the Academy in its mission, and appoint the Chair of such groups; (3) decide when and where the Annual Academy Meeting shall take place and elect a Program Chair for the meeting; and (4) transact all such other business in the interest of the membership.

The national office is comprised of an Executive Director and 24 office staff who work closely with the President, other board members, and volunteers from the membership to facilitate operational activities of the Academy. Examples of such activities include government relations, credentialing, public relations, marketing, publications, continuing education and professional education.

The Future

The AAA has experienced extraordinary growth and success the first two decades of its existence. The future of AAA, however, will depend on the ability of the Academy leadership to continue to meet the ever-changing needs of audiologists and the profession as well as to develop effective tools to measure progress. Indeed, those organizations that fail to define their goals and critical success factors for the future and then communicate the goals to their members will not be successful. To this end, AAA leadership has developed a comprehensive strategic plan that sets the course for the future of the profession. Goals, strategies, and action plans have been developed to help ensure that the Academy will achieve its vision of advancing the science and practice of audiology and achieving public recognition of audiologists as experts in hearing and balance. Some of the specific goals in the AAA strategic plan include (1) promote a member-driven environment that fosters involvement and provides services essential to their success; (2) partner with other organizations to advance hearing and balance initiatives; (3) shape the future of science and practice through effective leadership and advocacy and; (4) increase consumer and patient awareness of and access to optimal hearing and balance care.

RELATED PROFESSIONAL ORGANIZATIONS

Related Professional Organizations (RPOs) are available to individuals with research, clinical, or educational interests that may not be fully addressed within the scope of ASHA or AAA. Examples of these organizations are the Academy of Neurologic Communication Disorders and Sciences, an organization with professional clinical, educational, scientific and charitable interests directed toward the quality of life for adults and children with neurologic communication disorders; the Acoustical Society of America, an organization involved in the scientific pursuit of acoustics information, which includes members from diverse scientific professions, including physics, engineering, biology, psychology, and speech and hearing; and the Council for Exceptional Children, an organization dedicated to improving educational outcomes for students with exceptionalities such as developmental disabilities, learning disabilities, and communicative disabilities and deafness.

These are just a few of the many examples of related professional organizations that may engage the student or professional with special interests in a focused educational, clinical, or research area. A listing of some relevant related professional organizations is provided at the end of the chapter.

STATE ORGANIZATIONS

State organizations in speech-language pathology and audiology are often affiliated with a larger national organization and have similar purposes and structure when this is the case. For example, many state speech-language-hearing associations are recognized affiliates of ASHA. As such, they have access to ASHA's state-national relations resources, which provide informational and sometimes financial assistance with legislation, licensure, and other state-focused issues. The Council of State Association Presidents meets twice annually, once in the spring in conjunction with the ASHA State Policy Workshop and on the day prior to the annual ASHA convention. Audiology members in some states are also affiliated with AAA with similar benefits and connectivity.

State organizations have an opportunity to influence practice issues, regulations, funding decisions, and other aspects of the day-to-day practice of the professions within a locale. As such, these organizations offer students and professionals the opportunity to become engaged in activities of vital importance to their current or future livelihood.

Students are often provided reduced fees or even free memberships and convention registration if they assist with state activities. Assisting at the state association level is an excellent means to enter the volunteer workforce that is so essential to the viability of professional organizations. Students who affiliate with state associations while they are in their training programs have an opportunity to network with individuals who may ultimately be future employers or mentors when the students graduate.

STUDENT ORGANIZATIONS

Training programs in communication sciences and disorders typically have local chapters of the National Student Speech-Language-Hearing Association

(NSSLHA) and the National Association of Future Doctors of Audiology (NAFDA). Like the earlier model, NSSLHA, which is affiliated with ASHA, includes student members who are preparing for careers in audiology or in speech-language pathology. NAFDA, which is affiliated with AAA, includes student members preparing for careers in audiology.

NSSLHA

As the only student association formally recognized by ASHA, NSSLHA's President and Past-President sit as voting members on the ASHA Legislative Council. Additionally, NSSLHA has representatives to a number of the ASHA councils and boards. The requirements for membership in NSSLHA are that an undergraduate or graduate student has an interest in the study of normal and disordered human communication behavior and is enrolled either part- or full-time in a training program in communication sciences. Local chapters in university settings allow students opportunities for leadership development, volunteerism, philanthropic work, professional networking, educational events, reduced ASHA convention registration, and a reduction in ASHA certification fees if membership is maintained throughout the graduate training program.

NAFDA

The National Association of Future Doctors of Audiology is the only student organization committed to the advancement of the AuD degree. NAFDA was founded in October 1998 by an AuD student at the University of Louisville. NAFDA accepts AuD students for membership who are currently enrolled in a regionally accredited university. Some of the benefits of being a NAFDA member include the student newsletter, an academic journal, an online forum and chatroom, assistance with the 4th-year placement, and scholarships and writing contests. Moreover, NAFDA works closely with AAA to help ensure that students receive a student-oriented experience within the AAA annual meeting. Approximately 40 NAFDA chapters exist at university programs throughout the country and afford AuD students with excellent opportunities for professional development.

INTERNATIONAL PROFESSIONAL ORGANIZATIONS

For those who have an interest in international professional issues in speech-language pathology and audiology, affiliation with a number of professional organizations may be useful. For example, the International Society of Audiology and the International Association of Logopedics and Phoniatrics (IALPP) provide membership and education opportunities. In addition, you will read about professional organizations in other countries in Chapter 6, International Alliances. There you will read about associations in other English-speaking countries, including Australia, Canada, New Zealand, South Africa, and the United Kingdom.

SUMMARY

Students are encouraged to affiliate with national professional organizations as well as state organizations, special interest groups, and related professional organizations. Early involvement in these associations provide opportunities for volunteering, networking, advocacy, and learning. An excellent training ground for these experiences is active affiliation with a student organization affiliated with a national association, such as the National Student Speech-Language-Hearing Association or the National Association of Future Doctors of Audiology. Being a member of a larger group makes it more likely that problems can be solved and answers to questions can be obtained in a coordinated, consistent, and effective manner. Being aware of the history and governance of associations will also help students as they choose to affiliate with those associations that will continue to be the most effective in representing member interests and in relating to the larger global community.

CRITICAL THINKING

1. What benefits do student members of NSSLHA and NAFDA enjoy?

2. What are the advantages of membership in a national professional organization?

3. Refer to the opening scenarios. What specific kinds of assistance could these individuals expect to get from their national professional organization(s)?

4. Create scenarios specific to your own area of interest or a problem you might encounter as a professional and discuss resources your professional organization might provide to address the issue.

5. What valuable experiences are likely to be gained from affiliation with a state organization, a special interest division, or a related professional organization?

6. Should a graduate student in audiology affiliate with NSSLHA, NAFDA, or both? Should a practicing audiologist hold membership in AAA, ASHA, or both?

REFERENCES

American Academy of Audiology. (2005). Bylaws of the American Academy of Audiology. Available at http://www.audiology.org/

American Speech-Language-Hearing Association. (2004). Online desk reference: Volume I: Cardinal documents of the association, bylaws and policies associated with the bylaws of the American Speech-Language-Hearing Association (pp. 2, 207). Rockville, MD: Author. Available at http:// www.asha.org/

American Speech-Language-Hearing Association. (2005). Association governance structure. Rockville, MD: Author. Available at http:// www.asha.org/

American Speech-Language-Hearing Association. (2005). The strategic plan. Rockville, MD: Author. Retrieved from http://www.asha.org/

American Speech-Language-Hearing Association. (2006). Highlights and trends: ASHA counts for 2005. Rockville, MD: Author. Available at http://www.asha.org/

Schill, M. J., & Dublinske, S. (2005, March 1). Charting the course ahead: ASHA's strategic plan outlines future direction of the association. *AHSA Leader, 3*, 27.

Stach, B. (1998). In the beginning—1987–1988. *Audiology Today,* 6–11.

Uffen, E. (2005, August 16). Moving forward: ASHA's national office—Where we've been, where we're going. *ASHA Leader,* 10–11.

Williams, P. S. (2001). Professional organizations. In R. Lubinski & C. Frattali (Eds.), *Professional issues in speech-language pathology and audiology* (p. 26). San Diego, CA: Singular.

RESOURCES

American Academy of Audiology
8300 Greensboro Drive, Suite 750
McLean, VA 22102
702-790-8466, 800-AAA-2336
Web site: http://www.audiology.org

American Speech-Language-Hearing Association
10801 Rockville Pike
Rockville, MD 20852
301-897-5700
Web site: http://www.asha.org

National Student Speech-Language-Hearing Association
10801 Rockville Pike
Rockville, MD 20852
301-471-0481
Web site: http://www.nsslha.org

National Association of Future Doctors of Audiology
Myers Hall, School of Medicine, University of Louisville
Louisville, KY 40292
502-852-5274
Web site: http://www.nafda.org

Related Professional Organizations

Academy of Dispensing Audiologists (ADA)
http://www.audiology.org

Academy of Federal Audiologists and Speech-Language
Pathologists (AFASLP)
http://www.militaryaudiology.org/afaslp/index.html

Academy of Neurologic Communication Disorders and
Sciences (ANCDS)
http://www.ancds.org

Academy of Rehabilitative Audiology (ARA)
http://www. audrehab.org

Acoustical Society of America (ASA)
http://www.asa.aip.org

Alexander Graham Bell Association for the Deaf
http://www.agbell.org

American Academy of Private Practice in Speech-
Language Pathology & Audiology (AAPPSPA)
http://www.aappspa.org

American Auditory Society (AAS)
http://www.amauditorysoc.org

American Cleft Palate-Craniofacial Association (ACPA)
http://www.acpa-cpf.org

American Society for Deaf Children (ASDC)
http://www.deafchildren.org

American Tinnitus Association (ATA)
http://www.ata.org

Better Hearing Institute (BHI)
http://www.betterhearing.org

Brain Injury Association of America
http://www.biausa.org

Canadian Association of Speech-Language Pathologists
and Audiologists (CASLPA)
http://www.caslpa.ca

Council for Exceptional Children (CEC)
http://www.cec.sped.org

Council of Academic Programs in Communication
Sciences & Disorders (CAPCSD)
http://www.capcsd.org

Educational Audiology Association (EAA)
http:// www.edaud.org

International Association of Augmentative and
Alternative Communication (ISAAC)
http://www.isaac-online.org

International Association of Logopedics and
Phoniatrics (IALP)
http://www.ialp.info/index2_noflash.html

International Association of Orofacial Myology (IAOM)
http://www.iaom.com

The International Dyslexia Association (IDA) (formerly
Orton Dyslexia Society)
http://www.interdys.org

International Society of Audiology (ISA)
http://www.isa-audiology.org

Linguistic Society of America (LSA)
http://www.lsadc.org

National Aphasia Association (NAA)
http://www.aphasia.org

National Black Association for Speech, Language and
Hearing (NBASLH)
http://www.nbaslh.org

National Institute on Deafness and Other Communication Disorders (NIDCD)
http://www.nidcd.nih.gov

National Rehabilitation Association (NRA)
http://www.nationalrehab.org

National Stuttering Association (NSA)
http://www.nsastutter.org

Self-Help for Hard of Hearing People, Inc. (SHHH)
http://www.shhh.org

Stuttering Foundation of America
http://www.stutteringhelp.org

4

Professional Ethics

THOMAS D. MILLER, PHD, JD

SCOPE OF CHAPTER

No professional issue for audiologists and speech-language pathologists transcends more employment settings, levels of experience, or nature of clientele than ethical practice. The number of our professionals who intentionally commit unethical practice is extremely low. Professionals do, however, make mistakes, develop bad habits, or allow the motivations or constraints of their employment to lead them from preferred practice models. New technologies and practices may also challenge clinicians to review their ethical guidelines.

This chapter defines the role of a professional and explains regulation of the professions of audiology and speech-language pathology by professional organizations such as ASHA and AAA. Ethical standards of conduct are discussed and examples of unethical practice are presented. The chapter also suggests ways by which practicing professionals may decrease the risk of unethical practice complaints while improving the quality of their service. Professional liability is discussed in Chapter 5.

ROLE OF A PROFESSIONAL

The word *profession* comes from the Latin "bound by an oath" (Baker, 1999). Professionals render services to society as distinguished by their superior knowledge, training, and/or skill and have a special obligation to those they serve. Thus, they earn the respect of society for services provided. To maintain that respect, professionals are responsible for conforming to stated or implied minimum standards of conduct imposed by their particular profession. These standards are presented in a Code of Ethics that is designed by the profession itself. The professional assumes ethical or moral responsibility for demonstration of the ability and competence of an ordinary member in good standing in the profession.

REGULATION OF THE PROFESSIONS

When society seeks to have input regarding the practice of a profession, one route is to license the profession through minimum standards, rules, and regulations established by legislators or appointed administrative bodies. Standards are also established through appointed administrative bodies and the courts.

In contrast, ethical principles and standards of conduct are established by members of a profession and are relative to given practices, procedures, and circumstances experienced by members of the profession. Although members of society benefit from professional ethics, they do not have direct input into the formation of those ethics. Ethical standards may be determined by professional organizations at the national, state, or regional levels; by accrediting agencies; or by employers. See the ASHA Code of Ethics and the AAA Code of Ethics in the Appendix to this chapter.

One advantage (or disadvantage) of both legal and ethical regulation of a profession is that two distinct tracks are maintained. Each track performs a separate and unique purpose and serves different professional needs. In some states, for example, it is legal to provide speech-language services in public schools with a bachelor's degree. Although legal, this violates the ASHA Code of Ethics, Principles of Ethics II, Rule A., which requires that "Individuals shall engage in the provision of clinical services only when they hold the appropriate Certificate of Clinical Competence or when they are in the certification process and are supervised by an individual who holds the appropriate Certificate of Clinical Competence" (ASHA Code of Ethics (2003). A professional may perform a task that is illegal but ethical or may be perfectly legal but unethical. Ordinarily, conflicts concern the possession of appropriate credentials. For example, an audiologist who is otherwise ethical in holding certification to practice may be practicing illegally if he or she does not have a valid state license or registration. Likewise, an SLP may be practicing legally by holding a valid license but may be unethical if he or she is bound by a code of ethics that requires clinical certification to practice. However, many standards overlap or interact.

Audiologists and speech-language pathologists often seek practice advice from codes of professional ethics and/or from boards or committees that interpret and administer such codes. Codes of ethics generally try to strike a balance between presentation of proscriptions that may protect a professional from legal liability and proscriptions that set the highest internal standards for the profession (Boylan, 2000).

ETHICAL STANDARDS OF CONDUCT

Ethics are standards of conduct that guide your behavior as a professional. They define acceptable versus unacceptable behaviors and promote high and consistent standards of practice. Ethics are not feelings, are not law, are not religious, and are not scientific. Ethical standards across professions generally derive from five philosophical concepts (Santa Clara University, 2005).

1. The utilitarian approach: Do the most good and the least harm.

2. The right approach: Protect and respect the moral rights of those affected.

3. The fairness or justice approach: Treat all humans equally or fairly based on some defensible standard.

4. The common good approach: Our actions should enhance the community as a whole.

5. The virtue approach: Maintain the highest values, including truth, compassion, integrity, fairness, and prudence.

When standards reflective of these philosphies are compiled into a list by a professional organization, they are known as a professional code of ethics, a code of values, or a code of conduct. Baker (1999) in his history of ethics states that the first code of ethics for physicians and surgeons was proposed by Thomas Percival in Manchester, England, in 1794, followed by an expanded document in 1803. The first national professional association to adopt a code of ethics was the American Medical Association in 1847. Literally, thousands of codes of ethics have been created by professions from accountants to zookeepers. Today's ethics codes derive from these early documents, define standards for minimally acceptable professional conduct, and provide for the following of sanctions that determine who is included in or excluded from a profession.

Codes of ethics generally have three components arranged in a top-down or general-to-specific framework: a prologue or preamble, principles, and rules or guidelines. The preamble, or the vision statement, describes why the code is important, for whom it is relevant, if it is mandatory, how it will be enforced, and which principles and rules are fundamental. Principles delineate the goals to be maintained. Principles generally emanate from the concepts of impartiality, full disclosure, confidentiality, due diligence, fidelity to professional responsibilities, and avoiding conflict of interest (Colero, 2005). The rules of conduct are the specific do's and don'ts of each principle (Ethics Resource Center, 2005).

Codes of ethics are intended to be living documents that undergo periodic review and change as professions change. Codes must also be written to have some flexibility to meet changes in federal and state laws, scopes of practice, and new developments within the professions. In general, you will find that codes of ethics are user-friendly and avoid legal jargon. Remember that these are not laws, but professional guidelines.

Speech-Language Pathology and Audiology Codes of Ethics

The establishment and maintenance of a code of ethics has been a major function of ASHA since its founding in 1925. The ASHA Code of Ethics, as provided for by Article III, §1C of the association bylaws, was first issued in 1930 as part of the bylaws and then as an independent document published in 1952. The code is binding for all members, certified nonmembers, applicants, and/or clinical fellows. It was last revised in January 2003. It can be found on the ASHA Web site, in the ASHA membership application booklet, and periodically in the *ASHA Leader* and other supplements. See the Appendix to this chapter for the latest ASHA and AAA Codes of Ethics.

The ASHA Code of Ethics is reviewed periodically by the Board of Ethics. This group of 12 members includes one public member and others across various occupational settings (clinicians, administrators, researchers, teachers, etc.). The Board analyzes current practice trends and violations to determine if changes in the Code of Ethics are merited. Revisions are then circulated for peer review, finalization, and then approval by the Legislative Council. Thus, there are numerous levels of feedback to the Board of Ethics when revisions are proposed.

Although the ASHA Code of Ethics provides standards relating to important ethical precepts, such as holding paramount the welfare of persons served professionally, maintaining confidentiality, and professional competence, it is important to note a paragraph in the Preamble that provides for ethical questions that may not be specifically covered by the Code:

> Any violation of the spirit and purpose of this Code shall be considered unethical. Failure to specify any particular responsibility or practice in this Code of Ethics shall not be construed as denial of the existence of such responsibilities or practices. (ASHA, 2003)

State and regional professional associations also often have their own codes of ethics that may reflect variations in preferred practice models unique to the state or region. ASHA's policy recognizes the autonomy of these bodies and renders to them the responsibility for determining when or if violations of their codes occur. Only the ASHA Board of Ethics can make a determination of violations of the ASHA Code of Ethics (ASHA, 2004c).

If audiologists or speech-language pathologists are members of another professional organization (e.g., the Academy of Dispensing Audiologists, the American Academy of Audiology, the American Psychological Association, the Council for Exceptional Children), they should be aware these groups also have their own codes of ethics to which they may be bound. The Code of Ethics of the American Academy of Audiology is given in the Appendix of this chapter. In addition, with the establishment of the Quadrilateral Mutual Recognition agreement between ASHA, the Canadian Association of Speech-Language Pathologists and Audiologists (CASLPA), the Royal College of Speech and Language Therapists (RCSLT) in the United Kingdom, and the Speech Pathology Association of Australia Limited (Boswell, 2004), it may be necessary to be familiar with these international codes of ethics. Once an audiologist or SLP signs the agreement to follow the ASHA Code of Ethics and holds a current Certificate of Clinical Competence, he or she must abide by the ASHA Code regardless of other certification held or the location of services provided. See the ASHA Web site for membership certification and international rules.

The Center for the Study of Ethics in the Professions (CSEP) has been collecting codes of ethics of professional societies, corporations, governments, and academic institutions for more than 20 years. Currently, the CSEP has more than 850 codes of ethics in its archives (CSEP, 2005).

UNETHICAL PRACTICE COMPLAINT PROCESS

If you suspect that someone has violated a code of ethics, what should you do? The discussion here applies to violation of the ASHA Code of Ethics only. First, you should read the Code carefully, doing what is termed a *fair reading* whereby the evidence appears to suggest an ethical violation. Remember that the ASHA Code of Ethics applies to members, certificate holders, Clinical Fellows, and applicants for membership or certification only. Prepare your complaint in writing. Include all relevant information, supporting documentation, and corroborating witness statements. Sign your name to the letter of complaint, though under some circumstances, anonymous complaints may be accepted (Denton, 2002). Submit to the Board of Ethics or the Director of Ethics. E-mail or faxed complaints are not accepted. The Board of Ethics will adjudicate the alleged violations. Article III of the ASHA Bylaws establishes the Board of Ethics "to interpret, administer, and enforce the Code of Ethics of the Association" (ASHA, 1998, p. 46).

When a complaint of unethical practice is received by the ASHA Board of Ethics, the complaint is reviewed for subject matter and personal jurisdiction. The alleged offender (respondent) is notified of the complaint and is given 45 days to respond. The Board investigates the complaint and, if further proceedings are deemed warranted, prepares an "Initial Determination," which includes its findings, proposed sanctions (if any), the proposed extent of disclosure of the findings, and notice to the parties to the complaint.

Following the Initial Determination, the respondent may request a "Further Consideration" hearing during which he or she may appear before the Board, present witnesses, and be represented by counsel. After the hearing, the Board issues its decision. The respondent may then appeal the decision in writing to the ASHA Executive Board. The Executive Board will issue a final decision.

The complaint process for AAA, while similar, varies in some ways. The Ethical Practice Board reviews the complaint and determines whether a Notification of Potential Ethics Concern is warranted. If warranted, the respondent receives notification and has 60 days to respond. The respondent may request a hearing before the Board. The Board may find that no violation existed or that a violation occurred. If a violation has occurred, the board determines appropriate sanctions. The respondent may appeal the finding to the AAA Board of Directors, whose decision is final.

Types of Complaints

Although the true nature of each complaint of unethical practice is, of necessity, kept confidential, common complaints have been found in the following categories:

- Practicing without appropriate certification
- Practicing beyond the scope of certification
- Providing supervision beyond the scope of certification
- Failure to refer
- Failure to file a report or filing a false report
- Advertising extremes (Miller, 1983; Miller & Lubinski, 1986)

Sanctions

Sanctions for unethical practice by ASHA may include a Cease and Desist Order, a Reprimand, Censure, and Withholding, Suspending or Revoking Membership and/or Certification (ASHA, 2004 a, c). AAA sanctions may include an Educative Letter, a Cease and Desist order, Reprimand, Mandatory Continuing Education, Probation of Suspension, Suspension, or Revocation of Membership (AAA, 2002).

Disclosure

If the final decision of the ASHA Board of Ethics is a Censure or the Withholding, Suspension, or Revocation of Membership and/or Certificate(s) of Competence, this information will be published in an ASHA publication that is distributed to its membership. When a Reprimand is given, only the following are notified of the decision: the respondent and counsel, the Complainant, witnesses, and various ASHA staff members. This decision is strictly confidential (ASHA, 2004c). See the AAA Web site for further information on disclosure of ethical complaint decisions by that professional body.

Appeals

Respondents may appeal their ethical decision if they can demonstrate that the ASHA Board of Ethics did not follow process or the decision was "arbitrary and capricious and without any evidentiary basis" (ASHA, 2004c). The appeal may then go before the Executive Board. Guidelines regarding the process and time lines for this appeals process are outlined in the Statement of Practices and Procedures of the Board of Ethics (ASHA, 2004c).

PREPARING FOR FUTURE ETHICAL PRACTICE CONCERNS

The dynamic professions of audiology and speech-language pathology present constant changes and challenges for members to provide the best possible service to their clientele. Individuals working in health-care settings continue to adapt to the transition from fee-for-service models to managed care. The scope of practice has expanded to the use of telepractice, multiskilling, and intraoperative monitoring. The development of new technologies in both speech-language pathology and audiology also create ethical challenges. Emphasis on treatment outcomes requires objective measures of the value of services rendered. The increased delegation of services to speech-language pathology assistants and volunteers provides new opportunities as well as increased ethical concerns and possibly liability for supervising clinicians. The challenge to do a better job with fewer resources is increasing. These factors would seem to present growing obstacles to the

Examples of Professional Ethics Questions

The following are actual questions received by the author from students and practitioners. The answers suggested are the author's and represent one inter- pretation of ethical practice. Sections of the ASHA and AAA Codes of Ethics are included to reference portions of the codes used to address the questions.

Q1. I am a speech-language pathologist and own a small but growing private practice. I have devel- oped an inexpensive electronic listening aid for use in therapy. I plan to market the instrument and sell it to some of my clientele and am won- dering if it would be ethical for me to do so.

A1. The ASHA Code of Ethics prohibits misrepresenta- tion and/or fraud in dispensing of products or services (ASHA, Principle III, Rule D). If the device in question is used as a component of a compre- hensive treatment program and is not the focus of the treatment program and if the program can still be implemented without purchase of the device, it has traditionally been acceptable.

Q2. As a certified audiologist serving a rural commu- nity, I was asked by a parent if I could treat some speech-sound production problems in her child in addition to the central auditory processing ther- apy already being provided. I have an undergrad- uate degree in communication disorders and agreed to the additional therapy but later won- dered if it was ethical.

A2. Both ASHA and AAA codes prohibit the provision of services that fall beyond the competence or experience of the professional or beyond the scope of practice of the credential held. ASHA Principle of Ethics II states that "Individuals shall honor their responsibility to achieve and main- tain the highest level of professional compe- tence." The profession has determined that this level of competence is attained only after satis- factory completion of all of the requirements for the Certificate of Clinical Competence (CCC). In this case, the treatment of speech-sound produc- tion disorders falls within the scope, training, and experience of one who holds the CCC in Speech- Language Pathology and should be provided by one who holds that credential. The audiologist must make every effort to refer the parent to an SLP for that service. (ASHA, Principle II, Rules A and B; AAA, Principle 2, Rule 2a; and ASHA, 2004a).

Q3. I am a certified speech-language pathologist working in a rural area. The nearest audiologist is a two-hour drive away. I have nine graduate credits and over 100 hours of supervised practicum in audiology. Would I be in trouble if I gave a few air/bone conduction threshold tests to my students?

A3. Once again, this clinician could not only be "in trouble" but, more importantly, could put the integrity of the profession and the welfare of his/her clientele in question. (ASHA Principle II, Rules A and B; see also ASHA, 1996).

Q4. My husband says he doesn't want me working with patients who are HIV positive or who have AIDS. Am I unethical if I refuse to work with these patients?

A4. Numerous legal standards, as well as the ASHA and AAA Codes of Ethics, prohibit discrimination on the basis of disability. However, if the welfare of this clinician's patients would be jeopardized by her lack of academic preparation or practicum or by her own personal biases, she might do well to refer her HIV/AIDS patients to a more compe- tent clinician (ASHA, Principle I, Rule C; AAA, Principle 1, Rule 1b).

Q5. My administrator has hired another speech- language pathologist to help with the growing dysphagia caseload. The new person has had no coursework or practicum in feeding and swallow- ing disorders but has been told by my administra- tor to "wing it" until funds are available to obtain training. She really needs the job. What should I do?

A5. This speech-language pathologist should discuss with the administrator the ethical principle that limits practice to the scope of an individual's competence. Requiring a professional to "wing it" not only places the patient with dysphagia in danger, but creates substantial exposure to legal liability of all involved in the event of an undesir- able outcome (ASHA, Principle II, Rule B).

Q6. My supervisor has asked me to sign Medicaid claim forms for work completed by fellow speech-language "teachers" who are not licensed to practice speech-language pathology as I am. I have no knowledge of the service that was pro- vided other than what is briefly described on the forms. Am I required to do this? Do I incur any liability for signing these forms?

A6. Principle III, Rule C of the ASHA code warns against misrepresentation of any services or products to obtain funding or reimbursement for services. Professionals incur substantial legal liability when they "sign off" for services they have not adequately supervised (ASHA, Principle III, Rule C; ASHA, 2005).

Q7. My school district has replaced some speech-language pathologists with speech-language pathology assistants. I have been assigned to supervise six of them and feel that I cannot provide adequate supervision for their work with our students. Does the Code of Ethics address this?

A7. The Code permits delegation of duties to support personnel only when a certificate holder can provide "appropriate supervision." In this case, it would be reasonable to argue that supervision of six speech-language pathology assistants would exceed "appropriate" levels of effective supervision (ASHA, Principle II, Rule D; ASHA, 2004b).

Q8. I spoke with a fellow audiologist who also has her CCC about an incident during which she was clearly engaged in unethical conduct. She became indignant and threatened me with a lawsuit if I reported her. Should I just forget about it?

A8. Both ASHA and AAA Codes require professionals to inform the respective Board of Ethics of perceived violations of the Code. ASHA, Principle IV, Rule I and J, and AAA, Principle 8, Rules 8c and 8d also obligate individuals to cooperate with the boards in the investigation and adjudication of complaints of unethical practice.

Q9. A professional colleague submitted a paper for publication that contained entire sections of text lifted from other works that were neither quoted nor cited. Although the university has a plagiarism policy, do I have any ethical responsibility beyond the university policy?

A9. The Codes prohibit misrepresentation of research results and professional dishonesty. (ASHA Principles III, Rule D, and IV, Rule D; AAA, Principle 6, Rules 6a and 6b, and Principle 7, Rule 7b).

Q10. My professor is years behind the current research in my course. Isn't that unethical?

A10. ASHA Principle II, Rule C, and AAA Principle 2, Rule 2f, recognize the need for continued professional development throughout one's career. This concern may initially be addressed through established student evaluation of faculty processes or in consultation with the department chair. See also Chial (1998).

Q11. A hearing aid company offers incentives for the sales of particular models of hearing aids. Is it unethical for me to participate in the promotion of these aids?

A11. Any activity that could constitute a conflict of interest jeopardizes the professional's primary duty to hold paramount the welfare of persons served (ASHA, Principle III, Rule B; AAA, Principle 4, Rule 4). See also: American Academy of Audiolgy Guidelines on Financial Incentives from Hearing Instrument Manufacturers.

Q12. I have some patients in my caseload who are really not benefiting from treatment. I need the clinical hours, so I'm not planning to dismiss them until the end of the semester. That's OK ethically, isn't it?

A12. The Code of Ethics supports the provision of professional services for clients only when benefit can reasonably be expected. Artificial time boundaries such as semesters, marking periods, or payment periods must not be used to determine the length of therapy programs (ASHA, Principle I, Rule G; AAA, Principle 1, Rule 1a).

provision of ethical and professional quality service. Former ASHA President Kay Butler (1996) pointed out, however, that the changes may not actually present future ethical dilemmas since the ethical standards of conduct are already in place. The challenge is to apply the existing ethics principles the professions have developed to our efforts to provide new and cost–effective service.

The application of current standards of conduct also applies to the changing roles of audiologists and speech-language pathologists working in school settings. The emphasis on least restrictive environment has resulted in more severely disabled students receiving services in schools. Increased use of paraprofessionals, inclusion models, and outcomes measurement can present new ethical questions regarding caseload, delegation of service, and supervision liability. The present ethical standards of conduct held by the professions may be durable enough to address the changing nature of service delivery models.

ETHICAL PRACTICE RISK MANAGEMENT

Risk management involves routine, careful, and detailed evaluation of every component of assessment and therapeutic procedures used to determine whether they conform to established standards of ethical conduct. Most unethical practice complaints can be avoided through continued awareness of the quality of service provided in light of conduct standards. The following examples show inexpensive ways of reducing the risk of professional liability complaints.

1. Make every effort to ensure effective oral and written communication with your clientele, their parents, or spouses. Explain, to the degree necessary, the rationale for the use of individual procedures and techniques. Describe the program of therapy in such a way that the client, parents, or spouse know where he or she is in the progression of treatment at any time.

2. Strive to obtain truly informed consent. Informed consent requires not only that consent be obtained from the client or his or her parent or spouse but that the consent be based on reasonable understanding of procedures to be used, rationale, and expected outcomes. This may require the use of an interpreter for those who are hearing impaired or who speak other languages. It may also involve using graphics or a video presentation to explain procedures.

3. Review periodically the ASHA and/or AAA Codes of Ethics. Keep current on amended codes of ethics. ASHA, AAA, and state and regional associations are excellent resources for obtaining updated information regarding practice standards and trends through their publications, committees, and conference presentations. Volunteer to serve on an ethical practices committee.

4. Encourage your local associations to have informal discussions on ethical practices or formal presentations by leaders within the professions. This is a good setting in which to discuss *Issues in Ethics* statements published by ASHA on a regular basis. Such discussions help professionals engage in self-guided, ethical decision making.

5. Learn how to develop your "emotional intelligence" so that you are more aware of stressors that may compromise your ethical practice. For example, pressure to meet quotas from your administrator would be better dealt with through discussion than unethical practice.

6. Establish an ethical practices discussion group in your workplace. This may help to identify issues that present ethical challenges before they become problematic. Sharing resources on ethical practices in this informal format may provide support and education.

7. When in doubt, ask yourself, "How does this action or practice affect the welfare of my client?"

WHAT TO DO IF YOU FACE AN ETHICAL DILEMMA

Most clinicians will experience ethical predicaments at some point in their careers. While careful consideration of one's own professional judgment may sometimes be adequate, the following suggestions also may be of help:

1. Consult the current codes of ethics that apply to you.

2. Check with the Boards of Ethics of your local, state, and/or national professional associations.

3. Talk with a trusted colleague, supervisor, or former professor who is knowledgeable and willing to give confidential advice.

4. Retain an attorney who is experienced in professional liability issues, malpractice, contracts, or labor law. Most local bar associations can help with referrals.

SUMMARY

This chapter defined ethics, codes of ethics, and the process of what to do if you or a colleague is faced with an ethical dilemma. Numerous examples of possible ethical dilemmas are given for review and further discussion. The ASHA and AAA Codes of Ethics are provided in the Appendix for your review. Remember that these are living documents that undergo periodic revision as the professions change and face new challenges.

People do not usually set out to be unethical in their conduct. They are most often good people who have developed bad habits or have made poor decisions or who are faced with unreasonable constraints in their employment settings. Fellow professionals must routinely and vigilantly honor both ethical and legal standards of conduct. Former ASHA President Nancy Swigert (1998) reminded Association members, "Failing to follow the Code of Ethics puts patients in jeopardy because they are not receiving appropriate services. It puts our colleagues in jeopardy because it reflects badly on everyone in the professions" (p. 11). If we maintain a working knowledge of the ethical codes to which we are bound, the professions can only benefit in a time of reimbursement constraints and aggressive service delivery restructuring. Nothing will upgrade the professions more.

CRITICAL THINKING

1. What would you do if you faced an ethical dilemma that was not covered in your professional code of ethics? What steps are appropriate for reporting an ethical violation?

2. Suppose you have made an "honest mistake." Is this a violation of the Code of Ethics? What should you do?

3. How do the expanding scopes of practice in SLP and audiology affect our Codes of Practice? How will you keep abreast of changes in ASHA and/or AAA Codes of Practice?

4. After reading the next chapter on legal issues and professional liability, contrast the similarities and differences between ethics and liability. Why do we need both?

5. Read through the ASHA and/or AAA Codes of Ethics. Which principles are reflective of the philosophical concepts (a) do the most good and the least harm, (b) protect and respect the moral rights of those affected, (c) treat all equally, (d) enhance the community as a whole, and (e) maintain the highest values of truth, compassion, fairness, and prudence?

REFERENCES

American Academy of Audiology. (2002). Code of Ethics. Available at http://www.audiology.org

American Academy of Audiogy. (2005). Ethical practice guidelines on financial incentives from hearing instrument manufacturers. Available at http://www.audiology.org

American Speech-Language-Hearing Association. (1996). Issues in ethics: Clinical practice by certificate holders in the profession in which they are not certified. *ASHA, 38* (Suppl. 16), 62–63.

American Speech-Language-Hearing Association. (1998). Statement of practices and procedures of the Board of Ethics. *ASHA, 40* (Suppl. 18), 46–49.

American Speech-Language-Hearing Association. (2002). Ethics in research and professional practice. *ASHA Supplement 22.*

American Speech-Language-Hearing Association. (2003). Code of Ethics (revised). *ASHA Supplement 23,* pp. 13–15.

American Speech-Language-Hearing Association. (2004a). Clinical practice by certificate holders in the profession in which they are not certified. *ASHA Supplement 24,* 39–40.

American Speech-Language-Hearing Association. (2004b). Guidelines for the training, use, and supervision of speech-language pathology assistants. Available at http://www.asha.org/

American Speech-Language-Hearing Association. (2004c). Statement of practices and procedures of the Board of Ethics. Available at http://www.asha.org/

American Speech-Language-Hearing Association. (2005). Medicaid guidance for school-based speech-language pathology services: Addressing the "under the direction of" rule. Available at http://www.asha.org/

Baker, R. (1999). Codes of ethics: Some history. *Perspectives on the professions.* Available at http://www.iit.edu

Boswell, S. (2004, October 19). International agreement brings mutual recognition of certification. *ASHA Leader,* p. 1, 22.

Boylan, M. (2000). *Basic ethics* (pp. 152–164). Upper Saddle River, NJ: Prentice Hall.

Butler, K. (1996). Managed care: Emerging issues in clinical ethics. *ASHA, 38,* 7.

Center for the Study of Ethics in the Professions. (2005). Code of ethics introduction. Available at http://www.ethics.iit.edu/

Chial, M. (1998, October). Ethics, preferred practices and the professoriate. *ASHA Issues in Higher Education Newsletter* (Special Interest Division 10), *2*(2), 3–7.

Colero, L. (2005). A framework for universal principles of ethics. Available at http://www.ethics.ubc/

Denton, D. (2002, May 28). How to file an ethics complaint. *ASHA Leader,* p. 9.

Ethics Resource Center. (2005). Code construction and content. Available at http://www.ethics./org/

Miller, T. (1983). *Professional liability in speech-language pathology and audiology: Unprofessional conduct and unethical practice.* Unpublished doctoral dissertation, State University of New York at Buffalo.

Miller, T., & Lubinski, R. (1986). Professional liability in speech-language pathology and audiology. *ASHA, 28*(6), 45–47.

Santa Clara University. (2005). A framework for thinking ethically. Available at www.scu.edu/ethics/ practicing/decision/framework.html/

Swigert, N. (1998). Taking ethics seriously. *ASHA, 40*(3), 11.

RESOURCES

American Academy of Audiology Ethical Practices
http://www.audiology.org

American Speech-Language-Hearing Association Board of Ethics http://www.asha.org

Center for the Study of Ethics in the Professions (CSEP)
Illinois Institute of Technology
HUB Mezzanine, Room 204
3241 S. Federal Street

Chicago, IL 60616-3793
Phone: 312-567-3017
E-mail: csep@iit.edu

Ethics Resource Center
1747 Pennsylvania Avenue, Suite 400
Washington, DC 20006
Telephone: 202-737-7258
E-mail: ethics@ethics.org

APPENDIX 4–A

ASHA Code of Ethics

LAST REVISED JANUARY 1, 2003

PREAMBLE

The preservation of the highest standards of integrity and ethical principles is vital to the responsible discharge of obligations by speech-language pathologists, audiologists, and speech, language, and hearing scientists. This Code of Ethics sets forth the fundamental principles and rules considered essential to this purpose.

Every individual who is (a) a member of the American Speech-Language-Hearing Association, whether certified or not, (b) a nonmember holding the Certificate of Clinical Competence from the Association, (c) an applicant for membership or certification, or (d) a Clinical Fellow seeking to fulfill standards for certification shall abide by this Code of Ethics.

Any violation of the spirit and purpose of this Code shall be considered unethical. Failure to specify any particular responsibility or practice in this Code of Ethics shall not be construed as denial of the existence of such responsibilities or practices.

The fundamentals of ethical conduct are described by Principles of Ethics and by Rules of Ethics as they relate to the conduct of research and scholarly activities and responsibility to persons served, the public, and speech-language pathologists, audiologists, and speech, language, and hearing scientists.

Principles of Ethics, aspirational and inspirational in nature, form the underlying moral basis for the Code of Ethics. Individuals shall observe these principles as affirmative obligations under all conditions of professional activity.

Rules of Ethics are specific statements of minimally acceptable professional conduct or of prohibitions and are applicable to all individuals.

PRINCIPLE OF ETHICS I

Individuals shall honor their responsibility to hold paramount the welfare of persons they serve professionally or participants in research and scholarly activities and shall treat animals involved in research in a humane manner.

Rules of Ethics

A. Individuals shall provide all services competently.

B. Individuals shall use every resource, including referral when appropriate, to ensure that high-quality service is provided.

C. Individuals shall not discriminate in the delivery of professional services or the conduct of research and scholarly activities on the basis of race or ethnicity, gender, age, religion, national origin, sexual orientation, or disability.

D. Individuals shall not misrepresent the credentials of assistants, technicians, or support personnel and shall inform those they serve professionally of the name and professional credentials of persons providing services.

SOURCE: American Speech-Language-Hearing Association. (2003). *Code of Ethics,* Available at http://www.asha.org/about/publications/reference-library/. Reprinted with permission.

E.   Individuals who hold the Certificates of Clinical Competence shall not delegate tasks that require the unique skills, knowledge, and judgment that are within the scope of their profession to assistants, technicians, support personnel, students, or any nonprofessionals over whom they have supervisory responsibility. An individual may delegate support services to assistants, technicians, support personnel, students, or any other persons only if those services are adequately supervised by an individual who holds the appropriate Certificate of Clinical Competence.

F.   Individuals shall fully inform the persons they serve of the nature and possible effects of services rendered and products dispensed, and they shall inform participants in research about the possible effects of their participation in research conducted.

G.   Individuals shall evaluate the effectiveness of services rendered and of products dispensed and shall provide services or dispense products only when benefit can reasonably be expected.

H.   Individuals shall not guarantee the results of any treatment or procedure, directly or by implication; however, they may make a reasonable statement of prognosis.

I.   Individuals shall not provide clinical services solely by correspondence.

J.   Individuals may practice by telecommunication (for example, telehealth/e-health), where not prohibited by law.

K.   Individuals shall adequately maintain and appropriately secure records of professional services rendered, research and scholarly activities conducted, and products dispensed and shall allow access to these records only when authorized or when required by law.

L.   Individuals shall not reveal, without authorization, any professional or personal information about identified persons served professionally or identified participants involved in research and scholarly activities unless required by law to do so, or unless doing so is necessary to protect the welfare of the person or of the community or otherwise required by law.

M.   Individuals shall not charge for services not rendered, nor shall they misrepresent services rendered, products dispensed, or research and scholarly activities conducted.

N.   Individuals shall use persons in research or as subjects of teaching demonstrations only with their informed consent.

O.   Individuals whose professional services are adversely affected by substance abuse or other health-related conditions shall seek professional assistance and, where appropriate, withdraw from the affected areas of practice.

PRINCIPLE OF ETHICS II

Individuals shall honor their responsibility to achieve and maintain the highest level of professional competence.

Rules of Ethics

A.   Individuals shall engage in the provision of clinical services only when they hold the appropriate Certificate of Clinical Competence or when they are in the certification process and are supervised by an individual who holds the appropriate Certificate of Clinical Competence.

B.   Individuals shall engage in only those aspects of the professions that are within the scope of their competence, considering their level of education, training, and experience.

C.   Individuals shall continue their professional development throughout their careers.

D.   Individuals shall delegate the provision of clinical services only to: (1) persons who hold the appropriate Certificate of Clinical Competence; (2) persons in the education or certification process who are appropriately supervised by an individual who holds the appropriate Certificate of Clinical Competence; or (3) assistants, technicians, or support personnel who are adequately supervised by an individual who holds the appropriate Certificate of Clinical Competence.

E. Individuals shall not require or permit their professional staff to provide services or conduct research activities that exceed the staff member's competence, level of education, training, and experience.

F. Individuals shall ensure that all equipment used in the provision of services or to conduct research and scholarly activities is in proper working order and is properly calibrated.

PRINCIPLE OF ETHICS III

Individuals shall honor their responsibility to the public by promoting public understanding of the professions, by supporting the development of services designed to fulfill the unmet needs of the public, and by providing accurate information in all communications involving any aspect of the professions, including dissemination of research findings and scholarly activities.

Rules of Ethics

A. Individuals shall not misrepresent their credentials, competence, education, training, experience, or scholarly or research contributions.

B. Individuals shall not participate in professional activities that constitute a conflict of interest.

C. Individuals shall refer those served professionally solely on the basis of the interest of those being referred and not on any personal financial interest.

D. Individuals shall not misrepresent diagnostic information, research, services rendered, or products dispensed; neither shall they engage in any scheme to defraud in connection with obtaining payment or reimbursement for such services or products.

E. Individuals' statements to the public shall provide accurate information about the nature and management of communication disorders, about the professions, about professional services, and about research and scholarly activities.

F. Individuals' statements to the public— advertising, announcing, and marketing their professional services, reporting research results, and promoting products—shall adhere to prevailing professional standards and shall not contain misrepresentations.

PRINCIPLE OF ETHICS IV

Individuals shall honor their responsibilities to the professions and their relationships with colleagues, students, and members of allied professions. Individuals shall uphold the dignity and autonomy of the professions, maintain harmonious interprofessional and intraprofessional relationships, and accept the professions' self-imposed standards.

Rules of Ethics

A. Individuals shall prohibit anyone under their supervision from engaging in any practice that violates the Code of Ethics.

B. Individuals shall not engage in dishonesty, fraud, deceit, misrepresentation, sexual harrassment, or any other form of conduct that adversely reflects on the professions or on the individual's fitness to serve persons professionally.

C. Individuals shall not engage in sexual activities with clients or students over whom they exercise professional authority.

D. Individuals shall assign credit only to those who have contributed to a publication, presentation, or product. Credit shall be assigned in proportion to the contribution and only with the contributor's consent.

E. Individuals shall reference the source when using other persons' ideas, research, presentations, or products in written, oral, or any other media presentation or summary.

F. Individuals' statements to colleagues about professional services, research results, and products shall adhere to prevailing professional standards and shall contain no misrepresentations.

G. Individuals shall not provide professional services without exercising independent professional judgment, regardless of referral source or prescription.

H. Individuals shall not discriminate in their relationships with colleagues, students, and members of allied professions on the basis of race or ethnicity, gender, age, religion, national origin, sexual orientation, or disability.

I. Individuals who have reason to believe that the Code of Ethics has been violated shall inform the Board of Ethics.

J. Individuals shall comply fully with the policies of the Board of Ethics in its consideration and adjudication of complaints of violations of the Code of Ethics.

APPENDIX 4–B

Code of Ethics of American Academy of Audiology

PREAMBLE

The Code of Ethics of the American Academy of Audiology specifies professional standards that allow for the proper discharge of audiologists responsibilities to those served, and that protect the integrity of the profession. The Code of Ethics consists of two parts. The first part, the Statement of Principles and Rules, presents precepts that members of the Academy agree to uphold. The second part, the Procedures, provides the process that enables enforcement of the Principles and Rules.

PART I. STATEMENT OF PRINCIPLES AND RULES

PRINCIPLE 1: Members shall provide professional services and conduct research with honesty and compassion, and shall respect the dignity, worth, and rights of those served.

    Rule 1a: Individuals shall not limit the delivery of professional services on any basis that is unjustifiable or irrelevant to the need for the potential benefit from such services.

    Rule 1b: Individuals shall not provide services except in a professional relationship, and shall not discriminate in the provision of services to individuals on the basis of sex, race, religion, national origin, sexual orientation, or general health.

PRINCIPLE 2: Members shall maintain high standards of professional competence in rendering services.

    Rule 2a: Members shall provide only those professional services for which they are qualified by education and experience.

Rule 2b: Individuals shall use available resources, including referrals to other specialists, and shall not accept benefits or items of personal value for receiving or making referrals.

Rule 2c: Individuals shall exercise all reasonable precautions to avoid injury to persons in the delivery of professional services or execution of research.

Rule 2d: Individuals shall provide appropriate supervision and assume full responsibility for services delegated to supportive personnel. Individuals shall not delegate any service requiring professional competence to unqualified persons.

Rule 2e: Individuals shall not permit personnel to engage in any practice that is a violation of the Code of Ethics.

Rule 2f: Individuals shall maintain professional competence, including participation in continuing education.

PRINCIPLE 3: Members shall maintain the confidentiality of the information and records of those receiving services or involved in research.

Rule 3a: Individuals shall not reveal to unauthorized persons any professional or personal information obtained from the person served professionally, unless required by law.

PRINCIPLE 4: Members shall provide only services and products that are in the best interest of those served.

Rule 4a: Individuals shall not exploit persons in the delivery of professional services.

Rule 4b: Individuals shall not charge for services not rendered.

Rule 4c: Individuals shall not participate in activities that constitute a conflict of professional interest.

Rule 4d: Individuals using investigational procedures with patients, or prospectively collecting research data, shall first obtain full informed consent from the patient or guardian.

PRINCIPLE 5: Members shall provide accurate information about the nature and management of communicative disorders and about the services and products offered.

Rule 5a: Individuals shall provide persons served with the information a reasonable person would want to know about the nature and possible effects of services rendered, or products provided or research being conducted.

Rule 5b: Individuals may make a statement of prognosis, but shall not guarantee results, mislead, or misinform persons served or studied.

Rule 5c: Individuals shall conduct and report product-related research only according to accepted standards of research practice.

Rule 5d: Individuals shall not carry out teaching or research activities in a manner that constitutes an invasion of privacy, or that fails to inform persons fully about the nature and possible effects of these activities, affording all persons informed free choice of participation.

Rule 5e: Individuals shall maintain documentation of professional services rendered.

PRINCIPLE 6: Members shall comply with the ethical standards of the Academy with regard to public statements or publication.

Rule 6a: Individuals shall not misrepresent their educational degrees, training, credentials, or competence. Only degrees earned from regionally accredited institutions in which training was obtained in audiology, or a directly related discipline, may be used in public statements concerning professional services.

Rule 6b: Individuals' public statements about professional services, products, or research results shall not contain representations or claims that are false, misleading, or deceptive.

PRINCIPLE 7: Members shall honor their responsibilities to the public and to professional colleagues.

Rule 7a: Individuals shall not use professional or commercial affiliations in any way that would limit services to or mislead patients or colleagues.

Rule 7b: Individuals shall inform colleagues and the public in a manner consistent with the highest professional standards about products and services they have developed or research they have conducted.

PRINCIPLE 8: Members shall uphold the dignity of the profession and freely accept the Academy's self-imposed standards.

Rule 8a: Individuals shall not violate these Principles and Rules, nor attempt to circumvent them.

Rule 8b: Individuals shall not engage in dishonesty or illegal conduct that adversely reflects on the profession.

Rule 8c: Individuals shall inform the Ethical Practice Board when there are reasons to believe that a member of the Academy may have violated the Code of Ethics.

Rule 8d: Individuals shall cooperate with the Ethical Practice Board in any matter related to the Code of Ethics.

PART II. PROCEDURES FOR THE MANAGEMENT OF ALLEGED VIOLATIONS

Introduction

Members of the American Academy of Audiology are obligated to uphold the Code of Ethics of the Academy in their personal conduct and in the performance of their professional duties. To this end it is the responsibility of each Academy member to inform the Ethical Practice Board of possible Ethics Code violations. The processing of alleged violations of the Code of Ethics will follow the procedures specified below in an expeditious manner to ensure that violations of ethical conduct by members of the Academy are halted in the shortest time possible.

Procedures

1. Suspected violations of the Code of Ethics shall be reported in letter format giving documentation sufficient to support the alleged violation. Letters must be addressed to:

   Chair, Ethical Practice Board
   c/o Executive Director
   American Academy of Audiology
   11730 Plaza America Dr.
   Reston, VA 20190

2. Following receipt of a report of a suspected violation, at the discretion of the Chair, the Ethical Practices Board will request a signed Wavier of Confidentiality from the complainant indicating that the complainant will allow the Ethical Practices Board to disclose his/her name should this become necessary during investigation of the allegation.

   a. The Board may, under special circumstances, act in the absence of a signed Waiver of Confidentiality. For example, in cases where the Ethical Practice Board has received information from a state licensure or registration board of a member having his or her license or registration suspended or revoked, then the Ethical Practice Board will proceed without a complainant.

b. The Chair may communicate with other individuals, agencies, and/or programs for additional information as may be required for Board review at any time during the deliberation.

3. The Ethical Practice Board will convene to review the merit of the alleged violation as it relates to the Code of Ethics

a. The Chair of the Ethical Practice Board shall remove identifying information from the complaint and forward it to the members of this Board.

b. The Ethical Practice Board shall meet to discuss the case, either in person or by teleconference. The meeting will occur within 60 days of receipt of the waiver of confidentiality, or of notification by the complainant of refusal to sign the waiver. In cases where another form of notification brings the complaint to the attention of the Ethical Practice Board, the Board will convene within 60 days of notification.

c. If the alleged violation has a high probability of being legally actionable, the case may be referred to the appropriate agency. The Ethical Practice Board may postpone member notification and further deliberation until the legal process has been completed.

4. If there is sufficient evidence that indicates a violation of the Code of Ethics has occurred, upon majority vote, the member will be forwarded a Notification of Potential Ethics Concern.

a. The circumstances of the alleged violation will be described.

b. The member will be informed of the specific Code of Ethics rule that may conflict with member behavior.

c. Supporting AAA documents that may serve to further educate the member

about the ethical implications will be included, as appropriate.

d. The member will be asked to respond fully to the allegation and submit all supporting evidence within 30 calendar days.

5. The Ethical Practice Board will meet either in person or by teleconference:

a. within 60 calendar days of receiving a response from the member to the Notification of Potential Ethics Concern to review the response and all information pertaining to the alleged violation, or

b. within sixty (60) calendar days of notification to member if no response is received from the member to review the information received from the complainant.

6. If the Ethical Practice Board determines that the evidence supports the allegation of an ethical violation, then the member will be provided written notice containing the following information:

a. The right to a hearing in person or by teleconference before the Ethical Practice Board;

b. The date, time, and place of the hearing;

c. The ethical violation being charged and the potential sanction;

d. The right to present a defense to the charges.

At this time the member should provide any additional relevant information. As this is the final opportunity for a member to provide new information, the member should carefully prepare all documentation.

7. Potential Rulings.

a. When the board determines there is insufficient evidence of an ethical violation, the parties to the complaint will be notified that the case will be closed.

b. If the evidence supports the allegation of a Code violation, the rules(s) of the Code violated will be cited and sanction(s) will be specified.

8. The Board shall sanction members based on the severity of the violation and history of prior ethical violations. A simple majority of voting members is required to institute a sanction unless otherwise noted. Sanctions may include one or more of the following:

   a. Educative Letter. This sanction alone is appropriate when:
      1. The ethics violation appears to have been inadvertent.
      2. The member's response to Notification of Potential Ethics Concern indicates a new awareness of the problem and the member resolves to refrain from future ethical violations.

   b. Cease and Desist Order. The member signs a consent agreement to immediately halt the practice(s) which were found to be in violation of the Code of Ethics.

   c. Reprimand. The member will be formally reprimanded for the violation of the Code of Ethics.

   d. Mandatory continuing education.
      1. The EPB will determine the type of education needed to reduce chances of recurrence of violations.
      2. The member will be responsible for submitting documentation of continuing education within the period of time designated by the Ethical Practice Board.
      3. All costs associated with compliance will be borne by the member.

   e. Probation or Suspension. The member signs a consent agreement in acknowledgement of the Ethical Practice Board decision and is allowed to retain membership benefits during a defined probationary period.
      1. The duration of probation and the terms for avoiding suspension will be determined by the Ethical Practice Board.
      2. Failure of the member to meet the terms for probation will result in the suspension of membership.

   f. Suspension of Membership.
      1. The duration of suspension will be determined by the Ethical Practice Board.
      2. The member may not receive membership benefits during the period of suspension.
      3. Members suspended are not entitled to a refund of dues or fees.

   g. Revocation of Membership. Revocation of membership is considered the maximum punishment for a violation of the Code of Ethics.
      1. Revocation requires a two-thirds majority of the voting members of the EPB.
      2. Individuals whose memberships are revoked are not entitled to a refund of dues or fees.
      3. One year following the date of membership revocation, the individual may reapply for, but is not guaranteed, membership through normal channels and must meet the membership qualifications in effect at the time of application.

9. The member may appeal the Final Finding and Decision of the Ethical Practice Board to the Academy Board of Directors. The route of Appeal is by letter format through the Ethical Practice Board to the Board of Directors of the Academy. Requests for Appeal must:

   a. be received by the Chair, Ethical Practice Board, within 30 days of the Ethical Practice Board's notification of the Final Finding and Decision,

   b. state the basis for the appeal, and the reason(s) that the Final Finding and Decision of the Ethical Practice Board should be changed,

   c. not offer new documentation.

   The EPB chair will communicate with the Executive Director of the Association to schedule the appeal at the earliest feasible Board of Directors' meeting.

The member may attend the portion of the Board of Directors meeting that addresses the appeal, but will be prohibited from providing new information. The deliberation must be on the facts presented to the EPB, as introduction of new evidence would compel the Board of Directors to act as the adjudicating body, rather than the appeals body.

The decision of the Board of Directors regarding the member's appeal shall be final.

10. In order to educate the membership, upon majority vote of the Ethical Practice Board, the circumstances and nature of cases shall be presented in Audiology Today and in the Professional Resource area of the AAA website. The member's identity will not be made public.

11. No Ethical Practice Board member shall give access to records, act or speak independently, or on behalf of the Ethical Practice Board, without the expressed permission of the members then active. No member may impose the sanction of the Ethical Practice Board, or interpret the findings of the Board in any manner which may place members of the Ethical Practice Board or Board of Directors, collectively or singly, at financial, professional, or personal risk.

12. The Ethical Practice Board Chair shall maintain a Book of Precedents that shall form the basis for future findings of the Board.

Confidentiality and Records

Confidentiality shall be maintained in all Ethical Practice Board discussion, correspondence, communication, deliberation, and records pertaining to members reviewed by the Ethical Practice Board.

1. Complaints and suspected violations are assigned a case number.

2. Identity of members involved in complaints and suspected violations and access to EPB files is restricted to the following:
   a. EPB Chair
   b. EPB member designated by EPB Chair when the chair recuses him or herself from a case.
   c. AAA Executive Director
   d. Agent/s of the AAA Executive Director
   e. Other/s, following majority vote of EPB

3. Original records shall be maintained at the Central Records Repository at the Academy office in a locked cabinet.
   a. One copy will be sent to the Ethical Practices Board chair or member designated by the Chair.
   b. Redacted copies will be sent to members.

4. Communications shall be sent to the members involved in complaints by the Academy office via certified or registered mail, after review by Legal Counsel.

5. When a case is closed,
   a. The chair will forward all documentation to the Academy Central Records Repository.
   b. Members shall destroy all material pertaining to the case.

6. Complete records generally shall be maintained at the Academy Central Records Repository for a period of 5 years.
   a. Records will be destroyed five years after a member receives a sanction less than suspension, or five years after the end of a suspension, or after membership is reinstated.
   b. Records of membership revocations for persons who have not returned to membership status will be maintained indefinitely.

5

Professional Liability

JENNIFER HORNER, PHD, JD

SCOPE OF CHAPTER

The health professions, including speech-language pathology and audiology, govern themselves with relative autonomy (Frattali, 2001). Autonomy entails responsibilities and, in turn, duties and liabilities. A *responsibility* is: "The state of being answerable for an obligation, and includes judgment, skill, ability and capacity. The obligation to answer for an act done, and to repair or otherwise make restitution for any injury it may have caused" (Black, Nolan, & Nolan-Haley, 1990, p. 1312 [hereinafter, Black's]). The corresponding legal terms are *duty and liability*. According to Keeton and colleagues, a *duty is* ". . . an obligation, to which the law will give recognition and effect, to conform to a particular standard of conduct toward another" (Keeton, Dobbs, Keeton, & Owen, 1984, in Dickson, 1995, p. 523). A *liability* is a broad legal term referring to "all character of debts and obligations" (Black's, 1990, p. 914).

The liabilities of speech-language pathologists and audiologists arise from the promises they have made to abide by standards of practice and codes of ethics of their parent professional organization(s), such as the American Speech-Language-Hearing Association (ASHA, 2001, 2002, 2003, 2004, 2005a), the American Academy of Audiology (AAA, 2005), and the Academy of Neurologic Communication Disorders and Sciences (ANCDS, 2005). They also make promises to society by accepting a license to practice in their respective states. Liabilities also stem from the various codes of law (statutes) governing society-at-large, the provision of, or reimbursement for, health care services, and civil rights and commerce.

Lapses in professional judgment, carelessness when applying diagnostic or treatment methods, and/or failure to obey applicable laws all come with a cost.

According to a Technical Report by ASHA (1994), a review of insurance liability claims between January 1982 and June 1993 found a total of 129 claims—58 percent against audiologists and 20 percent against speech-language pathologists. The most frequent type of claim (25) was for improper treatment procedures and the second most frequent (23) involved hearing aids. Other types of claims involved physical injuries, improper diagnoses, errors during intraoperative monitoring, property damages, and false claims. Although the number of claims on average was only about 12 per year, the total dollars paid by the insurer for these claims over the 10-year period was $1,865,000. To the author's knowledge, there are no recent published reports summarizing the frequency of professional misconduct allegations, professional malpractice complaints, settlements, or litigated lawsuits regarding speech-language pathologists or audiologists; but see Tanner's forthcoming article (in press).

If the conduct of speech-language pathologists or audiologists falls below the legal standard of care or violates any other applicable legal standard, they may be liable for *professional misconduct*. In contrast, conduct that violates professional codes of ethics renders professionals liable for *unethical practices* (Miller, 2001, p. 66). Importantly, the same conduct can lead to liability in both forums. As ASHA (2004) points out, "the final decision of any state, federal, regulatory, or judicial body may be considered sufficient evidence that the Code was violated" (p. 190). In turn, ASHA's Board of Ethics may send its final decision to "any state agency that licenses or credentials speech-language pathologists or audiologists" (p. 190). Although this chapter focuses on professional liability, readers should recognize that the same alleged wrongdoing may implicate both ethical and legal norms. See Chapter 4 on Ethics for more detail.

The purposes of this chapter are to identify the sources of law that apply to our learned professions, to outline the correspondence between patients' rights and professional duties, to explain the duties of speech-language pathologists and audiologists under state licensure laws, and to identify an array of federal statutes that apply to our professional practices.

Finally, the law of negligence will be explained as it applies to both individual practitioners and health care institutions.

SOURCES OF LAW

The main sources of law at both the federal and state levels of government are constitutions, statutes, common law (case law), and regulations promulgated by legislatively authorized administrative agencies.

United States Constitution

The United States Constitution was approved September 17, 1787. This vibrant document articulates the structure and duties of the federal government, the relationship between federal and state governments, and the limits of federal authority over the states and their citizens. Article VI of the United States Constitution states:

> This Constitution, and the Laws of the United States which shall be made in Pursuance thereof; and all Treaties made, or which shall be made, under the Authority of the United States, shall be the supreme Law of the Land; and the Judges in every state shall be bound thereby, any Thing in the Constitution or Laws of any State to the contrary notwithstanding.

This article contains the *supremacy clause,* which means that the United States Constitution and federal laws are superior to, and binding on, states and their citizens.

Among the amendments to the United States Constitution, the Fourteenth Amendment, ratified in 1868, is especially important because it limits the authority of the state governments to infringe the rights of citizens:

> Section 1. All persons born or naturalized in the United States and subject to the jurisdiction thereof, are citizens of the United States and of the State wherein they reside. No State shall make or enforce any law which shall abridge the privileges or immunities of citizens of the

United States; nor shall any State deprive any person of life, liberty, or property, without due process of law; nor deny to any person within its jurisdiction the equal protection of the laws.

As interpreted by the United States Supreme Court, *liberty,* or "liberty interests," conveys the right to make personal decisions, including medical decisions (*Cruzan v. Director, Missouri Department of Health,* 1990). The *due process* clause, among other things, implies the right to notice, an opportunity to be heard, and the opportunity to appeal decisions affecting life, liberty, or property (e.g., due process rights under the Individuals with Disabilities Education Act). The *equal protection* clause provides the basis for numerous civil rights laws, including the Americans with Disabilities Act of 1990 (assuring the right of disabled persons to access public accommodations, such as hospitals and clinics), and the Individuals with Disabilities Education Act, based on the landmark case of *Brown v. Board of Education* (1954), assuring the right of disabled children to participate in the least restrictive learning environment, inclusively with nondisabled children. (See United States Department of Justice, 2001.)

State Government

State governments have the authority to protect the health, safety, and welfare of citizens within their geographic boundaries (jurisdictions) by virtue of their general "police powers." State legislatures enact laws, which are then administered by the executive (Governor) and the executive branch administrative agencies (e.g., Department of Health, Department of Labor). State laws ultimately are enforced by state attorneys general, subsidiary law enforcement officials, and the courts. Laws of a general nature (e.g., laws against theft, fraud, and other crimes) and those regulating insurance, health care institutions, and providers all affect the practice of speech-language pathology and audiology.

Legal controversies are handled by executive administrative agencies and the courts. The judicial system is tiered, with multiple trial courts at the base, courts of appeal in the middle, and supreme courts at the top. On matters involving only state law, the supreme court of the state has final jurisdiction; however, if the matter in state court involves a question of federal law, the decision may be subject to review, but only by the United States Supreme Court (Meador, 1991).

Federal Government

A separate source of laws affecting speech-language pathologists and audiologists originates at the federal level of government. The constitutional authority of Congress to regulate interstate commerce and to impose federal law on the states through its "conditional spending power" (United States Constitution, Article I, Section 8) allows Congress to enact laws for the general welfare of citizens (e.g., civil rights laws, food and drug laws, labor laws). In addition, for any agency or institution receiving federal funds through statutory entitlement programs (whereby the federal government functions as a buyer of health care services), Congress may enable executive branch administrative agencies (e.g., the United States Department of Health and Human Services) to establish "conditions of participation" (COPs). COPs demand that health care providers comply with specific laws to protect public monies (e.g., the False Claims Act as applied to Medicare and Medicaid providers). The President of the United States oversees the executive branch of the federal government.

Federal legal issues and controversies are handled by the United States Attorney and the Department of Justice, subsidiary law enforcement officials, executive administrative agencies, and, of course, the federal courts. The judicial system in the federal government, as in the states, is tiered. There are 94 federal judicial districts, each with a federal district court (the trial court) supplemented by subordinate federal magistrate judges (Meador, 1991). In addition, there are 12 geographically defined federal judicial circuits, each with a United States Circuit Court of Appeals. The 13th federal circuit court is the United States Court of Appeals for the Federal Circuit whose jurisdiction is defined by subject matter (e.g., international trade, patent laws, and damage suits against the federal government). When a dispute involves the constitutional legitimacy of federal statutes or the application of federal law, the United States Supreme Court has discretion to step in as the final arbiter.

> The Supreme Court has jurisdiction to review all decisions of the federal appellate courts. It also has jurisdiction over decisions of the highest state courts when those courts have decided a question of federal law. The power to review cases from both state and federal courts gives the Supreme Court a unique position in the American judiciary's firmament. (Meador, 1991, p. 27)

In some areas, such as professional malpractice litigation, the federal government historically has left the governing law entirely in the hands of state legislatures and state courts. In other areas (e.g., some criminal laws), state law may coexist peacefully with federal law. Alternatively, when there is a conflict between state and federal laws, federal law may completely "preempt," or supersede, state law (e.g., the law pertaining to the administration of employee benefit plans). Or, when there is a conflict between state and federal laws, federal law will preempt state law *unless* coexisting state law is more stringent (Meador, 1991). For example, states may enforce medical privacy rules more stringently than federal laws in this area.

In summary, the term *federalism* refers to the "interrelationships among the states and [the] relationship between the states and the federal government" (Black's, 1990, p. 612). In the United States, the state and federal governments—each with executive, legislative, and judicial branches—exist side by side. As citizens of both the United States and the state in which they reside, speech-language pathologists and audiologists are held to the standards of both federal and state law; in turn, patients in the health care system are protected by both federal and state law. The law is expressed in state and federal constitutions, state and federal statutes (codes of law), state and federal executive branch administrative regulations, and finally, judicial cases (common law) that decide legal controversies of all types—statutory, regulatory, and constitutional. When legal disputes involve questions of federal law (federal statutes, federal regulations, or questions of due process or equal protection under the United States Constitution), the United States Supreme Court has discretion to review lower court cases, and the Court's decisions are binding on all jurisdictions.

Rights and Duties

One purpose of our legal system is to adjudicate disputes or controversies involving the obligations of health professionals relative to the rights of individuals they serve. To say persons have "rights" implies that they have "claims" on others to behave in certain ways. In the health care arena, patients' *legal rights* place particular *legal duties* (obligations) on health professionals. For example, in the United States there is no right to health care under the United States Constitution (with the exception of prisoners, persons institutionalized by the state, or men and women in active military service). Patients' ability to hold health professionals responsible for providing services and for maintaining a standard of care, therefore, must emanate from different sources. These sources include general laws (both federal and state), statutory health care entitlement programs, employee benefit plans, practitioners' contracts with health care institutions, and private contracts between practitioners and patients.

For example, if persons are eligible for health care under a statute (e.g., the Social Security Act), then health professionals agreeing to participate have duties to provide health care under the terms of that statute. When individuals enroll in health plans through their employers (an employee benefit plan), this requires contracts between the employer and hospitals, health maintenance organizations, and other health care entities and providers. Health professionals employed by, or contractually related to, those health care entities accept legal obligations consistent with this web of contracts. These contracts incur responsibilities for health professionals, not only to third party payers, but also to enrollees. Finally, when health professionals accept patients into their practices, they form special legal relationships. Inherent in these relationships is the patient's right to receive (and pay for) clinical services and, in turn, the health professional's duties under common law to provide the standard of care.

In summary, even though there is no general "right" to health care in the United States, most individuals will receive health care by virtue of statutory entitlements, employee benefit plans, and contracts established among health care institutions, patients, and professionals. Health professionals' obligations arise from their participation in these arrangements (Scheutzow, 2004).

As summarized in Table 5–1, patients enjoy numerous rights or privileges, each of which incurs a corresponding duty or obligation on the part of health professionals. The table gives examples of governing law.

T A B L E 5–1 Duties of Health Professionals Corresponding with Rights of Patients

Rights	Legal Duties	Governing Law (example)
Right to health care (prisoners, institutionalized persons, servicemen)	Duty to provide health care	Eighth Amendment, United States Constitution "cruel and unusual punishment"
Right to services, per statutory entitlements (e.g., Medicare, Medicaid)	Duty to provide health care per conditions of participation	Social Security Act, Titles XVIII and XIX
Right to receive treatment without discrimination	Duty to treat individuals without regard to age, race, religion, gender, sexual preference, or disability	Constitutional law (Fourteenth Amendment of United States Constitution); Civil Rights Act of 1871, Section 1983; Civil Rights Act of 1964; Rehabilitation Act of 1973, Section 504; Americans with Disabilities Act of 1990
Right, per statutory entitlement, to special education or related services to assure free and appropriate education	Duty to provide health care under the statute	Individuals with Disabilities Education Act (IDEA)
Right to emergency care and to be stabilized before discharge or transfer	Duty to provide care in an emergency department	Emergency Medical Treatment and Labor Act (EMTALA)
Right to employee benefit plan benefits	Duty to provide health care under the terms of the contract	Employee Retirement Income Security Act of 1974 (ERISA)
Right to complete an advance directive	Duty to offer opportunity to complete an advance directive and to explain consent/refusal rights under state law	Federal Patient Self-Determination Act 1990
Right to medical privacy	Duty to safeguard confidential information	Health Insurance Portability and Accountability Act of 1996 (HIPAA) and state laws
Right by contract to health care (e.g., with a private practitioner or an insurer)	Duty to provide health care under the terms of the contract	State law, breach of contract
Right to continuing care	Duty to provide care or transfer to a qualified professional	Common law of "abandonment"; see continuity of care rule, Council on Ethical and Judicial Affairs, AMA. Code of Medical Ethics 10.01(5)

T A B L E 5–1 (continued)

Rights	Legal Duties	Governing Law (example)
Right to privacy in personal decisions	Duty of noninterference by the government	Constitutional law (e.g., *Griswold v. Connecticut*, 1965; *Cruzan v. Director, Missouri Department of Health*, 1990)
Right to informed consent	Duty to disclose risks, benefits, and alternatives	Common law of informed consent (e.g., *Canterbury v. Spence*, 1972)
Right to refuse	Duty to respect competent refusal	Common law; right to be informed of risks of refusal (e.g., *Truman v. Thomas*, 1980)
Right to bodily integrity, self-determination	Duty to refrain from touching or threatening to touch without consent	Assault and battery for unauthorized surgery (e.g., *Schloendorff v. Society of New York Hospitals*, 1914)
Right to be free from restraints	Duty to use care in administering chemical or physical restraints	Social Security Act, Title XVIII and XIX
Right to receive a level of care that is reasonable, skilled, and prudent	Duty to provide the degree of care and skill expected of the average practitioner in the class to which he or she belongs, acting in the same or similar circumstances.	Common law negligence (e.g., *Helling v. Carey*, 1974)
Right to personal security	Duty to warn of serious, imminent threat to health or safety	*Tarasoff v. Regents of University of California* (1976)
Right to accurate and truthful medical records	Duty to report timely, accurate, truthful, and legible clinical records in the regular course of business.	Paul-Brown, 1994; Horner, 2003

Duties of Health Professionals under State Licensure Laws The criteria for licensing speech-language pathologists and audiologists are determined by each state in which the professional practices. According to ASHA's Technical Report on telepractices, the National Council of State Boards of Examiners in Speech-Language Pathology and Audiology urges clinicians to "be licensed in the state in which the consumer is receiving the service" (ASHA, 2005b, p. 6). In a 2003 issue of *Seminars in Speech and Language* devoted to ethical and legal issues, Denton (2003) cited barriers to interstate use of telepractice and wrote: "The bottom-line rule of thumb is that speech-language pathologists must be licensed in the state where their client is receiving services *and* in the state from which they are providing services" (p. 315).

Without the option of holding a federal practice license (which would require an interstate legal compact among the states), speech-language pathologists and audiologists must practice within the geographic boundaries of the state in which they have a license to practice. The South Carolina Code of Laws, Section Title 40, Chapter 67 provides an exemplar of a licensure law (sometimes referred to as a "practice act"). This licensure law explains that the Board of Examiners in Speech-Language Pathology and Audiology is under the administration of the Department of Labor, Licensing and Regulation. Like comparable licensure laws in other states, South Carolina requires applicants to hold a master's degrees in the appropriate discipline, along with the ASHA CCC or its equivalent (§40-67-220).

If applicants falsify information for the purpose of obtaining a license, they may be found guilty of a misdemeanor, entailing a fine and/or imprisonment (§40-67-200). The licensure law further explains that the term *audiologist* "means an individual who practices audiology" (§40-67-20(2)), and the term *speech-language pathologist* "means an individual who practices speech-language pathology" (§40-67-20(11)). In each case, the scope of practice is defined. For example, *audiology* or *audiology service* is defined as:

> . . . screening, identifying, assessing, diagnosing, habilitating, and rehabilitating individuals with peripheral and central auditory and vestibular disorders; preventing hearing loss; researching normal and disordered auditory and vestibular functions; administering and interpreting behavioral and physiological measures of the peripheral and central auditory and vestibular systems; selecting, fitting, programming, and dispensing all types of amplification and assistive listening devices including hearing aids, and providing training in their use; providing aural habilitation, rehabilitation, and counseling to hearing impaired individuals and their families; designing, implementing, and coordinating industrial and community hearing conservation programs; training and supervising individuals not licensed in accordance with this chapter who perform air conduction threshold testing in the industrial setting; designing and coordinating infant hearing screening and supervising individuals not licensed in accordance with this chapter who perform infant hearing screenings; performing speech or language screening, limited to a pass-fail determination; screening of other skills for the purpose of audiological evaluation; and identifying individuals with other communication disorders. (§40-67-20(3))

The scope of practice for speech-language pathologists involves:

> . . . screening, identifying, assessing, interpreting, diagnosing, rehabilitating, researching, and preventing disorders of speech, language, voice, oral-pharyngeal function, and cognitive/communication skills; developing and dispensing augmentative and alternative communication systems and providing training in their use; providing aural rehabilitation and counseling services to hearing impaired individuals and their families; enhancing speech-language proficiency and communication effectiveness; screening of hearing, limited to a pass-fail determination; screening of other skills for the purpose of speech-language evaluation; and identifying individuals with other communication disorders. (§40-67-20(12))

No person may practice the professions without a license (§40-67-30), and the license "is a personal right and not transferable . . . [it] is the property of the State . . ." (§40-67-240). The list of actions warranting disciplinary actions under §40-67-110 of the South Carolina licensure law are listed in Table 5–2.

If the practitioner violates the licensure law, the board may impose monetary fines, refuse to issue a license, or demand surrender of the license (§§40-1-110 to 40-1-150). The Board has jurisdiction over licensees and prior licensees (§40-67-115). A person aggrieved by a Board decision has a right to appeal the decision (§40-67-160).

Duties of Health Professionals to the Public under State and Federal Law Licensure law is one method by which the state protects the health, safety, and welfare of its citizens. Another method is to adjudicate malpractice litigation, guided by the common law of torts (see discussion that follows).

Numerous federal statutes also apply to speech-language pathologists and audiologists, summarized in Table 5–3. These include the Medicare and Medicaid statutes (the Social Security Act) and related statutes to prevent fraud and abuse: the False Claims Act and the Anti-Kickback Act. The False Claims Act entails severe penalties for improper billing, billing for services not rendered, and inadequate documentation. The Anti-Kickback Act prohibits both bribes and kickbacks when referring patients or accepting patient referrals or dispensing products. The Ethics in Patient Referrals Act of 1989 (known as "Stark I" and "Stark II") prohibits health professionals from referring patients to entities in which they have a financial interest. In addition, many providers are subject to the Health Insurance Portability and Accountability Act (HIPAA)'s Privacy Rule pertaining to medical information, and severe penalties attach to individual and institutional

T A B L E 5–2 Duties of Health Professionals under the South Carolina Practice Acts (Types of Actions Warranting Disciplinary Actions) (§40-67-110)

(1) Violates federal, state, or local laws relating to speech-language pathology or audiology;

(2) Violates a provision of this chapter or an order issued under this chapter or a regulation promulgated under this chapter;

(3) Fraudulently or deceptively attempts to use, obtain, alter, sell, or barter a license;

(4) Aids or abets a person who is not a licensed audiologist or speech-language pathologist in illegally engaging in the practice of audiology or speech-language pathology within this State;

(5) Participates in the fraudulent procurement or renewal of a license for himself or another person or allows another person to use his license;

(6) Commits fraud or deceit in the practice of speech-language pathology or audiology including, but not limited to:

    (a) Misrepresenting an educational degree, training, credentials, competence, or any other material fact;

    (b) Using or promoting or causing the use of any misleading, deceiving, improbable, or untruthful advertising matter, promotional literature, testimonial guarantee, warranty, label, brand, insignia, or any other representation;

    (c) Willfully making or filing a false report or record in the practice of audiology or speech-language pathology or in satisfying requirements of this chapter;

    (d) Submitting a false statement to collect a fee or obtaining a fee through fraud or misrepresentation;

(7) Commits an act of dishonest, immoral, or unprofessional conduct while engaging in the practice of speech-language pathology or audiology including, but not limited to:

    (a) Engaging in illegal, incompetent, or negligent practice of speech-language pathology or audiology;

    (b) Providing professional services while mentally incompetent or under the influence of alcohol or drugs;

    (c) Providing services or promoting the sale of devices, appliances, or products to a person who cannot reasonably be expected to benefit from the services, devices, appliances, or products;

    (d) Diagnosing or treating individuals for speech or hearing disorders by mail or telephone unless the individual had been previously examined by the licensee and the diagnosis or treatment is related to the examination;

(8) Is convicted of or pleads guilty or nolo contendere to a felony or crime involving moral turpitude or a violation of a federal, state, or local alcohol or drug law, whether or not an appeal or other proceeding is pending to have the conviction or plea set aside;

(9) Is disciplined by a licensing or disciplinary authority of another state, country, or nationally recognized professional organization or convicted of or disciplined by a court of any state or country for an act that would be grounds for disciplinary action under this section;

(10) Fails to obtain informed consent when performing an invasive procedure or fails to obtain informed written consent when engaging in an experimental procedure;

(11) Violates the code of ethics promulgated in regulation by the board.

---

providers who breach medical confidentiality (see Horner & Wheeler, 2005a, 2005b). While perhaps less familiar to some readers, federal antitrust laws prohibiting anticompetitive business practices are also very important.

The Law of Negligence

The tort of negligence as applied to health professionals is referred to as *malpractice*. This section defines these terms, explains the legal meaning of *standard of care*, and uses hypothetical clinical cases to illustrate how speech-language pathologists and audiologists can be held liable for failing to administer appropriate tests, administering tests in a substandard manner, failing to interpret the tests accurately, and/or failing to recommend or implement appropriate interventions.

Tort A *tort* is a "wrong" experienced by one individual by the actions of another individual

T A B L E 5–3 Duties of Health Professionals to the Public under State and Federal Laws*

Topic	Legal Duties	Source of law
Licensure of professionals	To adhere to the scope of practice and all governing regulations	State licensure statutes
Participation in public health care programs	To adhere to federal conditions of participation (COPS)	State and federal statutory entitlements (e.g., Social Security Act; Title XVIII, Medicare, and Title XIX, Medicaid)
Safeguarding medical privacy	To adhere to medical privacy and security rules of HIPAA	Health Insurance Portability and Accountability Act of 1996 (HIPAA)
False Claims	To submit truthful claims for reimbursement of Medicare or Medicaid services; illegal to submit a false claim with specific intent to defraud or to knowingly or deliberately ignore or recklessly disregard the truth or falsity of the claim	False Claims Act
Kickbacks	To refrain from giving or receiving money or any other thing of value to induce someone to refer a patient or to purchase a good or service that is reimbursable under Medicare or Medicaid.	Anti-Kickback Act
Self-referral	To refrain from referring patients to facilities in which the health professional has an ownership interest.	Ethics in Patient Referrals Act (Stark I and II)
Antitrust law (restraint of trade; anticompetitive practices)	To avoid restraining trade or engaging in anticompetitive practices, because a free market is competitive, reduces price, and increases choice and quality. Price fixing: Unlawful for competitors to agree on a price (fee schedule). Boycotting: Unlawful for competitors to boycott a third competitor. Monopoly: Unlawful for competitors to allocate services to particular geographic regions, thereby creating monopolies.	Sherman Act: Section 1: conspiracy; effect on interstate commerce; restraint of trade; Section 2: possession of monopoly power; willful acquisition or maintenance of that monopoly power Clayton Antitrust Act: prohibits mergers and acquisitions that may reduce The level of competition

*Enforced by the United States Department of Justice in cooperation with other executive agencies such as the Office of Civil Rights, the United States Department of Health and Human Services, and the Federal Trade Commission.

(Harris, 2003) whereby the latter person has acted unlawfully (malfeasance) or has failed to act (nonfeasance) when he or she had a legal duty to act. The legal duty arises from the nature of the relationship between the parties as defined by common law or statute. The obligations arising from the law of torts is separate and distinct from obligations arising between parties by voluntary contracts (mutual promises). The law of torts as applied to professional malpractice arises after the patient and professional relationship has been established. This is a "special relationship" in the eyes of the law, which triggers a legal *duty of care.*

The Tort of Negligence One category of the law of torts is negligence (Glannon, 1995). Black's Law Dictionary defines negligence as: ". . . failure to use such care as a reasonably prudent and careful person would use under similar circumstances" (Black's, 1990, p. 1032). Liability for negligence rests on the bedrock of the *duty of care*.

There are gradations in the types of negligence. *Ordinary negligence* refers to "failure to exercise care of an ordinarily prudent person in same situation" (Black's, 1990, p. 1034); *gross negligence* is "the intentional failure to perform a manifest duty in reckless disregard of the consequences as affecting the life or property of another" (Black's, 1990, p. 1033); and *per se negligence* is "the unexcused violation of a statute which is applicable" (Black's, 1990, p. 1034). Finally, *malpractice* is a subcategory of the law governing negligence and is defined as:

> Professional misconduct or unreasonable lack of skill . . . Failure of one rendering professional services to exercise that degree of skill and learning commonly applied under all the circumstances in the community by the average prudent reputable member of the profession with the result of injury, loss or damage to the recipient of those services or to those entitled to rely upon them. It is any professional misconduct, unreasonable lack of skill or fidelity in professional or fiduciary duties, evil practice, or illegal or immoral conduct" (Black's, 1990, p. 959).

PROFESSIONAL NEGLIGENCE (MALPRACTICE)

For speech-language pathologists and audiologists, the duty of care arises from the patient-professional relationship itself; it is the formation of this "special relationship" that creates a heightened legal duty of care (i.e., a duty of care above and beyond what ordinary citizens engaged in ordinary activities owe one another). The tort of negligence applies to health professionals when behavior is careless and substandard. In the typical case, negligence is *unintentional*. A health professional may be held liable for harming a patient if the duty of care is breached; an *intent* to harm is *not* required for liability to attach. Liability can attach regardless of whether the professional was poorly trained, unprepared, distracted, rushed, fatigued, or ill. When credentialed professionals hold themselves out to the public as "prepared to do the job," they can be held liable for negligence that causes harm.

In 1881, Chief Justice Oliver Wendell Holmes wrote:

> The rule that the law does, in general, determine liability by blameworthiness, is subject to the limitation that minute differences of character are not allowed for. The law considers, in other words, what would be blameworthy in the average man, the man of ordinary intelligence and prudence, and determines liability by that. If we fall below the level in those gifts, it is our misfortune; so much as that we must have at our peril, for the reasons just given. But he who is intelligent and prudent does not act at his peril, in theory of law. On the contrary, it is only when he fails to exercise the foresight of which he is capable, or exercises it with evil intent, that he is answerable for the consequences. (pp. 108–109)

By way of background, consider an example of everyday behavior. The general rule is that ordinary citizens have a duty to act reasonably, particularly when harm is foreseeable. Their behavior is governed by the common law of (ordinary) negligence. If a neighbor plays softball in a backyard with no fence, and a pedestrian on the sidewalk is harmed by a fly ball, the neighbor will probably be liable to the pedestrian to pay him restitution for the injury. The reason for this is that the neighbor has a common law duty to act in a reasonable manner (to build a fence or to refrain from playing baseball in his backyard) in order to avoid foreseeable injuries to his neighbors. When such a case is heard by a jury, the jury must decide whether a "reasonable person," using an average degree of judgment and foresight, would have played softball in a fenceless yard adjacent to a busy sidewalk, or would have taken reasonable and prudent measures to prevent the risk of probable injury to pedestrians.

Health professionals are held to a higher duty of care than ordinary citizens. This higher duty stems from the fact that health professionals have specialized education, hold licenses to practice, and hold out their credentials to the public as skilled and qualified service providers. Health professionals are ethically and legally bound to exercise the level of care that similarly educated and skilled practitioners would provide in similar circumstances while exercising good judgment and acting prudently. Usually, the standard of care is established by the profession itself (and presented at a trial by an expert witness), but ultimately the jury, which decides the facts and the credibility of witnesses, and the judge, who applies the legal standards, will determine whether the *customary* clinical standard of care is adequate to satisfy the *legal* standard of care.

Two cases illustrate that the court has ultimate discretion in appraising whether the prevailing or customary standard of care is adequate as a matter of law (i.e., satisfies a *legal standard of care*). In 1932, Judge Learned Hand of the Second Circuit Court of Appeals opined that the captain of a tugboat named *The T.J. Hooper* was negligent by failing to equip his boat with a radio and thereby causing damage. Judge Hand wrote: "Courts must in the end say what is required; there are precautions so imperative that even their universal disregard will not excuse their omission" (*The T.J. Hooper,* 1932). In a controversial 1974 case, *Helling v. Carey,* the court (citing *The T.J. Hooper*) held an ophthalmologist liable for failing to diagnose a young woman's glaucoma, despite her persistent complaints of deteriorating vision over nine years. At the time, it was not common practice for ophthalmologists to test for glaucoma in individuals younger than age 40. Nevertheless, the court held that reasonable prudence was absent and that customary practice was insufficient as a matter of law.

Duty, Breach, Causation, and Damages

The common law of negligence as applied to health professionals engaged in their professional duties is known as the tort of malpractice. To hold the professional liable, the plaintiff (the person alleging harm who has brought the lawsuit) must prove four elements. With sufficient evidence, the professional will be held liable for the patient's injuries and be required to pay the patient money in damages.

> Duty: The duty required of the professional is the standard of care—the obligation shared by all similarly educated and skilled practitioners in similar circumstances exercising good judgment and prudence.
>
> Breach: The duty was breached (e.g., the practitioner failed to administer an intervention that was indicated or administered a customary intervention in a substandard manner).
>
> Damages: The patient experienced harm (e.g., misdiagnosis, physical injury, comorbidity).
>
> Causation: The harm experienced by the patient (plaintiff) was caused by the breach of the legal duty of care.

The element of causation is the most difficult for plaintiffs to prove. According to Glannon (1995), different jurisdictions embrace different methods of proving causation. For example, to attach liability, the defendant's conduct must be the *direct cause* of the injury, a *substantial factor* in causing the plaintiff's injury, the *natural and probable consequences* of the defendant's conduct, or a *foreseeable consequence of the defendant's conduct.* In the final analysis, to attach liability to the defendant, the jury must determine that conduct was the *proximate* cause of the injury—in essence, "but for" the defendant's conduct, the plaintiff would not have been harmed.

> Proximate cause means that cause which, in a natural and continuous sequence, unbroken by an effective intervening cause, produces an event, and without which cause such event would not have occurred (Glannon, 1995, p. 157).

Speech-Language Pathology. Imagine a middle-aged individual who experienced bilateral strokes and now presents a swallowing disorder. A speech-language pathologist, experienced and trained in the use of instrumental procedures, follows the established protocol for pharyngeal examination of swallowing function and consults with specialists in neurology, gastroenterology, and radiology. Following the examination, the speech-language pathologist recommends a non-oral nutritional method. The attending physician places the patient on NPO status (nothing by mouth) and orders insertion of a nasogastric tube. One week later, the patient experiences pneumonia with significant discomfort, a protracted hospital stay, and thousands of additional dollars in medical expenses. The family sues the speech-language pathologist (and all other attending health professionals).

In this hypothetical case, the plaintiff's lawyer will argue, "My client had dysphagia, the speech-language pathologist evaluated him, and her recommendations caused him to get pneumonia." To escape liability, the speech-language pathologist as a defendant will, first and foremost, try to prove to the court that she adhered to the standard of care. The court might, or might not, allow ASHA practice guidelines to be introduced into evidence, but probably will allow an expert witness, another speech-language pathologist with credentials in swallowing disorders, to testify as to the appropriate clinical standard of care. The defendant's lawyer will argue that the patient's underlying bilateral cerebral disease was the superseding (and legal) cause of the patient's injuries. In the end, the defendant speech-language pathologist will prevail if she adhered to the legal standard of care for this straightforward reason: The plaintiff's failure to prove breach of a legal duty precludes the possibility of proving a causal link between the defendant's conduct and the patient's medical condition. In other words, if no breach of a legal duty is found, the jury cannot by law conclude that a breach caused the harm.

Now imagine a slightly different scenario. The underlying facts are the same, *except* that the speech-language pathologist did not read the medical record thoroughly and missed the fact that the patient had a history of gastroesophageal reflux disease (GERD). Furthermore, the record shows that she did not consult with neurology or gastroenterology, nor did she advise the attending physician to place the patient on reflux precautions. When these facts come to light, the plaintiff's lawyer will

be in a stronger position to argue that "but for" the defendant's conduct (actions or inactions), the patient would have avoided the pneumonia and the protracted hospital stay.

Audiology. A young adult presents to an audiology clinic with progressive hearing loss. The audiologist's evaluation included an otoscopic examination, a pure-tone audiometric evaluation, and auditory brainstem evoked response (ABER) testing. The audiologist diagnosed a conductive hearing loss and referred the patient to an otolaryngologist for cerumen removal. Two years later, the audiologist is summoned to civil court by her former patient. Her patient alleges that he has been irreparably harmed by the audiologist's failure to diagnose his retrocochlear lesion (an acoustic neuroma). The patient has undergone surgery and now has a permanent hearing loss in one ear, in addition to paralysis of facial muscles on the same side. In this hypothetical case, the plaintiff's lawyer will argue, "my client had a progressive hearing loss, the audiologist evaluated him, and, her diagnosis was wrong. As a result of the delayed diagnosis, my patient has undergone surgery and suffers permanent hearing loss and facial disfigurement."

The audiologist (defendant) will, first and foremost, try to prove to the court that she adhered to the standard of care (i.e., recorded a thorough history, administered the appropriate diagnostic tests, and rendered an accurate diagnosis consistent with what a reasonable and prudent clinician in her circumstances would have provided). The court might, or might not allow ASHA or other practice guidelines and technical reports into evidence, but will probably allow an expert—another audiologist with credentials in differential diagnosis of hearing disorders—to testify as to the appropriate clinical standard of care. The plaintiff's lawyer will try to prove that the patient's hearing loss was only partly explained by cerumen and that the audiologist failed to interpret the ABER accurately. In the end, the plaintiff will win his civil malpractice lawsuit if the plaintiff convinces a jury that "but for" the audiologist's failure to correctly interpret the ABER, he would have received a timely diagnosis.

Now imagine a slightly different scenario. The underlying facts are the same, except that the audiologist performed *and interpreted* the audiometric tests appropriately and found no abnormality. Consistent with the audiologic evaluation, she referred the patient to an otolaryngologist, the cerumen was removed, and the patient experienced an improvement in hearing acuity. Nevertheless, at a later point in time, the patient experienced a decline in his hearing, and an acoustic neuroma was diagnosed. The plaintiff's lawyer will once again argue that the audiologist failed to diagnose the retrocochlear lesion. The defendant's lawyer will attempt to prove that the audiologist's evaluation was consistent with the prevailing standard of care and that the acoustic neuroma manifest itself after the evaluation. If the jury agrees, it will find that the acoustic neuroma was the superseding (and legal) cause of the patient's subsequent hearing loss, not substandard care. In the end, the defendant audiologist will prevail if she proves she adhered to the standard of care and there was no evidence of a retrocochlear lesion at the time of the evaluation.

Again, the first two elements of a malpractice lawsuit are: duty and breach. In a court of law, the duty of care must be established, typically by expert testimony, and then a breach of this duty of care must be proved (again, by expert testimony). If there is no breach of a legal duty of care, then any harm the patient experienced cannot be causally linked to the malfeasance (or nonfeasance) of the defendant clinician. In the absence of a breach of a legal duty, the patient has no remedy in a civil malpractice lawsuit. On the other hand, if the professional failed to administer the appropriate tests, administered the tests in a substandard manner, failed to interpret the tests accurately, and/or failed to recommend or implement appropriate interventions—*and the breach is causally linked to the patient's harm*—the professional will be held civilly liable to the patient and will be expected to compensate the patient by paying monetary damages.

In summary, this section has contrasted professional negligence (malpractice) in the conduct of clinical care with negligence in everyday affairs to illustrate that professionals have a heightened legal duty to conduct their clinical practices competently and prudently, commensurate with the knowledge and skills they portray to the public. This section identified duty, breach, causation, and damages as the four elements that must be proved in a court of law to sustain a finding of liability for substandard care. Issues relating to malpractice in the 21st century are complex, contentious, and beyond the scope of this chapter. Readers are referred to Studdert, Mello, and Brennan (2004) who discuss the prevalence of adverse events and negligence, the rise in health care costs, patient safety issues, and tort reform. These weighty policy issues aside, the best defense to any allegation of malpractice is diligent adherence to the standard of care.

Liability of Health Care Institutions

When health professionals incur legal liabilities, their supervisors or employers are also subject to legal liabilities. Misconduct by health professionals, whether intentional or not, may give rise to "vicarious liability" of health care institutions because (1) they are "agents" of the institutions; (2) they are selected, credentialed, supervised, and/or controlled by the institutions; and/or (3) they are acting within the scope of their employment on behalf of the institutions.

A fourth theory of corporate liability involves the idea that there are some duties an institution cannot delegate ("nondelegable duties"). These include, for example: providing adequate facilities and equipment; having sound hiring, credentialing, and retention practices; and maintaining safety standards. According to Glannon (1995), the institution "may delegate the *work* but cannot delegate away the *liability* for tortuous acts in the course of the work" (p. 380). The different legal theories of liability are identified in Table 5–4. Readers should note that the application of these theories of legal liability vary not only in relation to the facts of particular cases, but also depending on the statutes or case law in the governing jurisdiction (Furrow, Greany, Johnson, Jost, & Schwartz, 1997; Glannon, 1995; Harris, 2003).

T A B L E 5–4 Theories of Vicarious Liability and Direct Corporate Liability

Theory of Liability	Description
Captain of the Ship	An individual who exercises supervisory control and authority over health professionals may be liable for their misconduct.
Apparent Agency (Ostensible Agency)	A modern-day application of the Captain of the Ship doctrine, whereby a health care entity (the principal) may be held liable for the misconduct of health professionals (agents) who act on its behalf; a professional may be deemed "ostensibly" an agent of the health care entity even if not employed by the entity.
Respondeat Superior (Latin, "let the master respond")	When health professionals perform functions that are inherent to the operation of the health care entity, and the misconduct occurred within the scope of their employment, the entity may be held liable for their misconduct.
Direct corporate liability	The health care entity has legal duties independent of its employees, such as providing adequate facilities and equipment; having sound hiring, credentialing and retention practices; and maintaining safety standards. These are nondelegable duties for which the entity can be held directly liable.
Negligence per se	A health care entity may be per se liable for harm resulting from its failure to adhere to a statute or regulation or for negligent implementation of the statute or regulation.
Strict liability (products liability)	Some jurisdictions have held that service providers (individual practitioners or institutions) who regularly sell or dispense products may be held liable (along with manufacturers) for harm that results from defective products.

MANAGING RISK

The key to preparing for the possibility of a malpractice lawsuit is *prevention*. ASHA's 1994 Technical Report on risk management provides a useful, comprehensive summary of strategies that audiologists, speech-language pathologists, and their employers can employ. The strategies fall into three overlapping categories of activities: quality improvement, risk management, and insurance.

Professionals manage risks (and prevent errors) by embracing scope of practice and practice guidelines promulgated by ASHA and other authoritative professional organizations, by engaging in continuing education, and by establishing quality improvement projects for high-risk, high-volume, and problem-prone types of cases.

Quality improvement concentrates on maintaining optimal levels of client care; risk management focuses on meeting acceptable levels of care from a legal perspective. (ASHA, 1994, p. 243)

Finally, professionals should be sure they have adequate insurance. In many instances, state law will place caps on the tort liability exposure of duly licensed practitioners in the state. Typically, employers will provide insurance for the health care providers who are sued for mistakes that occur during the course of employment. In addition, professionals may purchase professional liability insurance either from their employer, through ASHA, or from independent insurance companies (ASHA, 1994, p. 244).

SUMMARY

This chapter explained that the United States Constitution and laws written by both state legislatures and Congress have a major role in defining the professional liabilities of speech-language pathologists and audiologists. The chapter identified numerous sources for professionals' legal obligations—to individual patients, to the state in which a license to practice is held, to public agencies that purchase health care services, and to the public at large. The chapter also outlined the law of negligence as applied to the professional arena (malpractice), and explained how health care institutions can also be held vicariously liable for the misconduct of their employees or can be held directly liable for failures to maintain requisite institutional standards of practice.

Although speech-language pathologists and audiologists have a daunting array of obligations, the bases of their legal liabilities lie ultimately in their moral responsibilities to their patients. This closing observation by Pellegrino (1983) emphasizes why speech-language pathologists and audiologists should be held accountable for the promises they made when they entered the professions.

> To be a professional is to make a promise to help, to keep that promise, and to do so in the best interests of the patient. It is to accept the trust the patient must place in us as a moral imperative . . .

> The nature of the relationships we have described are grounded in the human condition. They impose moral obligations that must transcend standards of moral behavior in society at large. A true professional is, in sum, an ordinary person called to extraordinary duties by the nature of the activities in which he or she has chosen to engage. (pp. 174–175)

CRITICAL THINKING

1. If a patient entered a speech-language pathology or audiology clinic and declared on the intake form that she was HIV+, would the clinician be permitted, under the law, to refuse to treat this individual? If yes, why? If not, why not?

2. If a child in the public school system was designated as needing speech-language pathology or audiology services, what issues would a clinician need to consider before deciding to treat the child on a one-to-one basis (rather than treating the child while engaged in classroom activities)?

3. If an employer demanded that the speech-language pathologist or audiologist change a billing code to maximize reimbursement, what law(s) would be implicated?

4. If a speech-language pathologist or audiologist had an ownership interest in a clinic, would it be appropriate to refer patients to his or her own clinic? If yes, why? If not, why not?

5. If a speech-language pathologist or audiologist was sued for professional malpractice due to allegedly providing substandard care to a patient (causing harm to the patient), what would be the clinician's best legal defense?

6. If a speech-language pathologist or audiologist was found by the American Speech-Language-Hearing Association's Board of Ethics to violate a provision of ASHA's Code of Ethics (2003), could the clinician avoid repercussions simply by changing employment or moving to another state? If yes, why? If not, why not?

7. If a speech-language pathologist or audiologist wishes to engage in telepractice diagnosis or treatment, may the clinician rely on his/her license to practice in his/her home state, or will she/he be required to seek licensure in other states?

8. Even though various health professionals strive to establish their own standards of care through

technical reports and practice guidelines, and even though the disciplines of speech-language pathology and audiology consider themselves to be relatively autonomous, should the professions be concerned about the legal standard of care? How does the law define *standard of care?*

REFERENCES

Academy of Neurologic Communication Sciences and Disorders. (2005). Mission statement of the ANCDS. Available at http://www.ancds.org

American Academy of Audiology. (2005). Code of Ethics of the American Academy of Audiology. Available at http://www.audiology.org/

American Speech-Language-Hearing Association. (1994, March). Professional liability and risk management for the audiology and speech-language pathology professions. *Asha,* 36 (Suppl. 12), 25–38.

American Speech-Language-Hearing Association. (2001, Spring). Practices and procedures for appeals of Board of Ethics decisions (p. 193). *ASHA Supplement.* Available at http://www.asha.org/

American Speech-Language-Hearing Association. (2002). Ethical practice inquiries: ASHA jurisdictions. *ASHA Supplement, 22,* 231–232.

American Speech-Language-Hearing Association. (2003). Code of Ethics. *ASHA Supplement, 23,* 13–15. Available at http://www.asha.org/

American Speech-Language-Hearing Association. (2004). Statement of practices and procedures of the Board of Ethics (pp. 189–192). Available at http://www.asha.org/

American Speech-Language-Hearing Association. (2005a). Background information and standards and implementation for the Certificate of Clinical Competence in Speech-Language Pathology. Available at http://www.asha.org/

American Speech-Language-Hearing Association. (2005b). Speech-language pathologists providing clinical services via telepractice: Technical report. *ASHA Supplement, 25,* in press. Available at http://www.asha.org/

Americans with Disabilities Act of 1990, 42 U.S.C. §§12101 et seq.

Anti-Kickback Act, 42 U.S.C. §1320a-7b(b)(1)-(2).

Black H. C., Nolan, J. R., & Nolan-Haley, J. M. (1990). *Black's law dictionary.* St. Paul, MN.: West Publishing.

Brown v. Board of Education, 347 U.S. 483 (1954).

Canterbury v. Spence, 464 F. 2d 772 (D.C. Cir., 1972).

Civil Rights Act of 1871 42 U.S.C. §1983.

Civil Rights Act of 1964, 42 U.S.C. §§2000 et seq.

Clayton Antitrust Act. (1914). 15 U.S.C. §§12-27, 52-53, Available at http://www.usdoj.gov/atr/foia/divisionmanual/ch2.htm

Council on Ethical and Judicial Affairs. (2002). *Code of medical ethics: Current opinions.* Chicago: American Medical Association.

Cruzan v. Director, Missouri Department of Health, 497 U.S. 261 (1990).

Denton, D. R. (2003, November). Ethical and legal issues related to telepractice. *Seminars in Speech and Language,* 24(4), 313–322.

Dickson, D. T. (1995). *Law in the health and human services: A guide for social workers, psychologists, psychiatrists, and related professionals.* New York: The Free Press.

Emergency Medical Treatment and Labor Act (EMTALA), 42 U.S.C. §1395dd.

Employee Retirement Income Security Act of 1974 (ERISA), 29 U.S.C. §§1001 et seq. Information available at U.S. Department of Labor: http://www.dol.gov/dol/topic/health-plans/erisa.htm

Ethics in Patient Referrals Act of 1989 (Stark I and II), 42 USC §1395nn.

False Claims Act, 31 U.S.C. §§3729 et seq.

Federal Patient Self-Determination Act 1990, 42 U.S.C. §1395 cc(a).

Federal Trade Commission. Available at http://www.ftc.gov/ogc/stat3.htm

Frattali, C. M. (2001). Professional autonomy and collaboration. In R. Lubinski & C. M. Frattali (eds.), *Professional issues in speech-language pathology and audiology* (2nd ed., pp. 173–182). San Diego, CA: Singular, Delmar.

Furrow, B. R., Greaney, T. L., Johnson, S. H., Jost, T. S., & Schwartz, R. L. (1997). *Health law: Cases, materials and problems* (3rd ed.). St. Paul, MN: West Publishing.

Glannon, J. W. (1995). *The law of torts: Examples and explanations.* Boston: Little, Brown.

Griswold v. Connecticut, 381 U.S. 479 (1965).

Harris, D. M. (2003). *Contemporary issues in healthcare law and ethics* (2nd ed., pp. 45–66). Chicago: Health Administration Press.

Health Insurance Portability and Accountability Act of 1996, Public Law 104-191 (August 21, 1995); Standards for Privacy of Individually Identifiable Health Information, 45 C.F.R. Parts 160 and 164 (December 28, 2000, as amended May 31, 2002 and August 14, 2002).

Helling v. Carey, 519 P.2d 981 (Wash. 1974).

Holmes, O. W. (1881). *The common law.* Available at Historic Law Books, Louisiana State University Law Center, Medical and Public Health Law Site, http://biotech.law.lsu.edu/

Horner, J. (2003). Legal implications of clinical documentation. *Perspectives on Swallowing and Swallowing Disorders, 13*(1), 10–16.

Horner, J., & Wheeler, M. (2005a, September 6). HIPAA: Impact on clinical practices. *ASHA Leader,* 10–11, 22–23.

Horner, J., & Wheeler, M. (2005b, November 8). HIPAA: Impact on Research Practices. *ASHA Leader,* 8–9, 26–27.

Individuals with Disabilities Education of 2004, Public Law 108-446, 118 Stat. 2647, 20 U.S.C. §§14000 et seq. Available at http://www.ed.gov/policy/speced/guid/idea/idea2004.html

Keeton, W. P., Dobbs, D. B., Keeton, R. E., & Owen, D. G. (1984). *Prosser and Keeton on torts* (5th ed.). St. Paul, MN.: West Publishing.

Meador, D. J. (1991). *American courts.* St. Paul, MN: West Publishing.

Miller, T. D. (2001). Professional liability in audiology and speech-language pathology: Ethical and legal considerations. In R. Lubinski & C. M. Frattali (Eds.), *Professional issues in speech-language pathology and audiology* (2nd ed., pp. 63–76). San Diego, CA: Singular, Delmar.

Paul-Brown, D. (1994). Clinical record keeping in audiology and speech-language pathology. *Asha, 36,* 40–43.

Pellegrino, Edmund. (1983). What is a profession? *Journal of Allied Health, 12,* 168–175.

Rehabilitation Act of 1973, Section 504, 29 U.S.C. §794.

Scheutzow, S. O. Patient care. In B. M. Broccolo, D. H., Caldwell, A. R., Daniels, et al., *Fundamentals of health law* (3rd ed., pp. 37–56). Chicago: American Health Lawyers Association.

Schloendorff v. Society of New York Hospitals, 105 N.E. 92, 93 (N.Y., 1914).

Sherman Act, 15 U.S.C. §§1, 2 (2002). Available at http://www.usdoj.gov/atr/foia/divisionmanual/ch2.htm

Social Security Act, Medicaid, Title XIX, 42 U.S.C. §§1396-1396v.

Social Security Act, Medicare, Title XVIII, 42 U.S.C. §§1395-1395ccc.

South Carolina Code of Laws, Speech-Language Pathologists and Audiologists, §§40-67-5 et seq. and §§40-1-110 to 40-1-150. Available at http://www.lawsource.com/also/

Studdert, D. M., Mello, M. M., & Brennan, T. A. (2004). Medical malpractice. *The New England Journal of Medicine, 350*(3), 283–292.

Tanner, D. C. (2006, in press). Dysphagia malpractice: litigation and the expert witness. *Journal of Medical Speech-Language Pathology.*

Tarasoff v. Regents of University of California, 551 P.2d 334 (Cal. 1976)

The T.J. Hooper, 60 F. 2nd 737 (2d Cir. 1932).

Truman v. Thomas, 611 P.2d 902 (Cal., 1980).

U.S. Constitution. (1787). Available at http://www.house.gov/Constitution/Constitution.html

U.S. Department of Health and Human Services. Available at http://www.hhs.gov

U.S. Department of Justice. Available at http://www.usdoj.gov

U.S. Department of Justice. (2001, August). A guide to disability rights laws. Available at http://www.doj.gov

6

International Alliances

LINDA WORRALL, PHD, AND
LOUISE HICKSON, PHD

SCOPE OF CHAPTER

International networks are increasingly a part of our work and social life (Harasim, 1993). The term *global village* was coined to promote discussion about the possibility of an interconnected world. The concept of a global village is becoming reality as the information age picks up speed in the new millennium. According to Cheng (1998), a global communicator is prepared "to learn and embrace cultural and individual diversity" (p. 283). Speech-language pathologists and audiologists have been swept up in the global communication revolution within both their social and professional lives. News broadcasts from all parts of the world are beamed into our homes 24 hours a day; telephone calls and e-mails instantaneously link people from all nations; Internet access provides a wealth of information from all over the globe; and jet travel is relatively commonplace. The global village has had an impact on the professional practice of speech-language pathologists and audiologists. International conferences are only a few hours travel away; relevant clinical information is accessible in minutes from the World Wide Web; and conversation with international colleagues via e-mail and telephone can be achieved in seconds.

This chapter has two aims. The first is to outline the benefits of creating and nurturing international alliances—benefits that include broadening one's knowledge base, developing skills, learning new procedures, and pooling resources to develop tests, resources, and/or standards that can be applied in a number of countries. Some of the barriers to developing international alliances (e.g., language barriers, ethnocentrism) are also discussed. The second aim is to examine the two main forms of transnational communication in the professions. Internet use is espoused as a means of forming international alliances, and practice in other countries is also encouraged.

Substantial information and resources necessary for speech-language pathologists and audiologists to practice in other countries are provided as an introduction on how to find jobs in other countries. The main emphasis in this chapter is on the practice requirements for Australia, Canada, Ireland, New Zealand, South Africa, and the United Kingdom. These countries were chosen because they are English speaking and represent the major destinations for English-speaking speech-language pathologists and audiologists. Since 2005, there has also been an agreement of mutual recognition of certification in speech-language pathology between the countries of Australia, Canada, United Kingdom, and the United States. The implications of this international agreement are discussed later in this chapter. A summary of information about working in developing countries is also included as well as a brief description of the international associations for speech-language pathologists and audiologists.

BENEFITS OF INTERNATIONAL ALLIANCES

Globalization has many advantages, and the benefits are beginning to influence the professions of speech-language pathology and audiology. Many clinicians and researchers are traveling to other countries to learn new perspectives and skills. They may also provide perspectives, skills, and services to the host country. The professions in many developing countries have been assisted by speech-language pathologists and audiologists from countries with established professional bases, such as the United States and the United Kingdom. Although information about opportunities for assisting developing countries is summarized in this chapter, we focus on the less-tangible benefits that international alliances can bring to those who want to interact with fellow professionals from other predominantly English-speaking countries.

Before discussing these benefits, some of the barriers need to be mentioned. First, the practice of speech-language pathology, and audiology to a lesser extent, requires that the clinician be a near native speaker of the home language in both its oral and written form. This therefore restricts the practice of speech-language pathologists and audiologists internationally. Hence, a monolingual clinician who was educated in an English-speaking country will find it difficult, if not impossible, to practice in non-English-speaking countries such as Japan or Germany. In addition, many students who have a non-English-speaking background and who choose to study in English-speaking countries such as Australia, the United Kingdom, Canada, or the United States may struggle to reach the English competency required to practice in that country or to graduate when clinical competency is part of the degree. It is often a requirement for registration or association membership in English-speaking countries (such as membership of Speech Pathology Australia and registration with the Health Professions Council in the UK), for people from non-English-speaking backgrounds to be proficient in English. English proficiency is measured by occupational English tests such as the International English Language Testing System. (See http://www.ielts.org for further information.)

There are also communication barriers between English-speaking countries. A good example of the differences among English-speaking countries is the use of the English language itself. Although English is the global language for international communication, and more than 80 percent of the world's research is published first in English, the language is diverse. Just as Afrikaans became a separate language from Dutch within a relatively short period of time, Stevenson (1994) concurs with the editor of the *Oxford English Dictionary* who predicts that American English and British English will drift into two distinct languages. Although American English is the language of the largest nation of speech-language pathologists and audiologists, other forms of English comprise the language of the professions in Australia, Canada, New Zealand, South Africa, and the United Kingdom. Some of these nations use a mix of both

American English and British English in their professional language.

Within speech-language pathology and audiology, differences are most noticeable in examples of written language emanating from each country. *Dysphasia* is still the term used most often in the United Kingdom, whereas *aphasia* is used in the United States. In audiology, *immittance audiometry* is the preferred term in the United States, whereas *impedance audiometry* is more commonly used in Australia and in the United Kingdom. The profession of speech-language pathology in the United States and Canada is called *speech pathology* in Australia and *speech and language therapy* in New Zealand, the United Kingdom, and Ireland. In South Africa, *speech and hearing therapist* has been the term for the combined professions of speech-language pathology and audiology (Bortz, Jardine, & Tshule, 1996; Tuomi, 1994). Overall however, *audiology* is the most commonly used term for the profession worldwide.

Denotative or dictionary meanings of words are well understood by the professional community; however, as Stevenson (1994) notes, the problem in cross-cultural communication (or miscommunication) is embedded in the connotative or subjective meaning of the word. These meanings are determined by the individual's experience within a culture, and for health professionals this experience includes their professional education. Stevenson (1994) gives the example of the word *house* in English', a dictionary translation would be *haus* in German, *maison* in French, and *casa* in Spanish. However, there are subtle differences between these words in a cultural sense, in that the concept of these "houses" is quite different. An example in speech-language pathology is found in the use of the terms *articulation disorders* and *phonological disorders*. Clinicians in the United States often interpret these terms differently than clinicians in Australia and the United Kingdom. The prevailing meanings in the United States are exemplified by Stone and Stoel-Gammon (1994), who use *phonological disorders* as the generic term that often includes articulation disorders due to structural characteristics or the control mechanism of the speech system (albeit having an impact on the phonological system). In the United Kingdom and

Australia, these terms are used to describe two discrete disorders, with *phonological disorders* implying an underlying cognitive-linguistic deficit and *articulation disorders* implying an underlying phonetic production deficit. Although connotative meanings of terms such as these may vary even within one country's profession, cross-cultural communication between professions in different countries may encounter difficulties caused by differences in the connotative meaning of professional terms.

The diverse nature of English is just one barrier in international alliances. Ethnocentric attitudes are another. The citation of local references is common to all disciplines, not just speech-language pathology and audiology. An increasing and contentious barrier is the American dominance of the two professions, which has the potential to marginalize the professions in other countries. The American Speech-Language-Hearing Association has the largest number of speech-language pathology and audiology members in the world. It represents some 11,684 certified audiologists and 98,334 speech-language pathologists (ASHA, 2005b). Given the power of numbers, the United States certainly exerts a large influence on speech-language pathology and audiology professions in other nations. There may be some advantages to this, such as the development of common professional terms; however, Americans need to be sensitive to this powerful influence. Many benefits can be gained from international alliances if cultural and communication barriers can be identified and overcome.

The Benefit of Learning New Skills, Procedures, and Perspectives

Speech-language pathologists and audiologists in various countries frequently use distinct theoretical frameworks and diverse practical techniques and work in very different policy environments. Gaining knowledge about these areas can enrich both the individual clinician and the professions as a whole. New ways are not always better, but it is possible to select particular aspects that will improve practice in another setting. An example is the innovative and exciting use of the social model of disability being used in aphasia rehabilitation in North York, Ontario, Canada (Kagan & Gailey, 1993) and the City University, London, England (Byng, Pound, & Parr, 2000). These approaches have founded many similar aphasia centers throughout the world, each a little different but reflecting the same principles.

The Benefit of Gaining New Perspectives of Cultural Diversity

As a preface to the introduction of the World View section of the *American Journal of Speech-Language Pathology,* Fey (1996) highlights the importance of evaluating trends in professional practice in the United States from the standpoint of the state of the art elsewhere. This is a welcome recognition of the benefits that a leading professional nation such as the United States can obtain from a flow of information into the country. Fey also states that "we cannot develop adequate theories of speech and language disorders or speech and language intervention unless we embrace an international perspective that takes into careful consideration the similarities and differences among cultures and languages across the world" (p. 2). Cultural diversity within a nation is a feature of everyday life in many countries. Hence, in addition to the influence of global communication networks, population mobility is shaping our future. Nations like Australia, Canada, New Zealand, South Africa, the United Kingdom, and the United States have a diversity of cultures within their own borders. The speech-language pathology and audiology professions are striving to provide relevant services to these populations and need to develop sensitivity to other cultures so they can best serve their clients. A benefit of international alliances is greater sensitivity to cultural and linguistic diversity.

The Benefit of Pooling Resources

Many resources produced in one country would be useful in other countries; however, only a few of these are distributed internationally, as they may have little commercial value within the local publishing industry. Such resources may nonetheless be extremely useful in other cultural settings. For example, the speech pathology department of a hospital in Australia produced an outcome scale, the Royal Brisbane Hospital Outcome Measure for Swallowing (1998), that has been widely accepted by speech pathologists across Australia. However, as the national market for the scale is relatively small and there is no specific speech-language pathology and audiology publishing company in Australia, this scale is unlikely to be distributed internationally. This is unfortunate because the scale is one of the only dysphagia outcome rating scales known to have substantial psychometric data (Ward & Conroy, 1999; Sonies, 2000).

An example of pooling international resources in speech-language pathology is seen in a project related to the ASHA Functional Assessment of Communication Skills for Adults (ASHA FACS; Frattali, Thompson, Holland, Wohl, & Ferketic, 1995), which has become a leading functional communication assessment around the world as well as in the United States. The ASHA FACS has gained greater recognition internationally because of the involvement of international contributors in the review process. Items that were not appropriate to other English-speaking countries were identified and discussed. The successful international alliance developed during the original ASHA FACS project has taken on an expanded role for the next phase of the project. The project has evolved into developing a measure of quality of communicative life, the ASHA Quality of Communication Life Scale (QCL) (Paul et al., 2005). International advisory group members have been able to offer theoretical perspectives on quality of life issues in their own countries, field-test the new measure in English-speaking countries outside the United States, and offer suggestions on how the tool might be accepted in countries outside the United States. Hence, a two-way information flow has developed. The end product will have a much wider application, and a new appreciation of international perspectives on functional communication and quality of life will have emerged in the process.

In audiology, a group of researchers and practitioners in the International Collegium of

Rehabilitative Audiology (ICRA) have worked on a number of projects from a global perspective. For example, they have developed the ICRA noise CD, which is a collection of noise signals that can be used as background noise in clinical tests of hearing aids and possibly for measuring characteristics of nonlinear instruments. It is hoped that these signals might become an international de facto standard. As another example, members of the collegium have developed and promoted the use of the International Outcome Inventory (Cox, Stephens, & Kramer, 2002) for measuring the outcomes of rehabilitation for adults with hearing impairment. The tool is available from the ICRA Web site in a number of different languages, and recent publications suggest that it is beginning to be used worldwide (e.g., Heuermann, Kinkel, & Tchorz, 2005).

Scholarship programs, such as the Fulbright program, encourage sharing knowledge and pooling resources between the United States and 140 other participating countries. The Fulbright program supports postgraduate students, researchers, and scholars to study or work in universities throughout the world. Joan Kosta, an American speech-language pathologist, recently traveled to Malaysia on the Fulbright Scholar Program and describes some of the benefits of collaborating with foreign countries as well as some language and cultural barriers (Kosta, 2005). Information about the Fulbright programs can be obtained online.

STRATEGIES FOR INTERNATIONAL ALLIANCES

We encourage professionals to begin appreciating the diversity of the profession across the world by becoming speech-language pathologists or audiologists of the world rather than professionals of their own specific country. There are two main types of professional transnational interaction. One is via mass communication system contacts such as those of the World Wide Web, and the other is person-to-person international contact, which often involves practicing professionally in another country (Mowlana, 1997). This section offers details about practice in other countries and about other strategies for transnational interaction that do not involve international travel.

Kuster and Poburka (1998) detail the advantages the Internet provides for bridging research and practice in speech-language pathology and audiology. In addition, Internet functions such as chat groups, e-journals, online bibliographies and journal services, Web sites that describe research and report findings, and simple e-mail can also be useful for bridging the gap between communication disorders professionals throughout the world. For example, in audiology, Balatsouras, Korres, Kandiloros, Ferekidis, and Economou (2003) detail newborn hearing screening resources available on the Internet. These include Web sites about hearing screening program guidelines and position statements, research laboratories, publications, related organizations and societies, equipment, and data management software, as well as online mailing lists and discussion groups. Addresses for 150 sites are listed. In addition to more specific Web sites, services such as Audiology Online and Speech Pathology Online are an excellent starting point for surfing the Web.

Opportunities to gather research on the Internet highlight the need for leadership by the international research community for cross-cultural communication in both professions (Kuster & Poburka, 1998). Individuals need to join discussion lists, post their own professional insights on Web sites, seek information about the profession in other countries via the Internet, request the Tables of Contents of international journals from publisher's Web sites, go to specific Web sites of speech-language pathologists or audiologists in other countries, and correspond if possible through e-mail. The Internet is fast becoming the most extensive communication and information system worldwide, and because of this, speech-language pathologists and audiologists should be keen to embrace it to develop international alliances.

Citing a United States commission on international studies by United States citizens, Mowlana (1997) concludes that study-abroad programs can have a lifelong impact on values and on understanding of other cultures: "Cross-cultural contact enables persons to understand the complexities of another society and empathize with persons of another culture" (p. 157). Experiencing the professions in another country provides a unique understanding of how cultural differences affect the practice of speech-language pathology or audiology. Sensitivity to cultural effects on clinical practice is a prized value of not only individuals, but also organizations.

PRACTICE IN OTHER COUNTRIES

The Internet can facilitate finding a job as a speech-language pathologist or audiologist in another country. Many of the larger professional associations now have Web sites and often provide information for professionals qualified outside their country. Some also have job vacancies listed on the site. The Resource section at the end of the chapter summarizes the speech-language pathology and audiology entry qualifications, practice requirements, and relevant professional associations in Australia, Canada, Ireland, New Zealand, South Africa, and the United Kingdom. Each country has different arrangements for the admission of people trained overseas to practice, and some reciprocity agreements are in place.

The best way to obtain information is to contact the country's professional association. The Web site addresses included in the Resources section are the most convenient way of accessing relevant up-to-date information. Further information about the features of professional practice in Australia, Canada, Hong Kong, South Africa, and the United Kingdom is contained in Pickering and colleagues (1998). For links to speech-language pathology and audiology professional associations and individual practitioners, see the section on Additional Resources at the end of this chapter.

Should the destination country not have a Web site, then contact information should be available through your own professional association. Further contact information for speech pathology and audiology associations outside the United States (including non-English-speaking countries) can also be obtained from ASHA's Web site.

As noted earlier, an agreement of mutual recognition of credentials between the four speech-language pathology professional associations of Australia, Canada, the United Kingdom, and the United States came into effect at the beginning of 2005. Boswell (2004) states that the agreement benefits include identifying common standards of clinical competence, facilitating ongoing exchange of knowledge, promoting greater international understanding of the role of speech-language pathologists, reducing trade barriers, improving mobility for employment abroad, and providing a process for countries interested in mutual recognition and qualifications and credentials. For speech-language pathologists wishing to work in countries covered by the agreement, this agreement does not mean automatic entry into the other countries' professional associations. Each professional association may still require additional certification. However, the agreement means that each applicant does not have to have his or her academic course work and clinical practicum evaluated as part of the application process. Further details about the specific requirements of each professional association under the agreement are contained on their Web sites (see Resources at the end of the chapter).

Australia

Speech Pathology Australia is the professional association that represents more than 3,250 speech pathologists in Australia. It is recognized as the national professional standards organization and provides services in representation, data collection and collation, public relations, publication, continuing education, member services, and government submissions.

The association has established educational and clinical standards that applicants are required to meet for admission to membership. For Practicing Membership, applicants are required to have an appropriate degree and to demonstrate participation in 300 hours of face-to-face clinical contact throughout the course. For applicants who graduated more than 5 years ago, evidence is required of at least 1,000 hours of speech pathology practice within the last 5 years. The eligibility for membership requirements has changed to a competency-based approach as contained in the Competency-Based Occupational Standards for Entry-Level Speech Pathologists (Speech Pathology Australia, 2001). The practice or licensing requirements for speech pathologists in Australia vary for the different states and territories. Queensland is the only state in Australia that requires mandatory registration through the Speech Pathologists Board of Queensland before practicing as a speech pathologist.

Membership in Speech Pathology Australia is not mandatory across Australia; however, employers usually require applicants for speech pathology positions to demonstrate eligibility for current practicing membership in Speech Pathology Australia. Some employers state that association membership is obligatory.

The Audiological Society of Australia is the professional association that maintains standards for audiology in Australia and represents more than 1,000 audiologists. To practice, an individual should be eligible for full membership in the society; that is, he or she must have completed a master's degree in an approved audiology program and 200 hours of supervised clinical contact during training. To obtain the society's Certificate of Clinical Practice, it is then necessary to complete a Graduate Clinical Internship of 12 months of supervised clinical practice. There are currently no official registration or licensing agreements for the practice of audiology in Australia. Although membership of the Audiological Society of Australia is not mandatory, most employers require applicants to have or be eligible for society membership.

Canada

The Canadian Association of Speech-Language Pathologists and Audiologists (CASLPA) represents the interests of both professions of speech-language pathology and audiology in Canada. In addition to the national association, there are provincial/territorial associations for speech-language pathologists and audiologists. These associations have varying practice requirements. CASLPA grants certification to speech-language pathologists and audiologists, and this involves both an examination and the fulfillment of the national standards. Continuing education is a necessary part of maintaining certification. Membership in the association is available without certification; however, the association encourages all members to undertake and maintain certification. Certification is recognized internationally and facilitates movement not only within Canada but also within the United States.

CASLPA requires a minimum academic requirement of a graduate university degree. The usual qualification is a master's degree in audiology and/or speech-language pathology or equivalent. Foreign-trained speech-language pathologists and audiologists who want to work in Canada are invited to become certified with CASLPA as the national association of the country. All applicants must also undergo an International Qualifications Assessment Service (IQAS) examination. A total minimum of 300 clinical hours in speech-language pathology or audiology is required to be a Full Member of CASLPA, while 350 hours is required to be a Full Member Certified. For speech-language pathology, the total minimum number of hours is specified according to distribution across disorders: developmental language disorders (40 hours), acquired language disorders (30 hours), fluency (15 hours), voice and resonance disorders (15 hours), articulation/phonology disorders (20 hours), dysphagia (10 hours), motor speech (10 hours), and minor audiology (20 hours). A minimum of 50 clinical hours must be with adults and 50 hours with children. A minimum of 100 hours must be spent in diagnostic activities and 100 hours in therapeutic activities.

For membership in the association as an audiologist, applicants must have obtained a master's degree in audiology and have completed 350 hours of clinical practice or 300 hours for noncertified full membership. These hours must be distributed according to diagnostic audiology (100 hours), amplification (65 hours), aural rehabilitation (25 hours), electrophysiological measurement (10 hours), and minor speech-language pathology (20 hours). Fifty hours must be spent with children, likewise for adults. A minimum of 100 hours must be spent in assessment and 100 hours in treatment activities. Some provincial associations have different clinical hour requirements than the national association, and these are listed separately on the association's Web site.

Practice requirements for registration and licensure differ from province to province, and these details can also be obtained from the CASLPA Web site. Information is available for British Columbia, Yukon, Alberta, Northwest Territories, Saskatchewan, Manitoba, Ontario, Quebec, New Brunswick, Nova Scotia, Prince Edward Island, and Newfoundland.

Ireland

All overseas graduates will need to apply for validation of qualifications through the National Validation Project before commencing work as an audiologist or a speech-language therapist in Ireland. Overseas graduates must submit details of their qualifications, along with course information (e.g., syllabus, subject content, hours of study, and practical placement details), details of professional memberships and professional experience. Validation of qualifications are assessed on a case-by-case basis. Speech-language therapists who have graduated from a British institute with accreditation by the Royal College of Speech and Language Therapy (RCSLT) do not need to submit course information or details of professional experience.

New Zealand

The New Zealand Speech-Language Therapists Association (NZSTA) asks that overseas graduates submit a certified copy of their qualifications and current association membership and a copy of their curriculum vitae to the President of the NZSTA. Provisional approval only may be given

to recent graduates with fewer than 2 years of experience. There are no licensing or registration requirements for New Zealand speech-language therapists. The entry-level qualification for the practice of audiology in New Zealand is a master's degree. The professional society representing audiologists is the New Zealand Audiological Society (NZAS). Requirements for entry to the society are a master's degree in audiology and a Certificate of Clinical Competence, which involves a year of supervised clinical practice. Although membership in the society is encouraged, it is not a prerequisite for working as an audiologist in New Zealand.

South Africa

To practice speech pathology and audiology in South Africa, it is necessary to register with the Health Professionals Council of South Africa (formerly the South African Medical and Dental Council). The requirements for registration are a degree from an accepted institution verified by academic transcripts. Speech pathology and audiology is a combined 4-year undergraduate degree in South Africa, and although postgraduate qualifications can be obtained, they are not necessary for practice. The professional association representing speech pathologists and audiologists is the South African Speech-Language-Hearing Association (SASLHA). Further details about the transition of both professions in this rapidly changing country are available in Bortz et al. (1996), Pickering et al. (1998), and Tuomi (1994).

United Kingdom

The Royal College of Speech and Language Therapists (RCSLT) is the regulating body for overseas speech and language therapists wanting to work in the United Kingdom. To work in the United Kingdom, applicants also need to be registered with the Health Professions Council. Under the Mutual Recognition of Credentials Agreement, applicants from Canada and Australia must have completed 12 months of post-qualification work experience to work in the United Kingdom. The national association of the applicant's country must also send a letter of good standing, confirming current certification.

The new professional society representing audiologists in the United Kingdom is the British Academy of Audiology (BAA). It replaces the British Association of Audiological Scientists (BAAS), the British Association of Audiologists (BAAT), and the British Society of Hearing Therapists (BSHT). Major changes have been underway in the United Kingdom over the past few years, and there are now three different ways to qualify as an audiologist. There are undergraduate programs (Bachelor of Science in Audiology), master's programs (Master of Science in Audiology) and some fast-track postgraduate diploma conversion programs for those with a bachelor of science in another relevant area of science. In addition to membership in the BAA, audiologists also need to register with the Health Professions Council.

INTERNATIONAL PROFESSIONAL ASSOCIATIONS

Membership in international associations for speech-language pathologists and audiologists can provide valuable opportunities for interaction with fellow professionals worldwide. Although there are many international associations in specialist areas of speech-language pathology and audiology, the major international association for speech-language pathology is the International Association of Logopedics and Phoniatrics (IALP), and the major international association for audiology is the International Society of Audiology (ISA).

International Association of Logopedics and Phoniatrics

The IALP is a nonprofit, nonpolitical, and nongovernmental organization whose purpose is to work for the benefit of people with a range of communication disorders (speech, language, voice, swallowing, and hearing). Founded in Vienna in 1924, the association now has more than 300 individual members from 54 countries and is affiliated with 56 national societies from 38 countries (including Australia, Canada, New Zealand, South Africa, United Kingdom, and the United States). The IALP has informative and consultative status with several United Nations offices, including UNESCO, UNICEF, and WHO. The association also publishes a journal, *Folia Phoniatrica et Logopaedica* (six issues annually).

International Society of Audiology (ISA)

The statutory purpose of the ISA is to facilitate knowledge, protection, and rehabilitation of human hearing. It also serves as an advocate for the profession and for people with hearing impairment throughout the world. The major activities of the ISA are publications of the *International Journal of Audiology*, newsletters (*Audinews*), organization of biannual congresses and other events, promotion of international standards in audiology, participation in the organization of affiliated societies, and representation of the multidisciplinary field of audiology in international organizations. Full membership requires a university degree in audiology or any related field, and associated membership includes anyone working in the field of Audiology without a university degree or having a professional interest in Audiology. Two current members of the ISA must support a membership application.

DEVELOPING AND OTHER NATIONS

In the first edition of this volume on professional issues, Wilson (1994) points out that appropriate speech-language pathology and audiology services are available in developed nations but not in many developing countries. This is particularly the case for speech and language disorders, as hearing impairment has received somewhat more attention internationally. For example, in 1991, the World Health Organization established a Division for the Prevention of Hearing Impairment, which aims to support the formation of organizations and committees in countries worldwide to address the prevention issue in hearing impairment.

Wilson suggests a number of possible roles for individual professionals who want to get involved with the evolution of the professions in developing countries. These roles include assisting with the development of training programs and services in other countries, acting as advocates for improved services for individuals with communication disorders around the world, joining an international professional association, building a local network of people with international interests, hosting international students, and being an advocate for the professions of speech-language pathology and audiology when traveling in developing countries. However, there is a danger that these practices promulgate Western imperialism in developing countries. It is suggested therefore that those who are interested in working abroad in developing countries are directed to specific agencies and programs, such as World Vision International, the Peace Corps, or Volunteer Services Overseas, that have bases in the home country.

Our focus in this edition is on the practice requirements for working in some of the major English-speaking nations. Opportunities do exist in many other countries, and various resources are available to assist the prospective traveler. Many of these countries also have audiology training programs. In a small number of countries, speech-language pathology and audiology are considered to be the same profession and therefore are taught conjointly (e.g., India, Brazil). Information about a range of countries is available in a number of journals such as the *American Journal of Speech-Language Pathology, American Journal of Audiology, International Journal of Audiology,* and *Folia Phoniatrica et Logopaedica.* For example, articles have appeared on speech-language pathology in the Dominican Republic (Meline, Penalo, & Oreste, 1996), Brazil (Ferreira, 2002), the Philippines (Cheng, Olea, & Marzan, 2002; Roseberry-McKibbin, 1997), Malaysia (Kosta, 2005; Lian & Abdullah, 2001), Taiwan (Tseng & Wen, 2002), Greece (Tsoukala & Tziorvas, 1995), Malta (Grech, 2002), Sri Lanka (Wickenden, Hartley, Kariyakaranawa, & Kodikara, 2003; Wickenden et al., 2001), India (D'Antonio & Nagarajan, 2003; Karanth, 2002), Iran (Nilipour, 2002), Israel (Korenbrot, Hertzano, & Ben Aroya, 2002), Uganda (Robinson, Afako, Wickenden, & Hartley, 2003), and Zimbabwe (Wolf-Schein, Afako, & Zondo, 1995), and articles on audiology in Trinidad and Tobago (Ali, 1992), Israel (Bergman & Hildesheimer, 1994), Nicaragua (Polich, 1995), Germany (Lenarz & Ernst, 1995), and Latin America (Madriz, 2001).

SUMMARY

This chapter has used the concept of the global village to illustrate how international alliances in speech-language pathology and audiology can be developed. It has emphasized the use of the Internet as a means for promoting greater international interaction, but it has also described the professions in six English-speaking countries of the world. Barriers to professional communication even within English-speaking countries abound; however, the advantages of international alliances are many. The forces that are driving globalization are powerful, and the professions of speech-language pathology and audiology are not exempt from such a global trend. Indeed, it is suggested that if the professions do not take advantage of international alliances, then they will not have the potency to serve those for whom we exist.

CRITICAL THINKING

1. What are the benefits of international alliances in the professions of speech-language pathology and audiology?

2. What are some of the barriers to international alliances?

3. What are some of the alternative names of the professions in other countries?

4. What are some strategies for developing international alliances that do not involve travel to other countries?

5. What are the international organizations that represent speech-language pathology and audiology?

6. How can you find out more about working as a speech pathologist or audiologist in another country? What would you need to learn about the culture and language of the country if you could work there?

REFERENCES

Ali, J. E. (1992). Audiology in Jamaica and Trinidad and Tobago. *American Journal of Speech-Language Pathology, 1*, 8–9.

American Speech-Language-Hearing Association. (2005a). *Audiology and speech-language pathology associations outside of the United States.* Available at http://www.asha.org/

American Speech-Language-Hearing Association. (2005b, July 21). Highlights and trends: ASHA counts for 2004. Available at http://www.asha.org/

Balatsouras, D., Korres, S., Kandiloros, D., Ferekidis, E., & Economou, C. (2003). Newborn hearing screening resources on the Internet. *International Journal of Pediatric Otorhinolaryngology, 67,* 333–340.

Bergman, M., & Hildesheimer, M. (1994). Forty years of audiology in Israel. *American Journal of Speech-Language Pathology, 3*, 11–15.

Bortz, M. A., Jardine, C. A., & Tshule, M. (1996). Training to meet the needs of the communicatively impaired population of South Africa: A project of the University of Witwatersrand. *European Journal of Disorders of Communication, 31*, 465–476.

Boswell, S. (2004, October 19). International agreement brings mutual recognition of certification. *ASHA Leader,* 1, 22.

Byng, S., Pound, C., & Parr, S. (2000). Living with aphasia: A framework for therapy interventions. In I. Papathanasiou (Ed.), *Acquired neurological communication disorders: A clinical perspective.* London: Whurr Publishers.

Cheng, L-R. L. (1998). Learning from multiple perspectives: Global implications for speech-language and hearing professionals. *Folia Phoniatrica et Logopaedica, 50*(5), 283–290.

Cheng, W. T., Olea, T. C. M., & Marzan, J. C. B. (2002). Speech-language pathology in the Philippines: Reflections on the past and present, perspectives for the future. *Folia Phoniatrica et Logopaedica, 54*(2), 79–82.

Cox, R. M., Stephens, D., & Kramer, S. E. (2002). Translations of the International Outcome Inventory for Hearing Aids (IOI-HA). *International Journal of Audiology, 41*(1), 3–26.

D'Antonio, L. L., & Nagarajan, R. (2003). Use of a consensus building approach to plan speech services for children with cleft palate in India. *Folia Phoniatrica et Logopaedica, 55*(6), 306–313.

Ferreira, L. P. (2002). Speech therapy in Brazil: Forty years of existence, two decades of recognition. *Folia Phoniatrica et Logopaedica, 54*(2), 103–105.

Fey, M. (1996). Inside. *American Journal of Speech-Language Pathology, 5*(2), 2.

Frattali, C. M., Thompson, C. K., Holland, A. L., Wohl, C. B., & Ferketic, M. M. (1995). *Functional assessment of communication skills for adults.* Rockville, MD: American Speech-Language-Hearing Association.

Fulbright Association. (n.d.). *Fulbright grant information.* Available at http://www.fulbrightalumni.org/

Grech, H. (2002). Speech-language pathology in Malta: Meeting local needs in a global perspective. *Folia Phoniatrica et Logopaedica, 54*(2), 91–94.

Harasim, L. M. (1993). *Global networks: Computers and international communication*. Cambridge, MA: MIT Press.

Heuermann, H., Kinkel, M., & Tchorz, J. (2005). Comparison of psychometric properties of the International Outcome Inventory for Hearing Aids (IOI-HA) in various studies. *International Journal of Audiology, 44*(2), 102–109.

Kagan, A., & Gailey, G. (1993). Functional is not enough: Training conversation partners for aphasic adults. In A. Holland & M. Forbes (Eds.), *Aphasia treatment: World perspectives* (pp. 199–225). San Diego, CA: Singular Publishing.

Karanth, P. (2002). Four decades of speech-language pathology in India: Changing perspectives and challenges of the future. *Folia Phoniatrica et Logopaedica, 54*(2), 69–71.

Korenbrot, F., Hertzano, T., & Ben Aroya, A. (2002). Emerging issues in Israel: Commentaries in a global context. *Folia Phoniatrica et Logopaedica, 54*(2), 72–74.

Kosta, J. C. (2005, August 16). An SLP in Malaysia. *ASHA Leader, 22,* 24.

Kuster, J. M., & Poburka, B. J. (1998). The Internet: A bridge between research and practice. *Topics in Language Disorders, 18*(2), 71–87.

Lenarz, T., & Ernst, A. (1995). Audiology in Germany: Before and since reunification. *American Journal of Speech-Language Pathology, 4*(1), 9–11.

Lian, C. H. T., & Abdullah, S. (2001). The education and practice of speech-language pathologists in Malaysia. *American Journal of Speech-Language Pathology, 10*(1), 3–9.

Madriz, J. J. (2001). Audiology in Latin America: Hearing impairment, resources and services. *Scandinavian Audiology, 30*(Suppl.53), 85–92.

Meline, T., Penalo, S., & Oreste, A. (1996). Speech-language pathology in the Dominican Republic. *American Journal of Speech-Language Pathology, 5*(3), 4–6.

Mowlana, H. (1997). *Global information and world communication: New frontiers in international relations*. London: Sage Publications.

Nilipour, R. (2002). Emerging issues in speech therapy in Iran. *Folia Phoniatrica et Logopaedica, 54*(2), 65–68.

Paul, D. R., Frattali, C.M., Holland, A.L., Thompson, C.K., Caperton, C.J., & Slater, S.C. (2005). *Quality of Communication Life Scale (ASHA QCL)*. Rockville, MD: American Speech-Language-Hearing Association.

Pickering, M., McAllister, L., Hagler, P., Whitehill, T. L., Penn, C., Robertson, S. J., & McCready, V. (1998). External factors influencing the profession in six societies. *American Journal of Speech-Language Pathology, 7*(4), 5–17.

Polich, L. (1995). Audiology in Nicaragua. *American Journal of Speech-Language Pathology, 4*(3), 6–9.

Robinson, H., Afako, R., Wickenden, M., & Hartley, S. (2003). Preliminary planning for training speech and language therapists in Uganda. *Folia Phoniatrica et Logopaedica, 55*(6), 322–328.

Roseberry-McKibbin, C. (1997). Understanding Filipino families: A foundation for effective service delivery. *American Journal of Speech-Language Pathology, 6*(3), 5–14.

Royal Brisbane Hospital Outcome Measure for Swallowing. (1998). (Available from Speech Pathology Department, Royal Brisbane Hospital, Herston, 4029, Queensland, Australia).

Sonies, B. C. (2000). Assessment and treatment of functional swallowing in dysphagia. In L. Worrall & C. Frattali (Eds.), *Neurogenic communication disorders: A functional approach*. New York: Thieme Publishers.

Speech Pathology Australia. (2001) *Competency-based standards for entry level speech pathologists*. Melbourne, Australia: Author.

Stevenson, R. L. (1994). *Global communication in the twenty-first century*. New York: Longman Publishing Group.

Stone, J. R., & Stoel-Gammon, C. (1994). Phonological development and disorders in children. In F. D. Minifie (Ed.), *Introduction to communication sciences and disorders* (pp. 149–187). San Diego, CA: Singular Publishing.

Tseng, C., & Wen, Y. (2002). Treatment program planning by speech therapists in Taiwan. *Folia Phoniatrica et Logopaedica, 54*(2), 83–86.

Tsoukala, M., & Tziorvas, R. (1995). The development of a new era of speech language pathology in Greece. *American Journal of Speech-Language Pathology, 4*(1), 5–7.

Tuomi, S. K. (1994). Speech-language pathology in South Africa: A profession in transition. *American Journal of Speech-Language Pathology, 3*, 5–8.

Ward, E. C., & Conroy, A-L. (1999). Validity, reliability and responsivity of the Royal Brisbane Hospital Outcome Measure for Swallowing. *Asia-Pacific Journal of Speech, Language, and Hearing*, 4, 109–129.

Wickenden, M., Hartley, S., Kariyakaranawa, S., & Kodikara, S. (2003). Teaching speech and language therapists in Sri Lanka: Issues in curriculum, culture and language. *Folia Phoniatrica et Logopaedica, 55*(6), 314–321.

Wickenden, M., Hartley, S., Kodikara, S., Mars, M., Sell, D., Sirimana, T., et al. (2001). Collaborative development of a new course and service in Sri Lanka. *International Journal of Language & Communication, 36*(Suppl. 2), 315–320.

Wilson, M. (1994). International perspectives. In R. Lubinski & C. Frattali (Eds.), *Professional issues in speech-language pathology and audiology: A textbook* (pp. 75–88). San Diego, CA: Singular Publishing.

Wolf-Schein, E. G., Afako, R., & Zondo, J. (1995). Sounds of Zimbabwe. *American Journal of Speech-Language Pathology, 4*(3), 5–14.

RESOURCES

Professional Practice in Australia, Canada, Ireland, New Zealand, South Africa, and the United Kingdom

Speech-Language Pathology

Australia

Speech Pathology Association of Australia
(Public Name: Speech Pathology Australia) 2nd Floor 11-19 Bank Place, Melbourne VIC 3000 Australia
Telephone: +61 3-9642-4899,
Fax: +61 3-9642-4922
E-mail: office@speechpathologyaustralia.org.au
Web site: http://www.speechpathologyaustralia.org.au
Four-year undergraduate bachelor's degree or 2-year postgraduate master's degree and 300 hours of face-to-face clinical experience. Competency assessed on the Competency-Based Occupational Standards for Speech Pathologists: Entry Level (Speech Pathology Australia, 2001).
Registration is compulsory in Queensland. Contact details are: Speech Pathologists Board of Queensland, GPO Box 2438 Brisbane, QLD 4001 Australia
Telephone: +61 7-3225-2508
Fax: +61 7-3225-2527
E-mail: speechpathology@healthregboards.qld.gov.au
Web site: http://www.speechpathboard.qld.gov.au

Eligibility for membership in Speech Pathology Australia is often a requirement of employers in other states and territories.

Canada

Canadian Association of Speech-Language Pathologists and Audiologists (CASLPA) 401-200 Elgin St., Ottawa, Ontario K2P 1L5 Canada
Telephone: +1 613-567-9968
Fax: +1 613-567-2859
E-mail: caslpa@caslpa.ca or sharon@caslpa.ca
(contact for queries regarding foreign trained SLPs and audiologist)
Web site: http://www.caslpa.ca/english/index.asp
(Information is also available on the Web in French: http://www.caslpa.ca/francais/index.asp)
Master's degree in speech-language pathology, including 300 clinical hours (or 350 clinical hours for certified members). Some provinces require 200–300 clinical hours.
Registration/licensure in each of the provinces and territories (see the CASLPA Web site for specific requirements for each province and territory, as follows: http://www.caslpa.ca/english/index.asp/.)

Ireland

Irish Association of Speech and Language Therapists (IASLT)
29 Gardiner Place Dublin 1 Ireland
Telephone/fax: +353-1-878-0215
E-mail: info@iaslt.com
Validation through the National Validation Project is compulsory, and each case is individually assessed.

Contact details are: National Validation Project, Northern Area Health Board, Swords Business Campus, Balheary Road Swords Co. Dublin Ireland
Telephone: +353-1-890-8741
Fax: +353-1-813-1873
E-mail: laura.kiernan@mailc.hse.ie

New Zealand

New Zealand Speech-Language Therapists Association (NZSTA)
Suite 369 63 Remuera Road Newmarket Auckland New Zealand
Telephone: +64-3-235-8257 Fax: +64-3-235-8850
E-mail: nzsta@nzsta-speech.org.nz
Four-year undergraduate degree or 2-year master's degree in speech and language therapy
Approval of qualifications by NZSTA is recommended.

South Africa

South African Speech-Language-Hearing Association
PO Box 5710 The Reeds 0158 South Africa
Telephone: +27-12-653-2114
Fax: +27-12-653-1351
Four-year professional bachelor's degree in speech pathology and audiology.
Registration is compulsory. Contact details are: The Registrar, Health Professions Council of South Africa, Professional Board for Speech, Language, and Hearing Professions, PO Box 205 Pretoria 0001 South Africa
Telephone: +27-12-338-9300
Fax: +27-12-328-5120
E-mail: hpcsa@hpcsa.co.za

United Kingdom

Royal College of Speech and Language Therapists (RCSLT)
2 White Hart Yard London SE1 1NX England UK
Telephone: +44-20-7378-1200
Fax: +44-20-7403-7254
E-mail: postmaster@rcslt.org
Web site: http://www.rcslt.org/
Three- or 4-year undergraduate degree in speech and language therapy, professional master's degree, or graduate entry 2-year bachelor's degree. One year of supervised membership before eligible for full membership. Registration with the RCSLT is not compulsory; however, registration with the Health Professions Council (HPC) is now compulsory. Contact details are: The Health Professions Council Park House 184 Kennington Park Road

London SE11 4BU England UK
Telephone: +44-20-7840-9804
Fax: +44-20-7840-9803
E-mail: international@hpc-uk.org
Web site: http://www.hpc-uk.org

Audiology

Australia

Audiological Society of Australia
Suite 7 476 Canterbury Road Forest Hill VIC 3131 Australia
Telephone: +61-3-9416-4606
Fax: +61-3-9416-4607
Two-year postgraduate master's degree and 200 hours of clinical contact. Eligibility for membership in the association.

Canada

Canadian Association of Speech-Language Pathologists and Audiologists (CASLPA) 401-200 Elgin St., Ottawa, Ontario K2P 1L5 Canada
Telephone: +1 613-567-9968
Fax: +1 613-567-2859
E-mail: caslpa@caslpa.ca or sharon@caslpa.ca (contact for queries regarding foreign trained SLPs and audiologist)
Web site: http://www.caslpa.ca/english/index.asp)
Master's degree in audiology, including 300 clinical hours (or 350 clinical hours for certified members). Registration and licensure differ according to province (see the CASLPA Web site for specific requirements for each province and territory, as follows: http://www.caslpa.ca/english/index.asp).

New Zealand

New Zealand Audiological Society
P.O. Box 9724 Newmarket Auckland New Zealand
Telephone/fax: +64-9-625-1664
E-mail: nzas@xtra.co.nz
Website: http://www.audiology.org.nz
Master's degree in audiology.

South Africa

South African Speech and Hearing and Language Association
P.O. Box 5710 The Reeds 0158 South Africa
Telephone: +27-12-653-2114
Fax: +27-12-653-1351
Four-year professional bachelor's degree in speech pathology and audiology.

Registration is compulsory. Contact details are: The Registrar, Health Professions Council of South Africa, Professional Board for Speech, Language, and Hearing Professions, P.O. Box 205 Pretoria 0001 South Africa
Telephone: +27-12-338-9300
Fax: +27-12-328-5120
E-mail: hpcsa@hpcsa.co.za

United Kingdom

British Academy of Audiology (BAA)
P.O. Box 346 Peterborough RM PE6 7EG England UK
Telephone: +44-1733-253-976
E-mail: admin@baaudiology.org
Web site: http://www.baaudiology.org
Master's degree in audiology. Membership in the association is not mandatory but recommended. Registration with the Health Professions Council (HPC) is compulsory. Contact details are: The Health Professions Council
Telephone 7840-9804
Fax: +44-20-7840-9803
E-mail: international@hpc-uk.org
Web site: http://www.hpc-uk.org

Additional Resources

Audiology Online, Inc.
http://www.audiologyonline.com
Caroline Bowen, PhD, Speech-Language Pathologist
http://members.tripod.com/Caroline_Bowen/home.html
International Collegium of Rehabilitative Audiology
http://ww.icra.nu/
International English Language Testing System
http://www.ielts.org/
Net Connections for Communication Disorders and Sciences (created by J. M. Kuster, Minnesota State University, Mankato)
http://www.mnsu.edu/comdis/kuster2/welcome.html
Rehab World
http://www.rehabworld.com/rwstdex.htm
Speech Language Pathology Web Site (created by S. Herring)
http://www.herring.org/speech.html
SpeechPathology.com
http://www.speechpathology.com/

Employment Issues

7

Workforce Issues in Communication Sciences and Disorders

SARAH C. SLATER, MS

SCOPE OF CHAPTER

This chapter describes the current status of the supply and demand of speech-language pathologists, audiologists, and communication science and disorders teachers/researchers in the United States. Data from the American Speech-Language-Hearing Association, Council of Academic Programs in Communication Sciences and Disorders (CAPSD), the United States Bureau of Labor Statistics, and other sources are presented to describe current demographics and employment characteristics of individuals in the professions and discipline. Next, enrollment and graduation trends in communication sciences and disorder programs are presented. The chapter concludes with a discussion of factors affecting the future employment of speech-language pathologists, audiologists, and teachers/scholars. Influential factors include federal policy and the impact of health care and reimbursement reform, advances in medical technology, technological change, and the changing demographics of the population.

A LOOK BACK

In 1988, a comprehensive study of the speech-language pathology and audiology workforce was conducted by ASHA (Shewan, 1988). In the years that followed the study, record numbers of enrollments and graduations in communication sciences and disorders programs were reported, and high-growth projections continued to be released by the United States Department of Labor's Bureau of Labor Statistics. The demand for health professionals was high overall, and the employment outlook for new graduates never looked brighter.

The 1988 ASHA workforce study (Shewan, 1988) concluded, in part, that the need for speech-language pathologists and audiologists would continue to grow and to outstrip supply, at least to the year 2000. How much this need will increase depends on the number of individuals with communication disorders in the population. However, need does not account for any of the political, professional, and economic aspects that operate in the workforce. The impact of these factors was to be realized in the mid- to late 1990s. Following the collapse of the Health Security Act, managed care had an impact on almost every health care professional. The federal government targeted Medicare and Medicaid as two major entitlements to be contained in an effort to balance the budget. In a trickle-down effect, employers attempted to control the costs of health benefits offered to employees. The health care environment continues to operate in a state of change. This chapter explores the possible impact these factors have had on the supply and demand of audiologists and speech-language pathologists and what we may expect the future to hold for these professionals. The shortage of doctorally prepared teachers/researchers also is addressed, as well as its potential impact on the discipline.

THE CURRENT WORKFORCE

In any discussion of a given profession, it is important to first define who is and who is not a part of the profession. Shewan (1988) indicated that the ASHA membership comprised about half of the speech-language-hearing workforce. The primary differences between the ASHA and non-ASHA personnel were reflected in educational attainment and primary employment facility. Non-ASHA personnel were more likely to hold a bachelor's degree and be employed in a school-based setting. Subsequent studies have suggested a much higher degree of overlap between the number of ASHA-certified providers and the audiology and speech-language pathology workforce. However, because ASHA currently recognizes the master's degree as the entry-level credential (note that the doctoral degree will become ASHA's recognized entry-level requirement for the profession of audiology beginning in 2012), this chapter focuses on the data and characteristics of professionals who affiliate with ASHA through certification and/or membership. Data from other relevant sources are introduced as they are available.

The ASHA Certificate of Clinical Competence (CCC) is the universally recognized credential in the professions of speech-language pathology and audiology. The CCC allows the holder to provide independent clinical services and to supervise the clinical practice of student trainees, clinicians who do not hold certification, and support personnel. The certificate can be obtained by an individual who meets specific requirements in terms of education degree, course work, practicum, and supervised professional experience, and who passes the national examination in speech-language pathology or audiology. Holders of the CCC must follow the ASHA's Code of Ethics, which incorporates the highest standards of integrity and ethical principles. Many hospitals, health care settings (including the U.S. military), educational programs, and private practices require the ASHA CCC for new hires and promotions. Many third party payers (including private insurance agencies) and publicly funded programs require the ASHA CCC for reimbursement for services rendered.

Licensure, unlike ASHA certification, is mandatory for those states that regulate the practice of audiology and/or speech-language pathology. In many states, licensure requirements parallel those of

ASHA certification. Further, ASHA certification often satisfies many of the requirements of state licensure. As of October 2005, 50 states regulated one or both professions (ASHA, 2005f).

ASHA MEMBERSHIP AND AFFILIATION DATA

As of year-end 2004, ASHA represented 118,437 speech-language pathologists, audiologists, and speech, language, and hearing scientists (ASHA, 2005a). Compared to year-end 2003, this number has increased by 4,402—a 3.9 percent increase (ASHA, 2004a). Figure 7–1 illustrates the growth of the ASHA membership and affiliation over the past 10 years. In 1994, 63,078 individuals held ASHA certification in speech-language pathology only; this number grew to 101,812 in 2004, a change of 61.4 percent over 10 years (ASHA, 1995, 2005a). The percent change in the number of ASHA certified audiologists over the same time period was

21.2 percent—from 10,640 certified audiologists in 1994 to 12,899 in 2004.

The lowest percent change was in the number of individuals who held ASHA certification in both audiology and speech-language pathology (individuals with dual certification). A total of 1,371 individuals held dual certification in 2004, compared to 1,451 individuals in 1994, a change of 5.5 percent (ASHA, 2005a, 1995). The lack of growth in the number of individuals who hold dual certification may be due, in part, to the increasing specialization of the professions. It may be more challenging to develop the broadening skills and knowledge base that each profession requires to work with individuals across the age, severity, and disorder spectrum.

Demographics

According to ASHA (2005a) males currently comprise 4.5 percent of speech-language pathologists and 18.7 percent of audiologists. These percentages

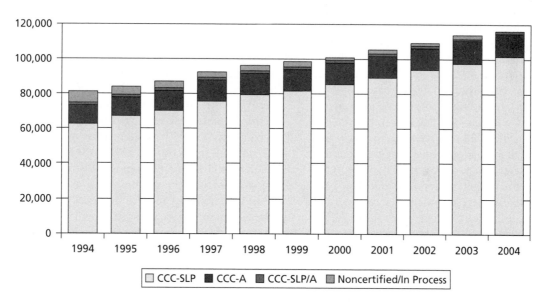

F I G U R E 7–1 American Speech-Language-Hearing Association Summary Membership and Affiliation Counts, 1994 to 2004

Adapted from American Speech-Language-Hearing Association, 2005. *American Speech-Language-Hearing Association Summary Membership and Affiliation Counts, 1994 to 2004.* Unpublished data. Rockville, MD: Author. Adapted by permission.

have decreased from 7.2 percent and 23.0 percent, respectively, over the past 10 years (ASHA, 1995).

As of year-end 2004, approximately 7.7 percent of audiologists, 7.0 percent of speech-language pathologists, and 8.0 percent of those with dual certification are members of a racial/ethnic minority group. These percentages have remained relatively constant over the years and are well below their distribution within the general population. Specifically, white non-Hispanics accounted for 77.1 percent of the total labor force in 1992. This figure is expected to decline to 65.5 percent by 2012 (United States Department of Labor, 2004a).

Employment Characteristics

In 2004, 73.1 percent of ASHA's membership and affiliation indicated they were employed on a full-time basis and 18.7 percent on a part-time basis (ASHA, 2005a). Only 1.7 percent was unemployed and seeking employment, well below the 2004 national unemployment rate of 5.5 percent reported by the United States Department of Labor (2005).

More than half (59.4 percent) of speech-language pathologists are employed in educational settings, including 3.9 percent in colleges or universities; an additional 35.4 percent are employed in health care facilities (ASHA, 2005a). Audiologists are generally employed in health care facilities (72.3 percent), including 47.3 percent in nonresidential health care facilities such as physicians' or audiologists' offices, 23.6 percent in hospitals, and the remainder in residential health care facilities. More than a fourth of audiologists (25.9 percent) are employed in private practice, compared to 16.7 percent of speech-language pathologists, rates that have remained relatively constant over previous years.

Most speech-language pathologists (82.3 percent) and audiologists (80.1 percent) report their primary employment function as clinical service provider, about the same as year-end 2003 and 2002 figures (ASHA, 2005a). The percentage of professionals holding administrative positions (i.e., executive officer, department chair, or supervisor) has remained stable as well—7.8 percent of speech-language pathologists and 8.8 percent of audiologists in 2004.

As of January 2004, the median number of years that workers across all occupations had been with their current employer was 4.0 years (United States Department of Labor, 2004c). Tenure increased with age, as almost one-third of employees (31.0 percent) age 25 and over had 10 or more years of service with their current employer. The 2001 ASHA Omnibus Survey found that 72.6 percent of respondents were in the same type of facility for three years or more. The percentage was similar for both audiologists and speech-language pathologists (ASHA, 2001).

Audiologists and speech-language pathologists are generally satisfied with their careers. According to the 1988 ASHA Omnibus Survey, approximately 79.0 percent of respondents reported that they were either very satisfied or satisfied with their career choice. An even higher percentage of satisfaction—approximately 85.0 percent—was reported by respondents to the 1995 ASHA Omnibus Survey (Zingeser, 2004). The most important factors for accepting or staying in a job included the type of clients and work setting, pay, collaborative relationships with others, administration's support, flexible schedule, and challenging work environment (ASHA, 2003b).

Audiologists' Salaries Most audiologists (72.2 percent) are paid on an annual—academic or calendar year basis—versus an hourly basis (27.8 percent) (ASHA, 2005h). The 2004 median annual salary for a certified audiologist employed on an academic-year basis was $51,000—a slight increase over the 2003 median salary of $50,000 (ASHA, 2005b, 2003a). In 2004, most audiologists paid on an annual salary-year basis were employed in a school or college/university setting. Audiologists employed on a calendar-year basis reported a median salary of $60,000 in 2004, up from $55,000 in 2003. Those paid on an hourly basis reported a median hourly salary of $29.00. Of audiologists paid on an hourly basis, most were employed in either a nonresidential health care facility (34.6 percent) or a hospital (31.9 percent) and worked an average (mean) of 26.7 hours per week.

Salaries for audiologists varied by geographic region, employment facility and function, number of years of experience, and highest educational degree. In 2004, the highest median calendar-year salaries were reported in the west ($66,890) and northeast ($65,000) regions of the United States (ASHA, 2005b). Median calendar-year salaries for audiologists were highest in hospital ($62,500) and college/university settings ($62,000), compared to $60,000 in school settings and $56,674 in nonresidential health care facilities. Clinical service providers reported a median salary of $60,000 compared to $78,274 for administrators and $78,000 for supervisors. The median entry-level (i.e., 1–3 years of experience) salary was $45,000 and reached $78,000 with 28 or more years of experience. The 2004 median calendar-year salary for individuals with a PhD was $82,606, compared to $65,000 for audiologists holding the AuD and $58,116 for those with a master's degree.

Salaries for Speech-Language Pathologists in Health Care Facilities According to the 2005 SLP Health Care Survey (ASHA, 2005d), almost half (48.6 percent) of speech-language pathologists in health care settings were paid on an hourly basis, 38.8 percent on an annual salary basis, and 12.7 percent on a variable salary basis depending on the type of service(s) provided. The median 2005 salary for a speech-language pathologist employed in a health care facility was $60,000. Median annual salaries

were highest in skilled nursing facilities ($68,200) and general medical hospitals ($61,250). Median annual (i.e., calendar year) and hourly salary data by type of health care setting are presented in Table 7-1.

Like audiologists, salaries for speech-language pathologists were influenced by a number of factors. Median annual salaries for speech-language pathologists were highest in the western region of the United States ($68,000) in 2005 and lowest in the south ($58,000) (ASHA, 2005g). Clinical service providers reported a median annual salary of $56,000 compared to $72,985 for administrators. A median annual salary of $95,000 was reported by individuals holding a doctoral degree in any field, compared to $60,000 for those with a master's degree. Years of experience also affected salaries. The median entry-level salary (i.e., 1–3 years of experience) for speech-language pathologists in health care settings was $52,694, versus $78,146 for individuals with 28 or more years of experience.

Salaries for Speech-Language Pathologists in School Settings Almost all (94.0 percent) speech-language pathologists employed in school settings are paid on an academic year (i.e., 9–10 month) salary basis (ASHA, 2004d). The median annual salary for a speech-language pathologist employed in a school setting on an academic year basis in 2004 was $50,000. Academic year salaries ranged from

T A B L E 7–1 2005 Median Annual (i.e., Calendar Year) and Hourly Salary for Speech-Language Pathologists by Type of Health Care Employment Facility

Employment Facility	Annual	Hourly Salary (25 or Fewer Hours)	Hourly Salary (26 or More Hours)
General Medical	$61,250	$30.00	$29.86
Rehab Hospital	$58,920	$30.33	$29.65
Pediatric Hospital	$60,000	$30.00	$27.92
Skilled Nursing Facility	$68,200	$35.00	$32.00
Home Health/ Client's Home	$53,000	$60.00	$45.00
Clinic	$60,000	$37.00	$33.00
All Types of Facilities	$60,000	$35.00	$30.84

SOURCE: Adapted from American Speech-Language-Hearing Association, 2005d. *SLP Health Care Survey: Frequency Report.* Rockville, MD: Author. Adapted by permission.

$46,000 in special day/residential schools to $53,000 in secondary schools. In elementary schools, the median academic year entry-level salary (i.e., 1–3 years of experience) was $38,669 compared to $60,000 for individuals with 28 or more years of experience. Those with 1–9 years of experience in secondary schools reported a median annual salary of $45,000; $58,900 for those with 22 or more years of experience. Salaries for speech-language pathologists in rural locations tended to be lower than for those in suburban or urban areas. In addition, almost 12 percent of the respondents who worked full- or part-time indicated that they received a salary supplement, a premium added to the wages of speech-language pathologists holding the ASHA Certificate of Clinical Competence.

Salaries in Colleges and Universities A recent salary study by the Council of Academic Programs in Communication Sciences and Disorders (Shinn, Kimelman, Currie, Goldberg, & Messick, 2004) reported that the average (mean) 9-month, full-time equivalency adjusted base salary across all faculty ranks and categories was $51,870; the median, $49,091. Salaries by professional area were virtually identical: an average (mean) of $52,914 for audiology and hearing science and $51,335 for speech-language pathology and speech-language science faculty. The mean percent salary change across all ranks between the 1998–1999 and 2003–2004 academic years was 9.0 percent. Individuals holding a research doctorate reported a mean salary of $60,565, compared to $47,790 for individuals with a clinical doctorate and $41,046 for those with a master's degree. Other factors influencing salaries in colleges and universities include type of institution (i.e., private or public), Carnegie classification, and tenure status.

U.S. Department of Education Data

As mentioned earlier, one of the challenges in describing the audiology and speech-language pathology workforce involves the identification of nonmembers (i.e., of ASHA), and, as noted earlier, data indicate that many of the nonmembers are employed in school settings. Public school employment data are collected by the United States Department of Education and disseminated through the Annual Reports to Congress on the Implementation of the Individuals with Disabilities Education Act (IDEA). States are allowed to use their own classification scheme in identifying special education teachers of students with speech-language impairments, special education teachers of students with hearing impairments, and for audiologists. In addition, both certified and noncertified personnel may be employed. Note, however, that the United States Department of Education's definition of *certified* differs from the ASHA definition.

According to the Twenty-Fifth Annual Report to Congress (United States Department of Education, 2005), 36,275 "fully certified" speech-language pathologists were employed to provide special education and related services to children and youth ages 3–21 with disabilities in the 50 states, District of Columbia, and Puerto Rico during the 2000–2001 school year. An additional 1,329 "not fully certified" speech-language pathologists were employed. A total of 1,137 "fully certified" audiologists and 48 "not fully certified" audiologists were reported for the same time academic year.

A Study of Personnel Needs in Special Education (SPeNSE) was conducted by the United States Office of Special Education Programs to address concerns about nationwide shortages in the number of personnel serving students with disabilities and the need for improvement in the qualifications of those employed in these capacities (United States Department of Education, 2004). School administrators and other personnel from a nationally representative sample of districts, intermediate education agencies, and state schools for students with vision and hearing impairments were surveyed during 1999–2000 for this study. Respondents reported 11,148 job openings for speech-language pathologists in school settings during the 1999–2000 academic year. Job openings were defined as positions for which personnel were actively recruited. Most of these job openings occurred in suburban areas (6,107), followed by urban (2,610) and rural (2,496) areas. School administrators were asked the extent to which specific factors created barriers to hiring qualified speech-language pathologists. From the respondents' perspective, the greatest barrier to recruiting speech-language pathologists was "shortage of qualified applicants;" 59 percent of respondents reported this factor as having the greatest impact on shortages. This percentage was highest in the western geographic division of the United States (82 percent), mountain plains division (78 percent), and southeast division (64 percent). Of particular note was the potential for shortages in the future. Almost half (49.0 percent) of school-based speech-language pathologists were 45 years of age or older and eligible for retirement during the next 15 years. As indicated in the report, "Unless the number of newly prepared speech-language pathologists increases substantially, a severe shortage seems unavoidable." The report concluded with several suggestions for increasing retention, including capping caseloads, increasing support from school administration, and inducing individuals to work beyond the typical retirement age.

ASHA implemented a focused initiative on personnel issues and IDEA personnel qualifications in 2005 (ASHA, 2005c). Strategies include initiating a data collection effort to increase the understanding of underlying factors that lead to persistent vacancies, developing plans to alleviate these persistent vacancies, lobbying state education and licensing agencies against any effort to reduce state certification and/or licensure standards for audiologists and speech-language pathologists in education and health care settings, and encouraging education and health care agencies to use enhanced salary and benefits packages to recruit and retain qualified audiologists and speech-language pathologists. These efforts are intended to decrease the number of reported vacancies for audiologists and speech-language pathologists in educational and health care employment facilities.

Enrollment and Graduation Data

The National Survey of Undergraduate and Graduate Programs in Communication Sciences and Disorders has been conducted since 1982–1983. The

biennial survey gathers data on the number of programs in the discipline, enrollments and graduations, and faculty and funding issues. Since the inception of the survey, the total number of communication sciences and disorders programs has remained relatively constant. The most recent report—presenting data for the 2000–2001 academic year—revealed several interesting findings (Shinn, Goldberg, Kimelman, & Messick, 2001).

Data for the 2000–2001 academic year revealed a significant decline in undergraduate enrollment in communication sciences and disorders programs—from 35,445 students in 1998–1999 to 16,397 in 2000–2001, a decrease of 53.7 percent. Undergraduate enrollment had seen an upward trend during the early 1990s, reported at 18,223 in 1990–1991 and peaking at 35,445 in 1998–1999. Subsequent data have yet to be released.

The number of master's level audiology students increased by 16.5 percent between 1998–1999 and 2000–2001, from 1,306 to 1,521 students. The number of audiology clinical doctorate students ($n = 124$) was first reported in the 2000–2001 reporting period. A slight decrease in the number of speech-language pathology students was reported between 1998–1999 and 2000–2001, from 12,075 to 11,616, respectively, a decrease of 3.8 percent. Enrollment at the research doctoral level decreased for audiology by 15.5 percent (from 239 in 1998–1999 to 202 in 2000–2001), but increased by 1.6 percent for speech-language pathology (from 443 to 450) and 26.5 percent for speech, language, and hearing science (from 113 to 143).

The number of bachelor's degrees awarded has fluctuated over the years, from a low of 3,923 in 1987–1988 to a high of 7,178 in 1993–1994. The number of master's degrees awarded continued an upward trend, at least up to the 1999–2000 academic year. The number of doctoral degrees granted decreased by almost half between 1981–1982 and 1991–1992. Subsequent years have shown no apparent trend.

The supply of teachers/researchers within the discipline presents a major predicament to the professions. A report issued by the Council of Academic Programs in Communication Sciences and

Disorders (Shinn et al., 2001) suggested that the number of doctoral graduates in speech-language pathology and audiology will not meet the anticipated needs for doctoral-level academic positions. Between 2000 and 2001, 120 doctoral-level faculty openings in speech-language pathology were anticipated, 34 in audiology, and 3 in speech/language/hearing science. A total of 131 doctoral degrees were granted in 1999–2000; however, only 45.0 percent of doctoral graduates accepted faculty positions in 1999–2000.

The Council of Academic Programs in Communication Sciences and Disorders formed a joint ad hoc committee to examine the shortage of PhD students and faculty in the discipline. Results from a 2002 survey revealed that the average (i.e., mean) age of doctoral faculty in PhD training programs was 49 years (Oller, Scott, & Goldstein, 2002). Programs indicated 333 unfilled slots available for PhD students during the 2001–2002 academic year. Funding was the most important factor seen in restricting enrollment. The report concluded with several recommendations to increase the successful recruitment and retention of doctoral candidates. ASHA also has recognized the critical nature of the discipline's doctoral shortage. One of the association's 2005 focused initiatives seeks to increase and promote the number of potential doctoral-level teachers/researchers (ASHA, 2005c). This initiative includes the development of a comprehensive, online higher education data system, coordinating the data-gathering efforts of the ASHA, Council of Academic Programs in Communication Sciences and Disorders, and the Council on Academic Accreditation in Audiology and Speech-Language Pathology.

Ensuring a solid foundation of teachers/researchers is a particular area of concern as the science of the discipline continues to play an increasingly important role in the education and day-to-day practice of audiologists, speech-language pathologists, and speech, language, and hearing scientists. A focus on evidence-based practice, research integrity, and other emerging areas is integral to the future role that the communication science and disorders professions and discipline play in service delivery and scientific research and publication. Doctorally prepared faculty are key in delivering this message to future practitioners and applying it to their research and publication practices.

A LOOK FORWARD: FACTORS AFFECTING EMPLOYMENT IN FUTURE YEARS

As a student or professional, you may be wondering what the employment forecast is for the next few years. This section discusses employment availability and factors affecting it.

U.S. Bureau of Labor Statistics Projections

Between 2002 and 2012, the BLS projects total employment—that is, across all employment sectors—to increase by 14.8 percent, a net employment growth of 21.3 million jobs (United States Department of Labor, 2004c). If both job openings due to net employment growth and net replacement needs are factored into the equation, the total number of job openings is projected to be 56.3 million. The number of new jobs anticipated in health care services—3.5 million jobs—is more than that projected for any other industry (United States Department of Labor, 2005). Health care cost containment, an aging population, technological advances, and advances in information technology serve as contributing factors to the increased demand. Much of the increased demand for health care personnel reflects service occupations (aides, assistants, etc.). The professional and related occupations subgroup of *healthcare practitioners and technical occupations,* under which both audiologists and speech-language pathologists are classified, is anticipated to grow rapidly and result in an additional 1.7 million jobs between 2002 and 2012 (United States Department of Labor, 2004c).

The total number of job openings for audiologists between 2002 and 2012 due to growth and net replacement is projected to be 6,000, a 29.0 percent increase. The projected employment of speech-language pathologists is anticipated to increase from 94,000 in 2002 to 120,000 in 2012, reflecting a 27.2 percent increase over the 10 years. Both professions remain on the list of occupations that were relatively high paying in 2002 and are projected to grow faster than average over the 2002–2012 projection period. The projections also suggest an increase in the number of self-employed speech-language pathologists. This trend may be influenced by a greater demand for contract services by schools, hospitals, and skilled nursing facilities.

Health Care and Reimbursement Reform

Managed care is one of the predominant forces in the health care marketplace today, controlling approximately 85 percent of the market, compared to only 30 percent just over a decade ago (ASHA, 1998). One of the most significant effects of health care reform on the audiology and speech-language pathology workforce has been the increased penetration of health maintenance organizations (HMOs) on the use of service providers. The effect of changes over time in HMO treatment patterns in and of themselves may initiate additional changes in the demand for health care professionals. More aggressive cost cutting by HMOs may further reduce the per capita demand for many specialists, including speech-language pathologists and audiologists.

Beginning in 1998, the Balanced Budget Act of 1997 required Medicare programs to implement a prospective payment method in various provider settings. The Prospective Payment System (PPS) was intended to promote efficiency in health care management by setting limits on reimbursement for care by establishing a set amount to be paid for each patient's case depending on his or her nursing and rehabilitation needs. In addition, speech-language pathology, occupational therapy, and physical therapy services provided to Medicare outpatients in skilled nursing facilities, rehabilitation agencies, public health agencies, clinics or comprehensive outpatient rehabilitation facilities were limited to $1,500 per patient, per year, as of January 1, 1999. Speech-language pathology services shared the $1,500 cap

with physical therapy. Once the $1,500 cap was exceeded, Medicare no longer covered the services.

Successful lobbying efforts by ASHA and other organizations resulted in a moratorium of this legislation. The moratorium temporarily eliminated the arbitrary $1,500 cap set on Medicare Part B outpatient speech-language pathology services that are deemed reasonable and necessary. ASHA continues to lobby for speech-language pathology to be included as an independent rehabilitation service and not combined with physical therapy. However, unless intervening legislation emerges, the caps may be reinstated in 2006. ASHA and other organizations are working with Congress to try to ensure that a more appropriate and equitable replacement is developed for outpatient Part B services under Medicare.

Health care and reimbursement reform may have several effects on the audiology and speech-language pathology workforce. Skilled nursing facilities may elect to renegotiate contracts or switch providers to reduce costs. Employers may decrease salaries of full-time staff, place professionals on an hourly wage schedule, implement hiring freezes, or downsize. In addition, patients may be directly affected through a move toward advanced discharge planning. Certainly, the aftershocks of health care and reimbursement reform will continue to be felt by all health care providers and the recipients of those services in coming years.

Competition

As professionals seek ways to expand their services and as administrators and health care providers attempt to maintain or reduce costs, increased attention has been placed on the use of assistants. Although assistants cannot replace qualified professionals, they can support the delivery of clinical services. Audiology and speech-language pathology assistants have been used and regulated by many states since the early 1970s. In a 2003 study (ASHA, 2003b), 16.4 percent of ASHA-certified speech-language pathologists indicated that at least one speech-language pathology assistant was employed at their facility. School-based speech-language pathologists were more likely to report the use of assistants than those in health care facilities.

There are two schools of thought on the use of assistant-level personnel. Some believe that assistants pose a threat to the audiology and speech-language pathology workforce—that assistants are competing for, and obtaining, jobs meant for graduate-level providers. Others, such as Kimbarow (1997), suggest that clinicians can provide more frequent treatment, longer sessions, and more timely screenings and evaluations to patients through the appropriate use of assistants. It is argued that more service providers will be needed to serve a growing and more diverse client base and an expanding scope of practice. In addition, some tasks may be more appropriate for support personnel than for professional-level providers, particularly within a current health care environment that focuses on cost containment. See Chapter 10 on paraprofessionals/assistants for greater depth on this topic.

Individuals from other professions also may be perceived as competitors for the audiology and speech-language pathology market share. Overlapping scopes of practice or a shift to multiskilling may allow other professionals to provide speech, language, hearing, and swallowing assessments and treatment. According to a 2005 survey (ASHA, 2005d), 12.9 percent of health care-based speech-language pathologists reported that professionals other than speech-language pathologists were providing primary swallowing services (e.g., assessment, treatment, instrumental studies) in their facility. This figure ranged from 4.1 percent of speech-language pathologists in skilled nursing facilities to 47.3 percent of those in pediatric hospitals. Additionally, 9.6 percent of respondents indicated that they had been asked to train or supervise other disciplines to provide primary swallowing services.

Federal Policy

The passage of federal laws and regulations addressing the needs of individuals with disabilities has resulted in a continued and growing demand for audiologists and speech-language pathologists. Federal law guarantees special education and related services to all eligible children with disabilities through IDEA. In 2004, new legislation, the Individuals with Disabilities Education Improvement Act of 2004, was signed into law. The legislation addressed several key issues surrounding the provision of services related to audiology and speech-language pathology, including personnel qualifications, early intervention, English language learners, assistive technology, learning disabilities, individual education programs (IEPs), and funding.

The United States Department of Education (2005) reported that, in the 2001–2002 academic year, 1,093,581 children, ages 6–21, were served primarily for speech and language impairments through the IDEA; an additional 71,222 children were served primarily for hearing impairments. Trend data suggest a continued emphasis on early intervention. More than 300,000 children ages 3–5 were served under IDEA, Part B, for speech-language pathology services during the 2001–2002 school year and almost 7,500 for hearing impairments (United States Department of Education, 2004). The report indicated that speech or language impairment accounted for 55.2 percent of all preschoolers served during the 2000–2001 school year and was the most prevalent disability category. It is anticipated that early intervention services will continue to grow as the nation places a higher priority on prevention and early intervention.

The early identification and diagnosis of hearing disorders in infants and toddlers is part of the national public health agenda. As of October 2005, 44 states and the District of Columbia had Early Hearing Detection and Intervention (EHDI) laws or voluntary compliance programs (ASHA, 2005b). As this issue continues to be brought before state legislatures, more states may enact mandates, thereby continuing to increase the demand for audiologists to oversee and perform these screenings.

The No Child Left Behind (NCLB) Act was enacted in January 2002. This program is designed to improve student achievement through greater accountability, personnel standards, and assessments. Specific sections of the act seek to improve academic achievement of disadvantaged students and language instruction for limited English proficient and immigrant students.

The Rehabilitation Act Amendments of 1998 assist Americans with disabilities to pursue careers through vocational training and rehabilitation. This act continues to serve as one of the most important laws for adult consumers of audiology and speech-language pathology services.

The Assistive Technology Act of 1998 has made individuals with speech, language, or hearing disabilities more aware of the availability and benefits of assistive technology devices, such as augmentative and alternative communication devices and assistive listening devices. It is anticipated that the act will also serve to bolster consumer access to assistive technology devices and assistive technology services, such as those provided by audiologists and speech-language pathologists, again adding to the demand for these professionals. See Chapter 12 on Health Care Regulation, Legislation, and Financing for more discussion of these issues.

Changing Demographics

The changing demographics of the United States population are a key influential factor in the workforce of communication sciences and disorders professionals. Americans over the age of 85 are the fastest growing segment of the population. As the baby boom generation reaches age 65, an elderly population explosion is inevitable. The 85 and older bracket is expected to increase by 43.5 percent between 2000 and 2010 and peak during 2030 and 2040, during which a 60.5 percent increase in the number of individuals age 85 and older is projected (United States Census Bureau, 2004).

The rapid growth in the population age 55 and over will cause the number of persons with hearing impairment to increase markedly. Baby boomers are now entering middle age, when the possibility of neurological disorders and associated speech, language, and hearing impairments increases. The incidence of many communication disorders such as hearing loss, swallowing disorders, aphasia, and the effects of chronic diseases such as Parkinson's disease or Alzheimer's disease, are associated with an older patient population. Lubinski and Masters discuss this issue in Chapter 11.

However, cost containment and reimbursement reform in the health care environment will continue to have an impact on the professions. As more restrictions are placed on coverage or reimbursement, audiology and speech-language pathology services may become unaffordable or unavailable, particularly to patients in older age brackets.

Earlier in the chapter, it was noted that the percentage of individuals in the professions from underrepresented racial/ethnic groups was below that for the general population. According to the United States Census Bureau (2004), the non-Hispanic white population is expected to only increase by 2.8 percent between 2000 and 2010 and 2.4 percent between 2010 and 2020. These percentages are far below those for all other racial/ethnic categories. Hispanics (of any race) are expected to increase by 34.1 percent between 2000 and 2010, and by 25.1 percent between 2010 and 2020; that translates to an increase of approximately 12 million individuals over each decade. The Asian segment of the United States population is expected to grow by 33.3 percent between 2000 and 2010, and by 26.3 percent between 2010 and 2020. The percentage of African Americans in the United States population is expected to increase by 12.9 percent and 12.1 percent, respectively, during the same periods.

To address the needs of a changing society, it is crucial to increase the number of professionals who are from underrepresented racial/ethnic groups. In its 1997 progress report, the Bureau of Health Professions emphasized the need to address the diversity of the health workforce to mirror that of the general population, so that health care professionals can understand and respond to the growing need for access to health care services by members of these communities (United States Department of Health and Human Services, 1998).

The ability to work with and to provide clinical services to individuals from diverse backgrounds is of utmost importance. As displayed in Figure 7–2, only 7.1 percent of audiologists felt that they were "very qualified" to provide services to multicultural populations, while 9.9 percent indicated that they were "not at all qualified" (ASHA, 2005h).

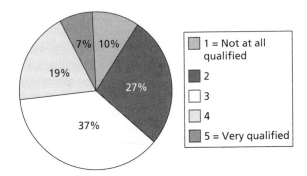

FIGURE 7–2 Audiologists' Self-Perception of Qualifications to Provide Services to Multicultural Populations

Adapted from American Speech-Language-Hearing Association, 2005. *2004 Audiology Survey: Frequency Report.* Rockville, MD: Author. Adapted by permission.

A high percentage of audiologists (61.6 percent) reported using interpreters/translators in the delivery of clinical service to individuals from culturally and linguistically diverse populations (ASHA, 2005h). More than one-third (37.0 percent) reported the use of alternate methods of speech audiometry assessment, and 26.4 percent indicated that they used translated written materials (e.g., consumer information, test instructions, etc.). An additional 13.2 percent of audiologists indicated that they provided a referral to a colleague (i.e., a bilingual service provider) in the provision of clinical services.

Speech-language pathologists in health care facilities reported that, on average, one-fourth of their caseload was comprised of individuals from a racial or ethnic minority group (ASHA, 2005d). An average of 7.0 percent of their patients required bilingual services and/or the use of an interpreter or translator. This percentage was highest in pediatric hospitals (12.4 percent) and lowest in skilled nursing facilities (4.4 percent).

School-based speech-language pathologists reported an average (mean) of 12.2 percent of their caseload as comprised of English language learners, or students for whom English is not their first language (ASHA, 2004b). These data suggest a need for education—both preparatory and continuing—for all audiologists and speech-language pathologists in working with individuals from racial, ethnic, and other diverse backgrounds. See Chapter 23 for more discussion of cultural diversity.

Technological Change

Advances in technology continue to have an impact on the supply and demand of audiologists and speech-language pathologists. Technology has enabled the audiology and speech-language pathology professional to deliver services in a more efficient and effective manner through the use of advanced instrumentation. Medical technology has improved the survival rate of premature infants and victims of trauma and stroke, who may then need assessment and possible intervention for communication, swallowing, and related disorders. The development and application of augmentative and alternative communication devices and systems also have served to expand the client and patient base.

Telehealth

Telehealth provides an example of how technology may affect the supply and demand of audiologists and speech-language pathologists; however, it is emerging as a factor in and of itself and its impact remains unknown. Telehealth comprises the delivery of services through remote means, such as computers, telephone, videoconferencing, or other technology. This service delivery model may allow clinicians to provide consultation, evaluation, and/or treatment more efficiently, more quickly and to more patients. Individuals in geographically rural and remote areas, as well as those who are homebound, also may benefit through greater access to audiology and speech-language pathology services.

A recent survey on telepractice use among audiologists and speech-language pathologists (ASHA, 2002a) found that 11.0 percent of the respondents used telepractice to deliver services. More audiologists (12.0 percent) used the technology compared to speech-language pathologists (9.0 percent). An additional 43.0 percent of respondents reported that they were interested in using telepractice in the future. A 2004 survey of audiologists (ASHA, 2005h) revealed that 34.9 percent of audiologists maintained products, 17.4 percent provided clinical services, and 9.7 percent provided products via the Internet.

The effect of telehealth on the audiology and speech-language pathology workforce may affect either end of the supply-demand spectrum. On one side, telehealth may result in decreased demand as fewer clinicians are needed to provide services. Conversely, an increased demand may result as individuals who previously did not have access to services seek the assistance of audiologists and speech-language pathologists through technology. Issues related to technology and telehealth, are discussed in Chapter 25.

ASHA Data

In recent years, a survey item has been included on several major ASHA data collection initiatives to assess the job market for audiologists and speech-language pathologists. The question and response categories were patterned after definitions used by the United States Bureau of Labor Statistics. The question reads as follows:

> *Based on your own observations and experiences, rate the current job market for your profession in your type of employment facility and in your geographic area.*

> 1. *Job openings more numerous than job seekers*
> 2. *Job openings in balance with job seekers*
> 3. *Job openings fewer than job seekers*

As shown in Figure 7–3, speech-language pathologists perceived greater shortages of personnel in both school and health care facilities compared to audiologists. Almost half (46.1 percent) of all audiologists responding to a 2004 survey (ASHA, 2005h) reported more job seekers than job openings, 34.5 percent indicated that the number of job openings were in balance with the number of job seekers, and 19.4 percent indicated

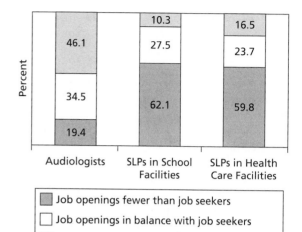

F I G U R E 7–3 Responses to ASHA Workforce-Related Questions by Profession/Facility, 2004–2005

Adapted from American Speech-Language-Hearing Association. *2004 Audiology Survey: Frequency Report 2005. SLP Health Care Survey: Frequency Report 2005. 2004 Schools Survey: Frequencies 2004.* Rockville, MD: Author. Adapted by permission.

that the number of job openings were more numerous than the number of job seekers. These figures are in contrast to 2003 data (ASHA, 2003b), in which more than half (53.3 percent) of all audiologists indicated that there were fewer job openings than job seekers, 30.7 percent indicated that the number of job openings were in balance with the number of job seekers, and 16.0 percent indicated that the number of job openings were more numerous than the number of job seekers. Responses to the 2004 survey varied by geographic region, geographic division, and state, as well as by the type of facility in which the respondent was employed. The greatest disparity between the number of job openings in audiology and job seekers appeared to be in college/ university settings, where 26.8 percent of respondents reported that the number of job openings exceeded the number of job seekers.

Almost two-thirds (59.8 percent) of speech-language pathologists in health care settings reported that job openings were more numerous than job seekers (ASHA, 2005e). An additional

23.7 percent indicated that the number of job openings was in balance with the number of job seekers, and 16.5 percent reported more job seekers than job openings. The largest gap between the number of job openings and job seekers appeared to be in home health/client home settings, skilled nursing facilities, and clinics, where 65.2 percent, 63.6 percent, and 62.2 percent of respondents, respectively, reported that the number of job openings exceeded the number of job seekers. More than half of the respondents in general medical hospitals (55.2 percent) also reported more job openings than speech-language pathologists to fill these positions. Across all facilities, more vacancies were reported by speech-language pathologists in rural areas (64.0 percent) compared to those in suburban (60.0 percent) or metropolitan/urban areas (58.0 percent). Overall, 40.5 percent of respondents further indicated that there were existing funded, unfilled positions for speech-language pathologists at their facility. This percentage ranged from 37.0 percent in skilled nursing facilities to 51.2 percent in pediatric hospitals. Speech-language pathologists in the Pacific (50.0 percent) and New England (48.6 percent) geographic divisions were most likely to indicate open positions, while those in the West South Central (31.5 percent) and Mountain (32.5 percent) divisions were least likely to report openings.

Earlier workforce data on speech-language pathologists in health care facilities were gathered through a 2002 survey (ASHA, 2002b). Results revealed that the largest percentages of unfilled positions were found in pediatric and rehabilitation hospitals, where 61.0 percent and 35.0 percent of respondents, respectively, indicated one or more speech-language pathology positions were unfilled. The largest percentage of respondents indicating their positions were unfilled for more than six months came from skilled nursing homes (72.0 percent) and home health facilities (69.0 percent). The majority of respondents across all health care-based settings reported having difficulty hiring qualified speech-language pathologists. This ranged from a low of 63.0 percent for respondents in general hospitals to a high of 79.0 percent from respondents in skilled nursing facilities. The most

frequently cited reasons for difficulty in hiring were a lack of qualified speech-language pathologists, noncompetitive salary and benefits, undesirable working conditions, and undesirable geographic location. Respondents from skilled nursing facilities appeared to have the greatest difficulty hiring qualified speech-language pathologists. Write-in comments confirmed the reasons cited previously and added concerns such as location was not close to a university, inefficient recruiting, and unavailability of bilingual speech-language pathologists. Overall, the majority of respondents reported that recruiting was conducted using local advertising and networking with professional contacts. A majority of respondents from pediatric hospitals reported they also use national advertising, while skilled nursing facilities were the largest users of professional recruiters.

In response to a 2004 ASHA Schools Survey (ASHA, 2004c), 62.0 percent of school-based speech-language pathologists reported that job openings were more numerous than job seekers. Note that this is a significant increase from 2000, in which 51.0 percent of respondents reported a shortage of qualified speech-language pathologists in their school district (ASHA, 2000). According to the most recent report (ASHA, 2004e), speech-language pathologists in the western geographic region of the United States were much more likely than those in other regions to report job openings than job seekers. The greatest impact of this shortage on the delivery of speech-language pathology services was increased caseload, followed by decreased opportunities for individual services and decreased quality of service. Responses were similar across all types of school settings (i.e., day/residential, preschool, elementary, secondary, combined, or other).

ASHA will continue to gather these data in future years to allow for the analysis of trend data and comparisons over time. The association anticipates that this type of data collection will more accurately represent what is occurring in the job market and be more sensitive to current conditions compared to long-term workforce studies conducted in previous years.

SUMMARY

This chapter provided a description of the demographics of individuals in the professions and discipline, data on employment characteristics, and trends in enrollment and graduation in communication science and disorders programs. Salary data and employment projections were presented. The chapter presented a discussion of factors that may affect the future employment of audiologists, speech-language pathologists, and teachers/researchers.

Factors included the impact of health care and reimbursement reform, technological change, federal policy, and changing demographics of the population. Data from ASHA and other organizations and agencies provided valuable information to assist in evaluating the impact of these factors on the future supply and demand of audiology and speech-language pathology professionals.

CRITICAL THINKING

1. How has the number of ASHA-certified audiologists, speech-language pathologists, and individuals with dual certification changed over the last decade?

2. How does the race/ethnicity of ASHA-certified audiologists and speech-language pathologists compare to that of the United States population as a whole? What strategies would you suggest to encourage more individuals from underrepresented racial/ethnic groups to enter the professions of audiology and speech-language pathology?

3. How might forthcoming changes in the general workforce (using information from the United States Department of Labor's Bureau of Labor Statistics) affect the future number of audiologists and speech-language pathologists?

4. Which federal laws or regulations might have an impact on the audiology and/or speech-language pathology workforce and in what way?

5. How might changes in the demographics of the United States population affect the supply of and demand for audiologists and speech-language pathologists in future years?

6. How will we meet the demand for academic/research professors in future years? What can we do to encourage individuals to seek advanced degrees and employment in academic settings?

REFERENCES

American Speech-Language-Hearing Association. (1995). *American Speech-Language-Hearing Association summary membership and affiliation counts for the period January 1, 1994, through December 31, 1994.* Rockville, MD: Author.

American Speech-Language-Hearing Association. (1998). *Issues brief: Private health plans issues and facts.* Rockville, MD: Author.

American Speech-Language-Hearing Association. (2000). *2000 schools survey special report: Work force and shortage information.* Rockville, MD: Author.

American Speech-Language-Hearing Association. (2001). *2001 ASHA Omnibus survey: Frequency report.* Rockville, MD: Author.

American Speech-Language-Hearing Association. (2002a). *Survey of telepractice use among audiologists and speech-language pathologists.* Rockville, MD: Author.

American Speech-Language-Hearing Association. (2002b). *2002 SLP health care survey.* Rockville, MD: Author.

American Speech-Language-Hearing Association. (2003a). *2003 ASHA Omnibus survey: Annual salaries.* Rockville, MD: Author.

American Speech-Language-Hearing Association. (2003b). *2003 ASHA omnibus survey: Frequency report.* Rockville, MD: Author.

American Speech-Language-Hearing Association. (2004a). *American Speech-Language-Hearing Association summary membership and affiliation counts for the period January 1, 2003, through December 31, 2003.* Rockville, MD: Author.

American Speech-Language-Hearing Association. (2004b). *2004 schools survey report: Caseload characteristics.* Rockville, MD: Author.

American Speech-Language-Hearing Association. (2004c). *2004 schools survey report: Frequencies.* Rockville, MD: Author.

American Speech-Language-Hearing Association. (2004d). *2004 schools survey report: Salaries.* Rockville, MD: Author.

American Speech-Language-Hearing Association. (2004e). *2004 schools survey report: Workforce.* Rockville, MD: Author.

American Speech-Language-Hearing Association. (2005a). *American Speech-Language-Hearing Association summary membership and affiliation counts for the period January 1, 2004, through December 31, 2004.* Rockville, MD: Author.

American Speech-Language-Hearing Association. (2005b). *Early hearing detection and intervention action center.* Available at http://www.asha.org/

American Speech-Language-Hearing Association. (2005c). *Focused initiatives: 2005.* Available at http://www.asha.org/

American Speech-Language-Hearing Association. (2005d). *SLP health care survey: Frequency report.* Rockville, MD: Author.

American Speech-Language-Hearing Association. (2005e). *SLP health care survey: Workforce report.* Rockville, MD: Author.

American Speech-Language-Hearing Association. (2005f). *State licensure trends: States regulating audiology and speech-language pathology.* Available at http://www.asha.org/

American Speech-Language-Hearing Association. (2005g). *2004 audiology survey report: Annual salaries.* Rockville, MD: Author.

American Speech-Language-Hearing Association. (2005h). *2004 audiology survey: Frequency report.* Rockville, MD: Author.

Kimbarow, K. (1997). *Ahead of the curve. Improving service with speech-language pathology assistants. Asha, 39*(4), 41–44.

Oller, K. D., Scott, C., & Goldstein, H. (2002). *PhD program survey results: 2002 executive summary.* Minneapolis, MN: Council of Academic Programs in Communication Sciences and Disorders.

Shewan, C. M. (1988). *ASHA work force study. Final report.* Rockville, MD: American Speech-Langauge-Hearing Association.

Shinn, R. E., Goldberg, D. M., Kimelman, M. D. Z. & Messick, C. M. (2001). *2000-01 demographic survey of undergraduate and graduate programs in communication sciences and disorders.* Minneapolis, MN: Council of Academic Programs in Communication Sciences and Disorders.

Shinn, R. E., Kimelman, M. D. Z., Currie, P. S., Goldberg, D. M., & Messick, C. M. (2004). *2003-04 salary survey of undergraduate and graduate programs.* Minneapolis, MN: Council of Academic Programs in Communication Sciences and Disorders.

U.S. Census Bureau. (2004). *U.S. interim projections by age, sex, race, and Hispanic origin.* Available at http://www.census.gov/ipc/

U.S. Department of Education. (2004). *24th annual (2002) report to Congress on the implementation of the Individuals with Disabilities Education Act, Vol. 2.* Washington, DC: U.S. Government Printing Office.

U.S. Department of Education. (2005). *25th annual (2003) report to Congress on the implementation of the Individuals with Disabilities Education Act, Vol. 2.* Washington, DC: U.S. Government Printing Office.

U.S. Department of Health and Human Services. (1998). *Health workforce newslink, 4*(1). Rockville, MD: Author.

U.S. Department of Labor. (2004a). Civilian labor force 16 and older by sex, age, race, and Hispanic origin. Available at http://www.bls.gov/emp/emplab2002-01.htm

U.S. Department of Labor. (2004b). Employee tenure in 2004. Available at ftp://ftp.bls.gov/pub/news.release/tenure.txt

U.S. Department of Labor. (2004c). *Employment outlook: 2002-12. Employment projections to 2012.* Monthly Labor Review, February 2004, 80–105. Washington, DC: Author.

Zingeser, L.. (2004, November 2). Career and job satisfaction: What ASHA surveys show. *ASHA Leader,* 4–5, 13–20.

RESOURCES

American Speech-Language-Hearing Association. (2005). *Learn about the professions.* Available at http://asha.org/

American Speech-Language-Hearing Association. (2005). *Start a career: Job search tips.* Available at http://asha.org/

Council of Academic Programs in Communication Sciences and Disorders available at http://www.capcsd.org/

U.S. Department of Health and Human Services Health Resources and Services Administration, Bureau of Health Professions available at http:// bhpr.hrsa.gov/

U.S. Department of Labor, Bureau of Labor Statistics available at http://www.bls.gov/

8

Preparing for Employment

ROSEMARY LUBINSKI, EDD

SCOPE OF CHAPTER

Professional employment is the natural and hoped-for culmination of several years of academic course work and clinical practicum in an area of specialty. This chapter discusses how you can undertake the important process of obtaining employment in a productive manner. The chapter begins with a discussion of the paths a career in speech-language pathology or audiology may take. The chapter focuses on how you can create a dynamic and individualized "game plan" for obtaining a clinical position. Major steps in this plan of action include creating a self-inventory, researching potential work settings, preparing a cover letter and resumé, and practicing interviewing techniques. Specific suggestions for accomplishing each stage are highlighted. The chapter concludes with a discussion of how to accept a job offer and how to approach a desired or imposed change in employment settings. New to the chapter is information on part-time employment, benefits, and retirement.

CAREER DEVELOPMENT

To reinforce the good news presented by Slater in the previous chapter, the United States Bureau of Labor Statistics (BLS) predicts that the employment rate for speech-language pathologists will expand at a faster rate than average for all occupations through 2010 (United States Dept. of Labor, 2001). The BLS estimates that between 2000 and 2010, there will be a need for an additional 34,000 speech-language pathologists. There is similar good news for audiologists, particularly because of the aging of the population (BLS, 2005). Thus, you are entering professions with good employment potential. Your search for professional employment as an audiologist or speech-language pathologist is actually the beginning of a career development ladder. An exciting and challenging aspect of becoming a communication disorders professional is that there are many settings in which to work, a variety of types of clients across the age span, and numerous opportunities for branching upward and outward within the professions. Although many of you will remain in your first professional position, it is likely that for a variety of reasons you will move vertically within your profession into supervisory positions; change jobs within your field and move to a different setting or client population; become self-employed; or continue your education and move into academia, research, or management. A small percentage of you will switch to a related field such as education or medical/rehabilitation administration or take off time for family care. In a study of career development characteristics within our professions, Shewan (1987) found that only 5 percent of professionals took extended leaves of absence after entering and working in the field for a time.

Most of you will work full time. More than 90 percent of SLPs employed in educational settings work between 36 and 38 hours per week (ASHA, 2004c). For SLPs employed as salaried employees in health care settings, 79 percent are employed full time (ASHA, 2002). Seventy-five percent of audiologists are employed full time

(ASHA, 2004a). This high rate of employment likely reflects the spectrum of potential employment settings and the number of positions available throughout the United States. According to ASHA's 2002 Health Care Survey, 25 percent of health care facilities had between one and three unfilled and funded SLP positions. Interestingly, 61 percent of pediatric hospitals had at least one unfilled position. The ASHA 2004 Schools Survey (2004c) identified a 51 percent shortage of SLPs in the schools with the greatest need, evident in urban areas and schools with a high percentage of student poverty.

The aging population will increase the need for professionals in all areas of the health care industry, including, hospitals, outpatient facilities, rehabilitation centers, long-term care facilities, physician's offices, home health care, and private practice. Positions in educational settings also remain strong in large urban areas and rural settings. Finally, professionals in communication disorders tend to remain in their positions and change jobs on an average of every 5 years. Shewan (1987) states that, "employment stability provides for continuity in the workplace, an environment conducive to continuous development, and a committed work force" (p. 29). It has also become more common for professionals to bridge two or more workplace settings. Increasing numbers of professionals work in educational settings and "moonlight" in home health care or early intervention during evenings, weekends, or summers. Some professionals who want to work on a part-time basis also look to per diem employment in home health care as a solution. These professionals need to be prepared to meet the assessment and intervention needs of children and adults with a wide variety of disorders. Funding difficulties in health care in the late 1990s precipitated some decrease in the availability of positions in health care settings and a move by some professionals to educational and private practice settings. It remains to be seen if this trend will continue and what long-term impact it may have on speech-language pathology and audiology services in health care settings.

EMPLOYMENT SETTINGS

Speech-language pathologists and audiologists work in a wide variety of employment settings. About 59 percent of ASHA-certified speech-language

T A B L E 8–1 Primary Employment Settings for Speech-Language Pathologists and Audiologists

Educational Facilities

- Public and private schools
- Preschools and day care
- Speech-language development programs
- Developmental centers
- Head Start programs
- Day care and treatment centers
- State schools and intermediate facilities for children with developmental disabilities

Health Care Facilities

- Acute care hospitals
- Subacute care facilities
- Inpatient rehabilitation centers
- Outpatient rehabilitation programs
- Hospital and clinic outpatient speech and hearing centers
- Residential health care facilities: nursing homes, adult care facilities, group homes, assisted living care
- Adult day care programs
- Nonresidential care facilities: home health, community speech and hearing centers, physician's offices
- Public health departments

Colleges and Universities

- Academic teaching
- Administration
- Clinical service delivery
- Research
- Supervision

Private Practice

Corporate Speech-Language Pathology

Industry

The Uniformed Services

Research Agencies

Other

pathologists are employed in educational settings, including public and private schools, developmental learning centers, specialized schools such as schools for the deaf, language development programs, state schools for those with developmental disabilities, and colleges or universities (ASHA, 2004b). Close to 36 percent of ASHA speech-language pathologists and 72 percent of audiologists are employed in health care facilities including hospitals, residential health care facilities, and nonresidential health care facilities. Thirty-seven percent of audiologists are employed in private practice settings as are about one quarter of speech-language pathologists. Table 8–1 delineates the variety of settings that employ professionals in our disciplines. See Chapter 7 for more specific demographics of workforce characteristics of speech-language pathologists and audiologists.

The majority (81 percent) of professionals in speech-language pathology and audiology are employed as clinical service providers (ASHA, 1999). Such professionals may be employed on a full-time basis, typically 35–40 hours per week for either the 12-month calendar or the 9- to 10-month school year, on a part-time basis, or by contract (PRN). PRN means that the professional is paid on an hourly or per service rate, generally with no fringe benefits and no guaranteed number of hours per week of employment. The compensation rate may appear high, but it may not include federal, state, or local deductions. In a time of budget cutbacks, a number of settings have turned to PRN employment, whereby the facility pays either a private contractor or an agency on an "as needed basis." School districts with large vacancy rates may also contract with private practice consultants to augment their workforce.

JOB SEARCH

Some of you will be fortunate to obtain a job through your practicum, externship, or clinical fellowship (CF) experiences. Most, however, will need to actively search for employment. Finding and securing the best job involves a strategic plan.

The process begins with self-assessment and job analysis and involves preparing a cover letter and resumé, and preparing for and participating in an interview. Hopefully, these steps will lead to a job offer for you.

Self-Assessment and Job Analysis

The first step begins with a self-assessment of skills, motivations, and constraints. This step is followed by an analysis of potential employment settings. Job candidates who know themselves and their target agency are better able to market themselves to a potential employer. Succeeding steps include preparing your resumé, going for an interview, and accepting a job offer.

Self-Analysis The search for employment is affected by personal, economic, and job availability factors. Some applicants are restricted geographically in the job search because of family circumstances, personal preference to remain in a particular area, or limited finances to support relocation. Others may live in areas that have few available employment settings and lack opportunities to complete a Clinical Fellowship (CF). Appropriate positions may not be available just when they are ready for employment. Such factors may necessitate a geographic move. Some new graduates may have a commitment to a financial sponsor of their graduate education to work in a particular setting or area. Others may desire and have the resources to relocate to what they perceive as a highly desirable area at this stage in their lives.

The search for first employment begins with answering several critical questions:

1. What is my career goal at this time? What do I see myself doing in the profession of audiology or speech-language pathology in 3, 5, and 10 years?

2. What type of setting(s) and clientele attracts me at this time?

3. How does my immediate career goal affect my long-range career aspirations?

4. What special skills, knowledge, and paid and unpaid experiences do I have that will make me attractive to employers of desired settings?

5. What special skills and experiences would I like to acquire?

6. What geographic areas are attractive to me as sites of employment?

7. What employment settings in those areas match my career goals?

8. What personal, economic, and job availability factors limit my search for employment either in my home area or in a relocation area?

9. What personal, economic factors, and job availability factors enhance my opportunities to seek employment away from my home area?

10. What factors will contribute to a feeling of job satisfaction?

Answering questions 4 and 10 is of particular importance in doing a critical self-analysis. Write down specific actions that describe your personal, clinical, and technical capabilities gained from academic and paid and unpaid employment experiences. For example, what tests and procedures have you *administered*? What programs have you *designed, managed*, or *supervised*? Employers will also be interested in skills and experiences you have had other than those related to speech and hearing. For example, do you speak and understand a foreign language? Do you have particular computer skills, business management or leadership skills, or specialized knowledge of areas such as geriatrics or pediatrics? Have you had research experiences that would be useful in the employment setting? All employers will be interested in your ability to work as a productive member of an educational or health care team. Finally, ask yourself what aspects of a job are likely to give you the greatest satisfaction. Are you interested in direct client care or more interested in program development and supervision? Are you interested in working with a variety of disorders, or would you prefer to specialize? Are you more comfortable with children or older adults?

Never forget that you may have gained valuable skills outside the workplace. For example, consider the skills you have gained from other types of activities such as those related to organization and implementation of programs and involvement with special populations. Individuals who have changed careers or who have managed their homes and families often have valuable skills that will be attractive to employers.

During serious consideration of these questions and others that arise during this pre-job analysis stage, some geographic areas and settings will be eliminated. One person may feel that options to relocate are limited until his or her spouse completes school. Another person may feel the need to work in an area geographically close to a frail and elderly parent. Some may have few personal restrictions regarding relocation but lack the finances needed to support a move to another area, to meet the costs of housing in that particular area, or simultaneously to repay outstanding loans while incurring the costs of relocation. Some may be willing to incur financial debt to pursue an especially challenging and professionally fulfilling position in a desired setting, with a special population, and/or in a geographically ideal area. Others may literally be in the "right place at the right time."

Targeting a Position As this pre-job self-analysis reveals your employment options, certain settings and geographical areas will emerge as best suited for you at this point in your career. The next step is to learn more about the reality of meeting individual personal employment goals in those settings and areas. This can be done in several ways. A first and basic resource in the early preemployment search is to discuss career goals and personal assets and limitations with graduate faculty. Faculty members are likely to be aware of the scope of positions that match your goals. In addition, through their participation in local, state, and national organizations and committees, faculty may know of positions available beyond the immediate area of the college or university setting. A similar discussion with off-campus graduate practicum supervisors may reveal present or potential employment opportunities. Sometimes these individuals will not know of specific positions available in other areas, but they may know of professionals in those areas who could be of assistance.

This is called *networking,* an invaluable means of entry into the professional world. Such discussions with faculty and supervisors serve as pre-interview practice and will also be helpful to these individuals in writing recommendations for you.

A second source of employment opportunities includes the employment listings in journals, bulletins, and publications such as *The ASHA Leader,* the monthly journal of the American Speech-Language-Hearing Association; *Advance for Speech-Language Pathologists and Audiologists,* a biweekly publication for speech-language pathologists and audiologists in health care settings; listings offered by local and state professional organizations; special employment bulletins posted in an academic department; national newspapers such as the *New York Times* (Sunday edition); and community newspapers. Some newspapers publish a special section devoted to employment on a weekday in addition to weekends. The annual conventions of the American Speech-Language-Hearing Association and the American Academy of Audiology offer special opportunities to peruse employment listings, list one's name under "Employment Wanted," and meet with potential employers on site. Similar employment opportunities occur at conventions of state speech-language-hearing associations and meetings of other related professional organizations. Check also listings posted at the ASHA Career Center. Be sure to review the employment section of professional journals in related areas such as education, physical therapy, occupational therapy, and hospital administration. Job seekers interested and prepared for a position in academia might review possible listings in the *Chronicle of Higher Education.* Listings of governmental job positions are available through individual city and state departments of labor and the United States Civil Service Commission.

The newest source for jobs is the Internet, which provides copious information about job search strategies and access to information about all types of settings from all over the United States and the world at any time. Numerous Web sites may include available positions in any type of setting. Remember to check these sites frequently as information change is rapid. See the Resources section at the end of this chapter for samples of Internet and other sources of employment.

A third option for identifying employment in a target geographic area is to do some preemployment research on settings that match your goals and skills. For example, if you are interested in working in an acute care hospital in Chicago: (1) obtain a list of hospitals accredited by the Joint Commission on Accreditation of Healthcare Organizations (JCAHO) or the Rehabilitation Accreditation Commission (CARF) (2) review the directory of hospitals published by the American Hospital Association or your state health department; (3) contact the local professional organization for a listing of hospitals; (4) obtain lists of hospitals from the local Chamber of Commerce; (5) check the Sunday edition of major metropolitan newspapers for position announcements; and finally (6) review the listings of hospitals in the phone book.

A final option for seeking potential employers is to sign with a search firm. Not common in the field of communication disorders, particularly at the entry level, this is a more likely avenue for professionals seeking high-level clinical or academic administration positions and those willing to change geographic areas. Two types of search firms are available: those that work specifically for you and those that are retained by client hospitals or agencies to fill specific vacancies. Should you choose to work with a search firm, it is prudent to have all details regarding expectations and results in writing before making any payment for this service. It is also wise to consult with an attorney or the Better Business Bureau before signing a contract with a search firm.

Preemployment Research Doing some preemployment research on potential employers will be invaluable in clarifying career goals, in preparing a resumé, and in asking for references to tailor recommendations to a potential employment setting. The primary goal of this research is to optimize a match between your skills, experiences, and career objectives with the particular institutional and departmental objectives, programs, and needs. Answer the following questions by reviewing agencies' Web sites and brochures and by talking to those familiar

with the setting. Begin by making a list of standard questions to be answered about each setting to make a careful analysis of options. Some areas to include on an analysis sheet are:

- Name of setting.

- Address.

- Phone number of setting, personnel department, and communication disorders department

- Full name of person(s) heading the communication disorders department (include degree, if possible)

- Number of positions currently filled within the communication disorders department and number of openings

- Description of the communication disorders program (e.g., pediatric head trauma, adult neurogenic disorders, central auditory processing disorders)

- Gaps in the program that you could fill, such as assessment of patients with dementia, dysphagia assessment and treatment, instrumental procedures to assess respiratory and laryngeal functioning, hearing aid assessments, balance system assessment, augmentative communication system selection and training

- Availability of a CF position with the necessary supervision to meet ASHA certification or state licensure requirements.

Although it will not be possible to visit all potential employers for a preapplication visit, inspection of the analysis sheet should reveal several settings that match your goals, skills, and experiences and that potentially have positions available. You may be able to arrange an informal site visit of these settings, thus providing more opportunities to know how to tailor an eventual cover letter and resumé to that particular institution (Baker, 1989). The site visit may also help eliminate the setting as a potential place of employment.

These site visits have a dual objective: You discover more about the program, and the program representative begins to know more about you as a potential job candidate. Even in times of economic constraints on communication disorders programs, there may be potential employment opportunities. It is essential to call ahead and make an appointment with the director/codirector of the communication disorders program, the director of rehabilitation, or the director of the specific division in which the communication disorders program is located. In educational settings, the director of speech-language pathology or the director of pupil personnel services is the likely professional to interview. In some large settings, communication disorders may be located in more than one branch of the setting. For example, in some hospitals speech-language pathology may be located in outpatient rehabilitation, neurology, and/or ENT; in educational settings, communication disorders may be a separate program or subsumed under special education, special services, or some other department. Audiology may be associated with speech-language pathology, ENT, or rehabilitation, or it may be its own department. You should never arrive unexpectedly, and after the visit, you should send a typed thank-you letter to the host.

Continued Self-Analysis After selecting a list of potential employers, you need to continue your preemployment self-analysis. This will involve objective, critical consideration of assets and deficits versus the needed skills to work successfully in the target setting(s). For example, if visitation to a large metropolitan hospital reveals that 50 percent of the current case load is dysphagia and you have no academic or clinical experience in that area, this setting should be eliminated as a potential place of employment until continuing education and further experience in that area can be fulfilled. Although potential employers generally realize that few applicants, particularly those entering their clinical fellowship, can be prepared in all areas, they will want to hire someone who can best fulfill the job requirements with minimal immediate on-the-job training. At this point, you have identified through advertisements, networking, or site visits a number of agencies that are potential employment settings. This is the time to prepare a cover letter and resume.

COVER LETTER

Your cover letter is equally important as the resumé in marketing yourself to a potential employer. This is the *first* impression an employer has of you as a job applicant, and it is a powerful persuasive tool in sparking interest in the resumé. A well-prepared cover letter and resumé are essential in obtaining an interview, the situation in which you actually "sell" yourself. Beatty (1989) maintains that the cover letter reflects an applicant's motivation, organization, and knowledge about the agency. Employers use the cover letter as a critical screening device even before reviewing a resumé. Considerable time should be spent in the preparation of each letter. In *The Perfect Cover Lette*r, Beatty (1989) suggests that applicants have between 20 and 40 seconds to attract the employer's attention and stimulate interest in the resumé. Detailed suggestions for preparing the cover letter can be found in numerous publications, in a library or bookstore, and in materials available through a college or university's career planning and placement office or Web sites. Many colleges have extensive materials, resources, and online examples to help you prepare your cover letter and resumé. These suggestions can be divided into those focusing on style and those focusing on content. Because this business letter is highly critical in projecting you as a potential employment candidate, spend extra time ensuring it is "letter perfect." See Appendix 8-A at the end of this chapter for a sample cover letter.

Style Suggestions

1. Confine the letter to one page. Individuals applying for college level teaching, administration, and research positions may find that they need a second page.

2. Professionally type the letter or use a word processor to guarantee that the layout and design are stylistically appropriate for a business letter.

3. Use good quality 20 pound 8.5 × 11-inch, neutral-color bond paper and matching envelopes.

4. All letters should be originals, never copies.

5. Use appropriate business letter style, such as, full or modified block style, including return address, date, agency address, salutation, body of letter, closing, signature, and typed name.

6. Each letter should be personalized to the person who is responsible for making hiring decisions in your target department. Be sure to have the correct full name, spelling, title, and address.

7. Address the person by the appropriate title: Dr., Mr., Mrs., Ms. Never send a letter addressed "To Whom It May Concern" or "Dear Sirs."

8. Use complete, well-constructed sentences in an active voice. Avoid overly lengthy or complex sentences.

9. Check grammar and spelling. Do not rely solely on Spell or Grammar Check of computer programs.

10. Put the cover letter aside for a few days and then recheck a printed version of the letter.

11. Keep and file appropriately a copy of all letters.

12. Check that you have the appropriate letter with its matching envelope.

Content Suggestions

Generally, the letter contains three or four paragraphs that complement the resumé:

Paragraph 1 introduces you, states the target position by name, mentions how you learned of the position, and excites the reader about you as a potential employee. If appropriate, include the name of a person who has suggested that you apply for the position. Specify why you are a desirable candidate for the position.

Paragraph 2 focuses on your experiences and assets and how these might meet or enhance the needs of the target department. Review your self-analysis and that of the agency to highlight how you can enhance the organization. Review your list

TABLE 8–2 Sample Action Verbs

administered	edited	organized
aided	enhanced	performed
analyzed	established	programmed
appraised	evaluated	provided
assessed	examined	rehabilitated
assisted	formed	recommended
communicated	generated	stimulated
created	implemented	submitted
demonstrated	interpreted	supervised
developed	managed	taught
designed	measured	trained
discussed	monitored	tested
documented	observed	utilized

of action verbs (see Table 8–2) that describe your skills and experiences and choose those that might provoke interest in your resumé. Include another paragraph if you must elaborate on some skill or experience that is of special importance to this job setting. Impart a confident tone without bragging.

Paragraph 3 is the "action" section in which you request an interview, tell the employer to expect a call to arrange an appointment for an interview at a convenient time, and state a willingness to provide additional information. State if you are enclosing additional information such as a resumé. Mention when you are available for an interview and how you can be reached.

Paragraph 4 offers appreciation for considering the letter and resumé.

RESUMÉ

The resumé or curriculum vitae (CV) is the second important tool for marketing yourself to a potential employer. The purpose of the resumé to get you an interview for a position. For job seekers entering first professional employment, this document will be an initial presentation of their academic and clinical background. Experienced professionals will need to review and update their resumés regularly to ensure that career developments such as additional clinical or administrative responsibilities, teaching, continuing education, and supervision are included. The major hallmarks of a quality resumé are that it is well organized, concise, prioritized, readable, truthful, and polished (Eubanks, 1991; Nazareth College of Rochester, 1994). Focus on both functional and chronological information, thus making your resumé a dynamic description of your history and accomplishments.

Again, as in the cover letter, the suggestions for preparing a resumé can be divided into style suggestions and content suggestions. Many bibliographic resources are available for more in-depth suggestions, and some are presented at the end of this chapter. Finally, the resumé should reflect you as an individual and not be a sterile, dull document. Avoid packaged resumés with "fill in the blank" formats. Several drafts will be necessary until one emerges that is clear, concise, creative, and reflective of you, the job seeker. Some suggestions for style and content standards are given next.

Style Suggestions

1. Some job applicants may want to work with a commercial resumé preparation expert to enhance resumé style. Job applicants should research and clarify the scope and quality of services provided and all expenses. The work done by someone else reflects only on the job applicant, not the preparer. Some colleges also provide such services in their career placement offices.

2. The resumé should be limited to one or two pages, particularly for individuals entering the field. Persons with extensive experience *may* require more space.

3. Preparation of an outline helps to organize the major information to be presented. The major words of the outline become the bold headings of the resumé. These headings easily alert the reader to important information.

4. A consistent chronological format should be used to present the history of education and employment. The advantage of listing the most recent data first is that the reader knows immediately where the applicant is and present qualifications.

5. A resumé must be "readable" (Eubanks, 1991). This means that font is of appropriate size; there are 1-inch margins on all sides; headings are in bold or all-capital type to focus the reader; and indentions are used to separate information and are consistent in style across the resumé. Bullets may be helpful in setting off information.

6. Prudent use of varying typefaces is crucial. Headings should stand out but not distract the reader. Bullets may be helpful in setting off information.

7. A resumé that is dense with information prevents the reader from quickly scanning the document and finding information.

8. Brief, jargon-free phrases are the best choice, and avoid the use of "I."

9. The resumé must be checked several times on separate days for typographical, grammatical, spelling, or content errors. There should be no erasures or corrections.

10. Someone else should proofread the resumé for both style and content. Qualified people to do this include faculty and supervisory staff, a college or university's career planning and placement office, previous employers, and colleagues. Check a grammar book or dictionary for additional help.

11. High-quality, 20 pound, neutral color, 8.5 × 11-inch paper, as in your cover letter, should be used. Unusual colors or border designs should be avoided as a means of attracting attention.

12. All copies prepared by commercial duplicating should be checked carefully. Ink smudges, shadows, jagged staples, and torn or missing pages reflect negatively on the job applicant.

Content Suggestions

1. **Identification Section:** The first section of the resumé should feature identifying information, including name, current and permanent address, phone number for the applicant to be reached during business hours of job search, and business address and phone number, if appropriate to be contacted at that setting. Brenner (2005) recommends including a straight forward e-mail address, not something "cutesie" like honeybunny@xyzmail.com. Also be sure that your voice answering machine has a professional greeting.

2. **Job/Career Objective:** Resources differ as to whether a career objective should be included in the resumé or cover letter. Some suggest that it is too restrictive, whereas others argue that it focuses the employer on your goals. If an objective is included, it should be brief but comprehensively describe the type of position you wish to obtain. You may need to customize your objective if you are applying to different types of settings. Limit your objective to one or two sentences.

3. **Education:** List in chronological or reverse order your earned degrees, full name of college or university where obtained, city and state, and dates. Education is listed first by recent graduates or those applying for college/university positions. Recent graduates may include their GPAs if they are especially outstanding—at least 3.5 on a 4-point scale.

4. **Certification and Licensure:** Briefly list any special certifications or licensures you hold or for which you have completed all requirements to date.

5. **Experience or Work History:** This section lists relevant paid professional positions, or in the case of new entrants to the workforce, practicum positions. The purpose of this section is to describe the quantitative and qualitative results of each accomplishment. For example, employers are interested in programs developed, skills learned, revenues generated, and individuals served. Information can be presented in chronological or reverse order: dates of employment/participation, setting name and address, and job title. You should list job duties, highlighting special components of the program (e.g., developed a kindergarten language screening program in an inner city public school, implemented an in-service program on hearing problems of elderly residents for nursing staff). Use your list of active verbs in this section.

6. **Publications:** Any published books, monographs, chapters, or articles should be included here with full bibliographic referencing as seen in professional journals, or what is commonly referred to as American Psychological Association (APA) format. This is the place to include the title of your dissertation or thesis.

7. **Honors:** Include here any professional or academic awards or scholarships/traineeships.

8. **Presentations:** This section focuses on presentations to professional associations, including title, copresenter(s) (if any), name of conference, date, location, and whether invited or competitive.

9. **Professional Affiliations:** This segment lists the name(s) of any professional local, state, national, or international associations to which the applicant belongs. Included also are special roles within such organizations, including committee chair or conference organizer.

10. **Continuing Education:** This section is reserved for professionals who have participated in postgraduate training or education. It is usually listed after Employment History.

11. **References:** The job applicant must decide ahead of time whether references will be included in a "College Credential File." Only the name of persons who have given explicit approval to serve in this capacity can be listed on the resumé. Recommendations for obtaining references will be discussed later in this chapter.

12. **Personal Data:** Resources differ on whether to include personal information such as age, ethnic background, marital status, and number of children. On the positive side, this information reflects the job applicant more personally and often is the "ice breaker" during an eventual interview for the employer. Conversely, such information may be used to discriminate in subtle ways. This is a good

topic to discuss with a faculty advisor or supervisor before you complete your resumé.

LETTERS OF RECOMMENDATION

Students and even professionals may be uncertain as to who serves as a good reference for employment and how to go about securing that recommendation. Good written or oral recommendations are essential in separating you from other applicants with similar or even superior backgrounds. In choosing references, you should consider what the employer wants to know. Although employers are interested in academic achievements, they are more interested in clinical and personal characteristics. Through these letters or conversations, the employer should see a well-rounded, multidimensional professional. Employers want to know the following types of information:

- Do you have the professional skills to carry out the target job? What professional or student experiences do you have that will support these statements?

- What particular professional skills do you have? How have they been exhibited? How have these skills enhanced your present employment/practicum?

- What will you be like as a professional? Employers want to know about your ability to communicate orally and in writing, your reliability and punctuality in completing tasks, your ability to initiate without direction, your creativity, and your commitment to your position. They want to know if you will easily "fit in" with the existing program and if you are willing to grow professionally as demands change.

- What is your self-initiative growth potential? Do you demonstrate a sense of independent career development, such as attendance at workshops, creative problem solving, and participating in journal groups?

- How flexible are you? Do you demonstrate adaptability to changes in schedule, cancellations, and client needs?

- How do you communicate verbally with clients and their families? How do you communicate with other professionals?

- Do you have professional writing skills for diagnostic reports, daily notes, and progress reports? How familiar are you with a variety of report writing styles appropriate to the setting? For example, can you complete Medicare reports or Individualized Educational Plans?

- What will you be like as a colleague? Are you appropriately assertive? Do you know how to work on a team? How well do you take direction and criticism?

- What are you like as a person? Some reference to family or personal background helps the potential employer know you better.

Thus, applicants need to carefully consider both the number and types of individuals who can serve as personal references. Students entering the employment field for the first time generally rely on academic and clinical faculty as well as outside placement supervisors. It is advantageous to have a balance of academic faculty and clinical supervisors who can reflect on both professional and personal skills. Generally, most applicants have between three and five references. Family or friend type references who attest to your positive qualities, but who have no credibility as a professional reference, should never be submitted.

Be prepared when approaching someone to be a reference. This involves calling ahead and, if necessary, making an appointment to discuss reference needs. You should provide the individual with a copy of your cover letter, your resumé, name of target agency(s) and intended individual(s) to whom the reference should be sent, and a brief description of the target position. This information helps individualize the reference letter for a particular agency. Students should generally include a listing of courses taken with a professor, grades earned in those courses, and overall grade point average. Clinical supervisors might like to see copies of semester clinical evaluations. This is the time to accentuate clinical and academic accomplishments.

If you are using a college or university's career placement reference forms, these should be given to your reference person. These forms usually have a place for the applicant to waive the right to see the reference. It is to your advantage to waive your right to the letter because the employer then perceives that the letter is an honest and frank opinion of you. If you are asking for letters to individual employers, provide typed full names, full addresses, and stamped envelopes. Politely ask your reference writers if they are prepared to offer positive recommendations.

Job applicants who are not currently in a college setting but who want to ask an academic or clinical faculty member for a recommendation may need to "refresh" the individual's memory. This can be done by describing any special experiences you had with the reference writer in class or clinical practicum. Employed professionals seeking new jobs may find it difficult to obtain references for several reasons. First, the applicant may not want supervisors or colleagues to know about the potential change of jobs. Second, colleagues may not be in a position to comment on all of your skills. Other sources of recommendations include former employers and other supervisory staff with the proviso that the current job search be kept confidential. If at all possible, references should be sought from your current supervisor, or you should be prepared to discuss in an interview why this information is not available.

Students frequently ask reference writers to give them the letters of recommendation to distribute to potential employers as they go for interviews. Not all will agree to this request. Some writers may prefer to send the letters individually as the need arises, and others may prefer to submit the letter to an on-file service in Career Services. Some will give you the letter in an envelope that has been signed across the sealed flap. Do not be discouraged if reference writers prefer to send individual letters as they may perceive that this is more professional and to your advantage.

Be sure to send a written thank-you note or e-mail to each person who has written a letter of recommendation for you as soon after the letters are sent or you have an interview. These persons have done you a professional courtesy, and you may need them to follow up with a phone call or a form to complete. It is also polite to let your recommenders know what job you have accepted.

INTERVIEW

If you have been called for an interview, it means you are likely one of several individuals whose cover letter and resumé have sparked an interest in the agency. Consider the interview a series of phases: the preinterview, the interview, and the follow-up.

Preinterview

Preparation for the interview is critical because this is when you really have the opportunity to sell yourself to a potential employer. Review of your preapplication analysis is essential, combined with information about the setting gathered from professors, supervisors, colleagues, or friends. Such an information base provides you with confidence to make knowledgeable and constructive comments about the program. Your preparation should lead you to answer both directly and indirectly the major question employers want answered during the interview," Why should we hire you?" You should critically review your clinical assets and deficits with a mind to the target position, leading to a clear concept of what you can or cannot do. Be prepared to answer questions about these areas in a pressure situation. Edis (1989b) states that overestimation of abilities is likely to encumber, although "openness about your faults may also suggest that you are a self-aware and honest person" (p. 55).You must be prepared to articulate how your skills and experiences can match or enhance the target position and setting. Although you do not want to present yourself as a false master of all skills, this is not the time to assume that the employer knows your special skills and assets. King (1993) recommends that applicants should use strong confident language without being aggressive and should highlight achievements without being arrogant.

Practice or rehearsal is the most important strategy of the preinterview phase. This step can involve writing out potential questions and answers, rehearsing them by yourself or, even better, with another person who has some knowledge of the potential position. Role playing with a fellow student or colleague is an excellent preparation and desensitizing strategy (Davis, 1989). Role playing gives you an opportunity to "think on your feet" and answer questions that might not have been considered otherwise. It also gives an opportunity to prepare questions for you to ask the employer during the interview. Role playing the employer gives you an opportunity to predict questions that might be asked. Your questions reveal a great deal about your preparation, interest in the position, and insight into the employer's programs. Video- or audio-taping the simulated interview provides opportunities to review and refine problem areas, particularly in nonverbal communication. On the other hand, you do not want to be so "programmed" for the interview that you appear robot-like and cannot easily adjust to unexpected questions. The interviewer is trying to get a sense of how quickly, logically, and insightfully you think, solve problems, and relate to people.

Types of Interview Questions Some interviewers will ask general open-ended questions that give you freedom to respond; for example, "Tell us about yourself." When responding to this question, focus on what qualifies you for this position, including academic and clinical experiences. Another interviewer might ask specific questions about particular skills such as, "How much clinical experience do you have in doing swallowing studies?" A third interviewer might present a case for you to analyze, for example, "We recently had a patient with a _____ diagnosis. How would you go about evaluating this individual?" One common interviewing technique is to ask applicants to provide examples of how they managed a situation similar to the job requirements. For example, you might be asked to describe a time when you worked on a team to develop a therapy plan. Try to respond with specific information that reflects positively on your skills and accomplishments whenever possible.

Be prepared to ask a few questions during the course of the interview or at its conclusion. Avoid questions that are obvious or purely self-centered, such as vacation and benefits. Employers cannot discriminate against any group (age, gender, disability, etc.) in their hiring practices, but it is hard to prove why someone is or is not hired for a given position. If you ask questions during the interview that are limited to vacation leave, maternity leave policies, health and disability benefits, sick leave, and accumulation of, the employer may surmise that you could have a medical condition, making you appear to be a potentially less reliable worker than another candidate. Asking a few insightful questions demonstrates that you are interested in the agency and the position and have been thinking critically during the interview.

The questions listed in the next section can be used as sample questions for role playing. This list is not exhaustive, but the act of role playing both the employer and interviewee is likely to generate more questions. Remember that the interviewer will not ask all of these questions but is likely to sample questions about your background, interests, specific abilities, and motivations. The Internet also offers sites that include possible types of interview questions; see the Resource section at the end of the chapter for some examples.

Possible Questions from Employer

1. Tell me about yourself.

2. How did you become interested in speech-language pathology? Audiology?

3. What are your primary professional interests? What clinical populations are you interested in? How did you develop these interests?

4. What are your long-term career goals? Where do you see yourself in 5 years? 10 years?

5. Why are you interested in the position of _____?

6. What types of clinical skills do you have that will fulfill this position?

7. How would you plan an assessment for _____?

8. What intervention methods do you find appropriate for a _____ case?

9. How much experience have you had with _____?

10. How would you handle a patient or family member who cried?

11. What experience do you have in completing reports for _____? (e.g., Medicare, insurance)

12. What computer experience do you have?

13. What would you do if . . .? Have you ever . . .?

14. In what ways might you make a contribution to our agency?

15. What do you see as your strengths? Weaknesses?

16. How would you describe your interpersonal skills?

17. How do you handle criticism?

18. Tell me about your most recent clinical placement/job?

19. What did you like most about that placement? The least?

20. What problems did you have to deal with in that placement/position? How did you handle the problem?

21. What were your greatest accomplishments during that placement/position?

22. Do you see yourself in a supervisory position?

23. What is your salary requirement?

24. What questions do you have for me?

Possible Questions to Employer

1. What are the responsibilities of this position?

2. What would my case load be like?

3. How does this position fit into the overall goals of the agency?

4. Who will supervise my CF?

5. Is the position permanent? What happens at the end of the CF?

6. How is the agency or department funded? How stable is this funding?

7. On what type of team will I work?

8. How is patient scheduling handled?

9. To whom would I report?

10. What problems might I encounter with this position?

11. Will I be required to work overtime? How is that time reimbursed?

12. Is there an orientation for new employees?

13. Does the agency have a continuing education program? Is there an education budget for each person?

14. What opportunities are there for advancement in this department?

15. May I observe a clinician today?

Polished Professionalism of Attire and Style

It is critical to project an image of polished professionalism during the interview. This involves tasteful, well-fitting, clean, and pressed classic clothing; polished, comfortable shoes; conservative accessories; and immaculate personal grooming. It is best to dress conservatively in a suit (skirted for women; tie for men) and to avoid conspicuous, trendy colors and patterns, ornate jewelry, heavy makeup, extremely high-heeled shoes or sandals, bare midriffs or legs, short skirts, and strong fragrances. Check your appearance standing and sitting. It is prudent to wear your interview outfit during one of your rehearsals, to check its fit, and to solicit a review from a colleague regarding its appropriateness. Remember to check seams, buttons, and other tailoring before wearing the outfit to the interview itself.

Before the interview, gather several extra sets of your resumé, pen and paper, and reference letters if not already sent to the agency. Carry these in a briefcase, leather folder, or portfolio. Avoid carrying both a purse and a briefcase if possible. A frequent question regarding style of attire is "What if the professionals in the setting wear casual clothes? Won't I look inappropriate in a suit or professional dress?" The answer is No. You are participating in an interview and should dress for that role. Many organizations have dress codes that prohibit visible tattoos and body piercing, acrylic nails, denim, Capri pants, sandals, T-shirts, sweatshirts, and so forth. If conforming to such a dress code would be personally difficult for you, then that is not the organization where you would want to work. Increasingly, hospital and clinic-based programs are allowing clinicians to wear scrubs, particularly if there is any risk of exposure of their clothing to body fluids. There are few professional settings in speech-language pathology or audiology where anything less than business attire would be allowable.

Location of Interview

Before the interview, you should check the location of the agency, parking availability and cost, or needed travel and time arrangements. *Never be late for an interview.* A 10- to 15-minute early arrival gives you time to refresh, greet, and introduce yourself to the receptionist; find the restroom; review materials about the agency; or complete further application forms provided at that time. Dispose of any cigarettes, chewing gum, candy, or breath mints before entering the building. All of these preparations for the interview will give you a sense of confidence to participate in the interview in a meaningful and positive manner.

Interview

The interview should be perceived as a conversation, dialogue, or information exchange between you and the employer. Consideration has already been given to the cover letter, resumé, and letters of reference; so this is your opportunity to convince the employer that you are the best person for the job and will "fit in" to the culture of the program. Krannich and Krannich (1990) state that impressions made of the applicant during the first 5 minutes of the interview are *critical* in obtaining the position. Remember that this is your opportunity to make a good impression and give yourself an "edge" over other applicants.

The interview itself will progress through stages. The first part of the interview, the greeting or introduction, is when the first impression of you is formed. It begins with a firm handshake, eye contact

between the interviewer and you, and a few preliminary remarks or "chit-chat" comments focusing on the weather, travel to the interview, common personal interests, and so on. Be sure to address the interviewer by his or her last name and if the interviewer has a "doctor" title, use that. If you are unsure of pronunciation of the interviewer's name, ask. Do not sit until offered a chair and take the one offered by the interviewer or the one closest to that person. Sit upright, comfortably, but not casually. The interviewer will lead with opening questions such as: "Tell me why you are interested in this position." Another direction an interviewer may take is to encourage you to talk about why you are interested in speech-language pathology or audiology in general. You may be asked to describe your relevant clinical experiences.

Some interviews may begin with the most open of comments "Tell me about yourself." The underlying agenda of the questions focuses on answering the questions: What kind of person are you? What kind of employee will you be? Edis (1989a) states that interviewees should be aware of the style of questions being presented and the focus of the interview. Do the questions tend to be open and allow you a great deal of freedom to answer? Are the questions closed, requiring yes or no responses with little room for elaboration or explanation. There may be some "leading questions" that suggest the expected response such as "How would you deal with a confrontational mother during an interview?"

Applicants should be aware that employers are not allowed by federal law to ask personal questions such as age, health, marital status, children, child care needs, and religion. "To be legally acceptable a question has to be related to the job and asked of all candidates, irrespective of sex" (Edis, 1989a, p. 47). You should be prepared to deal with such questions, however, because they may occur in both direct and indirect ways. For example, during the preliminary informal remarks, questions about personal life may appear in innocuous ways. Applicants should tailor their answer to their own advantage by discussing the job-related quality the interviewer is seeking. Unfortunately, not answering such a question may be subtly held against an applicant. Another tricky question centers on length of time between jobs. Do not say that you have missed out on other jobs, only that you are looking for the right position where you can contribute your skills. Refocus the question by returning to your qualifications. Keep all information truthful, open, and succinct without being terse.

During the interview, you should be sensitive to your own and the interviewer's nonverbal behavior. Interviewers will be aware of eye contact, body posture, gestures, tone of voice, and rate of speech. Firmly shaking the interviewer's hand on entrance along with clear articulation of the person's name and good eye contact tend to make a positive first impression. Active, careful listening skills during the interview are essential. You need to pay attention to both the overt question and what may be underlying the message. The interviewer expects appropriate feedback through nods and smiles and relevant responses and questions. This is not the time to let your mind wander from the topic or situation or allow yourself to be distracted by anything in the environment.

What Is the Interviewer Evaluating?

The interviewer is assessing simultaneously your professional and interpersonal qualities, including intelligence; motivational characteristics; interpersonal skills and personality strengths and weaknesses; competence, knowledge, and experience; and interest in the job (ASHA, nd; Krannich & Krannich, 1998). In addition to assessing your professional competence and problem-solving skills, employers are evaluating your appearance of honesty, responsibility, stability, confidence, enthusiasm, and ability to communicate ideas clearly, precisely, and sensitively. You are being evaluated as much on personal skills as on professional knowledge and experience. Employers are looking to see if you can do the job, will do the job, and are a good fit for the position (Golper & Brown, 2004).

Employers are likely to have numerous equally qualified applicants for a position. Thus, in addition to strong clinical skills, the interviewer will be searching for the best fit: an employee who will fit in well with existing staff and capably implement the agency's goals. At a time when many agencies are focusing on team care, the interviewer will be looking for your ability to share ideas, to act in a leadership role without being dominant, and to generate new ideas. The employer wants to hire an individual who will enhance the organization and will search for the individual who comes as close to the ideal as possible. The employer is seeking to determine not only professional interests and skills, but also longevity as an employee and desire for promotions. Having reasonable career aspirations increases an applicant's value as an employee. Thus, your goal is to project these qualities. It is not unusual for employers to involve a number of people in an interview, especially if the position is one that involves working on a team. This approach allows the group you will be working with to get a sense of how well you will fit with the team and permits you to ask questions of individuals with whom you could ultimately work. This is a great time to ask clinician-to-clinician questions (e.g., How are caseloads assigned? Is weekend coverage required? What kind of documentation system does the facility use, and are staff happy with that?) Even if you are given the opportunity to meet with clinicians or individuals other than the hiring manager, you will most likely still terminate the visit with a brief meeting with the interviewer you met with initially.

End of Interview

You will sense when the interview is coming to a close. The interviewer may have given you a timed agenda if you will be meeting with others. The interviewer will also send nonverbal signals that the interview is concluding, for example, by looking at a watch or asking if you have questions. Keep in mind throughout the interview that its purpose is to get an offer. Thus, during the closing of the interview clearly articulate your interest in the position. The closing of the interview also gives you an opportunity to express appreciation for the interview and briefly summarize your strengths as they relate to the target position. This is when you tell the interviewer where and when you can be reached for further discussion about the position. A student's permanent address may be more useful than a college address. Currently employed applicants must tell the employer the best methods for correspondence. For example, this applicant may want to give a home phone number for a message to be left on a telephone answering machine, cell phone, or an e-mail address. These methods allow the applicant to reply to the interviewer from a convenient location and time.

Should you feel that the interview has not gone well or that you did not feel that this setting was a good match for you at this time, it is still important to end the interview with a positive attitude. Never let your discouragement or lack of enthusiasm show. The interviewer may be a source for future positions or may know of opportunities in other settings that better fit your skills and needs. A polite and sincere exit is important.

Post Interview Follow-up

Within a week after the interview, you should send a typed thank-you letter to your interviewer. Again, appropriate business letter style should be used on 8.5 × 11-inch good quality bond. This letter gives the applicant a chance to express appreciation for the interview, to renew interest in the position, to briefly restate major qualifications, and to explain any unresolved issues raised during the interview. Be sure to carefully proofread the letter. Allen (1992) suggests that if an applicant has not heard from the employer within one week of sending a follow-up letter, a phone call to the interviewer is appropriate. This is actually a courtesy to the interviewer or hiring manager, as they may simply not have had time to contact you, and they can let you know the status of the hiring process. You should prepare for this phone call as carefully as you did for the interview through practice and role playing. This phone call shows that you are sincerely interested in the position and are willing to go a step further to obtain the job. Monday is not a good time to make such a call as it tends to be the busiest day of the week. The interviewer may tell

you the agency has selected another candidate. Should the interviewer state that the position has been given to someone else, express appreciation for the interview and ask the interviewer to keep your résumé on file for future consideration.

Second Interview

In some agencies, a second interview (or third) will be offered to those candidates who appear most qualified for the position, sometimes called the *short list*. It is likely the applicant will be called to schedule this appointment. This interview may be with the Program Director or another individual in an administrative capacity within the organization. For example, when applying to an educational setting, the applicant now may be interviewed by the director of pupil personnel services, principal of the school, or director of special education; in a hospital, the meeting may be with the director of rehabilitation or the head of otolaryngology. In some cases, the second interview will also include an opportunity to meet either formally or informally with a select group of current employees. You may be asked to have lunch with one or more staff members. Be sure to have enough money with you to pay for your lunch if it is not covered by the institution. In some settings such as academia, there may be a reception at a faculty home for you to meet other faculty and their families in a more informal context. Try to circulate during the event to meet as many faculty as you can. The same approach to rigorous preparation, conservative dress, grooming, dining and drinking etiquette, and on-time arrival should be applied to subsequent interviews and social events. Be sure to thank personally the host and hostess of any social events for their hospitality.

Is This Where I Want to Work?

Although it may seem that an interview is one-sided and the interviewee is the only person being judged, an interview ought to allow an applicant to judge the qualities of the organization that will influence his or her determination of *is this where I want to work?* (Golper & Brown, 2004). When making that determination, consider factors such as the following:

- What is the reputation of this program? Will I be proud to say I work here?
- What is the financial stability of the program?
- What are the program's vision, mission, and values?
- Is the facility clean and well maintained?
- Are there sufficient supplies and materials?
- Will I have my own computer?
- Will I have sufficient privacy to do my desk work?
- Do people seem happy?
- What is the staff turnover?
- Are the support and clinical staff friendly, respectful, and welcoming?
- Do people appear to behave and dress in a professional manner?
- Are there others in the program who are a part of my ethnic or cultural group?
- Does the staff work as a team or independently?
- Can I see myself making friends here?
- Is there someone who could be a good mentor for me?
- Is the supervisor someone I can trust? Does he or she demonstrate good leadership?

FORMAL OFFER

Once the decision to hire an applicant has been made, a formal offer will be made. Although many offers will be made by phone, a written offer is essential. Tammelleo (1989) states, "To avoid misconceptions, disappointments or possibly even a lawsuit, get the job offer in writing" (p. 74). The written offer should explicitly state the title of the position, the period of employment, the duties expected, the salary, steps for salary increments, the beginning date of employment, the benefits package, and any other conditions of employment. Such

conditions include appropriate supervision of the Clinical Fellowship, necessary certifications or licensure, preemployment physical, employee evaluation procedures, continuing education opportunities, and expectations. Some of this information will be presented in an employee manual or handbook. Details presented in this document serve as an agreement between the newly hired individual and the agency (Allen, 1992). The more you know about conditions of employment, the easier it will be to make an informed decision regarding acceptance or rejection of that position. Remember that the "cemetery of broken job dreams . . . is full of verbal hiring miscommunications" (Kennedy, 1998, p. A-14).

Consider the offer for a few days (not too long) before accepting. An offer should be accepted with a sense of confidence that this is the best position and that all aspects of the position are clear. You might discuss the offer with respected colleagues or individuals who wrote your letters of recommendation. Issues to consider at this time include salary, cost of relocation and living expenses in a new area, quality of life in the environment in which you will live and work, challenges inherent within the position, and opportunities for advancement and continuing education. These factors become even more important when an applicant has more than one offer at a time. Should you have more than one desirable job offer, you may decide to negotiate with both to obtain the best working conditions and salary.

ADVANCEMENT

Once employed, you may find that opportunities are possible for advancement within the current program, within the larger organization, or even within other settings. Individuals become aware of available positions through professional publications, networking, or direct solicitation to apply for a position. Advancement can take the form of moving upward to positions of more direct program responsibility such as supervisory roles, or it can be laterally in which the individual remains in a similar position but has new responsibilities or type of caseload. For example, in some programs, individuals may become team leaders or have special duties such as coordinator of quality improvement or continuing education. Increasingly, programs have "career ladders" intended to promote staff development and leadership and provide opportunities for new challenges, without having to be "promoted" to a supervisory position. Advancement both vertically and laterally can be challenging and contribute to a more fulfilling career.

Before advancement, some basic questions arise. What duties does the new position entail? What are prerequisite technical and personal skills and credentials for fulfilling the position? Will the new responsibilities be challenging or constitute a professional or personal burden? Will the prestige or financial reward be adequate to compensate for new responsibilities? For example, if promotion entails increased travel, is this be possible within your current lifestyle? What personal accommodations, such as the need for child care, would be required? Should an advanced position be attractive, the application process will be similar to that already described in this chapter: preapplication analysis, preinterview preparation, interview(s), and final offer. A major difference in seeking an advanced position within a present organization is that the interview will be with familiar individuals. Careful preparation is no less important for a longtime employee. In some cases, a current employee may be competing with individuals from both within and outside the organization whose credentials and experiences are equal to or superior to your own.

Should you decide to apply for advancement within your present organization, you need to be prepared psychologically for a rejection. Some individuals may perceive this as overwhelming personal rebuff by colleagues, and it may affect their ability to work productively in that setting. This is an important concept to consider as you apply for promotions within your setting. Having a positive support network is vital to helping you cope should such a rejection occur. While rejection does not usually mean that your current position is in jeopardy, this may be a good time to reevaluate your goals and have a frank discussion with trusted colleagues about your options at this time.

CHANGING EMPLOYMENT

An employee may change employment settings for any number of reasons. These reasons include job loss, relocation, unreasonable demands in current position, lack of opportunities for professional growth, infrequent raises, boredom or burnout, lack of employer appreciation, or readiness to assume new or increased responsibilities associated with a different position (Raudsepp, 1990). Recent changes in Medicare reimbursement for long-term care and outpatient rehabilitation services have seriously affected employment in medical settings. Thus, some professionals may make a job change by choice, whereas others will find this an unwelcome event in their lives.

The new job search may begin while you are employed at an agency, or the process may begin after resignation or termination from a position. Securing a new position while currently employed presents some challenges. If you are currently employed, you may not want your employer to know that a job search has begun. Should the job search become public, how will this knowledge affect your current position? How available can you be for interviews? Should you feel that you do not want your current employer to know about a potential move, options for references will change. You also must be prepared to take time off from work to attend an interview.

In the case of a relocation or a mutually agreeable job change, your current employer will be the best possible reference in securing new employment. In the situation in which a position has ended before beginning a job search, you again have to evaluate the helpfulness of a former employer. Target agencies will want to know the circumstances of why you left the last position and generally will want some reference from that employer. It is important to consider that a current employer is the most important reference for the future; therefore, conditions under which the applicant leaves should be positive—"a graceful exit" (Kroner, 1989). When an employee leaves, employers are sometimes asked to indicate on the termination documentation if they "would" or "would not" rehire this individual. That is a question often asked by future employers when calling for references on a terminated employee. An ungraceful exit, such as leaving with less than a month's notice, is not likely to get a "would rehire" response.

Before you resign from a current position, be sure to have the new offer in writing. Check your agency's policy and procedure manual for contractual information on what time period constitutes sufficient notice of termination. Your present employer must then receive notification of your departure. Include in this letter your exit date, the name of your new position and employer, and the last date of work. It is also dignified to inform your boss before telling coworkers and meet with this person in a formal exit interview. Exit interviews should be positively focused on making an orderly and courteous transition between you and your replacement (Kennedy, 1998). Before leaving a current position, all work should be summarized for a successor, and client reports must be completed and filed. Some applicants offer to help train a replacement. How a departure is handled can positively or negatively affect the tone of future references from the employer.

Many speech-language pathologists and audiologists have felt the impact of changes in Medicare and other insurance reimbursement in medical settings. Some have lost their jobs while others have had positions changed or hours reduced. Although this is likely to be a time of anger, despair, and frustration, it is also an important time to know what your options are financially and vocationally. Be sure to seek psychological support during this time of unwelcome transition. Some human resources departments will have such support available to assist you.

Financial Considerations

Should you be faced with an impending loss of a job, it is critical to plan for the time when you may be without a regular income. To be prepared: (1) know your financial assets and monthly expenses and make a realistic financial plan, (2) reduce all unnecessary expenses, (3) build a 3- to 6-month cash reserve, (4) reduce debt, (5) know the rules regarding any 401(k) or retirement plans to which you have contributed, (6) discuss mortgage and insurance coverage with qualified professionals, (7) investigate your agency's severance package options and negotiate the best one, (8) plan for health insurance while unemployed (e.g., COBRA option), and (9) claim your unemployment benefits.

The Between Jobs Interval

It may take you several months to find new employment. This is an important time to review your skills and update them as this demonstrates a commitment to learning and self-improvement. For applicants who have been unemployed for an extended time, the prospective employer will want to know why and how you have kept your clinical skills up to date. Applicants need to provide clear, concise, and honest answers to these questions. All attempts should be made to redirect the interviewer to the applicant's interest in and qualifications for the present position. It is prudent to maintain your professional certification, licensure, and continuing education requirements during any extended periods from active work. You should also use this opportunity to maintain contact with other professionals who may provide employment leads. Volunteering is a good way to maintain or create contacts and develop new organizational and leadership skills.

SALARY

Two frequent questions job seekers ask are: "Should I bring up the topic of salary during the interview?" and "What is a reasonable salary?" You should be prepared to discuss salary expectations and benefits, although interviewers differ on whether they will introduce this line of discussion during a first interview. It is best to secure the position before *you* bring up the topic. Challenger (1997) states that "bringing up money too early in the interviewing process is one of the main reasons prospective jobs are lost. (It) sends a negative message to the employer that you are more interested in yourself than the job"

(p. I-1). To gauge what is a fair salary, you should do some research in the area in which you are applying. Other professionals in the target geographical area may provide data on beginning or range of salaries. New employees are not likely to get salaries above the average for that position and geographical area. There can be a vast difference between geographical locations, but the cost of living may also be different. Individuals with more professional experience need to factor in their experience and expectations. Do not try to secure a job by naming a salary that is lower than what is considered fair for your educational level and experience in the particular setting and geographical area. This sends a negative message to the employer that you lack confidence in yourself. Similarly, naming a salary that is far higher than your background will price you out of the market. It is more important to impress the employer of your value and potential contributions to the agency before you enter into salary negotiations. It is also best to keep questions about vacations, bonuses, and other benefits until a job offer has been made.

PART-TIME EMPLOYMENT

Some of you may prefer a part-time position so you can devote time to your families or other professional or personal interests. New graduates must know the requirements for part-time work to meet the mandates of certification and/or licensure. Part-time positions, sometimes called *contracting,* have become popular in many settings as they usually pay only for direct clinical service and provide few or no benefits. Such positions may appear to have higher hourly salaries than full time positions. In fact, these positions are usually paid on a strict per hour or per session basis and do not include paid time for traveling to and from client homes, report writing, or conferencing with caregivers or others. There may be a different, usually lower, pay schedule for team or staffing meetings. Travel may be reimbursed at a specified rate per mile if you are providing home care. It is important to know the salary schedule for

services offered, reimbursement in the case of client cancellations, requirements for make-up sessions, travel compensation, and tax deductions from your paycheck. It is wise to consult with an accountant if you are doing part-time work to ensure that you are following federal and state tax guidelines. Part-time employers may require that you do a specific number of hours of continuing education per year. This may be provided through the agency, or it may be considered your own obligation to fulfill and document. Finally, clinical testing and therapy materials may or may not be available from part-time employers. This is an important question to pose during an interview so that you are prepared to provide comprehensive services requested. Again, discussion with an accountant is important so that you have appropriate documentation for any deductions you might be entitled to in contractual work.

BENEFITS

You likely will receive a variety of benefits while employed. The number and array of these depend on the setting, the position, your length of appointment, and full- or part-time status. Some settings offer a hiring or sign on bonus, ranging from a few hundred to several thousand dollars, as a means to entice you to join the agency. Find out when the bonus will be paid and if you must stay with the agency for a specified length of time to receive the bonus (Messmer, 1999). When considering salary, be sure to consider the entire benefits package, including the number of paid holidays, fringe benefits, continuing education benefits, paid professional development days, parking costs, reimbursement for licensure and certification fees, reimbursement for professional association dues and memberships, uniform allowances, flexible hours, opportunities for overtime, etc. In areas where housing is expensive, some agencies may offer corporate housing, a housing bonus, and/or a moving allowance. Some agencies have what are called "noncompete" clauses in their contracts, forbidding you from working for a competitor for a

TABLE 8–3 Possible Benefits Offered to Employees

Health plans	In-house services
Vision/dental plans	CF supervision
Retirement plans	Resource library
401(k) plans	24-hour support from consultants
Paid vacation/holidays	Licensure assistance
Paid sick leave	Direct deposit
Paid personal/ educational leave	Second language learning opportunities
State/national dues	Opportunities for bonuses
Certification/licensure	Opportunities for research
Moving allowance/ expenses	Travel reimbursement
Housing/housing allowance	Child care allowance/ dependent care
Uniform allowances	Parking
Accidental death insurance	Business travel insurance
Disability insurance	Tuition reimbursement
Health club membership	Employee assistance programs

specified amount of time after leaving the agency. An assortment of typical benefits is given in Table 8–3. Remember some of these benefits are for you alone and some may cover family. Increasingly, both employer and employee contribute to cover the cost of these benefits. Your benefits package may be valued at 20 percent to 40 percent of your salary, and some options may not be taxable. Check your employee handbook or the personnel office for specifics.

RETIREMENT

While discussion of retirement may appear incongruous in a chapter devoted to finding employment, both young and mature professionals need to be aware of the retirement plans available through their employers. Retirement plans may or may not be available for part-time employees. Check your employee handbook or raise this question after you have been offered a position so that you know the retirement program to which you are entitled. Retirement planning is a serious and lifelong process and involves new financial tools, including individual retirement accounts. While some settings offer traditional pension plans sponsored and managed by the agency, more are offering "self-directed" programs in which you will both contribute to and direct the investment (Kiplinger Washington Editors, 2005). Good questions to ask your employer include the amount of employer versus employee contributions, time to investiture, transferability, and opportunities for extra contributions and profit sharing. Again, discussion with an accountant or financial planner may be helpful in understanding your retirement options.

SUMMARY

The focus of this chapter has been on how to secure employment. Key concepts can be summarized in single words: know thyself, research, networking, preparation, practice, style, and follow-up. Securing fulfilling employment is a deliberate process that begins with self-evaluation and employment setting research. These analyses help you to tailor and prepare your cover letter and resumé —marketing tools that hopefully will solicit an interview. Careful preparation for the interview gives you confidence and helps you to project a winning image. Contacts made during interviews can serve as networks for future career moves. Leaving a current employment setting also entails careful planning and courtesy. Securing employment may be a challenging experience but will result in the fulfillment of your career aspirations.

CRITICAL THINKING

1. What steps will you take in securing a meaningful job?
2. What characteristics of a cover letter and resumé attract the attention of an employer?
3. What skills and experiences do you have that will be attractive to an employer?
4. What are the key ingredients in a successful interview?
5. Why and how should you follow up after an interview?
6. What are the differences in the job search process for someone seeking first employment versus an experienced professional?

7. What steps should a professional take if faced with sudden unemployment?
8. What are some important facts part-time employees should know about their positions?
9. What types of benefits are valuable to you at this stage of your life? What benefits might you want or need in 10 years?
10. A frequent question posed by graduate students is, "I'd like to work for a few years in a hospital and then when I have a family, switch to the schools. Is this realistic?" How would you answer this question?

REFERENCES

Allen, J. (1992). *The perfect follow-up method to get the job.* New York: John Wiley.

American Speech-Hearing-Language Association. (1992). *1992 update on personnel shortages.* Rockville, MD: Author.

American Speech-Hearing-Language Association. (1997). *Tools for a successful job search.* Rockville, MD: Author.

American Speech-Hearing-Language Association. (1999). *1999 Omnibus survey: Salary report.* Rockville, MD: Author.

American Speech-Hearing-Language Association. (2002). *Speech language pathology health care survey: Executive summary.* Available at http:// www.asha.org/

American Speech-Hearing-Language Association. (2004a). *Demographic profile of ASHA member and nonmember certificate holders certified in audiology only. Highlights and trends: ASHA counts for 2004.* Rockville, MD: Author.

American Speech-Hearing-Language Association. (2004b). *Demographic profile of ASHA member and nonmember certificate holders certified in speech-language pathology only. Highlights and trends: ASHA counts for 2004.* Rockville, MD: Author.

American Speech-Hearing-Language Association. (2004c). *2004 Schools survey.* Rockville, MD: Author.

Baker, J. (1989). Preparing a curriculum vitae. *Nursing Times, 85,* 56–58.

Beatty, R. (1989). *The perfect cover letter.* New York: John Wiley.

Brenner, L. (2005, June 12). How to land your first job. *Parade Magazine, 18.*

Bureau of Labor Statistics. (2005). *Audiologists.* Available at http://bls.gov/oco/ocos085.htm.

Challenger, J. (1997, September 14). How to negotiate salary: Don't settle for less than you have to. *Buffalo News,* I–1.

Davis, W. (1989). Simulated job interviews as learning devices. *Academic Medicine, 64,* 438–439.

Edis, M. (1989a). The interview: 2. Games people play. *Nursing Times, 85,* 45–47.

Edis, M. (1989b). The interview: 1. Rules of the game. *Nursing Times, 85,* 54–55.

Eubanks, P. (1991). Experts: Making your resumé an asset. *Hospitals, 65,* 74.

Golper, L. & Brown, J. (Eds.) (2004). Business matters: A guide to business practices for speech-language pathologist. Rockville, MD: ASHA Publication.

Kennedy, J. L. (1998, September 12). When it's time to resign, do it with savvy. *Buffalo News,* A–14.

King, J. (1993). *The smart woman's guide to interviewing and salary negotiation.* Franklin Lakes, NJ: Career Press.

Kiplinger Washington Editors. (2005). *Retire worry-free* (5th ed.). Chicago: Dearborn Trade Publishing.

Krannich, C., & Krannich, R. (1990). *Interview for success.* Woodbridge, VA: Impact Publications.

Krannich, C., & Krannich, R. (1998). *Interview for success: A practical guide to increasing job interviews, offers, and salaries* (7th ed.). Woodbridge, VA: Impact Publications.

Kroner, K. (1989). Take the gamble out of changing jobs. *Nursing, 20,* 111–118.

Messmer, M. (1999). *Job hunting for dummies* (2nd ed.). New York: Wiley.

Nazareth College of Rochester. (1994). *Guide to resumé writing.* Rochester, NY: Author.

Raudsepp, E. (1990). Knowing when to look for a new job. *Nursing, 20,* 136–140.

Shewan, C. (1987). Some characteristics of career development in the speech-language-hearing profession. *Asha, 29,* 27–29.

Shewan, C. (1989). ASHA work force study. *Asha, 31,* 63–67.

Tammelleo, A. D. (1989). Ways to pin down an employer's promise. *Registered Nurse, 52,* 74–78.

U.S. Department of Labor. (2001). *Occupational employment projections to 2010. November 2001.* Washington, D.C.: Author.

RESOURCES

Securing Employment

Check your local library or bookstore for the section on employment or business.

There are dozens of texts on topics such as interviewing, resumé preparation, and follow-up methods. Most college or university departments receive notices of job vacancies. These may be posted or available in a department administrator's office. Check your local communication disorders department for such information. The monthly publication *The ASHA Leader* has a section on employment opportunities.

ADVANCE. This free weekly publication of Merion Publications lists available employment positions by geographic area. For information, write to 2900 Horizon Drive, Box 61556, King of Prussia, PA 19406-0956. Web site: http://www.ADVANCE-forSPandA.com.

American Academy of Audiology. In addition to job listings and opportunities for interviews at the annual convention, check for current job listings at http://www.audiology.org. For information, write to 11730 Plaza America Drive, Suite 300, Reston, VA 20190, or call 800-AAA-2336.

ASHA Leader. This twice monthly publication of the American Speech-Language-Hearing Association lists job openings. Positions are updated weekly on ASHA's Web site.

ASHA and State Conventions. There is a Placement Center at the annual ASHA convention held each November. State conventions may also have the same service.

ASHA Career Center—the official career center for jobs in communicative disorders. http://www.asha.org/aboutcareer

Federal Government Uniformed Services Positions

U.S. Public Health Service Recruitment
500 Fishers Lane 4A-18
Rockville, MD 20857
Phone: 800-279-1605
Web site: http://www.usphs.gov

Navy
U.S. Navy Recruiting District Washington
Presidential Building, Room 285,
6525 Belcrest Road
Hyattsville, MD 20782-2082
Phone: 301-394-0500

Air Force (military position)
U.S. Air Force Health Professions
4815 Fredericksburg Road
San Antonio, TX 78229-3627
Phone: 210-341-6802

Air Force (civilian)
Civilian Personnel Headquarters
U.S. Air Force, The Pentagon
Washington, DC 20331
Phone: 703-697-3127

Dependent Schools on Military Bases
Department of Defense
Office of Dependent Schools
4040 N. Fairfax
Arlington, VA 22203
Phone: 703-696-3033

Internet Sources

NOTE that the following sources are fluid and should be checked periodically for their availability and current Internet addresses.

Advance Publications
http://www.ADVANCEforSPandA.com

America's Health Care Source
http://www.healthcaresource.com

American Hearing Aid Associations
http://www.ahaanet.com/

America's Job Bank
http://www.jobsearch.org

ASHA
http://www.asha.org/professionals/careers/resume.htm

Audiology Depot
http://www.audiologydepot.com

Audiologyonline.com
http://www.audiologyonline.com

Audiology Jobs
http://www.audiologyjobs.net

Audiology Job Web
http://www.audiologyinfo.com/websites/jobweb

Career Builder.com
http://www.careerbuilder.com

Career Path
http://www.careerpath.com

HireTherapy.com
http://www.hiretherapy.com

MedHunters
http://www.medhunters.com

MedSearch
http://www.medsearch.com

Monster.com
http://www.monster.com

Rehab.Career.com
http://www.rehabcareer.com

Rehab Quest
http://www.rehabquest.com

Rehabworld.com
http://rehabworld.com

SLPJOB.com
http://www.slpjob.com

Speech Pathology.com
http://www.speechpathology.com

Therapy Jobs
http://www.therapyjobs.com/speech

Sample Interview Questions

http://www.best-interview-strategies.com/questions.html

http://www.espan.com/docs/intprac.html

http://www.studentcenter.com/brief/virtual/virtual/htm

State and Local Association Resources

Contact your state or local professional association to determine if it has a job listing or matching service. For state association contact information, visit ASHA's Web site http://www.asha.org/professionals/governmental-affairs/state-associations.htm

APPENDIX 8–A

Sample Cover Letter

123 Prescote Avenue
Rochester, New York 14226
March 29, 2007

Rochelle Peteers, Ph.D.
Director Audiology Program,
Fairwell Rehabilitation Hospital
5342 Burroughs Way
Toronto, ON M3B 2R2
Canada

Dear Dr. Peteers:

I am very interested in the position of clinical audiologist at Fairwell Rehabilitation Hospital. I was informed of this position by my recent Clinical Fellowship supervisor, Dr. Bernard Trippe, who is in private audiology practice in Rochester, New York. I will receive my Au.D. from the University of Buffalo on June 1, 2007, by which time I will have met all requirements for CASLPA registration and New York State Licensure.

Given the cultural and linguistic diversity of your clientele, I understand your clinic's growing need for foreign language expertise. As a clinician proficient in six languages, including Spanish, Italian, French, Mandarin, and Cantonese, I am uniquely suited to helping the Fairwell Rehabilitation Hospital Audiology Program reach a higher level of client service—one that truly meets the needs of the multiethnic Greater Toronto area.

During my doctoral program at the University of Buffalo, I provided more than 2,000 hours of diagnostic and counseling services to children and adults in clinic, hospital, education, and private practice settings. I earned more than 200 hours in fitting digital hearing aids. My culminating project focused on follow-up audiololgy services for children who have received a cochlear implant. I presented the results of my study at a recent convention of the American Academy of Audiology in Baltimore, Maryland. I was also recipient of the Jack Katz Scholarship for my work with school-aged children with central auditory processing disorders.

I feel that my skills and experience would enable me to make a valuable contribution to the Fairwell Rehabilitation Hospital, and I would greatly appreciate an opportunity to discuss my qualifications with you in person. I will call within the coming week to arrange an appointment as your schedule allows. I can be reached by telephone at (716) 839-5555 at any time, or by e-mail at lincsmith21@abcd.edu.

Sincerely,

Linda Chau-Smith

APPENDIX 8–B

Sample Resumé

CATHERINA WILLIAMSON
cwlmsn@abcd.edu

25 Longview Court
Buffalo, NY 14226
(716) 555-6629

EDUCATION

University at Buffalo, Buffalo, NY
M.A. in Speech-Language Pathology, 2006
Member of National Student Speech-Language-Hearing Association
Research in Literacy Scholarship
Who's Who Among Students in American Universities and Colleges

Cornell University, Ithaca, NY
B.A. in Spanish and Linguistics, 2003
Graduated Summa Cum Laude, Phi Beta Kappa

PRACTICUM EXPERIENCES

Graduate Clinician Speech-Language Pathology

Waterville Elementary School, Buffalo, NY   February–May 2007

- Provided assessment and intervention services for severely impaired bilingual children
- Presented a 6-week communication enhancement education program for Spanish-speaking parents.
- Conducted hearing screenings for preschool program
- Developed Individual Education Programs for school-age children

Harwick Neurological Hospital, Buffalo, NY   September–December 2006

- Provided assessment and intervention clinical services for outpatient adult aphasia program
- Conducted weekly adult aphasia group program
- Provided assistive communication assessments for children with severe neurological impairments
- Assisted with bedside dysphagia evaluations

University at Buffalo Speech-Language and Hearing Clinic   January–August 2006

- Provided comprehensive diagnostic assessments and therapy for adults and children with aphasia, motor speech disorders, phonological disorders, voice disorders, and stuttering
- Conducted intensive 6-week group language/learning program for high school students
- Performed hearing screenings for elders at Amherst Senior Center
- Conducted weekly speech and language screenings at Bright Beginnings Head Start Program

VOLUNTEER

Literacy Volunteers of America Buffalo Branch   September 2005-present

PRESENTATION

Williamson, C. and Duncan, J. (April 2006). Techniques for Enhancing Language and Literacy of Older Students. Paper presented at the Annual Convention of New York State Speech-Language-Hearing Association, Saratoga Springs, New York.

SPECIAL ABILITIES

Fluent in Spanish and American Sign Language
Computer Skills in HTML, CSS, MS Office, Adobe Acrobat

REFERENCES WILL BE SENT UPON REQUEST

9

Professional Autonomy
and Collaboration

JANET E. BROWN, MA
JAYNEE A. HANDELSMAN, PHD

SCOPE OF CHAPTER

Autonomy is the foundation of our professional identity as audiologists and speech-language pathologists (SLPs), while collaboration connects us to the broader clinical community of service providers. Anyone receiving professional services expects to receive them from an individual who meets established standards as a qualified professional and who can provide independent judgment based on knowledge and experience. At the same time, we expect the professional treating us to consult and collaborate with individuals from other disciplines when it is appropriate. External factors such as national and state regulations, facility policies, and payer requirements now place additional constraints on professional decision making. This chapter defines and describes professional autonomy from an official standpoint and discusses some of the challenges of autonomy and collaboration in real-life situations.

DEFINITIONS OF AUTONOMY AND COLLABORATION

Autonomy simply means the ability of an individual or group to make independent decisions regarding behavior. According to Princeton University's WordNet® (2003), it is defined as freedom from the arbitrary exercise of authority, which includes political and personal independence, and is synonymous with liberty and self-direction. Being autonomous, then, means being independent in mind or judgment and being self-directed (American Heritage, 2000). When the word is used to apply to a group, it also refers to self-governance and being free from the control of outside forces.

Speech-language pathology and audiology are recognized to be autonomous professions devoted to clinical service delivery, education, and research in the areas of normal and disordered human communication (ASHA, 1986). ASHA defined an autonomous profession as "one in which the practitioner has the qualifications, responsibility, and authority for the provision of services which fall within its scope of practice" (p. 53). While being autonomous does not mean that an individual or group is free from being monitored or regulated by external bodies such as licensure boards, it does mean that individuals within the professions have the authority to define qualifications for practice, ethical standards, scopes of practice, and preferred practice patterns.

Collaboration refers to working together to accomplish a mutual goal. According to the dictionary, collaboration is particularly relevant to intellectual effort and includes cooperation (Princeton University, 2003). Collaboration, as it relates to the discipline of communication disorders, is important to providing optimal services to persons served and can occur between speech-language pathologists and audiologists. It could also occur between other professions. For example, in a medical setting, audiologists typically work with physicians to establish plans of care for individuals with balance system disorders. Similarly, speech-language pathologists may collaborate with physicians to establish plans of

care for clients being treated for head and neck cancer. Therefore, while collaboration, by definition, would appear to be at odds with autonomy, we know that both are important to the discipline as a whole, and to individuals within the professions of speech-language pathology and audiology. The following sections discuss the application of factors related to autonomy and collaboration in these professions.

Sources of Professional Autonomy

One of the factors related to establishing professional autonomy is the definition of qualifications for practice, which is covered in detail in Chapter 2. Historically, the criteria for obtaining the Certificate of Clinical Competence (CCC) have been used as to define the qualifications for entry into the professions. Specifically, the CCC-SLP is awarded to individuals in the profession of speech-language pathology who have met the minimum criteria specified by the Council for Clinical Certification, (CFCC), and the CCC-A is awarded to individuals in the profession of audiology meeting the specified criteria (ASHA, 2005b). The current criteria include the following requirements:

1. A minimum of 75 semester credit hours culminating in a master's, doctoral, or other recognized graduate degree within a program that is accredited by ASHA's Council on Academic Accreditation in Audiology and Speech-Language Pathology (CAA)

2. Demonstrated knowledge of ethical standards, research principles, applicable professional and regulatory issues, and skills in oral and written communication

3. A minimum of 400 clock hours of supervised clinical experiences that encompass the entire scope of practice throughout the age span, including 375 hours of direct client contact and 25 hours of observation

4. A 36-week clinical fellowship

5. Obtaining a passing score on the Praxis examination

Differences for audiologists:

1. Effective January, 2012, a doctoral degree (AuD or other doctoral degree) will be required for certification in audiology (ASHA, 2005b).

2. Effective 2007, instead of a clinical fellowship, graduate programs must include practicum experiences equivalent to a minimum of 12 months of full-time, supervised work spread over the course of the graduate study.

In both areas of practice, maintenance of clinical certification also includes continuing education requirements as specified.

Other qualifications for clinical practice are determined by the location and setting in which an individual practices. Most states now require state licensure. Generally, individuals within the professions are included on licensure boards and in so doing participate in crafting the rules for practice included in licensing bills. Similarly, individuals working in the schools may be required to hold teacher certification, and clinicians employed in hospital settings may be required to obtain specific credentialing. While other stakeholders may be included in determining the specific qualifications for practice in these cases, involvement of individuals within the professions is important to our professional autonomy.

Ethical standards for the professions are specified in the Codes of Ethics of our professional organizations. Specifically, ASHA's Code of Ethics (ASHA, 2003) sets forth the essential principles and rules necessary to preserve the highest standards of ethical behavior and integrity that are vital to the responsible practice of SLPs, audiologists, and speech, language, and hearing scientists. The ASHA Code of Ethics applies to individuals who are members, certificate holders, and in the certification process. Similarly, the Code of Ethics of the American Academy of Audiology specifies what that organization considers to be appropriate professional ethical standards for audiologists in an effort to protect the integrity of the profession (AAA, 2005).

The principles and rules specified by the ASHA Code of Ethics outline ethical behavior as it relates to professionals honoring their responsibility to persons served by holding their welfare paramount, honoring their responsibility to achieve and maintain the highest level of competence, honoring their responsibility to the public, and honoring their responsibilities to the professions, including relationships with colleagues, students, and members of allied professions.

While certification and licensure requirements specify the minimum qualifications to practice speech-language pathology and audiology, the Code of Ethics holds individuals within the professions to a higher standard. In addition to meeting the requirements of certification, the Code requires that "Individuals shall engage in only those aspects of the professions that are within the scope of their competence, considering their level of education, training, and experience" (Principle II, Rule B). Thus, while there may not be a legal constraint to accepting a job in any setting, the Code of Ethics mandates that an individual has adequate training in the specific area of practice and with a given population to provide services competently. For example, a speech-language pathologist may decide to accept a new job at a hospital because of increased professional opportunities and increased salary. While previous hospital experience may satisfy the potential employer in terms of credentials for practice, if the new job includes working in the Neonatal Intensive Care Unit (NICU), competence in the area of feeding disorders in infants would be a necessary prerequisite from an ethical perspective. Similarly, although vestibular assessment and rehabilitation are within the scope of practice of audiology and employers may expect audiologists to conduct vestibular testing and perform particle repositioning maneuvers when indicated, the Code of Ethics compels audiologists and SLPs to refrain from practicing in any area in which adequate knowledge and skills have not been acquired.

The areas of practice within the professions are outlined in scope of practice documents. The ASHA scope of practice document for audiology (ASHA, 2004d) describes the services provided by qualified audiologists serving in various roles, serving as a reference for interested parties about the profession, and informing ASHA members, certificate holders, and students of the professional activities for which the CCC-A is required. Similarly, the scope of practice document in speech-language pathology (ASHA, 2001b) specifies areas of practice within the profession and defines professional activities for which the CCC-SLP is required.

The preferred practice documents (ASHA, 2004c, 1997b) were created to enhance the quality of professional services in speech-language pathology and audiology by outlining procedural aspects of clinical service. The documents include "statements that define universally acceptable characteristics of activities directed toward individual clients, and that address structural requisites of the practice, processes to be carried out, and intended outcomes" (ASHA, 1997b, p. 4). The practice patterns are designed to be generic and apply to all practice settings; they are organized by procedure as defined by the scope of practice and other ASHA documents. The audiology preferred practice document includes 23 individual practice patterns, while the speech-language pathology document includes 47 practice patterns. Each practice pattern in both documents refers to fundamental components and guiding principles as specified.

The scope of practice and preferred pattern documents define the realm of speech-language pathologists' and audiologists' professional activities and the populations and disorders they serve. In combination with certification, licensure, and codes of ethical professional conduct, they serve the purpose of protecting consumers by defining the qualifications for practice and the scope of the professions. Not only do these guidelines provide information about what is within the scopes of the professions, they prevent SLPs and audiologists from performing procedures that fall into the scopes of other professionals. For example, it is clear that SLPs may not interpret magnetic resonance imaging (MRI) studies and audiologists may not place tympanostomy tubes. The documents are dynamic and subject to periodic review. Accordingly, new procedures or areas of practice are added when appropriate, just as dysphagia became part of the scope of practice for speech-language pathologists in the 1980s and audiologists have added cerumen management and intra-operative surgical monitoring to their practice. Ideally, individuals within the professions are responsible for defining the scopes of

practice and for articulating the preferred practice patterns. However, as speech-language pathologists and audiologists add areas of practice or when our scopes overlap with those of other professions, other stakeholders are likely to become more involved.

Legal Autonomy of the Professions

Being a certified and/or licensed professional allows SLPs and audiologists to work in the setting of their choice and to be in private practice as long as they comply with professional ethics and state regulations. As individuals practicing within autonomous professions, SLPs and audiologists may see clients without a physician's prescription or order. This is in direct contrast to physical therapists (PTs) and occupational therapists (OTs), who in many states must have a prescription from a physician in order to provide clinical services. State licensure boards, which exist to regulate practice and protect consumers within the state, have deemed that consumers can consult speech-language pathologists and audiologists without physician prescriptions. While the specific rules within the license may limit the scope of practice of audiologists or SLPs within a given state, or may require physician referral for the completion of certain types of services, audiologists and SLPs are able to practice independently. This means that they can independently determine which tests to administer, interpret results, make a communication diagnosis, and provide intervention without direction from a physician. Autonomy does not mean that clients are best served by having professionals operating in a vacuum without physician consultation, but it allows them to use independent judgment. Note that the term *prescription* is used specifically to refer to professions that can only provide services when prescribed by a physician. On the other hand, referrals are often part of the process required by payers to initiate SLP or audiology services.

Referrals

Institutional employment settings that provide clinical services, including hospitals, clinics, schools, and other settings, must have policies and procedures to ensure consistency and accountability for the manner in which the services are provided. Facilities are often accountable to government agencies such as the state department of health or state education agencies to be in compliance with state policies. Facilities may also seek accreditation by voluntary accrediting organizations such as the Joint Commission on Accreditation of Healthcare Organizations (JCAHO) or the Commission on Accreditation of Rehabilitation Facilities (CARF). Government agencies may audit client records and accounting practices, and accrediting organizations may perform periodic reviews to ensure that facilities are adhering to specified requirements or standards. Standards and procedures that are developed within institutions or facilities to comply with accrediting groups seek to ensure the quality and safety of the services to persons served and to establish administrative procedures for the facility's streamlined and efficient operation.

Within health care organizations, it is common for policies and procedures to require that physicians initiate referrals for services from other professions, including speech-language pathology and audiology evaluations or interventions. Typically, the "privilege" of admitting a client to the facility is limited to only members of the medical staff with certain credentials, such as licensed physicians. Essentially, the facility (hospital, rehabilitation inpatient facility, skilled nursing facility) provides a setting for the physician to admit and care for his/her client. The admitting physician, therefore, is legally responsible for decisions regarding the nature and extent of services provided and thus is required to "order" all services—from the level of nursing care required to the client's diet. In care settings managed under health maintenance organizations (HMOs), an outpatient referral from a primary care physician (PCP) is typically required for any specialty consultation or service (e.g., otolaryngology, radiology, audiology, speech-language pathology). This serves a dual purpose of ensuring that the primary care physician coordinates and participates in all aspects of the client's care, and it establishes a "gatekeeping" process for ensuring that physicians document their authorization for services for insurance purposes. While SLPs and audiologists have the right to practice independently, communication and collaboration with medical professions are often essential for optimal client care. Policies and procedures regarding how referrals are managed can be used to facilitate that collaboration.

In addition to complying with standards for quality and safety, health care providers are also responsible for meeting the bottom line—namely, generating sufficient revenue to pay for salaries, supplies, and operating costs of the facility. This financial reality means facilities and individual providers must meet requirements set by various payment sources, including Medicare, Medicaid, private health plans, HMOs, preferred provider organizations (PPOs), and private contracts. Inasmuch as the insurance providers and others are free to establish criteria for payment, it may be difficult for SLPs and audiologists to keep up with current standards. In reality, it often seems that professionals are asked to shoot at moving targets to obtain payment for services, and it is typical for physicians and insurance company administrators to be involved in making decisions about covered services. For example, payers for speech, language, and/or swallowing services typically require that a physician serve as a gatekeeper by attesting to the need for the services by signing a referral. In some cases, then, SLPs must advocate for authorization of services by persuading the primary care physician that specific services are needed. Similarly, an SLP in private practice may be required to obtain a referral from a physician to be paid for services for a child by a family's health insurance plan.

Increasingly, schools use medical reimbursement resources such as Medicaid to pay for services provided to eligible children. In addition to the introduction of the "medical model" of requiring a physician referral for the clinician to provide services that will be reimbursed, the involvement of Medicaid creates additional challenges within educational settings because of the definition of who is a "qualified provider." Although Medicaid's guidelines specify that only a certified and/or licensed professional can provide services, individual state regulations regarding the provision of SLP services in the schools may be less stringent and include individuals with a bachelor's degree or a teaching credential (ASHA, 2004a, 2004b). In this case, Medicaid's definition of *qualified provider* may exceed the requirements of the schools, leaving certified SLPs in the uncomfortable position of having to supervise individuals who are not certified but who are deemed qualifed by the state. ASHA has developed policy documents that provide guidance to SLPs in theses situations: "Medicaid Guidance for Speech-Language Pathology Services: Addressing the 'Under the Direction of' Rule" (2004a, 2004b).

In summary, while a physician's referral may be required for insurance purposes or to comply with an organization's policies and procedures, speech-language pathologists and audiologists are legally autonomous in terms of their ability to practice and make independent clinical decisions. Furthermore, SLPs and audiologists are bound by their ethical codes to make clinical decisions based upon independent clinical judgment within their scope of practice and professional competence.

Prescription and Threats to Professional Autonomy

As noted previously, health care facilities or educational settings develop policies and procedures that establish a process for delivering services. However, SLPs and audiologists must participate in the development of the policies and procedures affecting their services so they do not conflict with professional and ethical guidelines. For the same reasons that SLPs and audiologists must practice only in the areas in which they have knowledge and skills, the Code of Ethics also compels individuals to maintain independent clinical judgment (ASHA, 2003). Specifically, the Code states that "Individuals shall not provide professional services without exercising independent professional judgment, regardless of referral source or prescription" (Principle IV, Rule G). A challenge to both professional autonomy and ethical behavior can occur when working with physicians who provide referrals for services. As autonomous professionals, SLPs and audiologists conduct assessments and develop treatment plans. When a physician's referral includes prescriptive

requirements that conflict with a clinician's professional judgment, professional autonomy is compromised. Furthermore, the clinician is faced with an ethical dilemma. For example, despite a physician's referral order for treatment five times a week for four weeks for a client with severe dementia, the speech-language pathologist may determine that this intensity and length of treatment is inappropriate given the client's limited prognosis and functional goals. Similarly, while a physician might refer a client for amplification and may specify a particular amplification arrangement, the audiologist who ultimately fits the amplification must be responsible for determining what system is in the best interests of the persons served, including consideration of personal and situational variables as well as hearing status.

The Issues in Ethics Statement on *Prescription* by the Board of Ethics (ASHA, 2002) discusses the challenges to professionals whose professional responsibilities may be restricted by prescription: ". . . if a certificate holder [does] . . . not challenge prescriptive mandates where the welfare of the person served is at risk, the certificate holder could be held in violation of the Code of Ethics" (p. 59). Thus, certified professionals have an ethical obligation NOT to comply with prescriptions or team decisions that fail to serve the client's best interest.

Employer Challenges to Professional Autonomy

Audiologists and speech-language pathologists who are employees may also encounter institutional policies that can infringe on their professional autonomy. For example, many health care settings set productivity targets for staff (e.g., 10 patients per day, 24 billable units) (ASHA, 2005c). If these targets are presented as absolute requirements, clinicians might feel pressed to treat patients who are inappropriate for services or to treat them for a longer period than is clinically justifiable. They may even feel pressured to shade their clinical documentation to justify reimbursement. Similarly, when productivity guidelines are based on number of patients seen or number of procedures completed, audiologists or

SLPs may be pressed to spend an inadequate amount of time with any given patient. For example, many clinical settings allow 30 minutes for completion of a comprehensive audiological evaluation. While that time frame might be appropriate for cooperative adult patients, it might be inappropriate for patients with more complex needs. Any time professionals are asked to engage in practices that contradict their professional judgment or are otherwise unethical or illegal, they have an ethical obligation to refuse to comply. Furthermore, professionals should be involved in the establishment of clinical guidelines within the settings in which they are employed.

Employers who are not audiologists or speech-language pathologists may be unfamiliar with the scopes of practice, preferred practice patterns, and the Code of Ethics for audiologists and SLPs. They may be unaware that professionals who are both licensed and certified must adhere to the highest or most stringent standard of the state licensing law and ASHA. When supervisors are professionals such as otolaryngologists, nurses, or physical therapists, they form expectations about the practice and ethics of audiology and SLP based on their knowledge of their own profession. Some conflicts over professional judgment vs. facility policies can be resolved by educating the supervisor about audiology and SLP professional standards and providing relevant policy documents. In other situations, when financial pressures on a facility result in practices that place the client at risk for a poor outcome, professionals should raise the issue of potential liability for malpractice, negative publicity, or client dissatisfaction. Larger institutions appoint corporate compliance officers and risk managers to ensure quality of services and compliance with state and federal regulations

Being supervised by a member of another profession can also present challenges in terms of how audiologists and SLPs are evaluated on their individual performance. ASHA's policy on "Professional Performance Appraisal by Individuals Outside the Professions of Speech-Language Pathology and Audiology" stipulates that a supervisor from another profession may evaluate the performance of general responsibilities by an audiologist or SLP, but that a member of the same profession should evaluate clinical performance (ASHA, 1993). Where this is not feasible, the policy recommends the use of self-evaluation or peer review.

Autonomy and Liability

Autonomy comes with increased risk. As autonomous professionals, SLPs and audiologists who are engaged in clinical practice are vulnerable to liability claims in the event of injury or other unfavorable outcomes. Accordingly, an ASHA ad hoc committee was formed and charged with the task of investigating and reporting on the professional claims history of the profession and developing risk management procedures to limit the liability exposure for SLPs and audiologists (ASHA, 1993). Physicians pay large sums for malpractice insurance because their decisions and actions can result in serious and permanent injury to an individual. While SLPs and audiologists are much less likely to cause such serious harm directly, it is important to remember that individuals can be held liable for their clinical actions and client care decisions. Therefore, clinicians should exercise good judgment in deciding whether to confer with the primary care or other physician before treating a disorder related to a health condition (e.g., stroke, traumatic brain injury, cerebral palsy) as well as the timing of communication and consultation during and following treatment. Although consultation with other health care providers may not be strictly required, clinical judgment would dictate that clinicians be aware of any potentially complicating medical history before initiating treatment. In addition, complications that occur during treatment warrant additional communication.

MODELS OF COLLABORATION

In its broadest sense, collaboration simply means working with others. Applied to the practice of speech-language pathology and audiology, it could refer to working with a wide range of professionals from health care, education, and community services, as well as with members of the client's individual support network. According to current definitions of evidence-based practice, the persons served, including the client and designated family members or caregivers, are an essential part of the treatment team (see Chapter 28), in that their wishes need to be taken into account when making clinical decisions. ASHA's position statement on evidence-based practice emphasizes the role of the client in the following definition: "The term *evidence-based practice* refers to an approach in which current, high-quality research evidence is integrated with practitioner expertise and client preferences and values into the process of making clinical decisions" (ASHA, 2005a). Regardless of the professional setting, collaboration in clinical care includes the incorporation of the persons served into the diagnostic and treatment team.

Medical Model

In health care, collaboration can assume many forms, depending on a variety of factors, including the medical diagnosis and the health care setting. In some medical settings, formal multidisciplinary or interdisciplinary teams may be established to develop a structure and process to manage clients with complex problems. Payer requirements can either support or work against team evaluations and treatment. Payers seldom pay for two professional services billing for simultaneous procedure, typically only one provider can charge for a procedure when providers are "co-treating." However, collaboration is highly encouraged in certain care areas. For example, a stroke or traumatic brain injury team might include members representing various professions, including neurology, rehabilitation medicine, nursing, psychology, speech-language pathology, occupational therapy, physical therapy, and social work. Individual team members typically conduct an independent evaluation of each client, after which the team members confer to develop a plan of care that includes some or all of the professions represented. Similarly, cleft palate teams, at minimum, will consist of an otolaryngologist or plastic surgeon, a dentist or orthodontist, a speech-language pathologist, and an audiologist. A neonatal intensive care unit may have a feeding team comprised of a pediatric gastroenterologist, pulmonologist, nurse, lactation specialist, speech-language pathologist, dietitian, and occupational therapist. A balance and falls prevention team may consist of an audiologist and a physical therapist or occupational therapist along with a physician (otolaryngologist, geriatrician, neurologist, physiatrist). Because these multidisciplinary and interdisciplinary teams are formed to address specific client care needs, they are likely to establish procedures for conducting assessments, coordinating the treatment plan, and meeting periodically to review progress and update the plan.

Collaboration in a medical setting may also be less formal and still involve individuals from a variety of professions. For example, a client coming in to the emergency room with complaints of dizziness is likely to be seen initially by an emergency room physician and support personnel, who may consult with other physicians including neurologists, otolaryngologists, and radiologists. Following initial evaluations designed to rule out life-threatening conditions and the initiation of medical management, the client may be referred for additional outpatient testing or admitted into the hospital. Depending upon the initial medical diagnosis and the nature of the client's symptoms, audiologists may be called upon to provide assessment of hearing and vestibular system function and to provide recommendations regarding the need for audiologic and/or vestibular rehabilitation. In this instance, collaboration is essential to providing optimal care for the client, and the audiologist serves as an important member of the health care team and may ultimately direct the treatment decisions.

Educational Model

Participation in interdisciplinary teams is also an important role of SLPs and audiologists working in school settings. In fact, procedures for collaboration among various professional groups to plan and deliver services to identified students are legally mandated under the Individuals with Disabilities Education Act (IDEA) and other state guidelines. For example, students' Individualized Education

Program (IEP) teams consist of the parents, teacher(s), special education teacher(s), and professionals from other relevant disciplines who are working with the student. Various models of service delivery for the schools involve collaboration between the SLP, the classroom teacher, and other relevant professionals (ASHA, 2001a). For a detailed description, the reader is referred to Chapters 15 and 16.

As is the case in a medical environment, interdisciplinary teams may be formed to address specific disorders or client care needs. Examples of such teams include a dysphagia team and an augmentative and alternative communication (AAC) team. Teams are also appropriate for coordinating the educational services for children with hearing loss. These teams may be based in a single school or consist of specialists who provide evaluation and consultation within an entire school district. This type of collaboration may incorporate both the educational and medical model, as referrals for evaluation and/or treatment may include hospital or clinic-based services as well as school-based services. The role of the SLP or audiologist may be as team leader, team member, or consultant.

Collaboration and Scope of Practice

Collaboration can occur as joint diagnosis or treatment of the client or in the form of consultation to confirm that goals and treatment approaches complement one another. Each professional typically conducts an assessment focusing on those aspects of care that fall within his or her scope of practice. In some cases, the assessment or a portion of it can be conducted jointly so that simultaneous behavioral observations are made by more than one member of the team, which serves to facilitate later discussion among team members and to minimize the burden on the client. One application of this approach is in the completion of a developmental assessment on an infant by an interdisciplinary team. In other instances, it may be more efficient or informative for each professional to administer his or her own test battery separately and subsequently compare results.

Several challenges are associated with the evaluation and management of complex disorders when multiple disciplines are involved. To provide optimal care and to minimize problems with billing and reimbursement for services, professionals with overlapping scopes of practice should collaborate in advance to ensure that they are not duplicating assessments. For example, if both an SLP and an OT evaluate a client who has had a stroke, it is appropriate for the SLP to report on the speech, language, cognitive-communication, and swallowing aspects of the assessment, while the OT may report on the individual's ability to perform activities of daily living, including grooming, dressing, and feeding, with comments on how cognitive skills such as sequencing, problem solving, and safety awareness affect these activities. In this situation the SLP and OT may discuss their findings and collaborate to reinforce compensatory strategies for the client's cognitive-communication deficits while working on different tasks. On the other hand, if the client demonstrated only problems with swallowing and both professions remain involved in developing treatment plans for addressing swallowing problems, the overlap could result in a denial of payment for one of the services provided. Furthermore, the overlap may result in confusion for the persons served and for other members of the health care team.

MULTISKILLED PROVIDERS AND ENCROACHMENT ON THE SCOPE OF PRACTICE

As health care expenses began to soar in the 1990s, the possibility of training multiskilled rehabilitation professionals was discussed as a possible solution to provide more efficient and cost-effective services. After researching the issue, ASHA (1997a) issued a position statement on "Multiskilled Personnel" concluding that ". . . cross-training of clinical skills is not appropriate at the professional level of practice (i.e., audiologists or speech-language pathologists)."

Despite this conclusion, continued reimbursement pressures and perceptions of personnel shortages threaten the scope of practice of speech-language pathologists and audiologists. Encroachment occurs in situations in which a provider from one discipline delivers services across a range of clinical areas and responsibilities that overlap those of other professionals. Institutional pressures to "streamline" referrals to one type of professional or a less-qualified provider threaten collaboration and multidisciplinary teaming, in addition to potentially placing clients at risk.

Within health care settings, continuous tightening of reimbursement from federal, state, and private payers has induced administrators to cut costs. For example, Medicare's implementation of a Prospective Payment System (PPS) resulted in staff reductions in many skilled nursing facilities (SNFs). Specifically, SLP positions were eliminated or the hours of staff SLPs were reduced. As a result, some SLP services, particularly swallowing intervention, were picked up by full-time staff from other professions since swallowing services may be provided by SLPs, OTs, or PTs according to Medicare's definition of qualified provider.

Early Intervention (EI) programs, frequently funded by state Medicaid programs, have also given rise to concerns about encroachment in scope of practice. Many programs stipulate that a single provider (from the discipline in which the most intervention is needed or from "developmental interventionists") will deliver services to the child—which can range from motor skills to language stimulation—with input from other professionals. When these services are provided in the child's "natural environment" (e.g., the child's home), the provider delivering services must be keenly aware of the need to consult with other professionals monitoring the child's progress to ensure that the intervention is appropriate and to determine when reevaluation is needed. Such practices have given rise to concerns about the appropriateness of other professionals addressing language development and swallowing and the effectiveness of those services. When hearing loss in involved, concerns are also raised about the adequacy of knowledge and skills of the service provider related to aural habilitation. See Chapter 16 for more in-depth discussion of early intervention.

Adding Basic Client Care Skills

The "Multiskilled Personnel" position statement also addressed areas where SLPs and audiologists may be asked to acquire new client care skills that are outside of their respective scopes of practice. The document includes the statement that "Cross-training of basic client care skills, professional non-clinical skills, and/or administrative skills is a reasonable option that clinical practitioners at all levels of practice may need to consider depending on the service delivery setting, geographic location, client population, and clinical workforce resources" (ASHA, 1997b).

This statement responds to other concerns arising from cost-cutting efforts in both health care and education. In trying to achieve the greatest efficiency of services or reduce staff to a minimum, schools or health care organizations may ask speech-language pathologists and audiologists to perform tasks that they never before had considered to be within their purview as professionals.

ASHA concluded that SLPs and audiologists may perform basic client care skills if they have been trained and if they demonstrate competence in that skill, in accordance with the Code of Ethics. This can create some discomfort on the part of professionals who may not welcome these additional responsibilities. Examples of basic client care activities include taking blood pressure readings (which is frequently a routine part of home health visits), performing client transfers (such as from a wheelchair to a bed), and performing suctioning (which may be a frequent part of client care in a hospital specializing in tracheotomized and/or ventilator-dependent patients). While audiologists and SLPs may view the addition of these activities as burdensome, in some settings they may facilitate optimal client care and safety. For example, an audiologist may encounter a patient becoming less responsive during an evaluation, in which case being able to take a blood pressure reading is important. Similarly, when clients arrive for balance function testing in a wheelchair, they may need to be safely transferred to another chair for the evaluation. As is true with the provision of clinical services that are within the scopes of practice of the professions, SLPs and audiologists are compelled by their Code of Ethics to perform only those services for which they have adequate knowledge and skills. If professionals do not feel comfortable in performing a task after being trained, they should discuss the matter with their supervisor or consider seeking employment in another setting.

ADDITIONAL THREATS TO AUTONOMY

While many of the challenges to autonomy are common for audiology and speech-language pathology, audiology has faced some that are unique to that profession. Audiologists have struggled to become the point of entry for individuals with hearing and balance disorders and been met with opposition from many fronts. Physicians have argued that they should remain the gatekeepers of services to protect clients from potential harm, and physician groups have lobbied Congress to thwart legislative attempts to enable clients to initiate hearing care through audiologists. In addition, Medicare policies have historically restricted the payment for audiologic testing to those instances in which the testing is determined to be medically necessary. Furthermore, the Medicare fee schedule, which includes the procedures that fall within the scope of practice of audiology, and which is frequently used by private insurance companies to determine coverage for services, has not recognized the professional work of audiologists enables them to be reimbursed for interpretation of test data. While physicians can completely bill and be paid for the professional component for each of the procedures that are performed by audiologists, audiologists remain unable to directly collect for professional fees. Inasmuch as the billing codes that are used belong to the American Medical Association (AMA), physicians have been able to maintain fairly tight control over access to reimbursement by audiologists.

INTERDEPENDENCE OF AUDIOLOGY AND SPEECH-LANGUAGE PATHOLOGY

Audiology and speech-language pathology currently are viewed as separate professions within one discipline. Intuitively, that position makes sense since both professions address aspects of the discipline of human communication sciences and disorders. As the scopes of practice have expanded, each profession has added areas of practice that are more specialized, creating increased separation between the professions and giving rise to tensions. For example, AAA has espoused the position that it is and must be the primary professional home of audiologists and that audiology must separate itself from speech-language pathology to become an autonomous profession. Essentially, AAA is asserting that ASHA cannot rightfully represent the interests of audiologists. That position has created conflict within the profession of audiology and the discipline as a whole (see Chapter 4 for further discussion of ASHA and AAA as professional associations).

In reality, while there are clear areas of separation, there is a great deal of overlap in the knowledge that is required for the practice of audiology and the practice of speech-language pathology. For example, both professions require an understanding of normal anatomy and normal communication processes, including hearing, speech, and language. Audiologists must understand normal speech perception to make clinical decisions about the rehabilitation of hearing loss, including the fitting of hearing aids. Similarly, speech-language pathologists must appreciate the impact of hearing loss on language perception, including its impact on clients' performance on speech and language assessments. The management of infants and young children with hearing loss must include input from both professions. The overriding purpose of improving hearing is to facilitate better communication (listening, speech, and language). In addition, the diseases and disorders that cause clients to need SLP and audiology services frequently cross several domains: hearing, balance, speech, language, cognition, and swallowing. Optimal care of clients across the life span requires audiologists and SLPs to collaborate. For all of those reasons, regardless of whether the professions continue to be viewed as members of a single discipline, it is evident that the professions of audiology and speech-language pathology are interdependent.

COLLABORATION AND CONFIDENTIALITY

While collaboration is an important part of coordinating and maximizing treatment, clinicians must be sure they protect the client's privacy and confidentiality by not disclosing information without the client's permission. The Health Information Portability and Accountability Act (HIPAA) of 1996 and state laws establish guidelines about the privacy of protected medical information and impose sanctions against individuals or institutions that do not protect the client's privacy. For example, the client must give written permission to send a report or videotape for a second opinion from a colleague at another hospital. The client also must give consent for his or her case to be discussed with family members. For that reason, the manner in which professionals conduct business may be affected. For example, leaving detailed messages on an answering machine that include protected information is prohibited. Audiologists and SLPs must be vigilant in obtaining necessary consents before discussing any aspect of care with anyone in order to maintain client confidentiality.

SUMMARY

As professions, speech-language pathology and audiology are constantly evolving and the scopes of practice and preferred practice patterns within the discipline of communication sciences and disorders are periodically reviewed and modified. Professional autonomy depends upon the involvement of the professions in crafting those documents and in determining ethical practice standards and policies regarding reimbursement for services. Both autonomy and collaboration are subject to the influence of evolving practice and reimbursement trends. The complexity of disorders, populations, and service delivery systems can challenge the autonomy of the speech-language pathologist or audiologist in independent decision making. However, collaboration, when conducted with mutual respect and established procedures, can benefit and enhance outcomes for the persons served and for other stakeholders. The key to achieving a successful balance between professional autonomy and collaboration is involvement of audiologists and SLPs in self-determination by taking a leadership role in setting their own standards of practice and shaping the policies and procedures within their work settings that will affect their autonomy. Ultimately, professional autonomy and collaboration within and outside of the discipline strikes a balance to benefit both the persons served and the professionals themselves.

CRITICAL THINKING

1. What would you do if a physician orders a modified barium swallow but you think the client's dementia will make him unable to cooperate?
2. What referral or authorization (if any) would a licensed SLP need to work on accent modification with an individual in his home if he was paying privately?
3. How do institutional and reimbursement constraints affect the autonomy of SLPs and audiologists?
4. What is the difference between a multiskilled provider and a multidisciplinary team?
5. What unique challenges to autonomy have audiologists faced?
6. In what ways are audiology and speech-language pathology interdependent, and is that relationship helpful or harmful to the discipline and to persons served?

REFERENCES

American Academy of Audiology. (2005). Code of Ethics of the American Academy of Audiology. Available at http://www.audiology.org/

The American Heritage Dictionary of the English Language (4th ed.). (2000). New York: Houghton Mifflin.

American Speech-Language-Hearing Association. (1986). Autonomy of speech-language pathology and audiology. *Asha, 28,* 53–57.

American Speech-Language-Hearing Association. (1993). Professional performance appraisal by individuals outside the professions of speech-language pathology and audiology. *Asha, 35,* (Suppl. 10), 11–13.

American Speech-Language-Hearing Association. (1994). Professional liability and risk management for the audiology and speech-language pathology professions. *Asha 36,* (Suppl. 12), 25–38.

American Speech-Language-Hearing Association. (1997a, Spring). Position statement: Multiskilled personnel. *Asha, 39* (Suppl. 17), 13.

American Speech-Language-Hearing Association. (1997b). Preferred practice patterns for the profession of audiology. Rockville, MD: Author.

American Speech-Language-Hearing Association. (2000). Guidelines for the roles and responsibilities of the school-based speech-language pathologist. Rockville, MD: Author.

American Speech-Language-Hearing Association. (2001). Scope of practice in speech-language pathology. Rockville, MD: Author.

American Speech-Language-Hearing Association. (2002). Prescription. *ASHA Supplement, 22,* 59–60.

American Speech-Language-Hearing Association. (2003). Code of ethics (revised). *ASHA Supplement, 23,* 13–15.

American Speech-Language-Hearing Association. (2004a). Medicaid guidance for speech-language pathology services: Addressing the "under the direction of" rule. Available at http://www.asha.org/

American Speech-Language-Hearing Association. (2004b). Medicaid guidance for speech-language pathology services: Addressing the "under the direction of" rule. Available at http://www.asha.org/

American Speech-Language-Hearing Association. (2004c). Preferred practice patterns for the professional of speech-language pathology. Available at http://www.asha.org/

American Speech-Language-Hearing Association. (2004d). Scope of practice in audiology. *ASHA Supplement, 24,* 27–35.

American Speech-Language-Hearing Association. (2005a). Evidence-based practice in communication disorders. Available at http://www.asha.org/

American Speech-Language-Hearing Association. (2005b). New certification standards. Available at http://www.asha.org/

Princeton University, Cognitive Science Laboratory. (2003). WordNet® 2.0. Available at http://wordnet.princeton.edu/

10

Support Personnel in Communication Sciences and Disorders

DIANE R. PAUL, PHD, CCC-SLP

SUSAN SPARKS, MA, CCC-SLP

SCOPE OF CHAPTER

Support personnel have been used in the professions of speech-language pathology and audiology since the early 1970s. Their use has been a topic of debate with passionate views on both sides. Those favoring the use of support personnel believe that access to care is improved, frequency and intensity of service are increased, and the skills of professionals are better used. Those opposing argue that the quality of care may be compromised and the services of professionals devalued. Proponents say use of support personnel is in the best interest of consumers; opponents say consumers may be misled (Breakey, 1993; Werven, 1993). The dynamics of the service delivery system, in tandem with cost controls and personnel needs, have led to the development of new and changing state and national policies related to the training, supervision, and use of support personnel in the two professions (ASHA, 1992b).

In many health care and education settings across the country, speech-language pathologists (SLPs) and audiologists are experiencing escalating caseloads and increasing paperwork in conjunction with shrinking budgets and personnel shortages (ASHA, 2003a, 2004a). In response, some facilities and institutions have chosen to employ support personnel to assist their professional staff. Support personnel, known by a variety of terms (e.g., *aides, assistants, paraprofessionals, paratherapists,* and *technicians*), have been employed by audiologists and SLPs as a way to extend and expand services. They are considered support staff rather than substitutes or replacements for qualified professionals.

The purpose of this chapter is to provide information about the use, training, supervision, responsibilities, and effectiveness of support personnel in the professions of speech-language pathology and audiology. Specifically, the chapter includes information on the rationale, concerns, professional policies, state regulations, current use, training recommendations, supervision requirements, job responsibilities, reimbursement, research, and future directions related to speech-language pathology and audiology support personnel. A glossary of key terms used in this chapter is provided in Appendix 10-A.

RATIONALE FOR THE USE OF SUPPORT PERSONNEL

The growing and diverse needs of individuals with communication and related disorders are increasing the demand for speech-language pathology and audiology services (Bureau of Labor Statistics, 2004a, 2004b). This increasing demand for communication services is one of the converging factors leading to the use of support personnel in the professions of speech-language pathology and audiology. Other influences include federal legislation sustaining the education rights of students with disabilities (IDEA, 2004), including the right of students to be assessed in their native language, and increasing caseloads due to (1) recognition of the value and need for early intervention services (ASHA, in press; Feldman, 2004; Guralnick, 2005), (2) aging of the population with concomitant health needs (Administration on Aging, 2002), (3) need to care for individuals with hearing loss resulting from occupational noise (AAA, 2003; ASHA, 2004b), and (4) expanding scopes of services in audiology and speech-language pathology (AAA, 1997, 2004; ASHA, 1997, 2001, 2004f, 2004g). Thus, because of

the growing need for services, combined with the rising health care and education costs and personnel shortages, some SLPs and audiologists have identified roles for support personnel in the delivery of service for children and adults with communication disorders. Let's consider first the rationale for two of the roles, serving as interpreters/translators in bilingual/bicultural environments and working on collaborative teams in classrooms.

The need to use bilingual/bicultural support personnel in speech-language pathology and audiology has increased as the United States population continues to diversify with respect to language and culture (United States Bureau of the Census, 2000). Because only about 7 percent of ASHA members are from a racial/ethnic minority background and less than 6 percent are bilingual, it often is not possible to match a clinician to a client's cultural and linguistic background (ASHA, 2004d). Consequently, the assistance of professional interpreters and cultural brokers is often necessary to provide culturally and linguistically appropriate services. Facilities that receive any type of federal funds, including Medicaid/Medicare, must develop a plan to provide equal access to services for people with limited English proficiency. IDEA 2004 also requires that assessment be conducted in a child's native language. Support personnel who share the same language and/or culture with a client may fill these roles to help meet the needs of a multilingual population, provided there is ongoing training, planning, and communication (ASHA, 1985a, 2004d; Langdon & Cheng, 2002). Support personnel in speech-language pathology also have been used to provide services in developing countries (Landis, 1973).

IDEA 2004 recognizes the use of paraprofessionals and assistants as adjuncts to the team of service providers in the schools. In accordance with state law, paraprofessionals and assistants who are appropriately trained and supervised may be used to assist in the provision of special education and related services for children with disabilities. In addition, the state must adopt a policy that requires local educational agencies to take measures to recruit, hire, train, and retain highly qualified personnel, including paraprofessionals, to provide special education and related services to children with disabilities. Special education paraprofessionals who provide instructional support in Title I programs (Improving the Academic Achievement of the Disadvantaged) also must meet the requirements of the No Child Left Behind Act of 2001.

The use of alternative service delivery models for SLPs in the schools also has prompted the use of SLP assistants. The prevailing SLP service delivery model in the schools has been a "pull-out" model (ASHA, 1995c). In recent years, the recognition of the need for more functional outcomes has led to an extension of service into the classroom (Paul-Brown & Caperton, 2001). The use of SLP assistants who work directly in the classroom has been a means to integrate speech and language goals within the curriculum, generalize learned concepts, enhance carryover of functional skills, and reinforce SLP goals in the student's natural setting (Gerlach, 2000; Goldberg & Paul-Brown, 1999; Pickett, 1999; Pickett & Gerlach, 1997).

The appropriate use of trained, supervised, and less costly support personnel may be one way to meet the growing service needs of persons with communication disorders and still maintain the role of the fully qualified SLP and audiologist (Paul-Brown & Goldberg, 2001). The use of support personnel in various roles (e.g., interpreters/translators, classroom collaborators) may provide a means to supplement services for a diverse population, extend services in natural settings, free professionals to dedicate more time to those individuals with more complex conditions, and fulfill increasing managerial responsibilities (ASHA, 2004d).

CONCERNS ABOUT THE USE OF SUPPORT PERSONNEL

Some audiologists and SLPs have expressed concerns about the impact of using support personnel on service delivery. Some believe that support personnel (1) may be hired in lieu of qualified providers, (2) may be used to increase caseload size, (3) may be asked to provide services for which they are not trained, or (4) may receive inadequate supervision.

In many school settings, demand for SLPs and audiologists outweighs supply. Indeed, 62 percent of respondents to ASHA's (2004a) school survey workforce report indicated that job openings were more numerous than job seekers in their school. Employers may be tempted to hire assistants to fill a persistent SLP or audiologist vacancy. There is a concern about quality of services when the motivation for using support personnel is to respond to a personnel shortage rather than to extend and enhance service.

Another area of concern is when a bilingual assistant is asked to work with bilingual clients. Although this practice may be beneficial, there also is the potential for misuse or overuse if the assistant has not been trained appropriately or is asked to go beyond an assistant's job responsibilities (e.g., inappropriately expected to conduct evaluations for bilingual clients). The ability to speak a second language does not automatically qualify someone to be a translator or interpreter, nor does it mean that the individual has the skills necessary to serve as an SLP or audiology assistant (ASHA, 1985a, 2004e; Langdon & Cheng, 2002).

Clearly, inappropriate use of support personnel could have far-reaching and negative effects on the professions (ASHA, 1992b). One way to ensure that the quality of care is not compromised is for SLPs and audiologists to adhere to national and state laws and follow professional guidelines, so that support personnel receive appropriate training and supervision and only provide services within a limited scope of job responsibilities. Another way to promote the appropriate use of support personnel is through education and awareness initiatives, such as providing information to administrators, principals, school boards, hospital boards, and others responsible for personnel or hiring decisions about the role of supervised support personnel and their job responsibilities in comparison to the scope of practice of the supervising SLPs and audiologists.

EVOLVING PROFESSIONAL POLICIES AND PRACTICES

State licensure boards and professional organizations have responded to the concerns about misuse of support personnel by providing regulations, policies, and reports with specific guidance. ASHA (1998b, 2004d, 2004i), the American Academy of Audiology (AAA, 1997, 2005), the Council for Exceptional Children (Consortium of Organizations on the Preparation and Use of Speech-Language Paraprofessionals in Early Intervention and Education Settings, 1997), and the National Joint Committee on Learning Disabilities (1998) are among the professional organizations representing SLPs and/or audiologists that have developed documents to provide guidance for the appropriate use and supervision of support personnel in those education and health care settings in which support personnel are employed. All of the professional policies rely on the clinical judgment and ethics of qualified professionals. This includes decisions regarding the delegation of tasks and the amount and type of supervision to provide. Table 10–1 presents a chronology of the policies that professional organizations have developed over the last 35 years to guide the practice and performance of speech-language pathology and audiology support personnel.

T A B L E 10–1 Chronology of Ethical and Professional Practice Policies Related to the Use of Support Personnel in Audiology and Speech-Language Pathology

- 1969—ASHA developed guidelines for the use of communication aides.
- 1973—Council for Accreditation in Occupational Hearing Conservation started training and certifying hearing conservationists.
- 1979—ASHA referenced *supportive personnel* in the Code of Ethics and issued an Issues in Ethics statement highlighting the professional and ethical responsibilities of the supervising professionals and emphasizing the dependent role of the *communication aide.*
- 1981—ASHA revised its guidelines for supportive personnel.
- 1988—ASHA developed a technical report about the use of SLP support personnel with underserved populations.
- 1990—ASHA revised the Code of Ethics and included a proscription about service delegation.
- 1992—ASHA developed a technical report on issues and the impact of support personnel in speech-language pathology and audiology. The 1992 and 1994 revised Code of Ethics dealt with the delegation of support services.
- 1994—ASHA approved a position statement supporting the establishment and credentialing of categories of support personnel in speech-language pathology.
- 1995—ASHA approved guidelines for the training, credentialing, use, and supervision of SLP assistants.
- 1996—ASHA convened a consensus panel to develop a strategic plan for approving speech-language pathology assistant programs and credentialing SLP assistants. The plan was used as a framework to develop a training approval process and credentialing process for SLP assistants.
- 1997—Consortium of Organizations on the Preparation and Use of Speech-Language Paraprofessionals in Early Intervention and Education Settings developed guidelines for three levels of paraprofessionals in education settings: aides, assistants, and associates. The assistant category parallels the ASHA SLP assistant guidelines. Consorium organizations included ASHA; Council for Exceptional Children, Division for Children's Communication Development and Division for Early Childhood; Council of Administrators of Special Education; and Council of Language, Speech, and Hearing Consultants in State Education Agencies.
- 1997 and 1998—AAA and ASHA published separate position statements and guidelines for support personnel in audiology.
- 1998—National Joint Committee on Learning Disabilities developed a report on the use of paraprofessionals with students with learning disabilities.
- 2000—Council on Academic Accreditation in Audiology and Speech-Language Pathology developed criteria and procedures for approving technical training programs for SLP assistants, the Council on Professional Standards in Speech-Language Pathology and Audiology developed criteria for registering SLP assistants, and the Council for Clinical Certification in Audiology and Speech-Language Pathology developed the implementation program.
- 2001—ASHA revised its Code of Ethics, added the terms *assistants, technicians, or any nonprofessionals* to the term *support personnel,* and mandated informing persons served about the credentials of providers.

T A B L E 10–1 (continued)

- 2002—ASHA developed knowledge and skills statements for supervisors of SLP assistants.

- 2003—ASHA voted to discontinue the registration program for SLP assistants and the approval process for SLP assistant training programs as of December 31, 2003, due primarily to financial concerns.

- 2003—ASHA revised its Code of Ethics and elaborated on delegation and supervision of support personnel.

- 2004—ASHA issued a new Issues in Ethics Statement on support personnel.

- 2004—ASHA revised its position statement for support personnel in speech-language pathology and its guidelines for SLP assistants to remove references to SLP assistant credentialing.

- 2005—AAA developed a new position statement to define the function of the audiologist's assistant.

Ethical Responsibilities

ASHA's Code of Ethics and Issues in Ethics statements have provided the general framework for the supervision of support personnel in the professions of audiology and speech-language pathology. The first reference in the Code of Ethics was in the 1979 Code, specifically, Principle of Ethics II, Ethical Proscription 4, which stated that "Individuals must not offer clinical services by supportive personnel for whom they do not provide appropriate supervision and assume full responsibility." The first Issues in Ethics statements to address support personnel highlighted the professional and ethical responsibilities of the supervising professionals and emphasized the dependent role of the "communication aide" (ASHA, 1979). The 1990 Code of Ethics used the same language and also had the first reference to "delegation" with its proscription not to delegate "any service." The 1992 Code and its revision in 1994 both dealt with the delegation of "support services." The 2001 Code added the terms *assistants, technicians, or any nonprofessionals* to the term *support personnel* and mandated that members had an affirmative requirement to "not misrepresent the credentials of assistants, technicians, or support personnel and shall inform those they serve professionally of the name and professional credentials of persons providing services."

The 2003 revision of the Code maintains this requirement and indicates in Principle of Ethics I, Rule of Ethics E,

> Individuals who hold the Certificate of Clinical Competence shall not delegate tasks that require the unique skills, knowledge, and judgment that are within the scope of their profession to assistants, technicians, support personnel, students, or any nonprofessionals over whom they have supervisory responsibility. An individual may delegate support services to assistants, technicians support personnel, students, or any other persons only if those services are adequately supervised by an individual who holds the appropriate Certificate of Clinical Competence. (ASHA, 2003b, p. 185)

The revised Issues in Ethics statement (ASHA, 2004h) discusses a variety of training options and tasks and indicates that support personnel should be supervised by ASHA-certified audiologists and/or SLPs.

Chronology of Professional Practice Policies

In addition to the policies related to ethical use of support personnel, professional organizations also developed documents to guide professional practice. In 1970, ASHA published its first professional practice guidelines on the use of support personnel in audiology and speech-language pathology. These guidelines, revised in 1981, delineated training needs, scope of responsibilities, and amount of supervision for support personnel in audiology and speech-language pathology (ASHA, 1970, 1981). The following two sections address professional practice policies specific to either SLP or audiology support personnel.

SLP Support Personnel

In a 1995 position statement, ASHA endorsed the use of support personnel in speech-language pathology for the first time, rather than only providing guidance for their use (ASHA, 1995b). In 1996, the earlier ASHA guidelines from 1981 were revised to address one category of support personnel, *speech-language pathology assistants,* defined as "support personnel who perform tasks as prescribed, directed, and supervised by certified SLPs, after a program of academic and/or on-the-job training" (ASHA, 1996a, p. 22). SLP assistants were differentiated from SLP aides, who usually have a narrower training base and more limited responsibilities relative to the duties of assistants. Like the first two ASHA guideline documents, the 1996 guidelines specified a scope of responsibilities and outlined the type and amount of supervision required. Some of these decisons were informed, in part, by the less restrictive policies developed by other professions with a longer history using support personnel, such as occupational therapy and physical therapy (ASHA, 1992). The ASHA guidelines were more prescriptive than those of the other professions to avoid the risk of assistants working outside of their limited scope of responsibilities or being hired in the place of SLPs (ASHA, 1996a).

The ASHA guidelines also called for training at the associate degree level rather than just on-the-job training and recommended a credentialing program for assistants and for assistant-level training programs. ASHA's plan to credential SLP assistants and approve training programs started with the 1995 position statement supporting the establishment and credentialing of categories of SLP support personnel (ASHA, 1995b). In 2000, criteria for approving technical training programs and for registering SLP assistants were developed by the Council on Academic Accreditation in Audiology and Speech-Language Pathology (CAA) (ASHA, 2000a) and the Council on Professional Standards in Speech-Language Pathology, respectively (ASHA, 2000b). Recommendations for assistant-level tasks, knowledge required, and where this knowledge could and should be obtained were based in part on a job analysis of SLP assistants conducted by the

Educational Testing Service (Rosenfeld & Leung, 1999). ASHA established implementation dates of January 2002 for the approval process for training programs and January 2003 for the SLP assistant registry process. The CAA was responsible for implementation of the technical training approval process and the CFCC was responsible for implementation of the assistant registration program. ASHA's commitment to these programs was linked to the receipt of sufficient fees to cover administrative costs paid by training programs and individuals seeking registration. When those revenues fell well short of what was required, the decision was made to discontinue the approval process for SLP assistant training programs and the registration program for SLP assistants as of December 31, 2003. In 2004, the ASHA position statement for SLP support personnel and guidelines for SLP assistants were revised to remove references to SLP assistant credentialing. Relevant portions of the criteria for SLP assistant technical training programs and assistant registration that related to training, use, and supervision were folded into the revised SLP assistant guidelines (ASHA, 2004d, 2004i).

ASHA has developed other documents and products over the years to assist professionals who choose to employ support personnel in various settings. These include a report on using support personnel with underserved populations (ASHA, 1988), knowledge and skills for supervising SLP assistants (ASHA, 2002a), and practical tools and forms for supervising SLP assistants (ASHA, 1999) and for using and supervising SLP assistants working in school settings (ASHA, 2000d).

Audiology Support Personnel

Multiple professional organizations are involved in the issue of audiology support personnel. In 1997, a Consensus Panel on Support Personnel in Audiology was convened with members of the Academy of Dispensing Audiologists, AAA, Educational Audiology Association, Military Audiology Association, and National Hearing Conservation Association and developed a position statement and guidelines (AAA, 1997). ASHA developed its own audiology support personnel position statement and guidelines

(ASHA, 1998b), which differed only in its requirement for supervisors to hold the Certificate of Clinical Competence in Audiology. The policy documents leave decisions about specific activities and supervision to the discretion of the supervising audiologist: "Support personnel may assist audiologists in the delivery of services where appropriate" (ASHA, 1998b, p. 59). The supervising audiologist is expected to provide competency-based training specific to job needs. According to the ASHA guidelines, supervising audiologists have the full responsibility for determining the specific type of training activities, the assigned tasks, and the nature and amount of supervision provided for support personnel (ASHA, 1998b). The AAA recently developed a new position statement to guide audiologists on the education and job responsibilities of audiologist's assistants (AAA, 2005). The statement indicates that assistants may be assigned duties at the discretion of an audiologist, provided that the assistant has a minimum of a high school diploma and competency-based training.

Support personnel in audiology are trained and used in a variety of employment settings, such as industry, schools, private clinics, and Veterans Administration hospitals and other medical centers. In industrial settings, assistants may help with the prevention of hearing loss resulting from noise. Occupational hearing conservationists have been trained and certified by the Council for Accreditation in Occupational Hearing Conservation (CAOHC) since 1973. They may be audiometric technicians, occupational health nurses, engineers, and others who do audiometric testing and help to fit hearing protection devices for employees (Suter, 2002). The CAOHC is an interdisciplinary group that includes representatives from the American Academy of Otolaryngology–Head and Neck Surgery (AAO-HNS), American College of Occupational and Environmental Medicine, ASHA, American Association of Occupational Health Nurses, Military Audiology Association, Institute of Noise Control Engineering, American Industrial Hygiene Association, and the National Safety Council. Their mission is to provide education about noise in the workplace and to prevent noise-induced hearing loss in industry. CAOHC also certifies course directors, the majority of whom are audiologists (ASHA, 2004b).

A new certificate program for otolaryngology personnel (CPOP) has been promoted by AAO-HNS and the American Neurotology Society to train otolaryngology office personnel to become otologic technicians (OTO techs) and conduct hearing testing. The program includes a self-study reading component, a 2½-day workshop, and six months of supervision by an otolaryngologist. The list of tasks these groups delegate to an OTO tech closely matches the scope of practice of audiologists (e.g., performing otoscopic examinations, pure tone air and bone conduction tests with and without masking, speech recognition threshold and word recognition tests with and without masking, and tympanometry), causing concern to professional audiology organizations such as ASHA about the blurring of professional and technical level boundaries. Those endorsing the use of OTO techs suggest that their use can free up time for audiologists to work with more challenging patients and perform more complex tasks, such as advanced hearing and balance services.

Some audiologists have argued that the move to the doctoral level for the profession of audiology may lead to increased use of audiology support personnel to have a less-costly option for the more technical aspects of the profession (Thornton, 1993). One of the reasons that audiologists decided not to require a higher education degree or credential for support personnel is to have the educational level and scope of responsibilities as distinct as possible between technical-level and professional-level personnel. Rather than have prescriptive policies related to education and tasks, audiologists prefer to determine independently what support personnel should do and how they should be trained.

STATE REGULATION

Thirty-four states have laws or regulations governing the use of support personnel in speech-language pathology and/or audiology. Some states that regulate speech-language pathology and audiology do not permit the use of support personnel. Table 10–2 provides an overview of state regulation of support

T A B L E 10-2 State Regulation of Support Personnel: An Overview

Type of Regulation

There are 34 states that officially regulate the use of support personnel. Of the 34 states, there are 12 states that regulate support personnel through licensure, the most stringent form of regulation and 22 states regulate support personnel through registration.

Licensure (12 states)	Registration (22 states)
AZ, ID, IL, KY, LA, MA, MD, NM, OH, OR, SC, TX	AL, AK, AR, CA, FL, GA, IN, IA, KS, ME, MS, MO, MT, NE, NC, OK, PA, RI, TN, UT, WV, WY

Although not officially regulated, support personnel are acknowledged in 6 additional states. In 5 states (CT, DE, NH, VA, WI), support personnel are not directly regulated; however, licensed SLPs and audiologists who use support personnel are required to observe specific supervisory guidelines. Washington has included in regulations a statement that its regulatory board is aware that support personnel are being used and is committed to study the situation.

Education/Experience Required

The level of education required of support personnel varies from state to state. At one end of the range are those states that require a bachelor's degree plus enrollment in a master's degree program. At the other end are states that require a high school diploma plus additional training or are silent on the issue. A few states have several tiers of support personnel with different educational requirements for each tier; therefore, some states appear under more than one of the following categories.

Bachelor's degree + graduate credit hours/enrollment in a master's degree program (3 states)	Bachelor's degree + some practicum requirement (6 states)	Bachelor's degree (6 states)	Associate's degree (11 states)	Other specified coursework and practicum hours (1 state)	High school diploma + additional training as specified by board and/or supervisor (15 states)
MT (SLP Aide I), NM, RI (SLP aide)	AR (SLP asst.), KY, LA, RI (SLP aides), SC, TX	AL, FL (SLP asst.), ID (SLP aide), IN (SLP asst.), MT (SLP Aide II), WV	AK (assoc. or bachelor's), AZ, ID (SLP asst.), IL, IN (SLP assoc.), MD (assoc. or bachelor's), ME (SLP asst.), MA (assoc. or bachelor's), MO (assoc. or bachelor's), NC (assoc. or bachelor's), CA (SLP asst.)	OR (30 semester hours of speech-language pathology technical course work, 30 semester hours of general education credit, and 100 hours of clinical interaction)	AR (SLP aide), FL (audiology asst.), GA, IA, IN, KS, MS, NE, OH, OK, PA, RI (audiology aide) TN, UT, WY

Types of Support Personnel Regulated

Regulate both SLP and audiology support personnel (19 states)	Regulate only SLP support personnel (14 states)
AL, CA, FL, IA, KS, MA, MS, MO, MT, NE, OH, OK, PA, RI, TN, TX, UT, WV, WY	AK, AR, GA, ID, IL, IN, KY, LA, MD, ME, NM, NC, OR, SC

Title

The most common title for support personnel is *assistant*, used in 13 states. Ten states use the term *aide*, and 5 states use both *assistant and aide*. The state of New Mexico uses *apprentice*, and Nebraska uses *communication assistant*. In some states with several levels or tiers of support personnel, each level has its own educational requirements, title, and specified level of authorized practice.

Restricted to Public Schools (2 states)

KY	(SLP asst.)
AR	(SLP aide)

Continuing Education (10 states)

These 10 states have extended the continuing education requirements for fully licensed SLPs and audiologists to include continuing education requirements for support personnel:

AL—10 hours per year	AK—15 hours per biennium
AR—12 clock hours per year	CA—12 hours per biennium
FL—20 hours per biennium	LA—10 clock hours per year
MD—10 hours per biennium	SC—8 hours per biennium
TX—10 hours per year	WV—5 hours per year

Supervisory Requirements

To ensure that support personnel do not exceed the boundaries of their education and experience, most states have imposed one or more supervision requirements. Some states limit the number of support personnel that one licensed SLP or audiologist may supervise. Some states specifically prescribe the amount of direct and indirect supervision that a supervisor must provide to the support personnel. Some states specifically define what activities may or may not be performed by support personnel, and others that simply provide a general statement that support personnel are the responsibility of the licensed SLP or audiologist and should be appropriately supervised given their individual education and experience.

States that limit the number of assistants per supervisor. Limited to 3 assistants per supervisor (8 states)	Limited to 2 assistants per supervisor (10 states)	Limited to 3 part-time or 2 full-time assistants per supervisor (3 states)	States with different standards for SLP and audiologist supervisors (2 states)
CA, IN, LA, MS, MT, NH, UT, WY	AK, GA, KY, ME, MD, NC, OH, OK, OR, WV	AR, SC, FL	RI (licensed SLP may supervise 1 aide; licensed audiologist may supervise 3 aides) WI (licensed SLP may supervise 3 assistants; licensed audiologist may supervise 10 assistants)

States that Specify the Amount/Percentage of Direct/Indirect Supervision (25 states, including those that do not officially regulate support personnel)

AL, AR, CA, CT, FL, GA, IA, IN, KS, KY, LA, ME, MS, MT, NE, NH, NM, OH, RI, SC, TN, TX, UT, WV, WI

States with Specific Definitions of Acceptable and Unacceptable Activities for Support Personnel (22 states)

AL, AK, AR, FL, GA, KS, KY, LA, ME, MS, MO, MT, NE, NM, NC, OH, OR, PA, SC, TX, UT, WV

NOTE. SLP = speech-language pathologist; asst. = assistant; assoc. = associate.

SOURCE: Prepared by Susan Pilch, JD, ASHA Director, State Legislative and Regulatory Advocacy

Laws and regulations may change at any time, so always check with the actual state regulatory board for the most up-to-date information. See the ASHA Web site at www.asha.org/governmental_affairs/state_policy.htm (click on state overviews) for state licensing board contact information. (Updated 9/06)

personnel. Of the states that regulate the use of support personnel, a wide range of educational requirements is found. A few states have different requirements for different levels of support personnel, ranging from a high school diploma or equivalent to a bachelor's degree in communication disorders with enrollment in a master's degree. Continuing education for support personnel is required in 10 states. A variety of titles is used to designate support personnel in the professions, with *assistant* being the most common. State agencies (licensure boards) currently regulating support personnel also have a variety of differing supervision requirements (see Table 10–2).

In addition to state regulatory agencies, state education agencies may credential support personnel to work solely in schools to support service delivery provided by qualified professionals. Some school districts hire assistants under the classification of teacher assistants. If a state regulates support personnel (i.e., under the term of *assistant, aide, paraprofessional,* or *apprentice*), then individuals who wish to

become employed in that state must meet the state requirements for practice under a licensed professional. ASHA also requires that audiologists and SLPs hold the Certificate of Clinical Competence to supervise support personnel (ASHA, 2005a). Table 10–3 provides information about the regulation of support personnel in schools in all states. Addresses and phone numbers for state licensure boards or departments of education are available at the ASHA Web site.

State regulations may differ from professional policies. In those states where there is a conflict, ASHA guidelines indicate that professionals should abide by whichever legal mandates or professional policies are more stringent (ASHA, 2004d). ASHA and the National Council of State Boards of Examiners for Speech-Language Pathology and Audiology developed a set of guiding principles addressing state laws/regulations and ASHA standards, guidelines, and requirements to clarify the relationship to help professionals meet both their legal and ethical obligations (ASHA, 1998a).

T A B L E 10–3 Regulation of Support Personnel in Schools

The use of support personnel in schools falls in one of the following categories:

1. Same requirements for SLP assistants in health care and school settings (11 states): A state license or credential (registration) obtained from the state's audiology and speech-language pathology licensure board is required for all settings (including schools). Alaska, Delaware, Florida, Idaho, Indiana, Kansas, Kentucky, Louisiana, North Carolina, Oregon, Texas

2. Separate State Department of Education credential is required (7 states): Georgia, Hawaii, Missouri, Nebraska, North Dakota, Vermont, West Virginia

3. General education paraprofessionals are used, with no specific training in speech-language pathology (11 states): Alabama, Arizona, California, Iowa, Maine, Minnesota, New Hampshire, South Dakota, Virginia, Wisconsin, Wyoming

4. These states have a state-specific approach to the use of SLP support personnel (4 states):
   - Arkansas: Must be written agreement between Arkansas Department of Education Special Education Unit and the state licensure board to use SLP aides and assistants.
   - Colorado: Employing school district must apply for SLP Assistant Authorization.
   - Illinois: Two types of support personnel used—assistants credentialed by SLP licensure board and SLP paraprofessionals credentialed by Department of Education.
   - Missouri: Districts must request approval for use of SLP implementers—only allowed after advertising/recruitment effort has been made for fully qualified person.

Not Currently Used (17 states)

Connecticut, Maryland, Massachusetts, Michigan, Mississippi, Nevada, New Jersey, New Mexico, New York, Ohio, Oklahoma, Pennsylvania, Rhode Island, South Carolina, Utah, Washington, Tennessee

SOURCE: Prepared by Susan Pilch, JD, ASHA Director, State Legislative and Regulatory Advocacy (Updated 11/05)

CURRENT USE OF SUPPORT PERSONNEL

Survey data were reviewed to determine the current use of SLP and audiology support personnel in educational and health care settings. Changes in the employment rates of support personnel over time also were explored for each profession.

SLP Support Personnel

The use of SLP assistants in the schools appears to have remained stable over the last 12 years, with approximately 25 percent of SLPs reporting that they work with assistants (ASHA, 1992b, 2004a). Recent survey data suggest a decline in use of SLP support personnel in health care settings (ASHA, 2003a). The 1992 ASHA Omnibus Survey found that 25 percent to 31 percent of respondents were assisted by support personnel (ASHA, 1992a). In 2002, only 2 percent of SLPs in health care settings reported that they employ SLP assistants (ASHA, 2002b). Between 8 percent and 13 percent reported that they employ other support personnel, such as rehabilitation technicians (ASHA, 2002b). SLPs working in facilities that use assistants report that they employ approximately 5.2 assistants (ASHA, 2003a).

Audiology Support Personnel

The most recent data from ASHA regarding support personnel in audiology are from the 1993 and 1995 ASHA Omnibus Surveys. Data from the 1993 survey showed that 16.4 percent of the audiologists who responded employed "audiometric technicians" in their facility. The main services provided by these technicians were troubleshooting amplification devices (14.4 percent), hearing screening for children (14.2 percent), hearing screening for adults (13.4 percent), assistance with ear mold impressions (11.9 percent), hearing aid repair (11.9 percent), and hearing screening for industry (10.3 percent) (ASHA, 1993). In 1995, 42.9 percent of audiologists who responded indicated that they support the use of audiometric technicians/assistants for audiology

service delivery. These audiologists considered the following to be appropriate supervised activities for technicians/assistants to perform: pure-tone air conduction hearing screening (96.4 percent), minor repair of amplification devices or parts replacement (90.9 percent), administration of automated brainstem response management without interpretation (56.6 percent), and audiologic rehabilitation treatment assistance (55.6 percent) (ASHA, 1995a).

A 2001 survey of audiologists showed that 45 percent hired assistants or previously hired assistants in their practices (Hamill & Freeman, 2001). A 2004 AAA survey of AAA members showed that approximately 28.4 percent of audiologists employed assistants (AAA, 2005). A 2005 report from the United States Department of Veterans Affairs by Robert Dunlop revealed a 619 percent increase in the number of audiology support personnel in Veterans Administration hospitals from 1996 to 2004 with a decrease in the ratio of audiologists to support personnel from 24:1 in 1996 to 5.26:1 in 2004 (as cited in AAA, 2005).

TRAINING FOR SUPPORT PERSONNEL

It is the responsibility of the supervising SLP and audiologist to ensure that the support person is adequately trained. Support personnel should not be permitted to work with individuals unless the supervising professional is confident that the support person has obtained a reasonable amount of training and possesses the appropriate skills.

Training SLP Support Personnel

The training requirements for SLP support personnel vary across the country. ASHA's guidelines are national in scope and were developed to promote greater uniformity in training requirements (ASHA, 2004d). ASHA recommends completion of an associate's degree from a technical training program with a program of study designed to prepare the student to be an SLP assistant. The ASHA guidelines suggest that SLP assistants complete course work, field work, and on-the-job training. The guidelines also recommend that the assistant demonstrate necessary technical skills to fulfill the SLP assistant job responsibilities. The document includes a sample curriculum, field work recommendations, and a sample technical proficiency form (see Appendix 10-B at the end of this chapter for a copy of the technical proficiency form). As of September 2006, we are aware of 27 operational associate degree programs for SLP assistants. Some of these programs have training opportunities through distance learning and collaborations between community colleges and universities. The course work and field work experiences required in the SLP assistant training program typically differ from those at the bachelor's, preprofessional, or master's professional levels. It is a challenge for SLP assistant training programs in community colleges to locate textbooks that are written specifically for SLP assistants. Often the programs must use more advanced textbooks that are written for SLP students and omit the sections that do not apply, such as those related to assessment and diagnosis and detailed theoretical discussions.

Assistant-level training programs are not specifically intended to be the start of a career ladder to professional level positions; however, some programs lend themselves to such opportunities. Assistant training programs also may be another avenue for bilingual and bicultural students to seek their bachelor's and master's degrees in communication sciences and disorders. Universities do not always accept course work from the SLP assistant training program to transfer to the bachelor's degree programs. Knowledge and skills needed to be an SLP assistant are distinctly different from those needed to be an ASHA-certified SLP. Academic programs/institutions have the discretion to determine which academic course work completed in technical training programs will be accepted for transfer to a bachelor's degree program. Students interested in pursuing a career as an SLP are encouraged to verify the transferability of credits between assistant training programs and bachelor's programs. Students also are encouraged to investigate the requirements of graduate educational programs to ensure that basic science courses taken at the undergraduate level will be acceptable to the graduate program (ASHA, 2005a).

Training Audiology Support Personnel

Support personnel in audiology are expected to have at least a high school diploma or equivalent and are expected to have competency-based skills needed to perform assigned tasks (AAA, 2005; ASHA, 1998b). According to the professional policies, training for support personnel in audiology should be planned and implemented by the supervising audiologist. In addition, the training process needs to encompass all assigned tasks, include information on roles and functions, and be (1) well designed, (2) specific to the assigned task, (3) competency based, and (4) provided through a variety of formal and informal instructional methods (AAA, 2005; ASHA, 1998b). Training programs for audiology support personnel include a structured technician program provided by the military, formal training programs in colleges or universities, occupational hearing conservation technician programs, and on-the-job training programs by audiologists.

An example of training programs for audiology support personnel at colleges or universities is the program of study for audiologist's assistants at Nova Southeastern University. The program has two self-paced training modules. One module prepares the student to assist in diagnostic testing, including conducting tympanometry, pure-tone air conduction testing on patients with prior complete testing on file, and screenings, as well as assisting the audiologist with other diagnostic tests. The second module is geared toward hearing aids. The assistant learns to make ear mold impressions; teaches patients how to insert, remove, and use their hearing aids; and performs troubleshooting on aids. Much of the material is presented through slide shows, distributed on CD, with assignments to complete.

The training program offered by CAOHC for occupational hearing conservationists involves successful completion of a practical and written exam after a 20-hour course on a variety of topics (e.g., social and legal ramifications of noise on people; basic anatomy, physiology, and diseases of the human ear; basic acoustics, noise measurements, and monitoring of noise in the work environment; federal and state regulations relating to noise and hearing loss; pure-tone audiometric procedures; recording of test data and record keeping; calibration requirements of test equipment and troubleshooting equipment problems; educating employees about hearing conservation; selection and fitting of hearing protection devices). CAOHC also offers an 8-hour recertification course; recertification is required every 5 years.

SUPERVISION OF SUPPORT PERSONNEL

Audiologists and SLPs may delegate services to support personnel only with appropriate supervision (ASHA, 2003b). It is essential that the supervising professional has the knowledge and skills needed to provide such supervision (ASHA, 2002a). Table 10–4 shows the knowledge and skills identified for supervisors of SLP assistants.

Management and supervision skills are not synonymous with the skills needed to be a highly qualified SLP or audiologist. Many professionals have not received specific supervisory training during their preservice education programs. To become a competent supervisor and manager, professionals may consider taking continuing education courses that target these areas. The amount and type of supervision provided should be based on the skills and experience of the support person, the needs of patients/clients served, the service delivery setting, the tasks assigned, and other factors such as initiation of a new program, orientation of new staff, and change in patient/client status (ASHA, 1998b, 2004d). The goal for the supervising professional is to ensure that support personnel restrict their clinical activities to prescribed tasks in contrast with the goal of independent clinical practice for supervision of students and clinical fellows (ASHA, 1985b; Paul-Brown & Goldberg, 2001).

T A B L E 10–4 Knowledge and Skills for Supervisors of Speech-Language Pathology Assistants

According to ASHA (2002a), the supervisor of SLP assistants needs to have the knowledge and skills to

- select and assign appropriate patients/clients to the SLP assistant
- determine the nature of supervision that is appropriate for each SLP assistant
- establish and maintain an effective relationship with the SLP assistant
- direct the SLP assistant in how to follow screening protocols
- demonstrate for and participate in the clinical process with the SLP assistant
- direct the SLP assistant in following individualized treatment plans that have been developed by the SLP
- direct the SLP assistant in the maintenance of clinical records
- interact with the SLP assistant in planning and executing supervisory conferences
- provide feedback to the SLP assistant regarding skills
- help the SLP assistant to develop skills of verbal reporting and assigned informal written reporting
- assist the SLP assistant to effectively select, prepare, and present treatment materials and organize treatment environments
- share information regarding ethical, legal, regulatory, and reimbursement aspects of professional practice
- model and facilitate professional conduct
- direct the SLP assistant in the implementation of research procedures, in-service training, and public relations programs
- train the SLP assistant to check and maintain equipment and to observe universal precautions
- guide the SLP assistant to use appropriate language (oral and written) when interacting with patients/clients and others
- establish a system of accountability for document use and supervision of the SLP assistant

SOURCE: From American Speech-Language-Hearing Association (2002a). Knowledge and skills for supervisors of speech-language pathology assistants. *ASHA Supplement, 22,* 113–188.

The supervising SLP or audiologist is responsible for the actions of support personnel. Specifically, the SLP or audiology supervisor would be held responsible and could be subject to sanctions if an assistant performed activities beyond the scope of his or her job responsibilities. Thus, any alleged violation of the Code(s) of Ethics governing the supervising professionals should be reported to the AAA Ethical Practices Board or the ASHA Board of Ethics for adjudication. According to the revised Issues in Ethics Statement on Support Personnel (ASHA, 2004h), "It is the responsibility of ASHA members and certificate holders to ensure that support personnel under their supervision behave in an ethical manner . . ." Thus, although ASHA does not have jurisdiction over support personnel, ASHA members and certificate holders are vicariously liable for the unethical conduct of support personnel they supervise and can sanction them if they are found in violation.

State laws pertaining to supervision vary and may differ from professional policies. This means that SLPs and audiologists need to check specific state regulations to determine amount of supervision required and qualifications for supervisors of assistants in a particular state. ASHA (2004d) provides the following guidance to assist SLPs and audiologists when state laws are more or less stringent than ASHA policies regarding supervision of support personnel:

> Fully qualified professionals and support personnel are legally bound to follow licensure laws and rules that regulate them and their practice in the state in which they work. Use of support personnel is not permitted in every state. ASHA members also are ethically bound to follow ASHA guidelines. (p. 5)

Concerns are ever present about the potential for inappropriate actions by support personnel and the lack of consequences when there are no state regulations to govern the use of SLP or audiology support personnel. Currently, no professional organization has direct oversight of the actions of support personnel in audiology or speech-language pathology. This is of particular concern when an SLP assistant or audiology support personnel is working under the supervision of a professional who is not required to be ASHA-certified and/or is employed in a state where there is no law that addresses the use of SLP or audiology support personnel.

Supervision of SLP Assistants

ASHA provides specific guidance related to the amount and type of supervision for SLP support personnel. For an SLP assistant in training, ASHA recommends no less than 50 percent direct supervision (ASHA, 2004d). The minimum amount of supervision suggested for a trained assistant is 30 percent weekly (at least 20 percent direct) for the first 90 workdays and 20 percent (at least 10 percent direct) after the initial work period. Direct supervision means "onsite, in-view observation and guidance by the SLP while an assigned activity is performed by support personnel," and indirect supervision "may include demonstrations, record review, review and evaluation of audio- or videotaped sessions, and/or interactive television" (ASHA, 2004d, p. 3). The ASHA assistant guidelines recommend that an SLP supervise no more than three SLP assistants at the same time (ASHA, 2004d).

The supervising SLP has responsibility for establishing a means of documenting the supervision of the SLP assistant. Appendix 10-C at the end of this chapter includes a sample supervision log for recording direct and indirect observations. Even when faced with time and workload pressures, the SLP is expected to adhere to these supervision guidelines. Although national and state guidelines are available to guide decisions about the amount of direct and indirect supervision, it remains the supervising SLP's responsibility to determine the type and exact amount (beyond the minimum) of supervision that each SLP assistant requires. For example, some SLP assistants may require more guidance and oversight to complete the required documentation. Another SLP assistant may need mentoring to ensure adherence to the rules and regulations of the facility. The SLP makes these decisions on the basis of the SLP assistant's individual strengths and technical proficiency.

Supervision of Audiology Support Personnel

Neither ASHA nor AAA has prescribed supervisory requirements for training support personnel in audiology; nor are there professional policies that set a specific amount of supervision after training or that specify a maximum number of support personnel to be employed. The supervising audiologist has the sole responsibility for these decisions (AAA, 2005; ASHA, 1998b).

Regarding supervision of occupational hearing conservation personnel, the Hearing Conservation Amendment (HCA), administered by the United States Department of Labor's Occupational Safety and Health Administration (OSHA), specifies who may perform certain audiological procedures and indicates where the responsibility resides. According to section 1910.95(g) (3) of the HCA:

> Audiometric tests shall be performed by a licensed or certified audiologist, otolaryngologist, or other physician, or by a technician who is certified by the Council of Accreditation in Occupational Hearing Conservation, or who has satisfactorily demonstrated competence in administering audiometric examinations, obtaining valid audiograms, and properly using, maintaining and checking calibration and proper functioning of the audiometers being used. A technician who operates microprocessor audiometers does not need to be certified. A technician who performs audiometric tests must be responsible to an audiologist, otolaryngologist, or physician.

With regard to supervision of OTO techs, an otolaryngologist is responsible for providing supervision during the 6-month portion of the training period. Thereafter, the OTO tech works loosely under the supervision of the physician. However, this is similar to a physician providing supervision to anyone in the physician's office who provides patient care as governed by the state's medical practices act. Presumably, a credentialed audiologist also may provide supervision to the OTO tech consistent with the Code(s) of Ethics governing the audiologist and provided the physician accepts this role for the audiologist (American Academy of Otolaryngology–Head and Neck Surgery, 2006).

JOB RESPONSIBILITIES OF SLP ASSISTANTS

According to the ASHA guidelines, the SLP should be involved in the hiring of an assistant (ASHA, 2004d). Because the assistant must be supervised by a licensed and certified SLP, the supervising SLP should make decisions about the specific tasks and activities assigned to the SLP assistant. The SLP should advise the administrator of a facility or school principal that it is the supervising SLP's responsibility to select the clients/patients, assign responsibilities, and determine the amount and type of supervision needed. Viewed collectively across states, support personnel have a broad scope of responsibilities ranging from clerical duties to clinical activities. ASHA has delineated a restricted set of tasks that an SLP may delegate to an SLP assistant (see Table 10–5) and those services that only an SLP can provide (see Table 10–6; ASHA, 2004d). It is the responsibility of the supervising SLP to make certain that SLP assistants engage only in those activities that are within their job responsibilities. The SLP assigns students/clients to an SLP assistant on the basis of the student's needs and the SLP assistant's level of experience. The SLP assistant may be assigned to work with clients/students on previously learned, less clinically challenging, or more rote or repetitive skills. For example, the SLP may assign an SLP assistant to work with a student on increasing generalization after the SLP has worked with the student to establish a specific sound in words or a phonological process. This allows the SLP to devote more time to the most clinically challenging clients. Support personnel also may work as members of a team in health care and education settings (Longhurst, 1997). In schools, IDEA has institutionalized the practice of using teams to determine the most appropriate course of action for each student and to collaborate and develop the Individualized Family Service Plan or the Individualized Education Program (IEP).

T A B L E 10–5 Job Responsibilities for Speech-Language Pathology Assistants

According to ASHA's 2004 *Guidelines for the Training, Use, and Supervision of Speech-Language Pathology Assistants,* which apply across all practice settings, SLP assistants may conduct the following tasks under the supervision of an SLP:

- assist with speech-language and hearing screenings (without interpretation)
- assist with informal documentation as directed by the SLP
- follow documented treatment plans or protocols developed by the supervising SLP
- document patient/client performance (e.g., tallying data for the SLP; preparing charts, records, and graphs) and report this information to the supervising SLP
- assist the SLP during assessment of patients/clients
- assist with clerical duties such as preparing materials and scheduling activities as directed by the SLP
- perform checks and maintenance of equipment
- support the supervising SLP in research projects, in-service training, and public relations programs
- assist with departmental operations (scheduling, record keeping, safety/maintenance of supplies and equipment)
- collect data for monitoring quality improvement
- exhibit compliance with regulations, reimbursement requirements, and SLP assistant's job responsibilities

NOTE. State laws vary and may differ from ASHA guidelines. Certain tasks may be outside the scope of responsibilities for assistants in a particular state.

SOURCE: From *Guidelines for the Training, Use, and Supervision of Speech-Language Pathology Assistants, 2003.* Rockville, MD: American Speech-Language-Hearing Association. Available from http://www.asha.org/about/publications/reference-library/. Reprinted with permission.

T A B L E 10–6 Tasks Outside the Speech-Language Pathology Assistant's Scope of Responsibilities

According to ASHA's 2004 *Guidelines for the Training, Use, and Supervision of Speech-Language Pathology Assistants,* which apply across all practice settings, speech-language pathology assistants *may not* perform the following tasks:

- administer standardized or nonstandardized diagnostic tests, formal or informal evaluations, or clinical interpretation of test results
- screen or diagnose patients/clients for feeding/swallowing disorders
- participate in parent conferences, case conferences, or any interdisciplinary team without the presence of the supervising SLP or other certified SLP designated by the supervising SLP
- write, develop, or modify a patient/client's individualized treatment plan in any way
- assist with patients/clients without following the individualized treatment plan prepared by the SLP or without access to supervision
- sign any formal documents (e.g., treatment plans, reimbursement forms, or reports; the assistant should sign or initial informal treatment notes for review and cosignature by the supervising professional)
- select patients/clients for service
- discharge a patient/client from service
- disclose clinical or confidential information either orally or in writing to anyone other than the supervising SLP
- make referrals for additional service
- counsel or consult with the patient/client, family, or others regarding the patient/client status or service
- use a checklist or tabulate results of feeding or swallowing evaluations
- demonstrate swallowing strategies or precautions to patients, family, or staff
- represent himself or herself as an SLP

NOTE. State laws vary and may differ from ASHA guidelines. Certain tasks may be outside the scope of responsibilities for assistants in a particular state.

SOURCE: From Guidelines for the Training, Use, and Supervision of Speech-Language Pathology Assistants, 2004d. Rockville, MD: American Speech-Language-Hearing Association. Available at http://www.asha.org/about/publications/reference-library/. Reprinted with permission.

JOB RESPONSIBILITIES OF AUDIOLOGY SUPPORT PERSONNEL

The supervising audiologist is responsible for planning and delegating tasks that a support person may perform. Examples of tasks that have been delegated to support personnel by supervising audiologists included daily visual and listening checks on hearing aids and auditory trainers for children in public schools (Johnson, 1999); assisting with hearing screenings, hearing aid monitoring, and use of assistive listening devices in rehabilitation hospitals (Johnson, Clark-Lewis, & Griffin, 1998); learning ways to optimize communication during interactions with persons with hearing loss (Johnson et al., 1998); and assisting with hearing conservation programs at work sites (ASHA, 2004b; Suter, 2002).

The audiologist has exclusive responsibility for a variety of clinical activities. Audiology support personnel may not interpret data; determine case selection; transmit clinical information, either verbally or in writing, to anyone without the approval of the supervising audiologist; compose clinical reports; make referrals; sign any formal documents (e.g., treatment plans, reimbursement forms, or reports); discharge a patient/client from services; or communicate with the patient/client, family, or others regarding any aspect of the patient/client status or service without the specific consent of the supervising audiologist (ASHA, 1998b, p. 60).

REIMBURSEMENT OF SERVICES PROVIDED BY SUPPORT PERSONNEL

Medicare policy currently does not recognize SLP or audiology assistants, regardless of the level of supervision. Private insurers may cover licensed or registered SLP assistants. One must query each payer to verify coverage. Private insurers may or may not provide a different rate of reimbursement for services provided by an SLP or audiologist as opposed to an SLP or audiology assistant. Services provided by professionals and their assistants are considered skilled services, as the assistants are implementing the treatment devised by the SLP or audiologist. Most private insurers do not cover services that do not require the skills (directly or indirectly) of an SLP or audiologist. There are some clear definitions of what type of activity constitutes a skilled service in the "Model Medical Review Guidelines for Speech-Language Pathology Services" (ASHA, 2005b): "The services must be of such a level of complexity and sophistication, or the patient's condition must be such that the services required can be safely and effectively performed only by or under the supervision of a qualified speech pathologist." Nonskilled activities include: "Nondiagnostic, non-therapeutic, routine, and repetitive and reinforced procedures . . . which may effectively be carried out with the patient by any nonprofessional (e.g., family member, restorative nursing aide) after instruction and training is completed."

Each state has considerable latitude in administering its Medicaid program. The federal regulation states that services may be rendered "by or under the direction of" a qualified SLP, but the state may still prescribe the qualifications of the subordinate practitioners. The state would be more likely to assign a Medicaid provider number to SLP assistants if they were registered or licensed in the state.

The federal regulations for Medicaid specifically recognize services provided by audiology support personnel if such services are provided under the direction of a qualified audiologist. According to the regulations, the supervising audiologist must have face-to-face contact with the client in the beginning and periodically throughout the treatment. The audiologist must provide adequate supervision of support staff as well as keep documentation of the supervision and ongoing involvement in the case. If the audiologist is employed by a Medicaid agency, clinic, or school, the federal regulations require that the audiologist's employment terms allow for adequate supervision of support personnel. Although specific supervision ratios are not stated, the regulations do require that these ratios be "reasonable and ethical and in keeping with professioinal practice acts" (Preamble to Federal Regulations).

RESEARCH RELATED TO SUPPORT PERSONNEL

To determine the effectiveness of using support personnel to extend the clinical work of SLPs and audiologists, a systematic literature search of published English language studies was conducted using 22 electronic databases. The studies, which spanned several decades, needed to be relevant to various clinical questions and contain original data or purport to be systematic reviews of the literature. A summary of the studies is provided below for four clinical questions.

Have Any Studies Compared SLP or Audiology Assistants with Professionals?

No studies were identified that compared audiology assistants with professional service provision. Some studies compared treatment outcomes by SLP assistants and SLPs, primarily with elementary schoolchildren with articulation disorders and adults with aphasia.

Studies with Children Studies involving children, most conducted in the mid-1970s, found no significant differences in the articulation outcomes of children with mild-to-moderate speech disorders when comparing treatment by *trained paraprofessionals* (also called *supportive personnel* or *speech therapy aides*) and professional clinicians; children in both groups showed improvements in articulation (Alvord, 1977; Costello & Schoen, 1978; Gray & Barker, 1977). Sounds that were not targeted for treatment showed no change for children in either the aide or clinician group (Gray & Barker, 1977).

One study reported no significant differences between groups of children with learning disabilities with "perceptual deficits" treated by trained "perceptual-aides" and "therapists" (including occupational, physical, recreational, and language); improvements were noted in motor skills, visual, and somatosensory perception, language, and educations skills in children from both treatment groups (Gersten et al., 1975). One study reported that four out of five young children made more progress on computer-based language tasks when a parent volunteer provided the training compared with an SLP (Schery & O'Connor, 1997). Small sample size and lack of statistical comparison make these results difficult to interpret.

A mother–child home program administered by paraprofessionals was compared with interventions by professionals that were tailored to the cognitive and language needs of two-year-old children. Children in both groups showed similar improvements; however, the children were still delayed in cognitive and language functioning at age 4 in both groups (Scarr, McCartney, Miller, Hauenstein, & Ricciuti, 1996).

Studies with Adults Studies comparing nonprofessionals and professionals providing clinical services for adults focused primarily on volunteers working with individuals with aphasia. Patients showed improvement in communication, and no differences were found in the amount of progress made for adults who received services from professionals compared with those receiving services from untrained volunteers (David, Enderby, & Bainton, 1982; Meikle et al., 1979). In a study with trained volunteers (e.g., wife, friend, or relative), men with aphasia showed improvement in their communication during treatment but not when treatment was discontinued. These results were similar to patients with aphasia who received treatment from SLPs (Marshall et al., 1989). In a study that compared three different treatment approaches and a no-treatment condition, two of the treatments for patients with aphasia were administered by professionals, and one was administered by "trained nonprofessionals" (Shewan & Kertesz, 1984). The two approaches administered by professionals showed significant differences compared with the nontreatment condition; the treatment method used by nonprofessionals approached significance. It is not possible to determine whether the difference in significance level was due to the treatment approaches themselves or to differences between nonprofessionals and professionals. In another study with patients with aphasia, comparisons were made among clinic treatment by an SLP, home treatment by a trained volunteer, and deferred treatment. No significant differences were found among the three groups after the deferred-treatment group received treatment by a professional (Wertz et al., 1986).

Studies Comparing Service by Professionals and Support Personnel Ideally, supervising professionals should only assign tasks to support personnel that can be performed with the same level of quality as professionals. The studies available reveal no differences in treatment outcomes for children or adults when the services provided by assistants are compared with those provided by professionals. The consistency between outcomes for professionals and support personnel is encouraging for those who employ or wish to employ assistants. Clearly, more research, with a large enough sample for adequate statistical power and sound methodology, is needed (see summary by Greener, Enderby, & Whurr, 1999).

Do Any Studies Show the Effectiveness of SLP or Audiology Assistants?

The studies described for the first clinical question (i.e., comparing clinical service by assistants with professionals) also address the second question of the effectiveness of SLP or audiology assistants. All of the previously cited studies showed that children and adults made improvements when SLP assistants were used. Other studies have been conducted that show the effectiveness of SLP or audiology assistants but did not have a comparison group of professionals.

Effectiveness of Support Personnel in SLP The few studies conducted on the effectiveness of SLP support personnel focus primarily on their use with children with articulation and expressive language disorders and adults with aphasia or dementia.

Studies with Children SLP support personnel have been used to conduct speech and language screening programs for children. In a pilot program, existing school personnel serving as "aides" were trained to screen the speech and language skills of elementary-age children. The aides were reported to

administer the screening tests accurately to make appropriate referrals for those children with a high probability of having speech and language problems (Pickering & Dopheide, 1976). In another pilot screening program, "paraprofessionals" screened young children between 19 and 21 months during home visits for language delay. Screening data from the administration of a standardized screening test were found to be reliable, valid, and sensitive in identifying children for further assessment (Pickstone, 2003).

Children with speech sound disorders showed improvement when they received speech services from SLP support personnel. A study of articulation treatment for elementary-age children by trained paraprofessionals reported that 83.5 percent of the treated sounds were used correctly in a conversational sample (Galloway & Blue, 1975). Improvements in speech production were reported for children treated by students (Hall & Knutson, 1978), "communication aides" (Van Hattum et al., 1974), and paid aides and volunteers (Scalero & Eskenazi, 1976).

Studies focused on improving language skills in children also demonstrated improvements when services were provided by SLP support personnel. A single-participant study reported increases in communication (e.g., percentage of correct information and words per minute) when a "nonprofessional" provided a structured maintenance program for an individual with epilepsy and language and cognitive impairments (Wright, Shisler, & Rau, 2003). Teachers in another study reported that 41 percent of their 22 kindergarten students showed improvement after receiving computer-aided language enrichment by volunteers, although the outcomes were not quantified (Schetz, 1989). "Nonprofessional tutors" were used to help first-grade children develop phonological and early reading skills (Vadasy, Jenkins, & Pool, 2000). Tutors provided one-to-one instruction for 30 minutes, 4 days a week, for 1 school year in phonological skills, letter–sound correspondence, decoding, rhyming, writing, spelling, and reading. Tutored children received significantly better reading, spelling, and decoding scores than students who did not receive tutoring. The tutored children continued to do better than nontutored children in decoding and spelling after second grade.

Positive outcomes in speech and language also were shown when children with severe disabilities received services from SLP support personnel. In one study, two psychiatric aides who served as "para-professional teachers" were trained to use a structured language training program with children with severe disabilities. In this study, matched pairs of children were randomly assigned to an experimental or control condition. Results showed that the children in the experimental group who received language training by the aides for 2 months showed improvement in language (e.g., identifying and labeling objects) and social skills (Phillips, Liebert, & Poulos, 1973). Another study trained undergraduate students to use behavioral principles to develop the verbal behavior of young children with severe disabilities with limited verbal repertoires (Guralnick, 1972). Five of the eight children showed progress in their development of communication skills (e.g., imitation of sounds, sustaining eye contact, using gestures). Another article reported on the use of blind and partially sighted high school students who were trained and paid to serve as "speech assistants" in a residential school to provide extra class practice for younger children with visual impairments who had speech problems (Briggs, 1974). Although data were not collected on the speech outcomes of the students receiving services, the author reported that most appeared to benefit from the additional practice provided by the assistants.

Studies with Adults   Adults with aphasia showed communication improvements when treatment was provided by support personnel, including relatives (Lesser, Bryan, Anderson, & Hilton, 1986), untrained volunteers (Eaton Griffith, 1975; Griffith & Miller, 1980; Lesser & Watt, 1978), and "community volunteers" (Lyon et al., 1997). Similarly, adults with "communication handicaps" showed increased responsiveness, verbalizations, and social interactions when trained volunteers were used as an adjunct to professional treatment (Mueller, 1990). Trained volunteers were judged to be better conversational partners for adults with aphasia than were untrained

volunteers (Kagan, Black, Duchan, Simmons-Mackie, & Square, 2001). In this study, trained volunteers scored significantly higher on acknowledging and revealing the competence of adults with aphasia during conversational interactions. The individuals with aphasia showed significant improvements in social skills and message exchange skills when interacting with volunteers who received supported conversation training. These changes were not seen in the adults with aphasia who interacted with the untrained volunteers.

Support personnel also have been used successfully with adults with dementia. One article described a "partnered volunteering" language and memory stimulation program for adults with Alzheimer's disease. The study reported positive changes in language and memory on pre- and posttests after two semesters of service by student volunteers from speech-language pathology or psychology (Arkin, 1996). Another study used nursing assistants to enhance discourse skills of nursing home residents with dementia. In this study, one group of nursing assistants was trained and supervised using communication techniques and memory books with the residents. A control group paired nursing assistants with residents with dementia but did not use specific communication or memory tools. The conversational skills of residents in the treatment group were more coherent and had fewer vague "empty phrases" compared with the no-treatment control group. The nursing assistants in the treatment group also used more "facilitative discourse strategies" (e.g., encouragement, cuing) than assistants in the control group (Dijkstra, Bourgeois, Burgio, & Allen, 2002).

Effectiveness of Support Personnel in Audiology

Only one study was identified that addressed the use of support personnel for individuals with hearing loss. A Canadian consumer organization trained seniors with hearing loss to serve as peer models and provide support for other seniors with hearing loss in long-term health care facilities or in the community (Dahl, 1997). The volunteers were trained to assist with hearing aid care, use of assistive listening devices, and strategies for coping with hearing loss. Within a 5-month period, the volunteers totaled 288 weekly half-day visits. The seniors receiving support found the visitor program to be helpful. An informal follow-up evaluation one year after the project showed continued visits by some of the volunteers and the addition of new trained volunteers.

Four studies were identified that addressed whether audiometric technicians could determine which patients could be fitted with a hearing aid without the need for a medical referral. One study was conducted to determine if "physiological measurement technicians" could safely prescribe hearing aids without medical supervision. The technicians reportedly failed to mention the presence of active inflammatory ear disease in the referral letter for three of eight cases where middle ear disease was present. The authors concluded that review by ear, nose, and throat (ENT) medical staff was needed before prescription of a hearing aid (Bellini, Beesley, Perrett, & Pickles, 1989). In the other studies, the authors concluded that the audiology technicians made accurate assessments of patients to determine if they required a hearing aid referral to an ENT (Koay & Sutton, 1996; Swan & Browning, 1994; Zeitoun, Lesshafft, Begg, & East, 1995). For example, a "senior audiology technician or higher grade" working in a general practitioner's office determined that 23 percent of the 135 patients required medical referral before being fitted for a hearing aid. The ENT review of the same patients showed 100 percent agreement with the audiology technicians (Koay & Sutton, 1996).

Effectiveness of SLP and Audiology Support Personnel The effectiveness of SLP and audiology support personnel remains an open question. Only a few studies are available, and most of those were conducted in the 1970s and 1980s. The methodological quality of many of the studies was poor (e.g., no control group, few participants, no randomized groups, few statistical comparisons) or not accessible. The available studies appeared to show that the use of SLP assistants could be effective in improving speech production for children with

articulation disorders or conversational skills for adults with aphasia or dementia. Audiometric technicians appear capable of determining which patients need a medical referral before being fitted for a hearing aid.

Are There Any Studies on the Amount or Type of SLP or Audiology Assistant Supervision?

No studies were found that were designed to determine the amount or type of supervision that would be most effective for the use of SLP or audiology assistants.

Do Any Studies Show the Effectiveness of Training Programs for SLP or Audiology Assistants?

No articles were found through the literature search that provided data on the effectiveness of SLP or audiology assistant training programs. None were found that compared different types of training modules. A few articles described training programs to prepare SLP assistants. For example, two articles described statewide public school programs for support personnel working with children with articulation disorders (Blodgett & Miller, 1997; Scalero & Eskenazi, 1976). One article described four model preservice training programs for communication assistants working in the schools with students with language and hearing problems (Shinn-Strieker, 1984). Another article presented a university program for preprofessional undergraduate students working as communication aides in schools (Hall & Knutson, 1978), and one described a program based in a rehabilitation center to train support personnel in speech-language pathology to work with individuals with traumatic brain injury (Werven, 1992).

Future Research Issues

In 1977, Gray and Barker wrote that "there is little substantive information about whether or not [aides] can reliably and effectively provide services"

(p. 534). Almost 30 years later, this same statement can still be made. There is a paucity of high-quality efficacy research on the use of support personnel in audiology or speech-language pathology. Among the few studies conducted, there is some evidence of comparable outcomes between supervised SLP assistants and professionals, particularly when services are limited to more repetitive treatment activities. Although some studies demonstrate that SLP assistants and audiology support personnel can carry out assigned tasks, most are descriptive rather than empirical. Few research designs go beyond a low level of evidence using case studies with no randomization or control group (ASHA, 2004c).

Research also is needed pertaining to the optimal amount or type of supervision necessary for assistants with various amounts of experience and to determine the effectiveness of different types of training programs for support personnel. The use of appropriately trained and supervised support personnel may be a viable option in some settings as a means to enhance the frequency and intensity of service delivery in the professions of audiology and speech-language pathology. However, more evidence, and better quality evidence, is needed before the value of SLP and audiology support personnel can be ascertained.

SUMMARY

The intended use of support personnel is to supplement and not supplant the work of the qualified professional. The SLP and audiology assistant may be hired to increase the frequency, intensity, efficiency, and availability of services by following a specific set of job responsibilities. However, the licensed and certified professional ultimately remains responsible for the training, selection, management, and supervision of the assistant. It is also the professional's obligation to inform the consumer of the level of training and expertise of the assistant, so that at no time is the assistant represented as an SLP or audiologist. The professional retains the legal and ethical responsibility for all services provided or omitted.

The professional and the assistant need to work as a team to support the communication needs of the individuals they serve. Although ASHA currently does not credential assistants, a number of states regulate their use. In these states, the use of assistants can be monitored, ensuring that the assistants are used in a legal manner in terms of education and supervision. Adherence to professional guidelines also serves as a means of monitoring ethical clinical practice. The limited research available suggests that services provided by assistants are effective, although much more quality research is needed to determine the degree of effectiveness and to make comparisons with professional level of service.

CRITICAL THINKING

1. What are some of the factors that have led to the use of SLP and audiology assistants?

2. What specific job responsibilities are appropriate for SLP and audiology assistants? What are some activities/tasks that are not appropriate for assistants?

3. What are some of the possible advantages and risks to using assistants? How might the possible negative effects be alleviated?

4. How have our state laws and national associations addressed the issue of assistants? Consider issues such as training, regulating, certifying, supervising, and ensuring that standards and ethics are not being compromised.

5. How might the inclusion of SLP and audiology assistants in our professions help to address the needs of our culturally and linguistically diverse community? When using assistants as

interpreters or translators, how should training and supervision issues be addressed?

6. According to the available research, does the use of assistants diminish or enhance the effectiveness of treatment? What additional information do we need to make a more objective analysis of the effectiveness of assistants and ensure comparability with professional level service?

7. As the supervisor of an assistant, list and describe your responsibilities and necessary knowledge and skills.

8. Consider the following: As an SLP, you work in a school district with a large number of students whose primary language is Spanish. Your administrator hires and assigns an assistant to you. The assistant has a bachelor's degree in communication sciences and disorders and is fluent in Spanish. The administrator states that the assistant will be doing all of the Spanish language testing as well as writing and managing the IEPs and working with the families of all students on your caseload whose primary language is Spanish. What are the ethical and legal problems, and how might you address them in this scenario?

REFERENCES

Administration on Aging. (2002). *Statistics: A profile of older Americans: 2002. Future growth.* Available at http://www.aoa.gov/prof/statistics/profile/2.asp

Alvord, D. J. (1977). Innovation in speech therapy: A cost-effective program. *Exceptional Children, 43,* 520–525.

American Academy of Audiology. (1997, May/June). Position statement and guidelines of the consensus panel on support personnel in audiology. *Audiology Today, 9*(3), 27–28.

American Academy of Audiology. (2003, October). *Preventing noise-induced occupational hearing loss.* Available at http://www.audiology.org/

American Academy of Audiology. (2004, January). *Audiology: Scope of practice.* Available at http://www.audiology.org/

American Academy of Audiology. (2005). *Audiologist's assistant.* Available at http://www.audiology.org/

American Academy of Otolaryngology–Head and Neck Surgery. (2006). Certificate program for otolaryngology personnel launched. Available at http://entnet.org/education/CPOP.cfm

American Speech-Language-Hearing Association, Committee on Supportive Personnel. (1970). Guidelines on the role, training, and supervision of the communication aide. *Asha, 12,* 78–80.

American Speech-Language-Hearing Association. (1979). *ASHA policy regarding support personnel.* Rockville, MD: Author.

American Speech-Language-Hearing Association. (1981, March). Guidelines for the employment and utilization of support personnel. *Asha, 23,* 165–169.

American Speech-Language-Hearing Association. (1985a, June). Clinical management of communicatively handicapped minority language populations. *Asha, 27*(6), 3–7.

American Speech-Language-Hearing Association. (1985b, June). Clinical supervision in speech-language pathology and audiology. *Asha, 27*(6), 57–60.

American Speech-Language-Hearing Association. (1988, November). Utilization and employment of speech-language pathology supportive personnel with underserved populations. *Asha, 30,* 55–56.

American Speech-Language-Hearing Association. (1992a). *ASHA omnibus survey.* Rockville, MD: Author.

American Speech-Language-Hearing Association. (1992b). *Technical report: Support personnel: Issues and impact on the professions of speech-language pathology and audiology.* Rockville, MD: Author.

American Speech-Language-Hearing Association. (1993). *ASHA omnibus survey.* Rockville, MD: Author.

American Speech-Language-Hearing Association. (1994a, March). ASHA policy regarding support personnel. *Asha, 36*(Suppl. 13), 24.

American Speech-Language-Hearing Association. (1994b, March). Supervision of student clinicians. *Asha, 36*(Suppl. 13), 13–14.

American Speech-Language-Hearing Association. (1995a). *Asha omnibus survey.* Rockville, MD: Author.

American Speech-Language-Hearing Association. (1995b, March). Position statement for the training, credentialing, use, and supervision of support personnel in speech-language pathology. *Asha, 37*(Suppl. 14), 21.

American Speech-Language-Hearing Association. (1995c). *Survey of speech-language pathology services in school-based settings: Final report.* Rockville, MD: Author.

American Speech-Language-Hearing Association. (1996a, Spring). Guidelines for the training, credentialing, use, and supervision of speech-language pathology assistants. *Asha, 38*(Suppl. 16), 21–34.

American Speech-Language-Hearing Association. (1996b). *Strategic plan for credentialing speech-language pathology assistants.* Rockville, MD: Author.

American Speech-Language-Hearing Association. (1997). *Preferred practice patterns for the profession of audiology.* Rockville, MD: Author.

American Speech-Language-Hearing Association. (1998a, June). *Guidance principles addressing state law/regulations and ASHA standards/guidelines/requirements.* Rockville, MD, Author.

American Speech-Language-Hearing Association. (1998b). Position statement and guidelines on support personnel in audiology. *Asha, 40*(Suppl. 18), 59–61.

American Speech-Language-Hearing Association. (1999). *Practical tools and forms for supervising speech-language pathology assistants.* Rockville, MD: Author.

American Speech-Language-Hearing Association. (2000a). *Council on Academic Accreditation in Audiology and Speech-Language Pathology: Criteria for approval of associate degree technical training programs for speech-language pathology assistants.* Rockville, MD: Author.

American Speech-Language-Hearing Association. (2000b). *Council on Professional Standards in Speech-Language Pathology and Audiology: Background information and criteria for registration of speech-language pathology assistants.* Rockville, MD: Author.

American Speech-Language-Hearing Association. (2000d). *Working with speech-language pathology assistants in school settings.* Rockville, MD: Author.

American Speech-Language-Hearing Association. (2001). *Scope of practice in speech-language pathology.* Rockville, MD: Author.

American Speech-Language-Hearing Association. (2002a). Knowledge and skills for supervisors of speech-language pathology assistants. *Asha, 44* (Suppl. 22), 113–118.

American Speech-Language-Hearing Association. (2002b). *Speech-language pathology health care survey.* Available at http://www.asha.org/

American Speech-Language-Hearing Association. (2002c). *A workload analysis approach for establishing speech-language pathology caseload standards in the schools.* Rockville, MD: Author.

American Speech-Language-Hearing Association. (2003a). *ASHA omnibus survey.* Rockville, MD: Author.

American Speech-Language-Hearing Association. (2003b). *Code of ethics* (Rev. ed.). Rockville, MD: Author.

American Speech-Language-Hearing Association. (2004a). *ASHA survey of school-based speech-language pathologists.* Available at http://www.asha.org/

American Speech-Language-Hearing Association. (2004b). *The audiologist's role in occupational hearing conservation and hearing loss prevention programs: Technical report.* Rockville, MD: Author.

American Speech-Language-Hearing Association. (2004c). *Evidence-based practice in communication disorders: An introduction.* Available at http://www.asha.org/

American Speech-Language-Hearing Association. (2004d). *Guidelines for the training, use, and supervision of speech-language pathology assistants.* Available at http://www.asha.org/

American Speech-Language-Hearing Association. (2004e). *Knowledge and skills needed by speech-language pathologists and audiologists to provide culturally and linguistically appropriate services.* Rockville, MD: Author.

American Speech-Language-Hearing Association. (2004f, November). *Preferred practice patterns for the profession of speech-language pathology.* Rockville, MD: Author.

American Speech-Language-Hearing Association. (2004g). *Scope of practice in audiology.* Rockville, MD: Author.

American Speech-Language-Hearing Association. (2004h). *Support personnel.* Available at http://www.asha.org/

American Speech-Language-Hearing Association. (2004i). *Training, use, and supervision of support personnel in speech-language pathology.* Available at http://www.asha.org/

American Speech-Language-Hearing Association. (2005a). *Frequently asked questions: Speech-language pathology assistants.* Available at http://www.asha.org/

American Speech-Language-Hearing Association. (2005b). *Model medical review guidelines for speech-language pathology services.* Available at http://www.asha.org/

American Speech-Language-Hearing Association. (in press). *Roles and responsibilities of speech-language pathologists in early intervention: Technical report.* Rockville, MD: Author.

Arkin, S. (1996). Volunteers in partnership: An Alzheimer's rehabilitation program delivered by students. *American Journal of Alzheimer's Disease, 11,* 12–22.

Bellini, M. J., Beesley, P., Perrett, C., & Pickles, J. M. (1989). Hearing-aids: Can they be safely prescribed without medical supervision? An analysis of patients referred for hearing-aids. *Clinical Otolaryngology and Allied Sciences, 14,* 415–418.

Blodgett, E. G., &. Miller, J. M. (1997). Speech-language paraprofessionals working in Kentucky schools. *Journal of Children's Communication Development, 18,* 65–79.

Breakey, L. K. (1993, May). Support personnel: Times change. *American Journal of Speech-Language Pathology, 2*(2), 13–16.

Briggs, B. M. (1974). High school speech assistants in a residential school for the blind. *Education of the Visually Handicapped, 6*(4), 119–124.

Bureau of Labor Statistics. (2004a). Audiologists. In *Occupational outlook handbook* (2004–05 Ed.). Available at http://www.bls.gov/oco/ocos085.htm

Bureau of Labor Statistics. (2004b). Speech-language pathologists. In *Occupational outlook handbook* (2004–05 Ed.). Available at http://www.bls.gov/oco/ocos099.htm

Code of Federal Regulations, Title 42, Section 440.110(c)

Consortium of Organizations on the Preparation and Use of Speech-Language Paraprofessionals in Early Intervention and Education Settings. (1997, January). *Report of the consortium of organizations on the preparation and use of speech-language paraprofessionals in early intervention and education settings.* Reston, VA: Author.

Costello, J., & Schoen, J. (1978). The effectiveness of paraprofessionals and a speech clinician as agents of articulation intervention using programmed instruction. *Language, Speech, and Hearing Services in Schools, 9,* 118–128.

Dahl, M. O. (1997). To hear again: A volunteer program in hearing health care for hard-of-hearing seniors. *Journal of Speech-Language Pathology and Audiology, 21,* 153–159.

David, R., Enderby, P., & Bainton, D. (1982). Treatment of acquired aphasia: Speech therapists and volunteers compared. *Journal of Neurology, Neurosurgery, and Psychiatry, 45,* 957–961.

Dijkstra, K., Bourgeois, M., Burgio, L., & Allen, R. (2002). Effects of a communication intervention on the discourse of nursing home residents with dementia and their nursing assistants. *Journal of Medical Speech-Language Pathology, 10*(2), 143–157.

Eaton Griffith, V. (1975). Volunteer scheme for dysphasic and allied problems in stroke patients. *British Medical Journal, iii,* 633–635.

Feldman, M. A. (Ed). (2004). *Early intervention: The essential readings.* Malden, MA: Blackwell.

Galloway, H. F., & Blue, C. M. (1975). Paraprofessional personnel in articulation therapy. *Language, Speech, and Hearing Services in Schools, 6,* 125–130.

Gerlach, K. (2000). *The paraeducator and teacher team: Strategies for success.* Seattle, WA: Pacific Training Associates.

Gersten, J. W., Gersten, J. W., Foppe, K. B., Gersten, R., Maxwell, S., Mirrett, P., et al. (1975). Effectiveness of aides in a perceptual motor training program for children with learning disabilities. *Archives of Physical Medicine & Rehabilitation, 56,* 104–110.

Goldberg, L., & Paul-Brown, D. (1999). *Strategies for the effective use of speech-language pathology assistants in the classroom.* Proceedings of the Seventh Annual Comprehensive System of Personnel Development

Conference, National Association of State Directors of Special Education, Alexandria, VA.

Gray, B. B., & Barker, K. (1977). Use of aides in an articulation therapy program. *Exceptional Children, 43,* 534–536.

Greener, J., Enderby, P., & Whurr, R. (1999). Speech and language therapy for aphasia following stroke (Abstract No. CD000425). In *Cochrane Database of Systematic Reviews.* Available at http://www. update-software.com/abstracts/AB0000425.htm

Griffith, V. E., & Miller, C. L. (1980). Volunteer stroke scheme for dysphasic patients with stroke. *British Medical Journal, 281,* 1605–1607.

Guralnick, M. J. (1972). A language development program for severely handicapped children. *Exceptional Children, 39,* 45–49.

Guralnick, M. J. (Ed.). (2005). *The developmental systems approach to early intervention.* Baltimore, MD: Brookes.

Hall, P. K., & Knutson, C. L. (1978). The use of preprofessional students as communication aides in the schools. *Language, Speech, and Hearing Services in Schools, 9,* 162–168.

Hamill, T., & Freeman, B. (2001). Scope of practice for audiologists' assistants: Survey results. *Audiology Today, 13*(6), 34–35.

Individuals with Disabilities Education Improvement Act of 2004, Pub. L. No. 108-446, 20 U.S.C. § 1400 *et seq.*

Johnson, C. E. (1999). Dimensions of multiskilling: Considerations for educational audiology. *Language, Speech, and Hearing Services in Schools, 30,* 4–10.

Johnson, C. E., Clark-Lewis, S., & Griffin, D. (1998). Experience, attitudes, and competencies of audiologic support personnel in a rehabilitation hospital. *American Journal of Audiology, 7,* 1–6.

Kagan, A., Black, S. E, Duchan, J. F., Simmons-Mackie, N., & Square, P. (2001). Training volunteers as conversation partners using "supported conversation for adults with aphasia" (SCA): A controlled trial. *Journal of Speech, Language, and Hearing Research, 44,* 624–638.

Koay, C. B., & Sutton, G. J. (1996). Direct hearing aid referrals: A prospective study. *Clinical Otolaryngology and Allied Science, 21,* 142–146.

Landis, P. A. (1973). Training of a paraprofessional in speech pathology: A pilot project in South Vietnam. *Asha, 15,* 342–344.

Langdon, H. W., & Cheng, L. L. (2002). *Collaborating with interpreters and translators.* Eau Claire, WI: Thinking Publications.

Lesser, R., Bryan, K., Anderson, J., & Hilton, R. (1986). Involving relatives in aphasia therapy: An application of language enrichment therapy. *International Journal of Rehabilitation Research, 9,* 259–267.

Lesser, R., & Watt, M. (1978). Untrained community help in the rehabilitation of stroke sufferers with language disorder. *British Medical Journal, ii,* 1045–1048.

Longhurst, T. (1997). Team roles in therapy services. In A. L. Pickett & K. Gerlach (Eds.), *Supervising paraeducators in school settings: A team approach* (pp. 55–89). Austin, TX: Pro-Ed.

Lyon, J. G., Cariski, D., Keisler, L., Rosenbek, J., Levine, R., Kumpula, J., et al. (1997). Communication partners: Enhancing participation in life and communication for adults with aphasia in natural settings. *Aphasiology, 11,* 693–708.

Marshall, R. C., Wertz, R. T., Weiss, D. G., Aten, J. L., Brookshire, R. H., Garcia-Bunuel, L., et al. (1989). Home treatment for aphasic patients by trained nonprofessionals. *Journal of Speech and Hearing Disorders, 54,* 462–470.

Meikle, M., Wechsler, E., Tupper, A., Benenson, M., Butler, J., Mulhall, D., & Stern, G. (1979). Comparative trial of volunteer and professional treatments of dysphasia after stroke. *British Medical Journal, 2,* 87–89.

Mueller, P. B. (1990). A volunteer speech-language facilitation program for communicatively handicapped elders in long-term care facilities. *Adult Residential Care Journal, 4,* 217–225.

National Joint Committee on Learning Disabilities. (1998). Learning disabilities: Use of paraprofessionals. In *Collective perspectives on issues affecting learning disabilities* (2nd ed., pp. 79–98). Austin, TX: Pro-Ed.

No Child Left Behind Act of 2001, 20 U.S.C., §6311 *et seq.* (2002).

Paul-Brown, D., & Caperton, C. J. (2001). Inclusive practices for preschool children with specific language impairment. In M. J. Guralnick (Ed.), *Early childhood inclusion: Focus on change* (pp. 433–463). Baltimore, MD: Brookes.

Paul-Brown, D., & Goldberg, L. R. (2001). Current policies and new directions for speech-language pathology assistants. *Language, Speech, and Hearing Services in Schools, 32,* 4–17.

Phillips, S., Liebert, R. M., & Poulos, R. W. (1973). Employing paraprofessional teachers in a group language training program for severely and profoundly retarded children. *Perceptual and Motor Skills, 36,* 607–616.

Pickering, M., & Dopheide, W. R. (1976). Training aides to screen children for speech and language problems. *Language, Speech, and Hearing Services in Schools, 7,* 236–241.

Pickett, A. L. (1999). *Strengthening and supporting teacher/provider–paraeducator teams: Guidelines for paraeducator roles, supervision, and preparation.* New York: City University of New York Graduate Center.

Pickett, A. L., & Gerlach, K. (Eds.). (1997). *Supervising paraeducators in school settings: A team approach.* Austin, TX: Pro-Ed.

Pickstone, C. (2003). A pilot study of paraprofessional screening of child language in community settings. *Child Language Teaching & Therapy, 19,* 49–65.

Preamble to Federal Regulations. (2004, February 28). *Federal Register,* p. 30585.

Rosenfeld, M., & Leung, S. (1999, July). *A job analysis of speech-language pathology assistants: A study to aid in defining the job of speech-language pathology assistants. A job analysis study conducted on behalf of the American Speech-Language-Hearing Association.* Princeton, NJ: Educational Testing Service, Education Policy Research Division.

Scalero, A. M., & Eskenazi, C. (1976). The use of supportive personnel in a public school speech and language program. *Language, Speech, and Hearing Services in Schools, 7,* 150–158.

Scarr, S., McCartney, K., Miller, S., Hauenstein, E., & Ricciuti, A. (1996). Evaluation of an islandwide screening, assessment and treatment program. *Early Development & Parenting, 3,* 199–210.

Schery, T., & O'Connor, L. (1997). Language intervention: Computer training for young children with special needs. *British Journal of Educational Technology, 28,* 271–279.

Schetz, K. F. (1989). Computer-aided language/concept enrichment in kindergarten: Consultation program model. *Language, Speech, and Hearing Services in Schools, 20,* 2–10.

Shewan, C. M., & Kertesz, A. (1984). Effects of speech and language treatment on recovery from aphasia. *Brain and Language, 23,* 272–299.

Shinn-Strieker, T. K. (1984). Trained communication assistants in the public schools. *Language, Speech, and Hearing Services in Schools, 15,* 70–75.

Suter, A. H. (2002). *Hearing conservation manual* (4th ed.). Milwaukee, WI: Council for Accreditation in Occupational Hearing Conservation.

Swan, I. R., & Browning, G. G. (1994). A prospective evaluation of direct referral to audiology departments for hearing aids. *The Journal of Laryngology and Otololgy, 108,* 120–124.

Thornton, A. (1993). The Cheshire profession. *American Journal of Audiology, 2,* 5.

U.S. Bureau of the Census. (2000). Resident population estimates of the United States by sex, race, and Hispanic origin: April 1, 1990 to July 1, 1999, with short-term projection to November 1, 2000. Available at http://www.census.gov/population/estimates/nation/intfile3-1.txt

Vadasy, P. F., Jenkins, J. R., & Pool, K. (2000). Effects of tutoring in phonological and early reading skills on students at risk for reading disabilities. *Journal of Learning Disabilities, 33,* 579–590.

Van Hattum, R. J., Page, J. M., Baskervill, R. D., Duguay, M. J., Conway, L. S., & Davis, T. R. (1974). The Speech Improvement System (SIS) taped program for remediation of articulation problems in the schools. *Language, Speech, and Hearing Services in Schools, 5,* 91–97.

Wertz, R. T., Weiss, D. G., Aten, J. L., Brookshire, R. H., Garcia-Bunuel, L., Holland, A. L., et al. (1986). Comparison of clinic, home, and deferred language treatment for aphasia. A Veterans Administration cooperative study. *Archives of Neurology, 43,* 653–658.

Werven, G. (1992, August). Training support personnel to provide services to persons with head injury. *Asha,* 72–74.

Werven, G. (1993). Support personnel: An issue for our times. *American Journal of Speech-Language Pathology, 2*(2), 9–12.

Wright, H. H., Shisler, R. J., & Rau, B. (2003). Maintenance of communication abilities in epilepsy: A clinical report. *Journal of Medical Speech-Language Pathology, 11,* 157–167.

Zeitoun, H., Lesshafft, C., Begg, P. A., & East, D. M. (1995). Assessment of a direct referral hearing aid clinic. *British Journal of Audiology, 29,* 13–21.

APPENDIX 10–A

Support Personnel in Communication Sciences and Disorders: Key Word Definitions

Aides: Support personnel who have a narrower training base and more limited responsibilities relative to the duties of assistants.

Assistants: Support personnel who perform tasks as prescribed, directed, and supervised by certified and licensed (where applicable) professionals after a program of academic and/or on-the-job training.

Direct supervision: On-site, in-view observation and guidance by the professional while an assigned activity is performed by support personnel.

Indirect supervision: Activities performed by the professional that may include demonstrations, record review, review and evaluation of audio- or videotaped sessions, and/or interactive television.

Interpreter: Individual who conveys information from one language to another for oral messages.

Support personnel: Provide activities adjunct to the clinical efforts of certified and licensed (where applicable) professionals with appropriate training and supervision.

Translator: Individual who conveys information from one language to another for written messages.

APPENDIX 10–B

Verification of Technical Proficiency of a Speech-Language Pathology Assistant

Speech-Language Pathology Assistant Name: _____

Supervisor(s) Name: _____

Program/Facility Name: _____

SKILLS	ACHIEVEMENT OF SKILL	
	Yes	No
Clerical/Administrative Skills		
Assists with clerical duties and departmental operations (e.g., preparing materials, scheduling activities, keeping records)		
Participates in in-service training		
Performs checks, maintenance, and calibration of equipment		
Supports supervising SLP in research projects and public relations programs		
Collects data for quality improvement		
Prepares and maintains patient/client charts, records, graphs for displaying data		
Interpersonal Skills		
Uses appropriate forms of address with patient/client, family, caregivers, and professionals (e.g., Dr., Mr., Mrs.)		
Greets patient/client and family and identifies self as a speech-language pathology assistant		
Restates information/concerns to supervising SLP as expressed by patient/client, family, and caregivers as appropriate		
Directs patient/client, family, and caregivers to supervisor for clinical information		
Is courteous and respectful in various communication situations		
Uses language appropriate to a patient/client, family, or caregiver's education level, communication style, developmental age, communication disorder, and emotional state		
Demonstrates awareness of patient/client needs and cultural values		

Supervising SLP = ASHA-certified speech-language pathologist   *SLPA = speech-language pathology assistant*

SKILLS	ACHIEVEMENT OF SKILL	
	Yes	No
Conduct in Work Setting		
Recognizes own limitations within the ASHA-approved SLPA job responsibilities		
Upholds ethical behavior and maintains confidentiality as described in the ASHA-approved job responsibilities of an SLPA		
Maintains client records in accordance with confidentiality regulations/laws as prescribed by supervising SLP		
Discusses confidential patient/client information only at the direction of supervising SLP		
Identifies self as an assistant in all written and oral communication with client, family, caregivers, and staff		
Demonstrates ability to explain to supervising SLP the scope of information that should be discussed with the patient/client, family, caregivers, and professionals		
Arrives punctually and prepared for work-related activities		
Completes documentation and other tasks in a timely manner		
Maintains personal appearance and language expected for the specific work setting		
Evaluates own performance		
Uses screening instruments and implements treatment protocols only after appropriate training and only as prescribed by supervising SLP		
Seeks clarification from supervising SLP as needed to follow the prescribed treatment or screening protocols		
Actively participates in interaction with supervisor demonstrating use of supervisor's feedback		
Maintains accurate records representing assigned work time with patients/clients		
Implements appropriate infection control procedures and universal precautions consistent with the employer's standards and guidelines		
Implements injury prevention strategies consistent with employer's standards and guidelines		
Uses appropriate procedures for physical management of clients according to employer's standards and guidelines and state regulations		
Technical Skills as Prescribed by Supervising SLP		
Accurately administers screening instruments, calculates and reports the results of screening procedures to supervising SLP		
Provides instructions that are clear, concise, and appropriate to the client's developmental age, level of understanding, language use, and communication style		
Follows treatment protocol as developed and prescribed by supervising SLP		

SKILLS	ACHIEVEMENT OF SKILL	
	Yes	No
Provides appropriate feedback to patients/clients as to accuracy of their responses		
Identifies and describes relevant patient/client responses to supervising SLP		
Identifies and describes relevant patient/client, family, and caregiver behaviors to supervising SLP		
Uses appropriate stimuli, cues/prompts with the patient/client to elicit target behaviors as defined in the treatment protocol		
Maintains on-task or redirects off-task behavior of patients/clients in individual or group treatment consistent with the patient's/client's developmental age, communication style, and disorder		
Provides culturally appropriate behavioral reinforcement consistent with the patient's/client's developmental age and communication disorder		
Accurately reviews and summarizes patient/client performance		
Uses age-appropriate and culturally appropriate treatment materials appropriate to the patient's/client's developmental age and communication disorder		
Starts and ends the treatment session on time		
Obtains cosignature of supervising SLP on documentation		
Accurately records target behaviors as prescribed by supervising SLP		
Accurately calculates chronological age of the patient/client		
Correctly calculates and determines percentages, frequencies, averages, and standard scores		
Uses professional terminology correctly in communication with supervising SLP		
Maintains legible records, log notes, and written communication		
Appropriately paces treatment session to ensure maximum patient/client response		
Implements designated treatment objectives/goals in specific appropriate sequence		

From *Guidelines for the Training, Use, and Supervision of Speech-Language Pathology Assistants* (pp. 14–16), by the American Speech-Language-Hearing Association, 2004. Available from http://www.asha.org/about/publications/reference-library/ Reprinted with permission.

A P P E N D I X 10–C

Supervisor Log of Direct
and Indirect Observations

Week ending: _____

SLP-A: _____

Supervising SLP: _____

Patient	Monday	Tuesday	Wednesday	Thursday	Friday	Sat./Sun.
Other activities						
Billing						
Equipment maintenance						
Documentation						
Meetings/In-services						
Other clerical						

* Indicate DO for direct observation + time

* Indicate IDO for indirect observation + time

Comments:

From *Practical Tools and Forms for Supervising Speech-Language Pathology Assistants* (p. 49), by the American Speech-Language-Hearing Association, 1999, Rockville, MD: Author. Reprinted with permission.

Expanding Clinical Populations and Professional Settings

11

Working with Special Populations

ROSEMARY LUBINSKI, EDD

M. GAY MASTERS, PHD

SCOPE OF CHAPTER

Many of you were attracted to the professions of speech-language pathology and audiology by an interesting, gratifying, or perplexing experience with an individual who had some type of communication problem such as stuttering, aphasia, or hearing loss. You may have a family member with a communication problem who inspired you to learn more about communication rehabilitation and eventually to enter our professions. It is common to find professionals who even changed career paths because of their personal interest in communication disorders. You may have taken an introductory course in communication disorders and been amazed by the variety of clients with whom we work and the range of clinical settings in which you could be employed. Some of you might be fascinated by the innovative uses of technology and the broad scientific bases of our professions or motivated to contribute through basic and applied research. Each year we continue to carve out new and challenging roles with clients from infancy through old age in medical, educational, community, and private practice venues.

The purpose of this chapter is to introduce you to *some* of the special client populations served by speech-language pathologists and audiologists. Some of these are relatively rare, while others are growing in numbers on our caseloads. This introduction should expand your professional horizons to those beyond the more traditional areas. It is important to remember that the characteristics of these topics often overlap. For example, consider the elder from a different linguistic background who incurs a head trauma and has dysphagia, the foreign-born child with subtractive bilingualism who lives in a rural area, or the high-risk, medically fragile infant with fetal alcohol syndrome and a hearing loss who comes from an economically disadvantaged home.

DEFINITIONS OF INCIDENCE AND PREVALENCE

Epidemiology is the dynamic study of how widespread a characteristic or problem is among a particular population at a particular time and place. Incidence and prevalence statistics are among the most common epidemiological tools used to define populations. Incidence is the number of new onsets of an illness, condition, or disorder in a specific population in a defined time period. Incidence rates are usually stated per year. For example, it is estimated that 80,000 individuals acquire aphasia each year (National Institute on Deafness and Other Communication Disorders, 2004b). Prevalence is the total number of current cases of an illness, condition, or disorder at one point in time or over a longer period of time (Shewan, 1994). For example, the total number of individuals (prevalence) with aphasia in the United States is estimated to be 1 million persons (ASHA, 2004c).

SPECIAL POPULATIONS

Each of the following populations presents unique challenges for communication disorders specialists. The challenge begins at the preprofessional level where ideally there is some academic information and clinical experience with each of these groups. During graduate study you are likely to have course work and practicum experiences with a variety of special populations. Professionals realize that their caseloads are "all inclusive" and reflect the diversity of the general population. Quality service is directly related to clinical knowledge and skill, plus appreciation for the distinctiveness of clients and their environments. It is also related to the skillful inclusion of family and professional caregivers in the diagnostic process, treatment planning, and intervention for each of these special populations.

Educated Professionals and Consumers

Special populations with relatively low incidence and prevalence can present special challenges not only to students in communication disorders, but to experienced clinicians as well. In the past, one hallmark of a special population was the difficulty in obtaining information about it. Now it is easy to find information within a few minutes using a good Internet search engine. The accessibility of information makes it easier for clinicians to find relevant sources for diagnosis and intervention models. It is ironic that the ease of finding information may cause more work for professionals. Not only do we need to critique the wealth of available information, but we also need to be aware that our clients and their families have access to the same information. This enables consumers to take an active role in diagnosis and treatment that may affect how they approach and follow through on professional suggestions.

An educated consumer actively participates in the clinical process. Specialized electronic mailing lists, or "listservs," exist for many topics, and subscribers freely exchange information regarding diagnosis and treatment. Listservs exist for parents of children with fetal alcohol syndrome, auditory processing disorder, and spina bifida, to name a few. Some listservs are moderated, requiring subscribers to abide by rules, but many are not moderated. Opinions are freely stated and may often appear factual to consumers. Web logs, or "blogs," are another online source of opinions stated as fact. Thus, the search for answers may be influenced by anecdotal, unproven information. For example, the hypothesis that autism is related to childhood immunizations containing mercury has resulted in some parents rejecting childhood immunizations.

In a similar fashion, the popularity and accessibility of the Internet has both assisted and hindered the practice of speech-language pathology. Clinicians often encounter a well-informed client/family, as consumers readily investigate communication development and disorders. It is common for families to seek an evaluation to confirm a self-made diagnosis. Bellis, an audiologist with an expertise in auditory processing disorders, cautions parents about this in her book written for laypersons (2002). A similar discussion was presented in the opening session of an ASHA Schools Conference (Ehren, Fey & Gillam, 2005). Students and professionals are encouraged to supplement information from this chapter with their own search for information in published texts, refereed journals, and the Internet. Professionals need to remember that parents and clients may have the same, or even sometimes more, information than they have. Family members may question our choice of diagnostic or therapy techniques, and we must be prepared to support our choices with evidence-based practice measures.

Hearing Impaired

Children who are deaf or significantly hearing impaired represent a significant special population. A brief developed by ASHA in 2005 indicates that hearing loss is the most common birth defect in America, with about 33 children with hearing loss born daily. Currently, 1 child in 1,000 live births is deaf, and 2–3 children in 1,000 have a partial hearing loss. About half of these children with hearing loss are from a racial or ethnic minority (ASHA, 2005c). Universal newborn hearing screening is now mandated in 47 states and the District of Columbia (ASHA, 2005c), suggesting that our ability to diagnose and properly treat this population should be excellent. Follow-up on infants who have failed the newborn hearing screening remains problematic.

The Joint Committee on Infant Hearing (2000) suggests that a child who fails the newborn hearing screening should be evaluated by 3 months and, if hearing loss is found, should be placed in early intervention by 6 months of age (Mencher,

Davis, DeVoe, Beresford, & Bamford, 2001). In spite of these guidelines, difficulties exist regarding the follow-up evaluation and placement in early intervention. In fact, about 33% of children who fail this screening have not been evaluated by 3 months of age, and more than half of the children who have been diagnosed with a hearing loss have not received early intervention by 6 months of age (ASHA, 2005c). Early intervention guidelines allow for services to be provided to a child at risk of a delay or disorder due to the diagnosis, even though the child may not be demonstrating a delay. Funding decisions at the state level often fail to offer this preventative intervention.

Many speech-language pathologists can tell the story of a deaf infant who, despite having failed the newborn hearing screening, did not receive a full audiological evaluation until after the age of 2 years. Thus, early intervention for this child did not begin in the first 6 months, and the child became ineligible for access to the early intervention system. Although the audiological results indicated that this child was a good candidate for a cochlear implant, other factors, particularly parental comprehension of the loss and subsequent failure to follow up on speech and audiology decisions, made implantation an unlikely outcome.

Hearing loss and/or deafness have significant educational risks at school age (ASHA, 2005c). Children with mild hearing loss are unable to hear up to half of speech in the classroom. Children with a unilateral hearing loss are 10 times more likely than their peers to experience grade retention. A longitudinal study completed by Gallaudet University continues to indicate that most hearing impaired individuals read no better than a fourth-grade reading level upon graduation from high school (ASHA, 2005c).

Children with significant hearing loss, who are unable to benefit from traditional amplification measures, may have auditory input provided via a cochlear implant. A cochlear implant consists of both external and internal hardware that work together to provide auditory information via electrical signals. By early 2002, cochlear implants had been provided to more than 7,000 children (Ertmer,

2002). Cochlear implant is now approved for very young children. A child with profound deafness (pure tone average $\geq$90 dB HL) can receive an implant as early as 12 months of age. If the hearing loss is in the severe-profound range (pure tone average $\geq$70 dB HL), the child cannot receive an implant until 2 years of age (ASHA, 2004d). Technology continues to improve, expanding the number of channels activated and thus improving the range of auditory information available. Multiple programming methodologies, typically referred to as the "map," are available. Mapping a cochlear implant requires multiple visits to the audiologist. The speech-language pathologist typically assists in developing programs that facilitate the child in making sense of auditory information.

Controversy exists regarding the primary communication mode used by individuals with hearing loss. Families must choose between oral communication, sign language, or a combination of both, known as *total communication*. Research suggests that the oral communication mode may positively impact auditory, speech, language, and reading skills over total communication mode (Geers, 2002). The Geers study was a large study of 136 children who shared the following characteristics: prelingually deaf, long-term users (4–6 years) of the same implant (Nucleus 22-channel), and implanted before the age of 5 years. Earlier research that had less control over independent variables such as length of time using an implant suggest that children who receive total communication mode instruction may develop a larger vocabulary (Connor, Hieber, Arts & Zwolan, 2000). Overall, research suggests that most children demonstrate positive outcomes in speech, language, and learning with a cochlear implant.

Fetal Alcohol Exposure

Knowledge concerning fetal alcohol syndrome has increased significantly in the last few years. Guidelines for diagnosis and referral were developed by the National Center on Birth Defects and Disabilities (NCBDD), the Centers for Disease Control and Prevention (CDC), Department of Health and Human Services, and the National Task Force on Fetal Alcohol Syndrome and Fetal Alcohol Effect (Gerberding, Cordero & Floyd, 2005). Prevalence rates for the United States, as reported by various studies, range from a low of 0.2 to a high of 2.0 per 1,000 live births. The variability in prevalence is due, in *part,* to variation in subgroups of women. Women who are Native American or economically disadvantaged or who have a history of substance abuse have higher incidence of children born with alcohol effects. One infant per 1,000 live births is the reported incidence rate for fetal alcohol syndrome (FAS) or fetal alcohol effect (FAE) (Centers for Disease Control and Prevention, 2005). Studies that have investigated drinking in women of childbearing years suggest that 2 percent of women are at risk for this preventable birth defect (Gerberding et al., 2005). Children who are adopted internationally are also identified or are at risk for diagnosis of FAS and FAE (Johnson & Dole, 1999).

Beginning in 1996, the Institute of Medicine began to use the terminologies *alcohol-related neurodevelopmental disorder* (ARND) and *alcohol-related birth defects* (ARBD) to capture the full range of children affected by alcohol. Diagnosis of FAS is based on four factors: facial anomalies, growth retardation, known or suspected maternal alcohol consumption, and neurodevelopmental disorder (Gerberding et al., 2005). Because these four factors are not always present, the lesser diagnosis of FAE or perhaps ARND/ARBD may be used instead of FAS. Facial anomalies include thin upper lip, reduced or absent philtrum, and possible ear anomalies. Weight, height, and head circumference fall below the 10th percentile; brain imaging clearly shows reduced development of white matter tracts evident in the corpus callosum, basal ganglia damage, and smaller cerebrum or cerebellum.

The speech-language pathologist may be involved with alcohol-affected children either directly or as a related service. Some children with FAS, FAE, or ARND/ARBD demonstrate speech and language disorders. These children often have difficulties with social communication. Learning and behavioral impairments relevant to related service clients include learning disability, attention deficit hyperactivity disorder, impulsivity, mental retardation, and executive function disorder. The CDC reports five different projects addressing the communication and/or education needs of children with alcohol-related impairments (Centers on Disease Control, 2005).

In addition, children with FAS may exhibit auditory disorders, including intermittent conductive hearing loss secondary to recurrent otitis media, sensori neural hearing loss, delayed maturation of the auditory system, central hearing loss, microtia, Eustachian tube dysfunction, and other outer ear malformations (Dittmer, 2005). Thus, audiologists should be alert to this condition during infant, preschool, and school-age screenings and comprehensive audiological testing. The impact of hearing loss on communication development, academic learning, and socialization becomes vitally important in this special population.

Language Learning Disabilities

Previous editions of this chapter have focused on language learning disabilities (LLD) as a special population of interest to many students and professionals. LLD is the terminology used by ASHA (1997–2004), indicating the impact of a language disability upon academic performance. Children prior to school age are often considered to demonstrate specific language impairment; at school age, when academic needs enter the picture, the term LLD is more descriptive (Windsor, Scott & Street, 2000). Although the term was introduced in 1984 by Wallach & Liebergott, LLD is not a recognized disability category under Individuals with Disability Education Act nor a covered diagnosis for insurance purposes. Therefore, incidence and prevalence figures can only be estimated from IDEA eligibility categories and ICD diagnosis codes. This task is made even more difficult by the fact that children with LLD often have comorbid conditions, such as attention deficit hyperactivity disorder (ADHD), auditory processing disorder (APD), or learning disability. In addition, children in the public education system may have a nonspecific label, *developmental disability,* until age 8.

According to the National Center for Learning Disabilities (1999–2005), 2.9 million school-age children, or 5 percent of children enrolled in public schools, have learning disabilities. A disproportionate number of these children are nonwhite. It appears that economic considerations rather than race contribute to this statistic, with learning disabilities being linked to toxins such as lead and alcohol exposure. School-age children with LLD typically have academic difficulties, often first identified as a problem with reading decoding and/or comprehension (Cornett & Chabon, 1986). Word-finding difficulties, where a child has the vocabulary knowledge but often is unable to produce the word, are common, particularly with children who have reading impairments (cf. German & Simon, 1991). Reading problems have been attributed to both poor phonological awareness in young children and metalinguistic deficits in older children (Schuele & Dayton, 1999). Young children may also demonstrate difficulties in recognizing the metapragmatics of the classroom (Wilkinson & Milosky, 1987). Older children show problems with deriving inferences from reading passages and often fail to recognize figurative language (Wallach & Miller, 1988).

(Central) Auditory Processing Disorder

In addition to the specific language difficulties noted, children with LLD may have central auditory processing disorders that hamper their ability to function in the classroom (Chermak & Musiek, 1992; Masters, Stecker, & Katz, 1998). (Central) auditory processing disorder, referred to as (C)APD has been a controversial diagnostic category for more than 50 years. According to the Working Group on Auditory Processing Disorders (ASHA, 2005a), (C)APD is "a deficit in neural processing of auditory stimuli that is not due to higher order language, cognitive, or related factors" (p. 2). Typical symptoms of a central auditory processing disorder include disorders in processing time, hypersensitivity to noise, and difficulty in integration of auditory and visual information. Difficulties in auditory memory may be present, but according to the revised position statement and subsequent technical report (ASHA, 2005a), memory is more likely to be a coexisting cognitive disorder rather than (C)APD itself.

There are no clear statistics regarding the number and prevalence of children with (C)APD. As indicated earlier, (C)APD has been a controversial topic in the field, and it is not an educational label under the Individuals with Disabilities Education Act. One estimate is half of the children labeled LD have (C)APD and about 75 percent of elderly adults (Bellis, 2004). A good discussion of the overlap of the diagnoses of LD, (C)APD, and ADHD can be found in Keller (1998). It is estimated that at least 20 percent of the four million children with learning disabilities have an attention disorder (National Institutes of Health, 1993). Attention difficulties include excessive daydreaming and/or distractibility. Hyperactivity may be associated with an attention disorder. When attention difficulties co-occur with either a learning disability or a central auditory processing disorder, language issues are usually present.

The diagnosis of (central) auditory processing disorder may only be made by an audiologist. However, results of multidisciplinary assessment, particularly speech-language and educational, are critical in determining an intervention plan for individuals with (C)APD. Direct remediation may include both auditory training and specific training in related deficit areas such as language and memory. In addition, compensatory strategies may be taught during auditory training and/or for residual effects following auditory training. Compensatory strategies include executive functioning training, self-advocacy, and specific strategies to facilitate attention and memory. Environmental modifications are also a frequent factor in (C)APD intervention. Assistive listening devices and/or modifications to reduce noise in the environment are examples of environmental modifications.

Developmental Apraxia of Speech

Developmental apraxia of speech (DAS) is another controversial diagnosis that continues to gain more recognition within the field (Forest, 2003). Child-

hood apraxia of speech, or CAS, is also a label that may be used (Lewis, Freebairn, Hansen, Iyengar & Taylor, 2004). DAS is diagnosed from the presence of a cluster of characteristics describing the child's speech ability. There is no common set of characteristics on which professionals unanimously agree (Hall, 2000). The primary characteristics that suggest DAS may be present include difficulty sequencing sounds and syllables, inconsistent errors, difficulty producing vowels, and groping behaviors (Hall, 2000). Although there is no clear consensus in the field that DAS is a disorder separate and distinct from a severe phonological disorder, the Diagnostic and Statistical Manual of Mental Disorders-IV lists it as one of five possible speech delays (cf. Shriberg, Aram, & Kwiatkowski, 1997).

The controversy has contributed to the fact that prevalence and incidence figures are not known (Forrest, 2003). Prevalence and incidence are further difficult to determine in part due to the comorbidity of DAS. A child with DAS is likely to have a coexisting disorder, usually language, and that disorder may be reported instead of DAS (Lewis et al., 2004). It appears that more boys than girls are affected, with ratios as low as 3:1 and as high as 9:1 (cf. Shriberg et al., 1997). There appears to be a familial characteristic suggesting that DAS is inherited.

There is little consensus regarding the mechanism of DAS. A review by Shriberg and colleagues (1997) describes theoretical perspectives of DAS. Various processing difficulties have been suggested, including temporal, perceptual-memorial, and organizational. Some theories indicate grammatical factors surrounding phonological encoding of morphemes. Other theories suggest motor programming and/or pre-articulatory sequencing, consistent with the diagnostic factors listed previously. Recent research suggests motor programming deficits (Nijland, Maassen, & van der Meulen, 2003). Therapy approaches used depend on the theoretical perspective of the professional providing services.

Autism Spectrum Disorders

Autism and autism spectrum disorders (ASD) refer to a developmental disorder with a significant disability in social communication skills. A term that encompasses five subtypes of ASD is *pervasive developmental disability* (PDD). PDD/ASD includes autism, Asperger's Syndrome, childhood disintegrative disorder, Rett's Syndrome, and PDD-NOS (pervasive developmental disability-not specified) (ASHA, 2004). A concern in recent years has been the apparent increase in ASD. As mentioned earlier, one hypothesis is the effect of mercury in vaccines that infants and toddlers receive. This causal factor has been refuted (National Immunization Program, 2004). The cause for the increase in diagnosis relates to the broadening of types of ASD, as well as increased professional and public awareness (ASHA, 2004). The current prevalence of ASD, which is about 60 per 10,000, has increased three or four times the estimated prevalence rate from 30 years ago (Diehl, 2003). Review of all five types of ASD is beyond the scope of this chapter. Instead, Asperger's Syndrome, a relatively recent subtype, will be discussed.

Asperger's Syndrome was initially described in the 1940s but was not a diagnostic category in the DSM until 1994 (Winner, 2003). Asperger's is considered to fall in the high functioning end of ASD, with individuals typically demonstrating normal to above-average intelligence. As with other forms of ASD, the primary difficulty lies in social interaction for both cognitive and communication issues (Winner, 2003). Unlike autism, Asperger's does not present itself as a language disorder. Most individuals with Asperger's develop language at age-appropriate milestones and are not diagnosed until 3 years old or later, when difficulties in social communication are apparent. Eye contact is often impaired, as is the ability to make complex inferences about the world (Silliman et al., 2003). Inferences require the individual to integrate past experiences, current knowledge, and predictions about other individuals. That is, the individual must be able to demonstrate theory of mind skills, and individuals with Asperger's typically do not demonstrate this (Silliman et al., 2003).

In addition to social communication difficulties, individuals with Asperger's may demonstrate concomitant disorders such as ADHD, anxiety disorder, depression, and obsessive-compulsive disorder. One difficulty for the SLP is the evaluation of the communication difficulties demonstrated by individuals with Asperger's. Standardized tests do not typically address social pragmatics, making it difficult to quantify the difficulty demonstrated or improvement when therapy is effective (Winner, 2003).

Subtractive Bilingualism

ASHA has well-defined standards regarding the assessment of children and adults from multicultural backgrounds, including those who speak languages other than English as a first language (ASHA, 1993, 1998). Children who become family members following international adoption pose a special problem to the speech-language pathologist and audiologist. These children often demonstrate rapid attrition of their first language, so much so that English is a new first language for these children (Glennen & Masters, 2002). In addition, the pregnancy, birth, and developmental histories of these children are consistent with the at-risk factors for early intervention services even before first language loss is factored into the equation. Both the speech-language pathologist and audiologist need to be aware of these factors when asked to evaluate these children for speech-language development, basic hearing ability, and central auditory processing skills.

Internationally adopted children often demonstrate the same risk factors as adopted children born in the United States, including poor or absent prenatal care, poor nutrition, and substance abuse that result in low birth weight and other perinatal and postnatal issues (Johnson & Dole, 1999). In addition, a great number of the children adopted internationally are placed in institutional settings rather than foster care. A 1-month delay in developmental milestones (gross and fine motor, growth, cognitive, and language) for each 3–5 months in an institution has been documented (Johnson & Dole, 1999). Varying levels of stimulation and interaction have been noted in institutions, with even the best settings rated significantly poorer than familial interaction. Oral motor and speech development is often compromised by feeding practices that use large-holed nipples and table food that requires little chewing (Glennen & Masters, 2002).

Bilingual standards are based on the assumptions that either the child learns two languages simultaneously or the child learns languages in succession, first one language, then the second language. Critical to these two acquisition descriptions is the assumption that the child is proficient in the native language and acquires English as a second language in addition to the first. The native language fosters development of the second language, with parental or other communication in the first language often used to teach vocabulary and concepts in the second language. A third bilingual theory is the concept of subtractive language acquisition, where one language is learned and lost, and then a second language is learned. This idea of language loss best describes the English language acquisition of the majority of the internationally adopted children. These children are best described as limited English proficient (LEP) who now are acquiring a new first language (Glennen & Masters, 2002).

The literature on bilingualism provides two important distinctions in second (or, in the case of internationally adopted children, new first) language acquisition: basic interpersonal communication skills (BICS) and cognitive-academic language proficiency (CALP). BICS refers to conversational fluency in peer-peer and child-adult verbal interactions, whereas CALP refers to the highly abstract language needed for school success. In the bilingual literature, BICS is acquired within 2 years, whereas CALP requires 5–9 years to acquire (Teeters, 1998).

Glennen and Masters (2002) found that language attrition for children adopted from eastern Europe is dramatic, with most children losing expressive language skills within the first 6 weeks to 3 months following adoption. Receptive language seems to be maintained for a longer period, but the utility of this base for second language acquisition is minimal, as adoptive parents are rarely fluent in the first language. English language acquisition is rapid in most cases, with children adopted under the age of 3 demonstrating only slight expressive language delays relative to their native language peers by age 3. Glennen and Masters' data on more than 100 children suggest that children adopted before 18 months of age can be assessed by typical infant-toddler scales

at 24 months. Most internationally adopted older children demonstrate BICS within 6 months and rarely qualify for English as a second language services after 1 year. Similar data for children adopted from China suggest that they, too, rapidly acquire at least BICS (Roberts et al., 2005). Receptive language testing and school success, however, indicate that CALP is not complete in about 50 percent of these children within the first 3 years in their new home (Glennen & Masters, 1999; 2002).

Glennen and Masters (1999) suggest the following practice standards for internationally adopted children (1) recognize that bilingual standards and definitions are a poor match for this population; (2) establish the receptive and expressive language skills in the native language within the first 3 months to determine how much, if any, delay is present in the native language; (3) assess oral-motor skills to determine if oral-motor weakness or incoordination is present; (4) use English language assessment measures as criteria-based references to document strengths and weaknesses and to determine whether acquisition is progressing; (5) consider the rapid attrition of the native language and the unique challenges imposed by the acquisition of a new first language by children who are not infants; and (6) assist school-age children in obtaining academic modifications and support during the lengthy period of arrested language development before CALP is acquired.

Persons with Traumatic Brain Injuries

Survivors of traumatic brain injury (TBI) receive services from speech-language pathologists throughout their recovery, beginning in the emergency room and extending through many levels of rehabilitation programming. Estimates vary as to the number of individuals who sustain a TBI each year; however, according to the Centers for Disease Control and Prevention (2005b), each year 1.4 million Americans suffer a TBI; 50,000 die and about 90,000 have long-term disabilities. The Brain Injury Association (2000) estimates that more than 5.3 million Americans are living with disabilities from TBI. Those at highest risk are adolescents, young adults, and individuals older than 75 years. The most common causes of TBI are motor vehicle accidents and falls. Recreational accidents rank high as a cause of TBI for school-age children, and assault is a major cause for young adults (Beukelman & Yorkston, 1991). Those who have experienced one brain injury are at increased risk for a second or even third injury (Brain Injury Association, 2000).

A person who sustains a brain injury may display a wide range of physical, behavioral, emotional, cognitive, and communicative difficulties caused by the possible diffuse pathophysiology of the injury. Of particular interest to the speech-language pathologist are resultant cognitive and language impairments. Difficulties are likely to occur in attention, concentration, visual processing, language, memory, reasoning, problem solving, and executive functions (Sohlberg & Mateer, 1989). Other difficulties that fall within the purview of the speech-language pathologist include motor speech disorders and dysphagia (Lazarus, 1991; Yorkston & Beukelman 1991). In addition, audiologists may assess both peripheral and central auditory functioning as sequelae of TBI. Many of these problems manifest themselves long after the original injury and interfere with successful return to school, work, and community activities.

TBI has numerous negative and lingering effects on the individual's family and social network. TBI has been called a "family matter" because it affects the entire family system from the time of the injury through rehabilitation, reintegration to home and community, and possibly through institutionalization. Web sites posted by the Head Injury Foundation and the Brain Injury Association offer information for families on national and state policy issues, conferences, services, and national directories. See the Resources section at the end of the chapter for further information.

In general, interdisciplinary approaches to rehabilitation for individuals with TBI are the most effective. Team members include, but are not limited to, the speech-language pathologist, audiologist, neurologist, physician, physiatrist, neuropsychologist, physical therapist, occupational therapist, special educator, clinical psychologist, rehabilitation nurse,

social worker, and vocational counselor. ASHA's Working Group on Cognitive-Communication Disorders (ASHA, 2005d) proposed that the specific roles of the speech-language pathologist include identification of individuals at risk for or presenting with such problems, assessment, and intervention. In addition, SLPs should be prepared to counsel; collaborate with individuals, families, teachers, other professionals, and care providers; do case management and education regarding cognition and language; and participate in prevention programs. Their roles may also involve client advocacy and research. This working group also prepared a detailed list of knowledge and skills needed by SLPs to work effectively with those with cognitive-communication problems (ASHA, 1987b, 1988b, 2005d).

Services for individuals who incur head injury begin in the emergency room or in specialized head trauma centers within hospitals. The initial goal is to stabilize the patient medically and address primary and secondary medical problems. Comatose patients will undergo continued assessment of their level of consciousness and may participate in early stages of cognitive stimulation. Rehabilitation will likely continue on an inpatient basis, at which time decisions will be made about the best course of ongoing treatment. These may include one or a combination of residential long-term rehabilitation programs, outpatient programs, home care, or educational settings. Availability of services, severity of the problems, age, and health care insurance status will all contribute to programming decision making. Individuals who have incurred head injury, their families, and caregivers can expect a long period of rehabilitation and recovery, often extending into years of service and need. When possible, the family and individual are included in the decision-making and rehabilitation process.

Medically Fragile Children

Advances in medicine have contributed to the population that may be termed *medically fragile* children. In the area of premature birth alone, the rate has increased by 9 percent in the last 10 years (Woodnorth, 2004). Children who are medically fragile often require technology such as ventilators or oxygen and nutrition support. Other medical technologies, such as dialysis, may be necessary. The Office of Technology Assessment estimated the number of technologically dependent children at 100,000 in 1987 (ERIC, 2005). Ventilators are now about the size of a laptop computer (Woodnorth, 2004). Such advancements in technology allows medically fragile children the opportunity to attend public school and perhaps become a part of the speech-language pathologist's caseload in that setting.

Some individuals with tracheostomies, with or without ventilator dependence, can achieve oral communication. The SLP will require competencies in the types of speaking valves available to assist in oral communication. Some individuals will be unable to speak, regardless of advances in speaking valves. These individuals require augmentative and alternative communication systems. Again, the SLP must remain current regarding choices in devices, switches, and language systems.

The Elderly

Aging of the population is a visible phenomenon in developed nations around the world. Perhaps the fastest growing group of potential clients audiologists and speech-language pathologists will serve in the next 20 years are those older than 65 years of age. In 2003, the nearly 36 million individuals 65 years and older in the United States constituted 12.4 percent of the population (U. S. Census Bureau, 2005d). According to the National Council on Aging (2005), that number will increase by another 5 million in the next 10 years, and by 2030 this age group will comprise 71 million persons, or about 20 percent of the population. Elderly individuals 85 years and older are among the fastest growing segments of the population. In 2002 there were 4.6 million persons age 85 years and older, and this is expected to balloon to 9.6 million in 2030. There are also more than 50,000 centenarians in the United States, an increase of 35 percent between 1990 and 2002.

The aging population shows some other specific characteristics. First, there are more elderly women than men, and this discrepancy increases with age. Second, the number of elders from minority populations is also increasing rapidly. For example, Hispanics of any race are expected to nearly triple by the year 2050 (United States Census Bureau, 2005c) Third, the aging population is becoming increasingly better educated, with at least 72 percent of today's elders having a high school education and 17 percent a bachelor's degree (U.S. Census Bureau, 2003a). Asian elders are the most likely to have a college degree (29 percent). Next, 79 percent of elderly men live with a spouse or other family member, while only 59 percent of elderly women do so (United States Census Bureau, 2003a). These statistics likely reflect the fact that most elderly men are married even through very old age, while a majority of elderly women are widows by age 75 (United States Census Bureau, 2003a). Interestingly, 95 percent of the elderly reside in the community (Statistical Abstracts of the United States, 1992). About 25 percent of community-based elders aged 65 to 74 years indicate that they have some limitation of activity caused by chronic conditions, and this number increases to 45 percent for those 75 and older (Health, United States, 2004). Finally, about 10 percent of elders have incomes below the poverty level, though the percentages are at least double for minorities, those who have not finished high school, and the very old (American Gerontological Society, 2005b).

Few statistics are available regarding the incidence or prevalence of speech or language disorders among the elderly in the community. Communication changes may be related to the aging process itself, but disorders are most likely related to disease and chronic disorders, including stroke, Parkinson's disease, and dementia. An estimated 1 million people in the United States have aphasia, and about 75 percent of them are over age 65 (ASHA, 1999–2000). Dysphagia is also a common problem related to neurologically based disorders among the elderly, including stroke, TBI, Parkinson's disease, and dementia. About 14 percent of those over age 60 have dysphagia (ASHA, 2004a).

Statistics compiled through the National Health Interview Survey for 1989 reveal that hearing impairments rank third behind arthritis and hypertension as a chronic condition among elderly individuals residing in the community (Statistical Abstracts of the United States, 1992). The prevalence rate of hearing impairments was 23 percent for those 65–74 years of age, 33 percent for those older than 75 years, and 48 percent for those older than 85 years. The prevalence of hearing loss is consistently higher for males than for females (National Institute on Deafness and Other Communication Disorders, 2004). Epidemiological studies conducted by Gallaudet University predict that by the year 2015 there will be 13 million elders with a hearing impairment (Bebout, 1989). According to the National Institute on Aging estimates (1987), at least 11,800 audiologists will be needed in 2015 to serve the hearing needs of the elderly.

Most elders reside and receive care in the community in their own homes or some type of assisted care facility. Service is provided on an outpatient basis or through home health care. Rice (1992) states that "the current philosophy of home health care is to provide cost-effective and quality health care in a setting that is often more conducive to health restoration and patient contentment than a hospital setting" (p. 12). Such services focus on a prevention role to maintain the health of the individual and forestall further disabilities, dependence, and relocation to an institutional setting and on supportive and therapeutic services (Lubinski, 1981; May, 1993). In 2000, more than 5 million elders received home health care services (National Center for Health Statistics, 2004). Due to increases in costs for home care in the 1990s, this number is actually a 20 percent decrease in persons served (American Gerontological Society, 2005a). The majority of persons served were white, elderly females who lived in private residences and who had on average three major diagnoses. Frequently occurring primary diagnoses included heart disease, diabetes, and stroke (National Center for Health Statistics, 2004).

Although nursing care is the most prevalent service offered by home health care programs, rehabilitation also constitutes an important aspect of service delivery. Rehabilitation includes occupational therapy, physical therapy, and speech-language pathology services. About 7 percent of all home health care patients receive speech-language pathology services (May, 1993). The majority of the caseloads consist of individuals with neurological disorders or dysphagia. Audiology services are seldom offered by most home health care agencies other than on a contractual basis.

About 3 percent of men and 6 percent of women over age 65 reside in traditional nursing home settings, and 45 percent of these are 85 years or older (Hobbs & Damon, 1996). Note that long-term facilities traditionally include nursing homes and adult care facilities, although the number of community-based specialized assisted care facilities for elders is growing and is not included in most statistics on long-term care facilities. Residents of nursing care facilities tend to be very old, with an average age of 82 years. Women, usually widows, outnumber men 2 to 1. Most residents are white, reside in the long-term care facility for at least 1 year, and die there. A majority have four or more chronic disabilities, are mentally impaired (usually dementia), and are nonambulatory. In 2002, there were about 1.8 million residents in nearly 16,500 nursing facilities (Health, United States, 2004). Most of these facilities were located in the Mid-Atlantic, East North Central, and South Atlantic areas of the United States.

Current and reliable statistics regarding the number of nursing facility residents in the United States with communication problems are scarce. Mueller and Peters (1981), in a study of the prevalence of communication problems in Wisconsin nursing homes, found that approximately 60 percent of the population had a communication problem. In a retrospective study of the types of communication problems referred to the speech-language pathology program in a nursing home, O'Connell and O'Connell (1978) found that the most frequent problems included aphasia, dysarthria, oral and verbal apraxia, laryngeal pathology, confusion, and impaired memory. More current studies indicate that 40 percent to 50 percent of residents of long-term care facilities have a swallowing disorder (ASHA, 1999–2000). Schow and Nerbonne (1980) found that 70 percent to 90 percent of nursing facility residents had some degree of hearing impairment. ASHA(1988) delineates the roles of audiologists and speech-language pathologists in nursing homes in more depth.

Several pieces of federal legislation have influenced delivery of audiology and speech-language pathology services in nursing home settings. In 1987, the Omnibus Budget Reconciliation Act mandated that all persons in a nursing home setting receiving Medicare and Medicaid assistance have a comprehensive assessment of their needs. This legislation led to the development of the Resident Assessment Instrument (Morris et al., 1990). Sections of this instrument assess communication and swallowing (Lubinski & Frattali, 1993). This instrument has undergone revision, and a new version will be available soon.

Federal legislation in 1997 imposed a $1,500 annual cap on Part B Medicare-reimbursed outpatient rehabilitation services in skilled nursing facilities, rehabilitation agencies, public health agencies, clinic, or comprehensive outpatient rehabilitation programs. This amount was to be shared by speech-language pathology and physical therapy. In 1999, the Balanced Budget Amendment placed a moratorium on this cap as further study of the impact of the reimbursement cap was done and better ways of meeting the rehabilitation needs of elders were explored. Speech-language pathologists need to be vigilant to federal legislation changes, to advocate strongly with their federal legislators regarding the funding cap, and to be aware of the detrimental effects on service delivery if the cap is reinstated.

Speech-language pathologists and audiologists can provide a wide variety of communication services to elders, their families, and other caregivers (ASHA. 1987a). These include traditional assessment and treatment. Delivery of services may focus on assessing the physical and psychosocial environment, providing in-services to family members and facility staff, counseling elders and their families, using individual and environmental communication technologies, and increasing involvement with other clients such as those with dementia. Considering the funding limitations imposed by insurers on therapy for elders, innovative approaches need to be developed in both the community and long-term care facilities.

Individuals with Dementia

Dementia involves a decline in cognitive function from previously attained intellectual levels and is sustained over a period of months or years. The decline is manifest in at least three of five areas of mental activity (1) language, (2) memory, (3) visuospatial skills, (4) emotion or personality, and (5) abstraction, calculation, and judgment (Cummings & Benson, 1983). The most common form of dementia is Alzheimer's disease, which affects 1 in 10 persons over age 65, or over 4.5 million Americans (Alzheimer's Association, 2005). Although studies differ on the prevalence of dementia in the elderly population, two constants emerge. First, the number of individuals with dementia rises with increasing age. Perhaps as many as 50 percent of those older than age 85 have Alzheimer's disease (Alzheimer's Association, 2005). Second, the prevalence of dementia is higher for those residing in nursing care facilities than for those in the community. The Alzheimer's Association (2005) estimates that half of all nursing home residents have Alzheimer's disease and that Alzheimer's disease costs the United States economy more than $100 billion each year.

The changes in communication abilities for those with dementia have stimulated much interest from the field of communication disorders. Numerous studies have been done to delineate the cognitive, language, motor speech, and auditory changes that occur with dementia, as well as differential diagnosis of dementia from aphasia, primary progressive aphasia, and other cognitively based language disorders. Primary language difficulties involve word knowledge and pragmatics and the use of contextually appropriate language. Auditory changes may parallel those associated with aging but also include changes in central auditory processing (Grimes, 1995). Such research has led to new roles for speech-language pathologists, including participating in differential diagnoses, documenting communication changes with disease progression, developing individual and environmental intervention approaches, counseling family members, and educating professional staff. Audiologists find traditional office-based diagnostic and hearing aid fitting challenging with these individuals particularly as the disease progresses. Again, more innovative approaches to improving the sound environment and counseling caregivers regarding strategies to facilitate communication may be more innovative ways of enhancing the hearing of persons with dementia.

Individuals with Dysphagia

One area of assessment and treatment that has grown exponentially in recent years is that of dysphagia, swallowing disorders. Dysphagia may result from neurological dysfunction such as stroke, progressive neurological diseases, or from other conditions, such as surgery for head and neck cancer. Increasingly, high-risk infants and children with oral motor speech disorders also present with dysphagia. Although dysphagia may occur without a concomitant speech or language disorder, it is highly likely these problems will co-occur. Martin and Corlew (1990) found that 87 percent of patients identified with dysphagia also had speech, voice, language, or cognitive difficulties.

In 1986, ASHA published a position paper describing the role of the speech-language pathologist in dysphagia and followed this in 1990 with a description of the knowledge and skills speech-language pathologists need to provide service to persons with swallowing problems (ASHA, 1986, 1990). Among the specific roles delineated are the ability to (1) identify individuals at risk for dysphagia; (2) conduct clinical oral-pharyngeal and respiratory examination, with a detailed history; (3) conduct instrumental/structural physiologic examination with related professionals; (4) determine patient management strategies; (5) provide treatment with related professionals; (6) provide education and counseling to appropriate others; (7) manage and/or participate in an interdisciplinary team; (8) maintain quality control and risk management; and (9) provide discharge planning and follow-up care.

In 1992, to address the technological advances occurring in dysphagia assessment, ASHA published a position statement and guideline on instrumental diagnostic procedures for swallowing. Specific instrumental procedures with which a speech-language pathologist may be involved include video fluorography, ultrasonography, fiberoptic endoscopy, scintigraphy, electromyography, and manometry. These procedures require the speech-language pathologist to obtain competencies beyond that necessary for ASHA certification (ASHA, 1992a). Speech-language pathologists should be cognizant of the ethical and liability issues related to dysphagia assessment and treatment.

UNDERSERVED POPULATIONS

One of the most socially important issues faced by speech-language pathologists and audiologists is whether we truly are reaching the wide range of individuals who need our services. In 1985, ASHA convened a National Colloquium on Underserved Populations and identified six populations for whom service was either inaccessible or underutilized. These populations included those who are (1) linguistic minorities such as Hispanics and Asians and those with social dialects, (2) the economically disadvantaged, (3) the institutionalized in prisons and psychiatric settings, (4) those residing in remote/rural areas, including Appalachia and Micronesia, (5) Native Americans, and (6) those residing in developing regions (ASHA, 1985b).

Linguistic Minority Populations

In the year 2000, more than 11 percent of the United States population was foreign born (United States Census Bureau, 2003b). The influx of immigrants from Asia (26 percent) and Latin America (52 percent) in the last two decades underscores the need for communication disorders professionals to become highly sensitive to the special cultural and language issues of clients from linguistic minorities. The percentage of individuals who state that they speak a language other than English at home increased from 14 percent to 18 percent in the last decade of the 20th century (United States Census Bureau, 2003c). In 2000, nearly 12 million of these individuals (an increase from 8 million in 1990) consider themselves as linguistically isolated because no one aged 14 or over in the home speaks English at least "very well."

Many individuals speak a language other than English at home. Spanish is spoken by about 28 million persons in the United States and is the most common non-English language spoken here. About 42 million individuals of Hispanic origin in the United States constitute 14 percent of the population (United States Census Bureau, 2005c). The largest percentage of these individuals were born or have roots in Mexico and Central America. Chinese ranks second, reflective of the growth from 1.2 to 2 million people from 1990 to 2000. Other major languages spoken at home include French, German, Tagalog, Vietnamese, Italian, Korean, and Russian. Non-English is more frequently spoken in the home in the Western part of the United States (29 percent) and the Northeast (20 percent). The United States Census Bureau (2003c) also indicates that those individuals in the West were also more likely to have difficulty with English. Table 11-1 shows the states with the highest percentages of population who speak a language other than English.

In addition, about 80,000 African American immigrants come to the United States each year from the Caribbean, South America, Africa, and Central America (Cole, 1989). When the number of legal and undocumented immigrants is added to those of other racial/ethnic minorities who may have different languages and dialects, the actual population of those who constitute a linguistic minority increases. This growth is expected to continue well in this 21st century, with the number of minorities expected to increase to at least 79 million by the year 2080.

Cole (1989) described eight multicultural imperatives that potentially affect audiology and speech-language pathology service delivery to this population (1) there will be more minorities with communication disorders; (2) more minority children are born at risk; (3) these populations present different etiologies and prevalence of communication disorders; (4) the heterogeneity among these groups contributes to difficulty in establishing norms; (5) these populations have different cultural views on health and disorders; (6) there is more potential for cultural conflict in clinical settings; (7) these cultural groups may have different service delivery preferences; and (8) linguistic minority populations cannot be categorized automatically into racial/ethnic minority groups.

To help audiologists and speech-language pathologists understand and meet the unique needs of linguistic minority clients, the Educational Standards Board of ASHA mandated that, as of January 1, 1993, accredited graduate programs in speech-language pathology and audiology must offer course content pertaining to culturally diverse groups (ASHA, 1992b). This is reiterated in the latest educational standards that graduate students must meet to obtain ASHA certification.

There is also an effort to increase the number of minority professionals. Some college and university programs offer specialized multicultural-based programs. For further reading on the topic of multicultural issues, see Chapter 22.

Economically Disadvantaged Populations

The good news is that poverty in the United States decreased in the 1990s from 13.1 percent to 12.4 percent of the population. The bad news is that although poverty decreased across all age groups, poverty among children still surpasses those for adults (United States Census Bureau, 2003d). In 1999, poverty was defined as an income of less than $8,501 for an individual and $13,410 for a family of three. The highest poverty rates are in the South

T A B L E 11–1 States with High Non-English–Speaking Populations

California 39%
New Mexico 37%
Texas 31%
New York 28%
Hawaii 27%
Arizona 26%
New Jersey 26%

(13.9 percent); 40 percent of all of those in poverty are Southerners (United States Census Bureau, 2003d, 2005a). Mississippi, Louisiana, and New Mexico have the highest poverty rates, though some declines have been realized in those states. Poverty also is related to lower education, race, increased residential mobility, single marital status, and families without a father present (United States Census Bureau, 2005d). Further, many of the economically disadvantaged are also part of the linguistic minority population. Cole (1989) stated that economically disadvantaged populations are at greater risk for handicapping conditions related to environmental, nutritional, and traumatic factors.

In addition, at least 3 million persons are homeless in the United States, and 40 percent of these are families (National Law Center on Homelessness and Poverty, 2005). O'Neill-Pirozzi (2003) in her review of homelessness and children's language and education states that language delays and school failure are common. She also found that 60 percent of mothers residing in shelters and 69 percent of their children presented with overall language deficits and delay. Most of these children did not receive adequate educational programming.

The ASHA Colloquium on Underserved Populations (ASHA, 1985b) raised the issue of the economically disadvantaged as a target population for inclusion in professional academic course work, clinical experiences, and research and for increased service availability and delivery. Further, the recruitment and retention of individuals from economically disadvantaged populations into our professions should be a priority and may facilitate access to communication services by underserved groups. Changes in health care delivery and financing are needed to assure that the economically disadvantaged have full and equal access to quality communication services.

Prison Populations

In 2004, more than 2.1 million inmates were incarcerated in federal, state, and local prisons in the United States (Bureau of Justice Statistics, 2004). The majority of these inmates were males between the age of 18 and 34. What is known from the few studies available is that the incidence of communication and hearing impairments among adult male and female prisoners is significantly higher than the general population (e.g., Belenchia & Crowe, 1983; Wagner, Gray, & Potter, 1983). The Parchment Project, prison-based program in Mississippi, serves as a prototype for meeting the complex needs of this underserved population (Crowe, Byrne, & Henry, 1999). The authors appeal for studies on the relationship between improvement in communication and recidivism rate of inmates. A comprehensive approach to rehabilitation is obviously a necessary component to reducing recidivism rates and successful return to the community.

Remote/Rural Populations

In 2000, 21 percent of the United States population resided in rural areas (United States Census Bureau, 2000). This is a decrease from 25 percent in 1990. Those residing in rural areas as compared with urban areas tend to be poorer and older, with more health issues and a dearth of professional resources (Agency for Health Care Policy and Research, 1996). According to ASHA's Ad Hoc Committee on Services to Remote/Rural Populations (ASHA,1991b), such areas include the Appalachian region of West Virginia, Kentucky, and Tennessee; Alaska and Hawaii; and the United States Territories, including Puerto Rico, the United States Virgin Islands, American Samoa, and the Pacific Trust of Guam. Rural areas of other states also qualify as underserved.

Rural populations often overlap with other underserved populations such as Native Americans and linguistic minorities. There is a higher prevalence of speech, language, and hearing disorders and a paucity of communication disorders professionals serving this category. The REACH model was developed by ASHA's Ad Hoc Committee on Services to Remote/Rural Populations (1991b) to improve service delivery in remote/rural areas. REACH stands for remote, rural education, access, consultation, and habilitation. It focuses on six target areas: data, grant funding, training programs, continuing education, professional resource development, and consumer resources. Although service delivery in rural/remote areas can consist of traditional hospital/clinic- or school-based service, more creativity and flexibility are needed to meet the needs of clients in these areas.

Examples of innovative approaches to service delivery in remote areas include itinerant consultants, staff team approaches (Olmstead & Bergeron, 1993), telehealth, development of rural health centers, and Internet-based assessment and therapy (Carlucci, 1999; Clark & Scheideman-Miller, 1999). Read Chapter 25 on technology for more information on telemed and Web-based distance programs.

Native Americans

Native Americans are those persons who originate from any of the indigenous people of North America and who have a cultural identification through tribal association or community affinity (Robinson-Zanartu, 1996). In 2004, about 1.5 percent of the United States population, approximately 4.4 million persons, was classified as Native American, Eskimo, or Aleut residing in the United States (United States Census Bureau, 2005b). The highest percentage of these individuals live in California, Oklahoma, and Arizona. Seventy-eight percent reside in urban areas. About 24 percent of Native Americans and those of Alaska native heritage live in poverty, far above the national average of 12.4 percent. The 1 million Native Americans who live on reservations receive health services from the Indian Health Service (IHS). In addition

to serious health problems such as tuberculosis, alcoholism, diabetes mellitus, gastrointestinal disorders, head trauma, and cancer, otitis media ranks as one of the most prevalent conditions among this population. The IHS offers audiologic services usually on a part-time outreach basis by otolaryngologists, audiologists, and audiometric technicians. Hearing aids are dispensed to children and offered at cost to adults (Stewart, 1992).

It is estimated that the incidence of communication disorders in this population is between 5 and 15 times higher than in the general population (Friedlander, 1993; Toubbeh, 1982). Unfortunately, speech-language services are considered nonmedical and are not offered routinely through the IHS (Stewart, 1992). Toubbeh (1982) states that "amelioration of these and other disorders is further complicated by cultural and linguistic factors, lack of indigenous manpower and inefficient intervention strategies. The multiplicity of federal agencies which purport to serve Native Americans today further aggravates an already complex and disparate situation" (p. 396). Robinson-Zanartu (1996) maintains that schools, in particular, have underserved Native American children. She suggests that communication disorders specialists must develop a better understanding of Native American culture and belief systems, learning style and communication, and relationship between home and school. Comprehensive speech-language and hearing services to this population require that we provide dynamic assessments based on interaction with the Native American environment and collaboration with their tribal leaders, educators, and family members.

SUMMARY

This chapter discussed a wide variety of special populations from high-risk infants to elders who may incur a speech, language, and/or hearing disorder. The communication difficulties these persons may exhibit are usually only one of a constellation of problems. As a communication disorders specialist you will find that your caseload across settings contains individuals from these special populations. Your responsibility is to ensure that you are knowledgeable regarding the uniqueness of these populations and gain skills in meeting their diagnostic and intervention needs. Undoubtedly as our clinical expertise and technological advances increase, our ability to identify and serve these populations will improve.

CRITICAL THINKING

1. What clinical groups initially attracted you to the profession of speech-language pathology?

2. Describe some other nontraditional clientele with whom we work that were not detailed in this chapter. Why do these populations require the services of an audiologist or speech-language pathologist?

3. What knowledge and skills are needed to work with special populations? How will you prepare to work with special populations?

4. The use of the Internet to access a variety of information sources regarding special populations was raised in this chapter. Under what circumstances is Internet use positive, when might it be negative? How would you respond to a parent or client who had secured information from a dubious source and used that as a basis for decision making?

5. Not every client or family understands what we do or supports our intervention. How will you approach such clients and families if you believe that a communication disorder is present and that you can provide service to improve the problem?

6. Why is professional advocacy so important for speech-language pathologists and audiologists when working with these special populations?

REFERENCES

Agency for Health Care Policy and Research. (1996). *Improving health care for rural populations.* AHCPR Publication No. 96-P040. Available at http://www.ahrq.gov/research/rural.htm

Alzheimer's Association. (2005). About Alzheimer's disease statistics. Chicago: Author.

American Gerontological Society. (2005a). *Community based care.* Available at http://www.healthinaging.org/

American Gerontological Society. (2005b). *Trends in the elderly population.* Available at http://www.healthinaging.org/

American Speech-Language-Hearing Association. (1985a). Clinical management of communicatively handicapped minority language populations. *Asha, 27,* 29–32.

American Speech-Language-Hearing Association. (1985b). 1985 national colloquium on underserved populations report. *Asha, 27,* 31–35.

American Speech-Language-Hearing Association. (1986). Ad hoc committee on dysphagia report. *Asha, 29,* 57–58.

American Speech-Language-Hearing Association. (1987a). The delivery of speech, language and audiology services in home care. *Asha, 29,* 49–52.

American Speech-Language-Hearing Association. (1987b). The role of SLPs in the habilitation and rehabilitation of cognitively impaired individuals: A report of the Subcommittee on Language and Cognition. *Asha, 29,* 53–55.

American Speech-Language-Hearing Association. (1988a). Provision of audiology and speech-language pathology services to older persons in nursing homes. *Asha, 30,* 72–4.

American Speech-Language-Hearing Association. (1988b, March). The role of speech-language pathologists in identification, diagnosis and treatment of individuals with cognitive-communication impairment. *Asha, 30,* 79.

American Speech-Language-Hearing Association. (1989). Communication based services for infants, toddlers, and their families. *Asha, 31,* 32–34.

American Speech-Language-Hearing Association. (1990). Skills needed by SLPs providing services to dysphagic patients/clients. *Asha, 32* (Suppl. 2), 7–12.

American Speech-Language-Hearing Association. (1991a). Guidelines for speech-language pathologists serving persons with language, socio-communicative, and/or cognitive-communicative impairments. *Asha, 33* (Suppl. 5), 21–28.

American Speech-Language-Hearing Association. (1991b). REACH: A model for service delivery and professional development within remote/rural regions of the United States and U.S. territories. *Asha, 33* (Suppl. 6), 5–14.

American Speech-Language-Hearing Association. (1992a). Instrumental diagnostic procedures for swallowing. *Asha, 34* (Suppl. 7), 25–33.

American Speech-Language-Hearing Association. (1992b). *Professional certification standards.* Rockville, MD: Author.

American Speech-Language-Hearing Association. (1993). Preferred practice patterns for the professions of speech-language pathology and audiology. *Asha, 35,* (Suppl. 11), 1–102.

American Speech-Language-Hearing Association. (1997–2004). *Language-based learning disabilities.* Available at http://www.asha.org/

American Speech-Language-Hearing Association. (1998). Provision of English-as-a-second-language instruction by speech-language pathologists in school settings. *Asha, 40* (Suppl. 18).

American Speech-Language-Hearing Association. (1999–2000). *Communication facts special populations: Dysphagia.* Rockville, MD: Author.

American Speech-Language-Hearing Association. (2004a). *Communication facts: Special populations: Autism–2004 edition.* Available at http://www.asha.org/

American Speech-Language-Hearing Association. (2004b). *Communication facts: Special populations: Dysphagia–2004 edition.* Available at http://www.asha.org/

American Speech-Language-Hearing Association. (2004c). *Incidence and prevalence of speech, voice, and language disorders in adults in the United States–2004 edition.* Available at http://www.asha.org/

American Speech-Language-Hearing Association. (2004d). Cochlear implants. *ASHA Supplements, 24.*

American Speech-Language-Hearing Association. (2005a). (Central) auditory processing disorders. Available at http://www.asha.org/

American Speech-Language-Hearing Association. (2005b). (Central) auditory processing disorders— The role of the audiologist. Available at http://www.asha.org/

American Speech-Language-Hearing Association. (2005c). *Early hearing detection and intervention: Brief.* Available at http://www.asha.org/

American Speech-Language-Hearing Association. (2005d). Knowledge and skills needed by speech-language pathologists providing services to individuals with cognitive-communication disorders. *ASHA Supplement, 25.*

American Speech-Language-Hearing Association. (2005e). Roles of speech-language pathologists in the identification, diagnosis, and treatment of individuals with cognitive-communication disorders. *ASHA Supplement, 25.*

Bebout, J. (1989). The aging of America. *The Hearing Journal, 42,* 7–12.

Belenchia, T., & Crowe, T. (1983). Prevalence of speech and hearing disorders in a state penitentiary population. *Journal of Communication Disorders, 16,* 279–285.

Bellis, T.J. (2002). *When the brain can't hear: Unraveling the mystery of auditory processing disorder.* New York: Atria Books.

Bellis, T. J. (2004, March 30). Redefining auditory processing disorder: An audiologist's perspective. *ASHA Leader, 6,* 22–23.

Beukelman, D., & Yorkston, K. (1991). Traumatic brain injury changes the way we live. In D. Beukelman & K. Yorkston (Eds.), *Communication disorders following traumatic brain injury* (pp. 1–14). Austin, TX: Pro-Ed.

Brain Injury Association. (2000). *Brain injury association home page.* Available at http://www.biausa.org

Bureau of Justice. (2000). Bureau of justice statistics. Available at http://www.ojp.usdoj.gov/bjs/press.htm

Carlucci, D. (1999). Distance imaging: Assessing patients in remote locations. *Advance, 9,* 10–11.

Centers for Disease Control. (2005a). Fetal alcohol syndrome: Developing intervention strategies for children. Available at http://www.cdc.gov/ncbdd/fas/interventing.htm

Centers for Disease Control. (2005b). Traumatic brain injury incidence and distribution. Available at http://www.cdc.gov/

Chermak, G., & Musiek, F. (1992). Managing central auditory processing disorders in children and youth. *American Journal of Audiology, 1,* 61–65.

Clark, P., & Scheideman-Miller, C. (1999). Telehealth prepilot successful in Oklahoma. *Advance, 9,* 18–19.

Cole, L. (1989). E pluribus pluribus: Multicultural imperatives for the 1990s and beyond. *Asha, 31,* 65–70.

Connor, C., Hieber, S., Arts, H., & Zwolan, T. (2000). Speech, vocabulary and the education of children using cochlear implants: Oral or total communication. *Journal of Speech, Language and Hearing Research, 43,* 1185–1204.

Cornett, B., & Chabon, S. (1986). SLPs as language-learning disabilities specialists: Rites of passage. *Asha, 28,* 29–31.

Crowe, T., Byrne, M., & Henry, A. (1999). Providing speech, language, and hearing services to inmates. *Journal of the American Speech-Language-Hearing Association, 41,* 50–55.

Cummings, J., & Benson, D. F. (1983). *Dementia: A clinical approach.* Boston: Butterworth.

Diehl, S. F. (2003). Prologue: Autism spectrum disorder: The context of speech-language pathologist intervention. *Language, Speech, and Hearing Services in Schools, 34,* 177–179.

Dittmer, C. (2005). Fetal alcohol syndrome. Available at http://www.emedicine.com/ped/topic767.htm.

ERIC Digest # 458. (2005). Students with specialized health care needs. Available at www.thememory-hole.org/edu/eric/ed209590.html

Ehren, B. J., Fey, M. E., & Gillam, R. (2005). *SLPs, Start your engines! Evidence-based practice in schools.* Presented at ASHA Schools 2005, Indianapolis, IN.

Ertmer, D. J. (2002). Challenges in optimizing oral communication in children with cochlear implants. *Language Speech and Hearing Services in Schools, 33,* 149–152.

Forest, K. (2003). Diagnostic criteria of developmental apraxia of speech used by clinical speech-language pathologists. *American Journal of Speech-Language Pathology, 12,* 376–380.

Friedlander, R. (1993). BHSM comes to the Flathead Indian reservation. *Asha, 35,* 28–29.

Geers, A. E. (2002). Factors affecting the development of speech, language and literacy in children with early cochlear implants. *Language, Speech and Hearing Services in Schools, 33,* 172–183.

Gerberding, J. L., Cordero, J., & Floyd, R. L. (2005). Fetal alcohol syndrome: Guidelines for referral and diagnosis (3rd printing). Available at http://www.cod.gov/ncbddd/fas/documents/FAS_guidelines_accessible.pdf

German, D., & Simon, E. (1991). Analysis of children's word-finding skills in discourse. *Journal of Speech and Hearing Research, 34,* 309–316.

Glennen, S., & Masters, M. G. (1999, November). *Language development and delay in children adopted internationally.* Presented at ASHA Annual Convention, San Francisco.

Glennen, S. & Masters, M. G. (2002). Typical and atypical language development in infants and toddlers adopted from eastern Europe. *American Journal of Speech-Language Pathology, 44,* 417–433.

Grimes, A. (1995). Auditory changes. In R. Lubinski (Ed.), *Dementia and communication* (pp. 47–69). San Diego, CA: Singular Publishing Group.

Hall, P. K. (2000). A letter to the parents of a child with developmental apraxia of speech. Part I: Speech characteristics of the disorder. *Language, Speech, and Hearing Services in Schools, 31,* 169–172.

Health, United States, 2004. (2004). *Nursing homes, beds. Occupancy, and residents, according to geographic division and state: United States, 1995–2002.* Washington, DC: Author.

Hobbs, F., & Damon, B. (1996). *65+ in the United States.* Washington, DC: U.S. Bureau of the Census & National Institute of Aging.

Huntley, R., & Helfer, K. (Eds.). (1995). *Communication in later life.* Boston: Butterworth-Heinemann.

Johnson, D. E., & Dole, K. (1999). International adoptions: Implications for early intervention. *Infants and Young Children, 11,* 34–45.

Joint Committee on Infant Hearing. (2000). Year 2000 position statement: Principles and guidelines for early hearing detection and intervention programs. *American Journal of Audiology, 9,* 9–29.

Keller, W. (1998). The relationship between attention deficit hyperactivity disorders, central auditory processing disorders, and specific learning disorders. In M. G. Masters, N. Stecker, & J. Katz (Eds.), *Central auditory processing disorders: Mostly management.* Boston: Allyn & Bacon.

Lazarus, C. (1991). Diagnosis and management of swallowing disorders in traumatic brain injury. In

D. Beukelman & K. Yorkston (Eds.), *Communication disorders following traumatic brain injury* (pp. 367–418). Austin, TX: Pro-Ed.

Lewis, B. A., Freebairn, L. A., Hansen, A. J., Iyengar, S. K. & Taylor, H. G. (2004). School-age follow-up of children with childhood apraxia of speech. *Language, Speech and Hearing Services in Schools, 35,* 122–140.

Lubinski, R. (1981). Speech, language and audiology programs in home health care agencies and nursing homes. In D. Beasley & G. A. Davis (Eds.), *Speech, language and hearing: The aging process* (pp. 339–356). New York: Grune & Stratton.

Lubinski, R., & Frattali, C. (1993). Nursing home reform: The resident assessment instrument. *Asha, 35,* 59–62.

Martin, B., & Corlew, M. (1990). The incidence of communication disorders in dysphagic patients. *Journal of Speech and Hearing Disorders, 55,* 28–32.

Masters, M. G., Stecker, N., & Katz, J. (Eds.). (1998). *Central auditory processing disorders: Mostly management.* Boston: Allyn & Bacon.

May, B. (1993). *Home health and rehabilitation.* Philadelphia: F. A. Davis.

Mencher, G. T., Davis, A. C., DeVroe, S. J., Beresford, B. & Bamford, J. M. (2001). Universal neonatal hearing screening: Past, present, and future. *American Journal of Audiology, 10,* 3–12.

Morris, J., Hawes, C., Fries, B., Phillips, C., Mohr, V., Katz, S., Murphy, K., Drugovich, M., & Friedlob, A. (1990). Designing the national resident assessment instrument for nursing homes. *Gerontologist, 30,* 793–807.

Mueller, P., & Peters, T. (1981). Needs and services in geriatric speech-language pathology and audiology. *Asha, 23,* 627–632.

National Center for Health Statistics. (2004). National home and hospice care data. Available at http://www.cdc.gov/nchs/fastats

National Center for Learning Disabilities. (1999–2005). Available at http://www.ld.org/

National Immunization Program. (2004). Center for Disease Control and Prevention. FAQs about MMR vaccine & autism (measles, mumps, and rubella). Available at http://www.cdc.gov/nip

National Institute on Aging. (1987). *Personnel for health needs of the elderly through the year 2020.* Washington, DC: Author.

National Institute on Deafness and Other Communication Disorders. (2004a). *Statistics about hearing disorders, ear infections and deafness.* Available at http://www.nidcd.nih.gov/health/statistics/vsl.asp

National Institute on Deafness and Other Communication Disorders. (2004b). *Statistics on voice, speech, and language.* Available at http://www.nidcd.nih.gov/health/statistics/vsl.asp

National Law Center on Homelessness and Poverty. (2005). Homelessness and poverty in America. Available at http://www.nlchp.org

National Research Council. (2001). Executive summary. Available at http://www.ld.org/

Nijland, L., Maassen, B., & van der Meulen, S. (2003). Evidence of motor programming deficits in children diagnosed with DAS. *Journal of Speech, Language and Hearing Research, 46,* 437–450.

O'Connell, P., & O'Connell, E. (1978, November). *Speech language pathology services in a skilled nursing facility.* Paper presented at the Annual Convention of the American Speech and Hearing Association, San Francisco.

Olmstead, P., & Bergeron, L. (1993). A rural/remote perspective: Alaska. *Asha, 35,* 43–45.

O'Neill-Pirozzi (2003). Language functioning of residents in family homeless shelters. *American Journal of Speech-Language Pathology, 12,* 229–242.

Rice, R. (1992). *Home health nursing practice.* St. Louis, MO: Mosby Year Book.

Roberts, J. A., Pollack, K. E., Krakow, R., Price, J., Fulmer, K. C., & Wang, P. P. (2005). Language development in preschool-age children adopted from china. *Journal of Speech, Language, and Hearing Research, 48,* 93–107.

Robinson-Zanartu, C. (1996). Serving native American children and families: Considering cultural variables. *Language, Speech and Hearing Services in Schools, 27,* 373–384.

Schow, R., & Nerbonne, M. (1980). Hearing levels among elderly nursing home residents. *Journal of Speech and Hearing Disorders, 45,* 124–132.

Schuele, C. M., & Dayton, N. D. (1999, November). Intensive phonological awareness training: A program for children with language impairments. Presented at ASHA Annual Convention, San Francisco.

Shewan, C. (1994). Incidence and prevalence of communication disorders. In R. Lubinski & C. Frattali (Eds.), *Professional issues in speech-language pathology and audiology.* San Diego, CA: Singular Publishing Group.

Shriberg, L. D., Aram, D. M. & Kwiatkowski, J. (1997). Developmental apraxia of speech: I. Descriptive and theoretical perspectives. *Journal of Speech and Hearing Research, 40,* 273–285.

Silliman, E. R., Diehl, S. F., Bahr, R. H., Hnuth-Chisolm, T., Zenko, C. B., & Friedman, S.A. (2003). A new look at performance on theory-of-mind tasks by adolescents with autism spectrum disorder. *Language, Speech, and Hearing Services in Schools, 34,* 236–252.

Sohlberg, M., & Mateer, C. (1989). *Introduction to cognitive rehabilitation.* New York: Guilford Press.

Statistical Abstract of the United States. (1992). Washington, DC: U.S. Department of Commerce.

Stewart, J. (1992). Native American populations. *Asha, 34,* 40–42.

Teeters, C. (1998). Language acquisition and subtractive bilingualism. Eastern European Adoption Coalition Website. Available at http://ww.ceac/org

Toubbeh, J. (1982). Native Americans: A multi-dimensional challenge. *Asha, 24,* 395–398.

U.S. Census Bureau. (2000). Urban/rural and metropolitan/nonmetropolitan population: 2000. Available at http://factfinder.census.gov/

U.S. Census Bureau. (2003a). *Current population survey, annual social and economic supplement.* Washington, DC: Author.

U.S. Census Bureau. (2003b). *Current population survey, annual social and economic supplement.* Available at http://factfinder.census.gov/

U.S. Census Bureau. (2003c). The foreign-born population: 2000. Available at http://factfinder.census.gov

U.S. Census Bureau. (2003d). Language use and English-speaking ability: 2000. Washington, D.C: Author.

U.S. Census Bureau. (2003e). Poverty: 1999. Washington, DC: Author.

U.S. Census Bureau. (2005a). Areas with concentrated poverty: 1999. Available at http://www.census.gov/hhes/www/poverty.html

U.S. Census Bureau. (2005b). Facts for features: American Indian and Alaska native heritage month: November, 2005. Available at http://www.census.gov/PressRelease/www/releases/archives/facts_for_features-special

U.S. Census Bureau. (2005c). Facts for features. Hispanic heritage month 2005: September 15-October 15. Available at http://www/census gov/PressRelease/www/releases/archives/facts_for_features_special

U.S. Census Bureau. (2005d). USA statistics in brief: Population by sex, age, and region. Available at http://www.census.gov/statab/www/pop.html

U.S. Department of Commerce. (1997). *Census brief, Disabilities affect one-fifth of all Americans.* Washington, DC: Author.

Wagner, C., Gray, L., & Potter, R. (1983) Communicative disorders in a group of adult female offenders. *Journal of Communication Disorders, 16,* 269–277.

Wallach, G., & Liebergott, J. (1984) Who shall be called "learning disabled": Some new directions. In G. Wallach & K. Butler (Eds.), *Language learning disabilities in school-age children* (pp. 1–14). Baltimore, MD: Williams and Wilkins.

Wallach, G., & Miller, L. (1988). *Language intervention and academic success.* Gaithersburg, MD: Aspen Publishers.

Wilkinson, L., & Milosky, L. (1987). School-age children's metapragmatic knowledge of requests and responses in the classroom. *Topics in Language Disorders, 7,* 61–70.

Williams, J., & Kay, T. (1991). *Head injury: A family matter.* Baltimore, MD: Paul H. Brookes.

Windsor, J., Scott, C. M., & Street, C. K. (2000). Verb and noun morphology in the spoken and written language of children with language learning disabilities. *Journal of Speech, Language and Hearing Research, 43,* 1322–1336.

Winner, M. G. (2003). Asperger syndrome across the home and school day. *ASHA Leader* (July–September).

Woodnorth, G. H. (2004). Assessing and managing medically fragile children: Tracheostomy and ventilatory support. *Language, Speech, and Hearing Disorders in Schools, 35,* 363–372.

Yorkston, K., & Beukelman, D. (1991). Motor speech disorders. In D. Beukelman & K. Yorkston (Eds.), *Communication disorders following traumatic brain injury* (pp. 251–316). Austin, TX: Pro-Ed.

RESOURCES

Alzheimer's Association National Office
225 N. Michigan Ave., Fl. 17, Chicago, IL 60601
Phone: 800-272-3900
Web site: http://www.alz.org/

American Association of Mental Retardation
AAMR 444 Capitol St. NW, Ste. 846
Washington, DC 20001
Phone: 800-424-3688; 202-387-1968
Web site: http://www.aamr.org/

The American Institute of Stress
124 Park Avenue
Yonkers, New York 10703
Phone: 914-963-1200; fax: 914-965-6267
E-mail: stress125@optonline.net

Autism Society of America
7910 Woodmont Avenue, Suite 300
Bethesda, Maryland 20814-3067
Phone: 301-657-0881 or 800-3AUTISM

Brain Injury Association of America
8201 Greensboro Dr., Suite 611
McLean, VA 22102
Phone: 703-761-0750;
Family Helpline: 800-444-6443
Web site: http://www.biausa.org/Pages/home.html

Centers for Disease Control and Prevention
1600 Clifton Road
Atlanta, GA 30333
Phone: 404-639-3311;
Public Inquiries: 404-639-3534/800-311-3435
Web site: http://www.cdc.gov/

National Council on Aging
300 D Street, SW, Suite 801
Washington, DC 20024
Phone: 202-479-1200; fax: 202-479-0735;
TDD: 202-479-6674
E-mail: info@ncoa.org

U.S. Department of Health and Human Services
200 Independence Avenue, S.W.
Washington, D.C. 20201
Phone: 202-619-0257; 877-696-6775
Web site: http://www.hhs.gov/

National Organization on Fetal Alcohol Syndrome
900 17th Street, NW, Suite 910
Washington, DC 20006
Phone: 202-785-4585/800-66NOFAS;
fax: 202-466-6456
Web site: http://www.nofas.org/contactus.aspx

12

Health Care Legislation, Regulation, and Financing

STEVEN WHITE, PHD

SCOPE OF CHAPTER

The evolutionary changes occurring in health care legislation and regulation in the early 21st century affect both speech-language pathology and audiology services. New clinical procedures for the professions were added to the American Medical Association's *Current Procedural Terminology* (American Medical Association, 2005) while reimbursement rates fluctuated as Medicare annually revised the outpatient payment system. The federal government continued to search for new ways to slow Medicare and Medicaid spending, and regulation of privacy and security regarding patient communications was instituted. The Centers for Medicare and Medicaid Services (CMS), formerly the Health Care Financing Administration, an agency in the United States Department of Health and Human Services, creates Medicare regulations based on federal law that affect the practices of speech-language pathology and audiology by both establishing reimbursement levels and requiring specific elements in documentation such as physician referral. The speech-language pathology and audiology community continued to adjust to the negative impact of federal legislation of the 1990s. The payment systems for outpatient and many inpatient Medicare settings had been remarkably altered with passage of the Balanced Budget Act (BBA) of 1997, a landmark bill that changed the rules for Medicare payment in most rehabilitation provider settings. Consequently, reimbursement based on the cost of rendering inpatient care became prospectively determined. Other Medicare laws further altered how health care services are paid.

The most positive aspect of the Medicare system has been its ability to ensure care for older individuals and those with severe disabilities who have communication and related disorders. Correspondingly, the growth of the numbers of speech-language pathologists in health care over the past 20 years may be attributed, at least in part, to the coverage of services in the Medicare program. This chapter, while providing a chronological account and summaries of pertinent health care legislation, regulations, and financing excerpted from the first edition version of this chapter (Frattali, Curl, & Bevan, 1994), expands the focus by emphasizing recent changes in the Medicare statute and its impact on speech-language pathology and audiology services. New to this chapter is discussion of HIPAA, private health care insurance, and the future of health care. Other forces affecting reimbursement and coverage such as the advocacy efforts by the American Speech-Language-Hearing Association are now included. Commonly used health care acronyms and abbreviations are found at the end of the chapter in the Appendix.

HEALTH CARE LEGISLATION

The creation of Medicare, Medicaid, and other federal health care programs is mandated by Congress through laws enacted to provide the most vulnerable Americans with improved access to health care. The following laws illustrate how the federal government develops and revises programs that have a remarkable impact on medical care.

Social Security Act Amendments of 1965

Title XVIII of the Social Security Act, Medicare, which provides health insurance for individuals age 65 and older as well as individuals with disabilities under age 65, was established by the Social Security Amendments of 1965. Congress has amended Medicare to add new benefits and create new payment approaches. The Amendments of 1965 also created Title XIX, Medicaid, the federal-state partnership of health insurance for people living in poverty.

Medicare covers individuals with disabilities under age 65 including people who have been receiving Social Security disability benefits for at least 2 years. Disability benefits are paid to people who cannot work because they have a severe medical condition that is expected to last at least 1 year or result in death. Children are covered under Medicare if they have chronic renal disease and need a kidney transplant or maintenance dialysis or if they have amyotrophic lateral sclerosis.

The Medicare program has several distinct parts. Medicare Part A, the hospital insurance benefit, covers the costs of inpatient hospital services, skilled nursing facility services, and most home health services. It is financed by the Medicare payroll tax. Medicare Part B, supplemental medical insurance, is a voluntary program financed by premium payments by enrollees and matching payments from general revenues. Part B benefits include physician services, independent practice diagnostic audiology services, and most outpatient rehabilitation services provided by hospitals, rehabilitation agencies, and comprehensive outpatient rehabilitation facilities. Medicare Part C allows beneficiaries access to managed care programs (e.g., health maintenance organizations) called Medicare Advantage. The Medicare Advantage programs are required to cover standard Medicare benefits such as speech-language pathology and audiology services. A new prescription drug benefit that went into effect on January 1, 2006, is described in Medicare Part D.

Medicaid also extended eligibility to include medically indigent persons not on welfare. Under this program, states are to provide at least some of each of five basic services: inpatient hospital services, outpatient hospital services, other laboratory and X-ray services, skilled nursing facility services, and physicians' services. A range of additional benefits, including audiology and speech-language pathology services and assistive technology, also can be offered as optional services by the states. The federal share of the program's cost is 50 percent to 83 percent, according to the state's per capita income.

Social Security Act Amendments of 1967

These amendments added outpatient physical therapy services under Part B of the Medicare program. They also eliminated the requirement that a physician certify the medical necessity of outpatient hospital services. However, periodic examinations by physicians after admission remain for hospitalized patients.

Social Security Act Amendments of 1972

The 1972 amendments expanded Medicare to include another vulnerable population: people with severe disabilities. Persons who have received cash benefits under the disability provisions of the Social Security Act for at least 2 years would be eligible for health care benefits under Medicare. Thus, Medicare became the health insurance program for individuals who are 65 and older and individuals who are under 65 and have a severe disability. The amendments of 1972 also added coverage of speech-language pathology services as part of a subsection of the outpatient physical therapy section pertaining to rehabilitation agencies.

As a result of these amendments, regulations were promulgated (effective in 1976) specifying conditions of participation for clinics, rehabilitation agencies, and public health agencies as providers of outpatient speech-language pathology services under Part B. Subsequently, speech-language pathologists independently can obtain a Medicare provider number if they meet the requirements for certification as a rehabilitation agency.

In addition, the Early and Periodic, Screening, Diagnosis, and Treatment (EPSDT) program under Medicaid was established. This program provides for child health screening, including hearing, speech, and language; hearing aids; augmentative and assistive communication devices; and subsequent treatment.

Social Security Act Amendments of 1982

Concern over rapidly rising health care costs led to amendments that changed the way in which Medicare reimbursed hospitals for costs. The Tax Equity and Fiscal Responsibility Act (TEFRA) marked the beginning of a new era in Medicare reimbursement. For the first time, hospitals were paid according to fixed payment levels rather than what they reported as their actual costs. The TEFRA limits were applied to all routine operating costs, costs of special care units, and costs of inpatient services such as speech-language pathology and audiology. Further, the TEFRA limits capped the reimbursement rate of increase for a hospital's Medicare reimbursement per discharge from one fiscal year to the next.

TEFRA offered a strong incentive to providers to contain costs, although Medicare's Prospective Payment System (PPS) that would be enacted in 1983 would offer a stronger incentive. As TEFRA continued and rehabilitation services have remained under its limits, providers became increasingly dissatisfied with the effect of the system (National Association of Rehabilitation Facilities, 1990). According to the National Association of Rehabilitation Facilities (now the American Medical Rehabilitation Providers Association) (NARF, 1990), increases in TEFRA limits were not sufficient to pay for the increasing costs of as many as half of all rehabilitation facilities, leading providers to propose changes to the way in which rehabilitation services are reimbursed. Not until 1997 did Congress require a new approach to paying rehabilitation hospitals and rehabilitation units in general hospitals.

TEFRA also added a new Medicare provider setting. Section 122 established coverage for hospice care. The new benefit specifically covers speech-language pathology services for the terminally ill. Section 418.92, Title 42 of the *Code of Federal Regulations* (Office of the Federal Register, 1996) states, "Physical therapy services, occupational therapy services, and speech-language pathology services must be available, and when provided, offered in a manner consistent with accepted standards of practice" (p. 783).

Social Security Act Amendments of 1983

In reaction to predictions that the Medicare program would go bankrupt by the year 2000 without drastic cost controls, the payment methodology of fixed payment levels or cost limits begun under

TEFRA was strengthened dramatically in 1983. The Social Security Amendments of 1983 created a new approach to paying for health services, the prospective payment system (PPS), in which a flat payment was determined prior to treatment and based on a patient's principal diagnosis or diagnosis-related group (DRG).

PPS was considered to provide strong incentives for hospitals to provide efficient services. Hospitals could keep any savings realized under Medicare DRGs. If the hospital's actual costs to treat a patient were less than the flat amount assigned to that particular DRG, the hospital kept the difference. However, if the hospital's actual costs exceeded the payment assigned, the hospital absorbed the loss.

Although such incentive reimbursement offered strong encouragement to providers for efficiency, it also raised concerns regarding a number of less positive effects. Health care professionals reported that PPS compromised quality of care. They alleged patients were being discharged after shorter lengths of stay and while still ill. Others raised the concern that hospitals struggling to survive in the health market would learn to "game the system" and simply shift costs to other areas.

Although anecdotal, the fallout of PPS for inpatient speech-language pathology and audiology services has reportedly been late or reduced inpatient referrals, fewer inpatient sessions, downsizing of staff, and reluctance to contract for new services. Moreover, a shift occurred for speech-language pathology inpatient services from language-based disorder services to assessing and treating patients with dysphagia. Physicians and hospital administrators knew the dysphagia services would assist in an earlier discharge.

Rehabilitation hospitals and rehabilitation units were exempt from Medicare PPS (as were children's, psychiatric, and long-term care hospitals), but remained subject to the TEFRA cost limits because of the unique case mix of patients. During the early period of PPS, the exempt rehabilitation hospitals and units enjoyed unprecedented growth (Wilkerson, Batavia, & DeJong, 1992).

United States Public Health Services Act (1944)

The Public Health Service Act of 1944 revised and brought together in one statute all existing legislation concerning the U.S. Public Health Service. It set forth provisions for the organization, staffing, and activities of the service. There have been many amendments to this act, including the Health Maintenance Organization Act.

The Health Maintenance Organization Act of 1973

This act amended the Public Health Service Act to provide assistance and encouragement for the establishment and expansion of health maintenance organizations (HMOs). The act added a new title, XIII, Health Maintenance Organizations, to the Public Health Service Act. It required the provision of the following basic medical services for a set, periodic payment fixed under a community rating system: physician services, inpatient and outpatient services, medically necessary emergency health services, short-term outpatient evaluative and crisis intervention mental health services (not over 20 visits), medical treatment and referral for alcohol and drug abuse, laboratory and X-ray services, home health services, and preventive services. Supplemental health services were also to be made available to enrolled members who wished to contract for them. They were intermediate and long-term care, vision care, and dental and mental health services not included under basic services, plus provision of prescription drugs.

Numerous amendments designed to make the requirements under the act less stringent were added to the act over the years. In 1976, an additional provision in the amendments required that HMOs receiving reimbursement from Medicare or Medicaid must be federally qualified. The regulatory language resulting from these provisions also resulted in clarification for the provision of speech-language pathology and audiology services:

Federally qualified HMOs must provide or arrange for outpatient service and inpatient hospital services (which) shall include short term rehabilitation and physical therapy, the provision of which the HMO determines can be expected to result in the significant improvement of a member's condition within a period of two months. (*Code of Federal Regulations*, Title 42, Section 110.102, 1990)

This section has reportedly had an apparently unintended effect on the length of treatment allowable for speech-language pathology services in HMOs. The regulatory language designates 2 months or 60 days as a *minimum* limit, at least for rehabilitation services such as speech-language pathology. However, it appears to be used by HMOs as a *maximum* limit, at least for speech-language pathology services. In a 1986 survey of HMOs (Cornett & Chabon), most reported limitations on speech-language pathology services to a maximum of 2 months or 60 days.

Technology-Related Assistance for Individuals with Disabilities Act of 1988

The purpose of this act is to provide financial assistance to states for developing and implementing a consumer-responsive statewide program of technology-related assistance for individuals with disabilities. Such programs must be designed, in part, to increase the availability of and funding for the provision of assistive technology devices and services. ASHA worked to include a broad definition of "assistive device" in the act (ASHA, 1990). The term refers to any item, piece of equipment, or product system—whether acquired commercially off the shelf, modified, or customized—that is used to increase, maintain, or improve functional capabilities of individuals with disabilities. The term *assistive technology service* refers to any service that directly assists an individual with a disability in the selection, acquisition, or use of an assistive technology device. It includes evaluation of needs, acquisition of devices, repairing/replacing devices, coordinating services, and training or technical assistance.

The Assistive Technology Act of 1998 reauthorizes the Technology-Related Assistance for Individuals with Disabilities Act of 1988 and includes provisions for low-interest loans for purchasing assistive technology (ASHA, 1998). The 1998 law also supports a national public Internet site and provides training in the needs for assistive technology and the rights of people with disabilities to such technology.

Health Insurance Portability and Accountability Act of 1996

When the Health Insurance Portability and Accountability Act of 1996 (P.L. 104-191) (HIPAA) amended the Internal Revenue Code of 1986, it was first constructed by Congress to protect the availability of health insurance coverage for workers and their families when they moved from one employer to another. That is, the purpose was to ensure that employees' health insurance was portable, particularly if they changed jobs or a family member had a preexisiting medical condition. There were, however, concerns on Capitol Hill with health care record keeping now that the country was in the cyberspace age. As a result, HIPAA has become better known by health care providers for the regulations regarding patient confidentiality and record storage and electronic transmissions of protected health information. Three major regulations have since been developed by agencies within the U.S. Department of Health and Human Services (HHS) as part of the Administrative Simplification section of HIPAA. Those rules are the electronic data interchange (EDI) rule, the privacy rule, and the security rule. Another section of HIPAA was recently released as part of the EDI rule: the National Security Identification Number.

HIPAA was implemented over a period of time. The first transaction standards for the EDI rule of HIPAA had a compliance deadline of October 16, 2002. The deadline for meeting the privacy rule was April 14, 2003, and the deadline for conforming to the security rule was April 2005.

In general, the EDI rule states that any health care provider or insurance entity that maintains or transmits "individually identifiable health information," referred to as *protected information* about a patient, is deemed a "covered entity" and is subject to HIPAA. In addition, business associates who view, manipulate, or otherwise handle this protected information on behalf of a covered entity are also subject to HIPAA. The final HIPAA privacy rule covers all individually identifiable health care information in any form, electronic or nonelectronic, that is held or transmitted by a covered entity. An entity that collects, stores, or transmits data electronically, orally, in writing, or through any form of communication, including fax, is covered under the HIPAA privacy rule, as is the information itself. The electronic transmission of this information is governed by the HIPAA EDI format standards. Conversely, if an entity uses a paper-only format, it is not governed by the EDI rules. However, once electronic data interchange is used, there is no going back to escape HIPAA rules.

All identifiable health information generated and transmitted by those in private practice and those practicing in rehabilitation agencies, schools, nursing homes, hospitals, and other institutional settings is considered protected information. Those professionals practicing as employees of covered entities are subject to the policies and procedures of those entities, which must be in full compliance with HIPAA rules. It also includes any provider under contract with a covered entity such as a nursing home or rehabilitation facility. In this situation, the speech-language pathologist or audiologist is a business associate of the facility and is therefore subject to the business associates provisions of HIPAA.

HIPAA is clear regarding the privacy rule and the role of speech-language pathology and audiology students participating in clinical services. Students are among those who are prohibited from disclosing individually identifiable information in any form. If the provider is a covered entity, the student must be educated on and comply with the privacy and security requirements of HIPAA. University clinics are among those providers, and the best approach is to educate students regarding HIPAA before they begin their clinical practicum (White, 2002).

In contrast to the privacy rule, which applies to all forms of protected health information, the security rule applies only to electronic protected health information (EPHI). This includes information that a covered entity creates, maintains, transmits, or receives. All methods of electronic information are covered by the rule, including records on computer hard drives, servers, and CDs. However, the security rule does not mandate the use of any specific technologies.

The new National Provider Identifier (NPI) is required for use by providers that bill electronically, but any health care provider is eligible to apply and receive one (Lusis, 2005). Health plans will be required to accept and use NPIs by May 23, 2007.

The security rule has three components. The first component includes the administrative safeguards that assign responsibility of training those who work in the entity about security of information within the entity and ensuring that the entity is secure. The second involves physical safeguards that relate to the actual mechanisms that protect the information. The third focuses on technical safeguards for processes that protect information such as encryption.

Penalties are to be imposed if the HHS Office of Civil Rights determines that an individual's right to privacy has been violated. EDI rule violations will be reported to the Secretary of HHS. The rule provides for civil penalties of $100 per violation up to a maximum of $25,000 per year. When violations are with the intent to sell, transfer, or use individually identifiable information for commercial advantage, personal gain, or malicious harm, criminal penalties ranging from $50,000 and 1 year in prison to $250,000 and 10 years in prison may be imposed.

OMNIBUS BUDGET RECONCILIATION ACTS (OBRAS)

Although many important pieces of legislation for health care have been authorizing statutes, much has also resulted from budget reconciliation. Traditionally, the budget process involved setting dollar outlays for broad budget categories or "functions," such as health and education. Specific programmatic changes to achieve those outlays were left to authorizing and appropriate legislation.

However, in the 96th Congress, the "reconciliation" procedure of the Congressional Budget and Impoundment Control Act of 1974 was used to "instruct" the authorizing committees to cut spending in numerous health programs. Since then, reconciliation has become an integral part of the budget process (National Health Council, 1993). Provisions in the following reconciliation laws are of interest to speech-language pathologists and audiologists.

Omnibus Budget Reconciliation Act of 1980

A component in the new law had a notable impact on speech-language pathologists providing services to Medicare beneficiaries. ASHA lobbied for legislation that was incorporated into OBRA 1980 that amended Medicare to eliminate the physician-only development of a patient's plan of treatment requirement for outpatient speech-language pathology services. Effective January 1, 1981, speech-language pathologists could write their own plans of treatment for Medicare beneficiaries.

In their 1979 reports on the Medicare Amendments legislation, the Senate Finance Committee and the House Ways and Means Committee stated that, "since speech (-language) pathology services involves highly specialized knowledge and training, physicians generally do not specify in detail the services needed when referring a patient for such services" (House Report 96-588 at p. 15; Senate Report 96-471 at p. 37).

Consolidated Omnibus Budget Reconciliation Act of 1985

Provisions of this act, which contained amendments to the Medicare and Medicaid programs, established the Physician Payment Review Commission. This commission was required to make recommendations to Congress regarding changes in the methodology for determining the rates of payment for Medicare Part B services. This legislation led to the implementation of the Resource-Based Relative Value Scale (RBRVS). The RBRVS is the foundation of the Medicare Fee Schedule that will be described later in more detail because of its implications for audiologists and speech-language pathologists.

Omnibus Budget Reconciliation Act of 1986

Section 9305 of the Omnibus Budget Reconciliation Act of 1986 (OBRA) required the development of a Uniform Needs Assessment Instrument (UNAI) to evaluate the functional capacity and health care needs of an inpatient upon discharge from the hospital. The legislation was a response to the increased anxiety and alarm expressed by health care consumers at the decreasing length of the average hospital stay. It was thought to be a safeguard to ensure the quality of care provided to Medicare beneficiaries (United States Department of Health and Human Services, 1992).

According to the law, the tool can be used by discharge planners, hospitals, nursing facilities, other health care providers, and fiscal intermediaries in evaluating an individual's need for post-hospital extended-care services, home health services, and long-term care services of a health-related or supportive nature. These services would include speech-language pathology and audiology services. The tool was developed and tested, but never implemented. A report submitted by then-Secretary of Health and Human Services Louis Sullivan indicated Congress should investigate unnecessary duplication of effort and wasteful expenditures that the UNAI may create (United States Department of Health and Human Services, 1992).

The tool, Form HCFA-32 (titled the Assessment of Needs for Continuing Care), addressed communication among those factors that may affect post-discharge care needs. A draft of the tool can be found in the *Report of the Secretary's Advisory Panel on the Development of Uniform Needs Assessment Instrument(s)* (United States Department of Health and Human Services, 1992).

OBRA 1986 also directed HCFA to proceed with research on a new system of Medicare Part B payment to physicians and other practitioners. It led to implementation of the Medicare Physician Fee Schedule.

Omnibus Budget Reconciliation Act of 1987

OBRA 1987, in response to the pervasiveness of substandard conditions in the nation's nursing homes, made sweeping reforms on the care provided by all nursing homes participating in the Medicare and Medicaid programs. This legislation mandates Medicare- or Medicaid-certified nursing facilities provide each resident the necessary care and services to "attain or maintain the highest practicable physical, mental and psychosocial well-being, in accordance with the comprehensive assessment and plan of care" (*Code of Federal Regulations,* Title 42, Section 483.25, Office of the Federal Register, 1996). The regulations resulting from this legislation further specify that the comprehensive assessment include an assessment of functional status, including the ability to use speech, language, or other functional communication systems (Lubinski & Frattali, 1993; White, 1989).

OBRA 1987 holds great potential for improving access to quality care for nursing facility residents with communication disorders and related disorders, such as dysphagia, cognitive deficits, and balance disorders. As a result of this legislation, the Resident Assessment Instrument (RAI) was developed (Morris, Hawes, Fries, & Mor, 1991). The RAI contains a minimum data set (MDS) that requires information on communication/hearing. It was developed with input from ASHA (Lubinski & Frattali, 1993).

Three years after the tool was established in the nation's nursing facilities, survey data collected by the research consortium involved in the development of the RAI documented a 31 percent increase in referrals to speech-language pathology (audiology data were not reported at the time) (Lubinski, personal communication, 1993). The MDS has just undergone another revision under the guidance of the Rand Corporation.

Omnibus Budget Reconciliation Act of 1989

OBRA 1989 established the Agency for Health Care Policy and Research, renamed the Agency for Healthcare Research and Quality (AHRQ) in 2000. It is one of eight agencies of the U.S. Public Health Service within the Department of Health and Human Services and replaced the National Center for Health Services Research and Health Care Technology Assessment. AHRQ supports studies on the outcomes of health care services and procedures used to prevent, diagnose, treat, and manage illness and disability (AHRQ, 1990b). An arm of AHRQ, the National Advisory Council for Health Care Policy, Research, and Evaluation is charged with improving the quality, safety, efficiency, and effectiveness of health care for all Americans (AHRQ, 2005).

OBRA 1989 also required Medicare to begin paying for charge-based Part B services by January 1992 based on an RBRVS with geographic adjustments for differences in costs of practice. This legislation replaced the reasonable charge payment mechanism with a fee schedule based on national uniform relative values for all "physician services," including outpatient physician services. The system was phased in during a 4-year period beginning in 1992.

The RBRVS caused concern among audiologists and speech-language pathologists (ASHA, 1992). The RBRVS does not recognize the interpretation of tests by audiologists or speech-language pathologists in the professional component also known as "physician work," but rather under the "technical" component or "practice expense." Thus, physicians and other practitioners have an approach that renders a value to their services based on intensity of service, stress, clinical judgment, and other factors. The value is determined based on a survey of those who perform the procedure with the results submitted by the specialty society and, subsequently, reviewed by a committee of experts known as the Relative Value Unit (RVU) Update Committee (RUC) of the American Medical Association. The RUC in turn submits the final values to the Centers for Medicare and Medicaid Services for consideration in the Medicare Physician Fee Schedule. The value of the professional component is added to practice expense and the malpractice expense (or professional liability) to give a total RVU. Conversely, services such as audiology and speech-language pathology have only time values. The time includes preparation for the service before the patient arrives; all time spent with the patient, including preparing the room and counseling the patient and family; report writing; and phone calls. However, it does not take into account the factors included for the professional component. Outpatient Medicare speech-language pathology services were included for reimbursement under the RBRVS in 1999 when the provisions of the BBA 1997 went into effect. A separate review of audiology and speech-language pathology relative value units in the MFS is produced by ASHA and updated annually. The RBRVS is discussed further in the Medicare Physician Fee Schedule section.

Finally, OBRA 1989 improved the Medicaid EPSDT program so that proper treatment for communication disorders discovered during screening must be provided. Prior to the law, states avoided providing needed services such as speech-language pathology services, audiology services, and assistive technology (White, 1990). OBRA 1989 mandated coverage of all medically necessary services for children enrolled in the Medicaid program.

Omnibus Budget Reconciliation Act of 1990

OBRA 1990 (Omnibus Budget and Reconciliation Act, 1990) includes Section 4005(b)(1), which states:

> The Secretary of Health and Human Services shall develop a proposal to modify the current system under which [excluded] hospitals receive payment . . . or a proposal to replace such system with a system under which such payment would be made on the basis of nationally determined average standardized amounts.

Through this provision, Congress made clear its intent to develop a more appropriate payment system for rehabilitation under Medicare (Wilkerson et al., 1992). Interestingly, through the Balanced Budget Act of 1997, Congress had to direct HHS to

implement the system. The 1990 OBRA legislation, as an interim measure, also provided some relief to hospitals in the form of partial payment for differences between the TEFRA cap and actual hospital costs (Wilkerson et al., 1992).

SOCIAL SECURITY ACT AMENDMENTS OF 1993

Unlike speech-language pathology services, audiology services were not mentioned in the Medicare statute until the Social Security Act Amendments of 1993. The amendments changed that by defining, in law, the definitions of audiology and audiologists as they related to Medicare services. Diagnostic audiology was, and is, covered as a diagnostic benefit. The type of coverage was defined by the Centers for Medicare and Medicaid Services (CMS, then HCFA) and provided a foundation for seeking a legislative remedy to include audiology as a Medicare benefit. The definitions that became part of the Medicare statute were consistent with contemporary coverage and ensured a placeholder for future improvements for audiology in the Medicare program. The definitions in the Social Security Act Amendments were taken from legislation introduced by Representative James Moody of Wisconsin. His bill, the Medicare Communication Disorders and Services Amendments Act of 1992, introduced during the 102nd Congress on June 3, 1992, would also have broadened audiology services to include aural rehabilitation. A section of the *Medicare Benefit Policy Manual* briefly describes the extent of audiology coverage in Medicare (Chapter 15, Section 80.3–Otologic Evaluations). Consequently, uneven medical review of Medicare claims occurs nationally.

CMS was not concerned about the almost cryptic description of covered audiology services because it left considerable discretion regarding appropriate coverage with the local reviewers who have a better understanding of an individual's need and the medical community's practice patterns. Local Coverage Decisions (LCDs) are developed by local Medicare contractors that are known as *fiscal intermediaries and carriers*. These contractors are usually health insurance plans such as local Blue Cross and Blue Shield plans and Mutual of Omaha but have separate bureaucracies for their Medicare services. CMS and the contractors—in essence, Medicare—*will* reimburse for audiology services when they assist a physician in the development of a treatment protocol or surgery. Medicare *will not* cover the service if it is related to determining the need for a hearing aid. The same holds true for services that are considered routine. Medicare, however, will not deny coverage if the hearing assessment results in the recommendation of a hearing aid evaluation (*Carriers Program Memorandum,* Transmittal B-01-34, April 30, 2001). Therefore, if a Medicare beneficiary did not complain of other symptoms related to an illness or syndrome other than a hearing loss, Medicare would not cover the audiology services. If the patient exhibits an asymmetrical or unilateral hearing loss and other symptoms of an illness such as Meniere's disease, then the audiologic services would be covered.

The Social Security Amendments of 1993 also defined speech-language pathology services and speech-language pathologists for the first time. Medicare regulations regarding the provision of speech-language pathology services and audiology services must be consistent with the following section of the United States Code for Title XVIII of the Social Security Act:

Sec. 1395x. Definitions

(II) Speech-language pathology services; audiology services

(1) The term "speech-language pathology services" means such speech, language, and related function assessment and rehabilitation services furnished by a qualified speech-language pathologist as the speech-language pathologist is legally authorized to perform under State law (or the State regulatory mechanism provided by State law) as would otherwise be covered if furnished by a physician.

(2) The term "audiology services" means such hearing and balance assessment services furnished by a qualified audiologist as the audiologist is legally authorized to perform under State law (or the State regulatory mechanism provided by State law), as would otherwise be covered if furnished by a physician.

(3) In this subsection:

(A) The term "qualified speech-language pathologist" means an individual with a master's or doctoral degree in speech-language pathology who—

(i) is licensed as a speech-language pathologist by the State in which the individual furnishes such services, or

(ii) in the case of an individual who furnishes services in a State which does not license speech-language pathologists, has successfully completed 350 clock hours of supervised clinical practicum (or is in the process of accumulating such supervised clinical experience), performed not less than 9 months of supervised full-time speech-language pathology services after obtaining a master's or doctoral degree in speech-language pathology or a related field, and successfully completed a national examination in speech-language pathology approved by the Secretary.

(B) The term "qualified audiologist" means an individual with a master's or doctoral degree in audiology who—

(i) is licensed as an audiologist by the State in which the individual furnishes such services, or

(ii) in the case of an individual who furnishes services in a State which does not license audiologists, has successfully completed 350 clock hours of supervised clinical practicum (or is in the process of accumulating such supervised clinical experience), performed not less than 9 months of supervised full-time audiology services after obtaining a master's or doctoral degree in audiology or a related field, and successfully completed a national examination in audiology approved by the Secretary.

HEALTH CARE CODING

HIPAA established the *International Classification of Diseases, 9th Edition, Clinical Modification* (ICD-9-CM) and the American Medical Association *Current Procedural Terminology* (CPT) as recognized code sets. Reporting of diseases and disorders is required using the ICD-9-CM while procedures must be identified using the CPT. The five audiologists and five speech-language pathologists of the ASHA Health Care Economics Committee (HCEC) monitor these code sets and make recommendations for additions and revisions. The work of the HCEC has resulted in new codes that are found in Table 12–1.

The HCEC has also advocated for equitable reimbursement of speech-language pathology and audiology procedures. Most of the audiology procedures and many of the speech-language pathology procedures only reflect practice expense.

T A B L E 12–1 Speech-Language Pathology and Audiology CPT[1] Codes Revised or Established 2003–2006

CPT Code	Descriptor
92506	Evaluation of speech, language, voice, communication, and/or auditory processing
92507	Treatment of speech, language, voice, communication, and/or auditory processing disorder; individual
92568	Acoustic reflex testing; threshold
92569	Acoustic reflex testing; decay
92601	Diagnostic analysis of cochlear implant, patient under 7 years of age; with programming
92602	Subsequent reprogramming
92603	Diagnostic analysis of cochlear implant, patient 7 years of age or older; with programming
92604	Subsequent reprogramming
92605	Evaluation for prescription of non-speech-generating augmentative and alternative communication device
92606	Therapeutic service(s) for the use of non-speech-generating augmentative and alternative communication device
92607	Evaluation for prescription of speech-generating augmentative and alternative communication device, face-to-face with the patient; first hour
92608	Each additional 30 minutes
92609	Therapeutic services for the use of speech-generating device, including programming and modification
92610	Evaluation of oral and pharyngeal swallow function
92611	Motion fluoroscopic evaluation of swallowing function by cine or video recording
92612	Flexible fiberoptic endoscopic evaluation of swallowing by cine or video recording
92614	Flexible fiberoptic endoscopic evaluation, laryngeal sensory testing by cine or video recording
92616	Flexible fiberoptic endoscopic evaluation of swallowing and laryngeal sensory testing by cine or video recording
92620	Evaluation of central auditory function, with report; initial 60 minutes
92621	Each additional 15 minutes
92625	Assessment of tinnitus (includes pitch, loudness matching, and masking)
92626	Evaluation of auditory rehabilitation status; first hour
92627	Each additional 15 minutes
92630	Auditory rehabilitation; pre-lingual hearing loss
92633	Post-lingual hearing loss

[1]CPT codes and descriptors are copyright 2004 American Medical Association

MEDICARE PHYSICIAN FEE SCHEDULE

In 1992, audiology underwent a major payment change with the advent of the resource- based relative value scale (RBRVS) (ASHA, 2005b). The system is the basis for the Medicare Physician Fee Schedule (MPFS). As mentioned earlier, the RBRVS assigns a relative value to each clinical procedure performed. A relative weighting value is derived from the scale. The components of the RBRVS for each procedure are:

1. The relative value unit (RVU) of the professional component, or physician work, that entails the amount of work for physicians and other practitioners with work defined as time, technical skill, physical effort, stress, and judgment;

2. The technical component or practice expense RVU composed of the overhead costs including the practice expense of nonphysician practitioners and the cost of supplies and equipment; and

3. The malpractice RVU representing the cost of professional liability coverage.

In 1999, one of the more dramatic changes that occurred in Medicare was the application of the MPFS to institutional providers for speech-language pathology services, physical therapy services, and occupational therapy services. Previously the MPFS had been confined to billing from physician and audiologist offices or group practices. Table 12–2 provides examples of some of the more common audiology and speech-language pathology procedures and their values for nonfacilities and facilities such as skilled nursing facilities, hospitals, and comprehensive outpatient rehabilitation facilities. The 2005 conversion factor of $37.8975 is applied to establish the national fee schedule used by Medicare. Geographical cost indices modify the values to account for state and local cost variations.

Table 12–3 illustrates how the reimbursement rates varied over 10 years as CMS revised the RVUs and the conversion factor (a multiplier used for all procedures used to establish the Medicare fee to conform with federal budget requirements) was changed to reflect medical inflation by Congress. Curiously, while the reimbursement rate increased from $49.52 in 1996 to $131.88 in 2005 for speech-language evaluation, the rate for speech-language treatment went from $30.47 to $62.53 during the same period. A high point of $77.25 occurred in 2003, but a reduction in the practice expense in 2004 negatively affected the rate. The lowering of the rate is a consequence of Medicare restricting the services of a speech-language pathologist to the technical component and not reflecting new data presented by ASHA in the professional component. A survey and a subsequent consensus panel

TABLE 12–2 Common Speech-Language Pathology and Audiology Procedures and Approximate 2005 Medicare Relative Value Units (RVUs) and Fees

Procedure	Work RVU	Practice Expense RVU	Malpractice RVU	Total RVU	Fee
Speech-language treatment, individual	0.52	1.11	0.02	1.65	$62.53
Speech-language treatment, group	0.26	0.51	0.01	0.78	$29.56
Swallowing evaluation	0.00	3.43	0.08	3.51	$123.02
Comprehensive hearing test	0.00	1.19	0.12	1.31	$49.65
Auditory evoked potential	0.50	2.06	0.17	2.73	$103.46

SOURCE: ASHA, *2005 Medicare Fee Schedule and Hospital Outpatient Prospective Payment System for Audiologists.* Rockville, MD: Author and ASHA, *2005 Medicare Fee Schedule for Speech-Language Pathologists.* Rockville, MD: Author.

T A B L E 12–3 Impact of MPFS Total RVU and Conversion Factor on Fee for Speech-Language Evaluation Reimbursement Level

Year	Total RVU	Conversion Factor	National Fee
1996	1.43	34.63	$49.52
1997	1.43	33.84	$45.98
1998	1.43	36.69	$52.47
1999	1.32	34.73	$45.85
2000	1.74	36.61	$63.71
2001	2.14	38.26	$81.87
2002	2.62	36.20	$94.84
2003	2.53	36.79	$93.07
2004	3.52	37.34	$131.43
2005	3.48	37.90	$131.88

T A B L E 12–4 Impact of MPFS Total RVU and Conversion Factor on Fee for Comprehensive Audiometry Threshold Evaluation and Speech Recognition

Year	Total RVU	Conversion Factor	National Fee
1996	1.26	34.63	$43.63
1997	1.26	33.84	$42.64
1998	1.26	36.69	$46.23
1999	1.33	34.73	$46.19
2000	1.32	36.61	$48.33
2001	1.29	38.26	$49.35
2002	1.23	36.20	$44.53
2003	1.28	36.79	$47.09
2004	1.31	37.34	$48.91
2005	1.31	37.90	$49.65

convened by the ASHA Health Care Economics Committee determined the revised figures.

Conversely, Table 12–4 shows a lack of impact on a common audiology procedure, comprehensive audiometry, during 1996–2005. The major difference is that the audiology procedure does not have a value for the professional component and CMS has placed it in the nonphysician work pool, a category of procedures that CMS considers primarily technical in nature. Please note how the national fee has remained fairly constant over 10 years. CMS proposed to eliminate the nonphysician work pool beginning in 2006 (CMS) but decided against the change due to the severe impact it would have on many of the procedures. CMS predicted that audiology would suffer up to a 21 percent loss in fees by the time the nonphysician work pool was totally eliminated over 4 years ending in 2009.

THE BALANCED BUDGET ACT OF 1997

A Republican Congress and a promise from the Clinton administration to bring the federal budget under control drove the most sweeping changes in the Medicare statute since its inception in 1965. As reported by the Medicare Payment Advisory Commission (MedPAC) of Congress (1998):

The Balanced Budget Act of 1997 (BBA) enacted substantial changes in Medicare's payment policies. Outpatient rehabilitation providers will be paid according to the physician fee schedule beginning January 1, 1999, and outpatient rehabilitation furnished by non-hospital providers will be subject to annual coverage limits. Skilled nursing facilities (SNFs) will begin transition to a per diem prospective payment system on July 1, 1998. Prospective payment for home health agencies and for inpatient rehabilitation facilities also is scheduled to be implemented on October 1, 1999, although the units of payment for those systems have not been finalized. (p. 79)

Although there was no mention of "outpatient rehabilitation" as a particular provider in the Medicare statute, there were various rehabilitation providers under the law. Hospital outpatient departments, rehabilitation agencies, and comprehensive outpatient rehabilitation facilities (CORFs) are all providers of rehabilitation services, as are independent practitioners of physical therapy and occupational therapy. Nevertheless, the three major rehabilitation professions are all separately described in the Medicare statute.

The two major areas of the BBA that most affected the practice of speech-language pathology were the requirement to impose a $1,500 annual financial limitation on each Medicare beneficiary for outpatient speech-language pathology and physical therapy combined and the change to prospective payment systems for inpatient services.

RECENT CHANGES TO THE MEDICARE STATUTE AND IMPACT ON SLP AND AUDIOLOGY

Three major laws that contained Medicare and Medicaid provisions were passed during the turn of the century in 1999, 2000, and 2003. Each has an impact on the professions of speech-language pathology and audiology. Privacy, electronic security of personal medical information, and new payment approaches for the private health plan market emerged.

The Medicare, Medicaid, and SCHIP Balanced Budget Refinement Act of 1999 (BBRA)

The BBRA was the first law that responded to the concerns of the beneficiary and provider communities about the problems caused by the Medicare therapy cap. It placed a two-year moratorium on the cap covering calendar years 2000 and 2001. The law also called for CMS to submit a report to Congress about the utilization patterns of outpatient therapy.

The Medicare, Medicaid, and SCHIP Benefits Improvement and Protection Act of 2000 (BIPA)

This federal statute was signed into law in December 2002 and became known as BIPA. BIPA had a positive effect on the provision of speech-language pathology services under Medicare by extending the moratorium on the annual financial cap for outpatient physical, occupational, and speech-language pathology services. Remember that the BBA established a $1,500 cap on the amount of outpatient physical, occupational, and speech therapy services that are reimbursable per calendar year. Congress never liked the cap after it was instituted and, as with BBRA and future laws, BIPA extended the moratorium on the cap through 2002 to add to the 2 years from the BBRA.

The Medicare Prescription Drug, Improvement, and Modernization Act of 2003 (MMA)

The MMA contains a number of provisions that affect speech-language pathology and audiology services. The most immediate effect of the MMA was a 1.5 percent increase in the Medicare payment schedule for services paid under the MPFS provided on or after January 1, 2004. The rates were set to be cut by 4.5 percent in 2004, and again in 2005, but the MMA reversed the cuts and provided an increase of 1.5 percent in the conversion factor of the MPFS for each of these years.

A new concept was introduced in the law—a "Welcome to Medicare" preventive screening examination. The new benefit is meant to promote health and detect disease. New beneficiaries of Medicare are eligible for an initial preventive screening examination known as a "Welcome to Medicare" examination. It includes a measurement of height, weight, and blood pressure; a screening electrocardiogram; a review of the patient's medical and social history; and a review of the individual's risk factors for depression, functional ability, and level of safety. It also includes education, counseling, and referral with respect to screening and preventive services currently covered under Medicare Part B. Hearing screening is part of the examination but only in an interview format. ASHA recommended that pure-tone screening be used, but CMS stated that a discussion between the beneficiary and physician is sufficient for the purpose of the Welcome to Medicare.

$1,500 Financial Limitation

The BBA created the arbitrary annual beneficiary cap in response to rapidly escalating expenditures in the Medicare outpatient rehabilitation benefits. Costs to the Medicare program for rehabilitation agency services went from $151 million in 1990 to $524 million in 1996 (Medicare Payment Assessment Commission, 1998, p. 80). Corresponding growth in cost for comprehensive outpatient rehabilitation facilities (CORFs) went from $19 million to $115 million in the same time period. Congress chose the cap as a quick fix for a complex issue.

Previously, physical therapists and occupational therapists in independent practice had a $900 cap, and this served as the model for all outpatient services. The outpatient financial limitation became effective on January 1, 1999, for speech-language pathology services, physical therapy services, and occupational therapy services in all Medicare-certified outpatient settings except for hospitals. Occupational therapy has a separate $1,500 cap from the combined cap for speech-language pathology and physical therapy. Advocacy efforts by ASHA and other rehabilitation organizations such as the American Occupational Therapy Association and the American Physical Therapy Association resulted in a revision of the rehabilitation cap. On November 29, 1999, the Medicare, Medicaid, and SCHIP Balanced Budget bill became law (Public Law 106-113). The Balanced Budget Refinement Act (BBRA) placed a 2-year moratorium on the $1,500 cap and required the Secretary of Health and Human Services to report to Congress on a new payment limitation method for outpatient rehabilitation services and on the utilization of services. The moratorium on the cap was a major victory for ASHA and the other professional associations.

CMS contracted with AdvanceMed to review billing practices and investigate the establishment of a payment system related to Medicare Part B rehabilitation services that would obviate the need for a therapy cap. AdvanceMed's Ciolek and Whang (2004) recommended a global approach to achieve a long-term outpatient therapy payment system solution in the second AdvanceMed report. The global approach would maintain the use of the MPFS, eliminate the therapy cap, continue medical review to identify targets for utilization review, create utilization thresholds for "medically unbelievable services," use national rather than local coverage decisions, develop a standardized outpatient therapy assessment instrument, and develop a condition-based outpatient therapy payment system.

The therapy cap issue refuses to recede completely, although federal legislation to repeal the cap has been popular. Legislation for repealing the cap has been introduced by members of Congress who sit on Medicare oversight committees. However, because of the negative budget impact of repealing the cap, the threat of its return persists. Table 12–5 highlights the law that created the cap, those laws that placed a delay in its implementation, court action that briefly delayed the implementation of the cap, and program memoranda from CMS that instruct Medicare contractors how to enforce the cap.

The Deficit Reduction Act of 2005 (DRA) was signed into law by President George W. Bush on February 8, 2006. The DRA required that CMS develop an exception process that allows Medicare beneficiaries access to medically necessary outpatient therapy services above the therapy cap for calendar year 2006. Speech-language pathologists can use the exceptions process for conditions such as those that require both speech-language pathology and physical therapy services. Moreover, CMS can use the approach to collect data that may demonstrate the necessity of functional outcomes–based data from providers. Details of the exceptions process are found on the ASHA Web site.

Prospective Payment Systems

In 1983, Medicare began its first prospective payment system (PPS) for inpatient hospital services. Reimbursement had been based on the cost of rendering care, but the PPS revised the approach by affixing rates according to the principle diagnosis of the patient. This diagnosis-related grouping (DRG) of patients altered inpatient care so that patients were being discharged early, or "quicker and sicker." Administrators of skilled nursing facilities (SNFs)

T A B L E 12–5 Chronologic History of the Medicare Therapy Caps

Law/Action	Date	Therapy cap impact
BBA 97	1997	Imposes $1,500 cap on outpatient therapy services in skilled nursing facilities (Part B), physician offices, Part B home health agencies (Part B); outpatient hospital services are excluded; speech-language pathology & physical therapy share $1,500 cap and occupational therapy has own $1,500 cap; effective date–January 1, 1999
BBRA	November 1, 1999	Places 2-year moratorium on therapy cap during calendar years 2000 and 2001
BIPA	December 2000	Extends moratorium through 2002
CMS PM	February 7, 2003	Program memorandum (PM) delays implementation through July 1, 2003
U.S. Court	May 2, 2003	Consumer groups sue U.S. Department of Health and Human Services arguing that insufficient notice has been given; judge delays implementation for 60 days or until September 1, 2003
CMS PM	September 1, 2003	Caps go into effect at a $1,590 level
U.S. Court	September 4, 2003	Consumer groups argue that there still has been insufficient notice to Medicare beneficiaries
U.S. Court	September 22, 2003	Judge states CMS can enforce therapy caps
MMA	2003	Places moratorium on caps from December 8, 2003 through December 31, 2005

and home health agencies (HHAs) had to revise their approach to patient care and place more emphasis on rehabilitation services such as speech-language pathology.

It was not until 1997 that the United States Congress and the Clinton administration instituted new PPSs. The BBA placed both SNFs and home health agencies (HHAs) under unique and, at that time, somewhat unknown PPSs. SNFs began the transition from a cost-based system to a per-diem approach on July 1, 1998, depending on the cost-reporting period to Medicare. HHAs began an interim payment system for cost-reporting periods beginning on or after October 1, 1999. The HHA PPS is based on an assessment instrument known as the Outcome and Assessment Information set, or OASIS. The SNF PPS system is based on resource utilization groups (RUGs). Other providers scheduled to go under a form of prospective payment system include rehabilitation hospitals and hospital outpatient departments.

The SNF PPS interim final regulations were published by the Health Care Financing Administration (now CMS) in the May 12, 1998 *Federal Register* and are based on the Nursing Home Case Mix and Quality System, a PPS demonstration project that had been funded by HCFA since 1989. The hallmark of the system is the RUG, which is composed of an assessment, Minimum Data Set (MDS), wage-weighted staff time measurements, and self-performance in activities of daily living (ADLs). SNF patients are assigned to one of 53 RUGs, of which 23 require intensive rehabilitation services. Patients in the 23 rehabilitation RUGs require from 45 minutes to 720 minutes per week of speech-language pathology, physical therapy, or occupational therapy services.

The Balanced Budget Act of 1997 was an attempt to bring fiscal controls to the Medicare program. A review of the development of Medicare through a series of amendments to the Social Security Act demonstrates the piecemeal approach to revising the program over the last 32 years. Further, the difficulties in creating a logical financing system are compounded by the various settings in which health care is delivered in the United States.

ROLE OF STATE GOVERNMENTS

Historically, the states have played an important role in shaping the structure, delivery, and reimbursement of health care services. One of the ways in which states affect change derives from their ability to receive a waiver from a federally prescribed system of implementing a program. Under such a waiver, states can enact systems that are more responsive to the specific needs of their residents while maintaining compliance with the overall goals of the federal program. This action often has an impact far beyond the individual states.

For example, New Jersey sought and received such a waiver from HCFA for the administration of Medicare within the state. As a result of that waiver, the state developed and implemented an alternative payment program that used diagnosis-related groups for reimbursement of hospital costs. In its health care cost containment efforts, the Reagan administration used the New Jersey system as a prototype in developing the federal DRGs for the Medicare inpatient hospital PPS. States also affect the structuring and delivery of health care services and the reimbursement for those services through direct authority over a number of health care issues. Those issues include the licensing of health care professionals, health insurance regulation, public health, health care for low-income families, rate setting, and access to health care services within the state. For example, states have considerable latitude for the administration of the Medicaid program. In fact, provider setting, procedures, and assistive technology find considerable variation from state to state in coverage of audiology and speech-language pathology services. Coverage should be consistent for children because of the EPSDT program, but the statewide use of managed care organizations by some states has an impact on the extent of speech-language pathology and audiology services.

The role of the states is expected to increase because of the call by some in Washington, DC, for more local control. Interest in extending considerable latitude to the states in providing and managing health care services has been expressed by players on all fronts, including Congress and CMS.

PRIVATE HEALTH INSURANCE

Speech-language pathology and audiology services have suffered from variable coverage by private health plans. Nevertheless, coverage does exist and knowledge of the different kinds of private health plans is necessary for clinical practice. A good source of information that discusses the relationship of speech-language pathology and audiology coverage and health plans is the ASHA *Health Plan Coding & Claims Guide* (McCarty & White, 2003).

Managed care organizations (MCOs) dominate American health plans today. There are two major types of MCOs: preferred provider organizations (PPOs) and health maintenance organizations (HMOs). According the Kaiser Family Foundation and Health Research Educational Trust (2005), PPOs now account for 61 percent of employees with health insurance coverage. PPOs contract with networks of providers, predominately hospitals and physicians, that agree to provide their services according to negotiated reduced payment rates. Most PPOs allow their members to go outside of the network but penalize this behavior with higher copayments (the enrollee's portion of the payment) and deductibles (the amount spent before the health plan pays for services). HMOs were a force in the health care market because they allowed purchasers to receive a broad range of services, including preventive care, at reasonable premium rates in exchange for a restricted network of providers or a clinical or staff model where the enrolled goes to specific facilities for care. HMO enrollment fell from 25 percent of covered workers in 2004 to 21 percent in 2005. The remainder of employees, 15 percent, remained constant for the past year in point of service (POS) plans. These plans, usually an HMO hybrid, allow the enrollee to choose providers outside of the network but with strong PPO-like incentives to stay within the point of service plans. The advantage for providers to become a provider for an MCO is inclusion on a restricted provider network list that will improve the number of referrals to your practice.

Speech-language pathologists and audiologists face several problems when claims are submitted to health plans. Most health plans limit coverage to services for health problems related to an accident or illness. They use this limitation to deny coverage of services provided to infants and children with development disorders such as a developmental speech disorder. They also limit coverage to physical disorders, thus creating a problem for coverage of speech-language pathology for services rendered to an individual with a fluency disorder. ASHA developed a product to assist speech-language pathologists and their patients facing these types of denials. *Appealing Health Plan Denials* (McCarty, Thompson, & White, 2004) includes sample appeal letters and efficacy papers that assist speech-language pathologists and audiologists in overturning unfair denials. Of course, these may not be successful if the plan has clear language excluding coverage to these services but the health plan may make an exception if the services have a clear point for termination of treatment.

Audiologists can have other concerns with health plans. Some plans deny coverage of hearing assessment services to physicians and hospitals. The state speech-language-hearing association and ASHA can assist the audiologist in presenting a case to the health plan so that private practice audiologists are included in their provider networks.

Private health plan coverage and reimbursement are such a major issues that ASHA has made them a focused issue since 2003. Strategies have been developed to improve private health plan coverage of speech-language pathology and audiology services. ASHA's 2006 issue and outcomes for the focused initiative are:

ISSUE: Coverage rules, reimbursement rates, and federal, state, and local funding streams are increasingly affecting access to and scope of services provided by audiologists and speech-language pathologists in health and education settings. (ASHA, 2006. Focussed Initiatives: 2006)

ASHA set out a list of goals for 2006 to help alleviate this problem. They are as follows:

OUTCOME 1: ASHA members will have access to information and tools to effectively negotiate with private health plans to ensure appropriate coverage criteria and equitable reimbursement rates.

OUTCOME 2: Increased number of employers that cover comprehensive speech-language pathology and audiology services in their health benefits package.

OUTCOME 3: ASHA members will have access to information and tools to help them effectively navigate state funded insurance programs (e.g., Medicaid, [Children's Health Insurance Programs] CHIPs) at the state and local level to ensure appropriate coverage criteria and equitable reimbursement rates.

OUTCOME 4: Increased advocacy for and use of public and private reimbursement systems/insurance programs that enhance the ability of consumers to receive quality programs and services by audiologists and speech-language pathologists.

OUTCOME 5: Increased reimbursement for audiologic rehabilitation services in federal and private insurance programs.

OUTCOME 6: Increased availability of information related to access for federal, state, and local funding streams for programs and services in the schools.

SOURCE: ASHA, 2006. Focussed Initiative: 2006.

FUTURE OF HEALTH CARE

There has been considerable discussion and debate in Washington, DC, over two major issues: the reform of the Medicare program and the establishment of federal standards for managed care organizations. Increased costs continue to dominate the concerns by all that pay for group health care benefits, both public and private. The concern over limited access to health care because of a lack of health insurance waned in the late 1990s. Nevertheless, there is little doubt it will return because it has been an issue since the early 20th century during the Theodore Roosevelt administration.

The impact of the MMA will be felt for some time because of the dramatic changes in coverage for pharmaceuticals and changes in payment to managed care organizations (MCOs). Many provider associations, including ASHA, continue to pursue legislation that will provide relief from the Medicare outpatient rehabilitation cap. The ASHA Government Relations and Public Policies (GRPP) Board established three top priority issues for 1999, and seeking a remedy for the cap was one of them (ASHA, 1999b). Unfortunately, the 2004 GRPP Board had to have a similar priority in the 2005 ASHA Public Policy Agenda as Congress and CMS continue to search for alternatives to the cap (ASHA, 2005c).

The highest priorities for ASHA are to:

■ Promote direct patient access to audiology and speech-language pathology services for Medicare beneficiaries, including direct billing and ensuring that both the work component and the technical component for these services are included in Medicare fee schedule payment rates.

■ Promote reauthorization, full funding, and implementation of the Individuals with Disabilities Education Act (IDEA), with emphasis on the recruitment and retention of highly qualified personnel, reducing caseloads/workloads, promoting effective early intervention and outcomes-based practices, and providing services to culturally and linguistically diverse children.

■ Promote federal financial aid policies and priorities that support recruitment of students to doctoral programs and retention of Ph.D. faculty and researchers in communications sciences and disorders graduate programs, with emphasis on culturally/linguistically diverse candidates.

General health care reform has taken a lower priority in Congress, and attention continues to be paid to containing costs. Nevertheless, when health care reform proposals return, Congress, the administration, consumers, states, and others are likely to include certain fundamental factors for health care reform. Universal concerns will most likely result in a national health care package that:

■ Controls costs

■ Enhances quality

■ Expands access

■ Encourages local responsibility

■ Focuses on patient outcomes

■ Increases accountability

■ Emphasizes health promotion and disease prevention.

Consistent with these fundamental principles, the ASHA Ad Hoc Committee on National Health Policy prepared a position statement on health care reform to be used in ASHA's advocacy efforts (ASHA, 1993c). According to this position statement, any national health policy must adhere to the following 12 principles:

1. Provide universal access to all consumers.
2. Recognize individual needs.
3. Ensure quality of life.
4. Ensure consumer and professional representation for policy development and implementation.
5. Support consumer education.
6. Allow consumers to choose provider settings.
7. Cover comprehensive services.
8. Provide cost-effective services.
9. Ensure broad-based financing.
10. Support research.
11. Recognize the autonomy of the audiology and speech-language pathology professions.
12. Provide access to necessary assistive and augmentative technology.

Similarly, the disability community, through the work of the Consortium for Citizens with Disabilities (1992), drafted a disability perspective on health care reform. The perspective included a number of key features. Health care reform must be nondiscriminatory (e.g., ensure that all persons have access to needed services), comprehensive (e.g., include audiology and speech-language pathology among benefits), appropriate (e.g., ensure appropriate amount, scope, and duration of services, ensure the availability of trained personnel), and efficient (e.g., reduce administrative complexity, maintain effective cost controls).

Beyond the fundamental principles articulated by a variety of players, one could expect to see a number of specific elements that will be in some health care reform efforts. A standard benefits package may be created to define exactly which services each individual is entitled to by law. The only means by which this can be bypassed is to create an independent agency to develop the standard benefits.

Although speech-language pathology and audiology services may be included, there may be limits imposed on length of service based on expectations of functional gain. Reimbursement may be linked directly to evidence that services provided are beneficial and cost-efficient. Health care providers will be held accountable for the quality and cost-efficiency of their services.

The professions of speech-language pathology and audiology, through the efforts of ASHA, are preparing now for this restructuring. ASHA's efforts include advocacy activities (ASHA 1993a, 1999b), work with national coalitions (National Rehabilitation Caucus, Patients Access to Responsible Care Alliance, and Consortium for Citizens with Disabilities), the National Outcomes Measurement System (NOMS), preferred practice patterns, the Health-Net grassroots network, input to the procedural coding systems, and continuous revisions on the ASHA Web site.

Advocacy for coverage and reimbursement of speech-language pathology services, audiology services, hearing aids, and assistive technology by private health plans is now encompassed in ASHA-focused initiatives. New documents have been produced to assist the requests of speech-language pathologists, audiologists, and patients that private health plan cover these essential services and products. Among the new materials are efficacy reports, health plan report card, checklists, and Web sites for members, consumers, and employers. A strategy of the focused initiative was the implementation of a new network of ASHA members in the states who will serve as leaders for local efforts. The State Advocates for Reimbursement (STAR) network has a listserv, holds periodic conference calls, and assists state associations in efforts to improve private health plan coverage (Jacobson & Thompson, 2005). The Florida STAR member has conducted workshops across the state to enlist more state association members in advocacy (Johnson, 2004). More speech-language pathologists and audiologists will have to become involved in communicating with health plan officials if coverage speech-language pathology and audiology services are to improve. Medicare remains a major focus of advocacy and educational efforts.

The reader is referred to the *Medicare Handbook for Speech-Language Pathologists* (Kander, Lusis & White, 2004) and the *Medicare Handbook for Audiologists* (Kander, Lusis & White, 2004) for a complete explanation of the Medicare program as it relates to either audiology services or speech-language pathology services. The Health Care Economics and Advocacy team at the ASHA national office can assist speech-language pathologists and audiologists in understanding and interpreting coverage under Medicare and Medicaid. The Health Care Economics and Advocacy team maintains and updates the Medicare, Medicaid, private health plan, and coding reimbursement pages on the ASHA Web site, and readers are advised to periodically check the site.

SUMMARY

The health care legislation and regulations summarized in this chapter have led to the creation of a complex health care maze that has fallen short of meeting the needs of all Americans. More specifically, reimbursement for audiology and speech-language pathology services is dependent on the variations of major payment systems. The current system has imposed layers of both public and private bureaucracies and program limitations that have fed into often-arbitrary decisions about who will provide the services, to whom, and at what cost. Soon one will be competing in yet a new system, most definitely on the basis of the cost, quality, and availability of your services.

Thus, one must collect and use objective and convincing evidence that what you do makes a difference and is cost-effective and convenient. Change will always be on the horizon. Consequently, both obstacles and opportunities will face speech-language pathologists and audiologists. The professions will continue to prepare for the future of health care. You are, however, well advised that the true measure of your success in a reformed health care system will be the ability to compete individually by acting collaboratively and beyond the boundaries of your own discipline.

CRITICAL THINKING

1. How does Medicare cover speech-language pathology services and audiology services in an outpatient setting versus in hospital?

2. Why did Medicare change from a retrospective to prospective payment system?

3. Describe the chronology of legislation that affects reimbursement of speech-language pathology or audiology services.

4. When does an audiologist or speech-language pathologist report CPT codes?

5. What are the three components of the RBRVS?

6. How does ASHA affect the public policy agenda?

7. How does the Medicaid program cover children's services?

8. How can a speech-language pathologist or audiologist have an impact on the legislative or regulatory process?

9. How has HIPAA affected documentation of our audiology or speech-language pathology services?

10. How do federal laws affect individuals in private practice?

11. How can you as a professional keep abreast of changes in federal and state legislation and their impact on your delivery of clinical services?

REFERENCES

Agency for Healthcare Policy and Research. (1990, March). Medical treatment effectiveness research, *AHCPR program note.* Rockville, MD: U.S. Department of Health and Human Services.

Agency for Healthcare Policy and Research. (2005). *AHRQ Profile.* Rockville, MD: Author.

American Medical Association (2005). *CPT 2006.* Chicago: Author.

American Speech-Language-Hearing Association. (1990, March). *Federal legislative issues: Current issues of interest to speech-language pathologists, audiologists, and persons with communication disorders* (ASHA Congressional Relations Division Report). Rockville, MD: Author.

American Speech-Language-Hearing Association. (1992). Strategies for responding to the Medicare resource-based relative value scale (RBRVS). *Asha, 34,* 63–68.

American Speech-Language-Hearing Association. (1993a). Health care reform: ASHA takes action. *Asha, 35,* 23–24.

American Speech-Language-Hearing Association. (1993b). Ad Hoc Committee on National Health Policy. Position statement on national health policy. *Asha, 35* (Suppl. 10), 1.

American Speech-Language-Hearing Association. (1993c). Report of the Task Force on Health Care. *Asha, 35,* 53–54.

American Speech-Language-Hearing Association. (1998). *Assistive Technology Act of 1998*. Rockville, MD: Author.

American Speech-Language-Hearing Association. (1999a). *2005 Medicare fee schedule and hospital outpatient prospective payment system for audiologists*. Rockville, MD: Author.

American Speech-Language-Hearing Association. (1999b). *2005 Medicare fee schedule for speech-language pathologists*. Rockville, MD: Author.

American Speech-Language-Hearing Association. (2005a). *2005 Medicare fee schedule and hospital outpatient prospective payment system for audiologists*. Rockville, MD: Author.

American Speech-Language-Hearing Association. (2005b). *2005 Medicare fee schedule for speech-language pathologists*. Rockville, MD: Author.

American Speech-Language-Hearing Association. (2005c). *2005 public policy agenda*. Rockville, MD: Author.

American Speech-Language-Hearing Association, 2006. Focused Initiative: 2006. http://www.asha.org/about/leadership-projects/national-office/focused-initiative.

Centers for Medicare and Medicaid Services (2001, April 30). Carriers program memorandum, transmittal B–01–34. Subject: *Payment for Services Furnished by Audiologists*. Baltimore, MD: Author.

Ciolek, D. E., & Whang, W. (2004, October 25). *Final project report*. Program Safeguard Contractor (PSC), Outpatient Rehabilitation Services Payment System Evaluation.

Consortium for Citizens with Disabilities. (1992, November). Principles for health care reform from a disability perspective. Washington, DC: Author.

Cornett, B., & Chabon, S. (1986). *Speech-language pathologists: Winners or losers in the health care revolution?* Paper presented at the meeting of the American Speech-Language-Hearing Association, Detroit, MI.

Frattali, C., Curl, B., & Bevan, M. (1994). Health care legislation: Implications for financing and service delivery. In R. Lubinski & C. Frattali (Eds.), *Professional issues in speech-language pathology and audiology* (pp. 173–187). San Diego, CA: Singular Publishing Group.

General Accounting Office. (1999). *Medicare home health agencies—Closures continue with little evidence beneficiary access is impaired*. Washington, DC: Author.

Health Care Financing Administration. (1998). Medicare program: Prospective payment system and consolidated billing for skilled nursing facilities. *Federal Register, 63,* 26252–26316.

Jacobsen, C., & Thompson, M. (2005, March 1). Advocate for fair reimbursement through the STAR network. *ASHA Leader, 2,* 14.

Johnson, P. (2004, February 17). Developing a statewide strategy to improve reimbursement. *ASHA Leader, 2*.

Kaiser Family Foundation and Health Research and Educational Trust. (2005). *Employer health benefits: 2005 summary of findings*. Available at http://www.kff.org/

Kander, M., Lusis, I., & White, S. (2004a). *Medicare handbook for audiologists*. Rockville, MD: American Speech-Language-Hearing Association.

Kander, M., Lusis, I., & White, S. (2004b). *Medicare handbook for speech-language pathologists*. Rockville, MD: American Speech-Language-Hearing Association.

Lubinski, R., & Frattali, C. (1993). Nursing home reform: The resident assessment instrument. *Asha, 35,* 59–62.

Lusis, I. (2005). Apply for your national provider identification number. *ASHA Leader, 10*(14), 3.

Medicare Payment Advisory Commission. (1998, June). *Report to the Congress for a changing Medicare program*. Washington, DC: Author.

McCarty, J., Thompson, M., & White, S. C. (2004). *Appealing health plan denials*. Rockville, MD: American Speech-Language-Hearing Association.

McCarty, J., & White, S. C. (2003). *Health plan coding & claims guide*. Rockville, MD: American Speech-Language-Hearing Association.

Morris, J. N., Hawes, C., Fries, B. E., & Mor, V. (1991). *Resident assessment instrument training manual and resource guide*. Natick, MA: Eliot Press.

National Association of Rehabilitation Facilities. (1990). ProPAC examines excluded facilities. *Medical Rehabilitation Review, 7,* 1–2.

National Health Council. (1993, July). *Congress and health*. New York: National Health Council.

Office of the Federal Register. (1990). *Code of federal regulations.* Washington, DC: U.S. Government Printing Office.

Office of the Federal Register. (1996). *Code of federal regulations.* Washington, DC: U.S. Government Printing Office.

Omnibus Budget and Reconciliation Act, Pub. L. No. 101-508, Section 4005(b)(1) (1990).

Social Security Amendments of 1993, 42 USC §1395x.

U.S. Department of Health and Human Services. (1992, December). *Report of the Secretary's Advisory Panel on the development of uniform needs assessment instrument(s): Report to Congress.* Washington, DC: Health Care Financing Administration.

White, S. (1989, April). Medicare and nursing home services. *Asha, 31,* 75, 59.

White, S. (1990, June/July). EPSDT: A program you should know. *Asha, 32,* 77–78.

White, S. (2002, July 23). HIPAA essentials: College and university clinics prepare for privacy rule. *ASHA Leader, 7,* 12.

Wilkerson, D. L., Batavia, A. J., & DeJong, G. (1992). Use of functional status measures for payment of medical rehabilitation services. *Archives of Physical Medicine and Rehabilitation, 73,* 111–120.

RESOURCES

Alliance for Health Reform
http://www.allhealth.org/

American Medical Association
http://www.ama-assn.org/

American Speech-Language-Hearing Association. Reimbursement pages on the ASHA website:
http://www.asha.org/

Blue Cross and Blue Shield
http://www.bcbs.com/

Health Affairs: The Policy Journal of the Health Sphere
http://www.healthaffairs.org/

Henry J. Kaiser Family Foundation
http://www.kff.org/

International Classification of Diseases (9th and 10th Eds.)
http://www.cdc.gov/nchs/icd9.htm

Medicare and Medicaid on the Centers for Medicare and Medicaid Services Web site:
http://www.cms.hhs.gov/

Medicare therapy pages on the Centers for Medicare and Medicaid Services Web site:
http://new.cms.hhs.gov/TherapyServices/01_overview.asp

News about private health plans from the industry's perspective:
http://www.ahip.org/

Common Health Care

Acronyms and Abbreviations

CMS: Centers for Medicare and Medicaid Services. The federal agency that administers the Medicare and the Medicaid programs' aspects not regulated by the states. CMS was previously known as the Health Care Financing Administration (HCFA).

CORF: Comprehensive Outpatient Rehabilitation Facility. A Medicare provider type that includes coverage for a number of outpatient rehabilitation services, including speech-language pathology, occupational therapy, physical therapy, psychology, and medicine.

CPT: Common Procedural Terminology. A listing of codes and corresponding medical procedures published and maintained by the American Medical Association and used by third-party payers for establishing reimbursement rates.

HCPCS: Healthcare Common Procedural Coding System. The federal government's listing of procedures that incorporates the CPT codes at level one, codes for devices and durable medical equipment and some procedures used by Medicare and Medicaid not found in the CPT list at level two.

HIPAA: Health Insurance Portability and Accountability Act. A statute that established requirements for employee mobility without loss of insurance coverage and uniform standards for patient privacy, especially via electronic communications.

HMO: Health Maintenance Organization: A prepaid health plan that includes wellness services; enrollees are required to see a closed panel of providers.

ICD-9-CM: International Classification of Diseases, Ninth Edition, Clinical Modification. A comprehensive list and corresponding codes for diseases and disorders. HCFA and other payers use these codes for identifying the need for medical procedures.

MPFS: Medicare Physician Fee Schedule. The listing of reimbursement rates by procedural codes for Medicare services billed by physicians and other practitioners. The MPFS was extended to institutional providers for speech-language pathology, occupational therapy, and physical therapy services only.

MedPAC: Medicare Payment Advisory Commission. A deliberative body comprised of appointed experts in Medicare reimbursement and government staff that researches and advises Congress on payment policies and their effect on the budget and patient care.

PPO: Preferred Provider Organization: A health plan that allows enrollees to see providers out-of-network but with higher cost sharing responsibilities.

PPS: Prospective Payment System. The federal government's system for determining reimbursement rates based on previous charges and costs rather than current and individual provider charges or costs.

RBRVS: Resource-Based Relative Value Scale. The method for determining payment rates for outpatient medical procedures by comparing the value of procedures with the value of a common procedure. The MPFS uses the RBRVS.

SNF: Skilled Nursing Facility. A Medicare-certified nursing facility that meets the conditions of participation developed by HCFA and is reimbursed by Medicare using a PPS. For example, a SNF uses a required patient health and disability screening tool (the Minimum Data Set, MDS) to determine the services required for each patient. The results of the MDS are a major factor in determining the per diem rate that Medicare will pay.

13

Service Delivery
in Health Care Settings

BECKY SUTHERLAND CORNETT, PHD

SCOPE OF CHAPTER

The work of audiologists and speech-language pathologists in health care settings is quite diverse and is determined by the mission and goals of specific organizations or programs. According to the membership statistics section of the American Speech-Language-Hearing Association's Web site, 35.6 percent of speech-language pathologists and 72 percent of audiologists work in health care settings. These settings include acute-care hospitals, skilled nursing facilities, rehabilitation hospitals, specialty hospitals (e.g., psychiatric, pediatric, cancer, eye and ear centers), home care agencies, hospices, transitional living facilities, and numerous hospital-based and community outpatient programs. Individuals in private practice also may specialize in providing health care services.

The roles of speech-language pathologists (SLPs) and audiologists across these numerous settings are defined by requirements and practices of specific work settings. For example, one SLP may specialize in the evaluation and treatment of swallowing disorders, leading a dysphagia team in a large urban teaching hospital. Another SLP in the same facility may evaluate and treat persons who need augmentative or alternative communication (AAC) systems. Still another staff member may be the community integration specialist for the brain injury (BI) team. Other practitioners in smaller hospitals or clinics may be generalists responsible for treating persons of all ages who have a variety of communication and related disorders. Table 13–1 outlines the clinical roles of speech-language pathologists in health care settings.

T A B L E 13–1 Clinical Roles of Speech-Language Pathologists in Health Care Settings

1. Assessment and treatment of
   - Dysphagia and other disorders of oral-pharyngeal function
   - Aphasia
   - Dysarthria
   - Apraxia
   - Right-hemisphere dysfunction
   - Cognitive-communicative disorders associated with brain injuries or dementias
   - Organic and nonorganic vocal pathologies
   - Fluency disorders
   - Speech, language, and swallowing disorders associated with cleft palate or other oral and oropharyngeal anomalies

2. Providing preoperative counseling, postsurgical evaluation and selection of communication methods, and rehabilitation for persons who have undergone oral, velopharyngeal, or laryngeal surgery

3. Specialized collaborative roles with medical and other health care staff in emergency departments, operative suites, and intensive care units in functions such as brain and language mapping, assessment of hyperacute stroke, and management of ventilator-dependent patients

4. Use of high-technology modes of service delivery such as telehealth/telemedicine, virtual reality software, and other computer-based assessment and treatment options

5. Participation in the evaluation, selection, and use of voice prostheses ("talking trach" tubes, one-way speaking valves) in persons with a tracheostomy

6. Participation in health care continuum strategies (e.g., prevention, disease management, and demand management)

7. Counseling patients, families, and caregivers regarding communication and swallowing assessment and treatment, progress, prognosis, facilitating techniques, coping, and adjustment strategies

8. Consultation with other professionals and agencies regarding patient management issues

Audiologists who work in health care settings also have varied roles. The audiologist who works in the hospital newborn nursery and neonatal intensive care unit (NICU) identifies and provides early intervention for infants who are at risk for communication disorders resulting from hearing impairments. Another audiologist may conduct comprehensive audiologic assessment and special tests, whereas another colleague may specialize in hearing aid and assistive device assessments, selection, dispensing, fitting, and orientation. Examples of the clinical roles of audiologists are presented in Table 13–2.

This chapter discusses trends and issues that impact the practice of audiology and speech-language pathology in health care settings. It focuses on major

T A B L E 13–2 Clinical Roles of Audiologists in Health Care Settings

1. Evaluation and diagnosis of peripheral and central auditory nervous system dysfunctions. Examples of high-technology evaluations include use of ABR, ENG, transient evoked otoacoustic emissions, and power reflectance

2. Hearing aid and assistive device or system assessment, selection, dispensing, fitting, orientation, and monitoring

3. Assessment and monitoring of the vestibular system

4. Aural rehabilitation assessment and provision of aural rehabilitation services

5. Collaborative roles with medical staff, including tests or procedures to assist in medical diagnosis and monitoring (e.g., neurophysiologic intraoperative monitoring, high-frequency ototoxicity tests, identification of vascular compression)

6. Audiologic assessment of central auditory processing

7. Participation in cochlear implant assessment, selection, placement, orientation, and follow-up

8. Participation in telehealth/telemedicine modes of service delivery

9. Participation in health care continuum strategies (e.g., prevention, disease management, and demand management)

10. Counseling patients, families, and caregivers regarding auditory and vestibular system assessment, treatment, progress, prognosis, facilitating techniques, and coping and adjustment strategies

11. Consultation with other professionals and agencies regarding patient management issues related to auditory and vestibular system functions and disorders and communication interactions and environments

health care initiatives, regulations, and administrative requirements as well as activities of everyday life such as making decisions about service delivery and documenting patient care.

CLINICAL PRACTICE IN CONTEXT: THE BUSINESS OF HEALTH CARE

In the previous edition of this text, we discussed the impact of "fiscal turmoil" in health care. It was a time of hospital budget reductions, layoffs, reengineering, restructuring, consolidation, managed care, and a focus on multiskilled practitioners who could assume additional responsibilities to achieve high productivity targets. Unfortunately, despite all the changes, health care costs continue to rise; hospital systems have been involved in some of the most publicized corporate scandals, and landmark reports on medical errors and health care quality have revealed alarming failures across the country. Consequently, the health care industry is moving back to basics. We are focusing on basic elements of the health care infrastructure: patient safety, improving clinical and service quality, documenting the results of care; evaluating and upgrading accreditation programs; regulatory compliance; and scrutiny of business and clinical ethics. Not long ago, clinicians could leave tasks such as Joint Commission on Accreditation of Health Care Organziations (JCAHO) accreditation survey preparation, development of organizational business strategies, analysis of quality indicators and outcome measurements, and scrutiny of the costs of providing services to departmental managers and organizational administrators. Today, clinicians must be thoroughly familiar with all aspects of the health care infrastructure. Each employee is responsible for managing his or her services within the context of the larger organization's goals, objectives, and business practices.

In 2003, an ASHA committee developed the policy statement "Knowledge and Skills in Business Practices Needed by Speech-Language Pathologists in Health Care Settings." This document provides detailed guidance to clinicians in understanding the business practice mechanisms underlying service delivery in health care: "Clinicians must understand their individual responsibility for adhering to practice standards that financially support their organization" (p. 87). The following roles are outlined:

Role 1: Provide appropriate services that meet the business needs of the organization.

Role 2: Ensure compliance and professional practice.

Role 3: Achieve quality outcomes and performance improvement.

Role 4: Provide advocacy.

Role 5: Promote and market professional services.

Role 6: Use technology.

Role 7: Obtain payment for services.

Much of this chapter presents information that supports the roles emphasized in the ASHA policy statement. Readers are also referred to Golper and Brown (2005) for additional information about business practices. Table 13–3 outlines the clinician's roles in the business of health care.

The following sections provide detailed information about health care accreditation; regulatory

T A B L E 13–3 The Clinician's Roles in the Business of Health Care

1. Participate in a range of outcomes measurement and management activities:
   - Measures of function, activity, and participation
   - Measures of health status
   - Health-related quality of life (HRQL) assessments
   - Customer satisfaction and patient experience of care surveys (patient/payer/referral sources)
   - Development and use of clinical guidelines, pathways, and protocols
   - Development and implementation of outcome-oriented models of patient care
   - Integration of clinical, functional, financial, administrative, social, and customer satisfaction outcome data

(Continued)

T A B L E 13-3 (Continued)

2. Develop, implement, and monitor clinical and service quality indicators:
   - Efficiency, effectiveness, appropriateness, timeliness, continuity, accessibility of patient care

3. Meet departmental and organizational targets for units of service, productivity, and cost per unit of service.

4. Assist in developing and implementing clinical competency programs.

5. Serve in case management and discharge planning roles as part of the treatment team.

6. Participate in clinical, outcomes, and evaluation research activities.

7. Participate in accreditation, regulatory compliance, and ethics activities:
   - Conditions of participation—CMS requirements for clinical services
   - Clinical documentation and record-keeping
   - Management of information
   - Coding, billing, and payment
   - Risk assessment and risk management
   - JCAHO & CARF
   - Professional licensure and certification
   - ASHA Code of Ethics and organizational codes of conduct
   - Patient safety Environmental and medical waste disposal
   - Emergency, disaster preparedness, and life safety
   - Human resources laws and regulations

8. Participate in and/or lead diagnostic and treatment teams.

9. Serve on organizational and departmental task forces, teams, and committees.

10. Supervise support personnel, clinical practicum students, clinical fellows.

11. Provide and participate in formal and informal continuing education and staff development activities for professional and support personnel.

compliance; patient safety and quality improvement; federal regulations pertaining to the use and disclosure of health care information (HIPAA); clinical accountability; and clinical documentation, coding systems, and billing for patient care services.

HEALTH CARE ACCREDITATION

Health care accreditation has always been a major concern of health professionals because the traditional process of preparing for site surveys has created considerable organizational and individual stress. However, government reports that questioned the value of accreditation in ensuring safe and effective patient care created a new, different set of concerns for the health care community. Now, the accreditation process focuses much less on written material, management meetings, and other structural issues and much more on actual patient care and what staff members actually do every day. Moreover, accreditation has become closely tied to compliance. This section addresses the activities of two major accrediting entities—JCAHO and CARF.

Joint Commission on Accreditation of Health Care Organizations (JCAHO)

Accreditation of health care organizations is the corollary to certification of health care professionals. JCAHO evaluates and accredits more than 15,000 health care organizations and programs in the United States. The mission of this independent, nonprofit organization is "to continuously improve the safety and quality of care provided to the public through the provision of health care accreditation and related services that support performance improvement in health care organizations." Accreditation services are provided for acute-care, rehabilitation, psychiatric, and children's hospitals; health care networks; home care organizations; skilled nursing and other long-term care facilities; behavioral health organizations; ambulatory care providers; and clinical laboratories. Disease-specific certification (DSC) is also awarded to hospitals, health plans, and other companies that provide disease management and chronic care services such as primary stroke care, congestive heart failure, coronary artery disease, and skin/wound management. Certification is available for other specific programs, including health care staffing services, lung volume reduction surgery (LVRS), and Left-Ventricular Assist Device (LVAD) services (JCAHO, 2005).

The JCAHO accreditation process has changed dramatically over the last decade, evolving from an emphasis on policies and procedures to evaluating patients' actual experience of care, focusing on safety, clinical quality, and service issues. Implemented in 2004, the new survey process, *Shared Visions, New Pathways,* promotes the practice of Continuous Survey Readiness (CSR) instead of "ramping up" for triennial surveys that were scheduled well in advance. By maintaining continuous compliance with the standards, organizations can use the standards as a management tool for doing business—that is, improving all aspects of patient care. Unannounced surveys also help to support the credibility of the survey process by increasing the likelihood that the survey is an accurate picture of what is happening under everyday circumstances, not just when the facility has been scrubbed and staff members have been rehearsed.

JCAHO measures an organization's level of performance according to standards that address priority focus areas such as patient care team communication, patient rights and ethics, quality improvement, physical environment, medication management, and information management.

According to JCAHO, the *priority focus process* (PFP) helps focus survey activity on issues most relevant to patient safety and quality of care at the specific health care organization being surveyed. Using automation, presurvey data are gathered from multiple sources (JCAHO, the health care organization itself, and public sources). Rules logic is applied to identify areas of priority focus for the organization and to facilitate surveyor selection of "tracers." *Tracer methodology* is the primary way that JCAHO surveyors now assess an organization's compliance with standards.

There are two types of tracers: *patient care tracers* and *patient system tracers.* During the site visit, surveyors select patients and "follow" their actual care experiences. The medical record is used as the roadmap to move through the organization's services, processes, and systems. Interviews and observations are used to supplement document reviews (which can include personnel records, specific policies, marketing, and educational materials, etc.). Patient system tracers assess the organization's overall systems by focusing on high-risk processes: data use, infection control, and medication management (note: other system tracers may be added in the future).

JCAHO is also a leader in establishing patient safety standards and ongoing monitoring activities. National Patient Safety Goals (NPSG) are published annually. JCAHO has also instituted the International Center for Patient Safety (in partnership with the World Health Organization). Readers are referred to the section in this chapter on patient safety and quality improvement for additional information.

CARF: The Rehabilitation Accreditation Commission

CARF is an international nonprofit entity that offers accreditation to human services organizations in the following areas: aging services. behavioral health, child and youth services, employment and community services, medical rehabilitation, and opioid (narcotics) treatment. Accreditation surveys are conducted using a consultative approach to standards conformance and focus on quality and service to persons served. Standards are consumer focused and are developed with the involvement of representatives of service areas participating in the survey process. CARF emphasizes that programs must actively involve consumers in selecting, planning, and using services (CARF, 2005).

Medical rehabilitation accreditation is offered for a wide variety of program types. Some of the accreditation options are: comprehensive integrated inpatient rehabilitation, spinal cord system of care, four types of brain injury settings, outpatient medical rehabilitation, and medical rehabilitation case management.

A closer look at CARF's Web site description of the Comprehensive Integrated Inpatient Rehabilitation. Program (CIIRP) provides insight about the commission's goals for medical rehabilitation programs:

> CIIRP is a program of coordinated and integrated medical and rehabilitation services that is provided 24 hours per day and endorses the active participation and choice of the persons served throughout the entire program. The

persons served, in collaboration with the inter-disciplinary team members, identify and address their medical and rehabilitation needs. The individual needs of the persons served drive the appropriate use of the rehabilitation con-tinuum of care, the establishment of predicted outcomes, the provision of care, the composi-tion of the interdisciplinary team, and discharge to the community of choice. An integrated interdisciplinary team approach is reflected throughout all activities.

CARF introduced standards for Stroke Specialty Programs in July 2005 and began accrediting stroke programs in January 2006. Note: JCAHO also offers a specialized stroke care accreditation program.

CARF's Strategic Outcomes Initiative (as part of the Quality and Accountability Initiative) focuses on outcomes research and continuous quality improvement goals in accredited programs and the larger rehabilitation field. The Research and Quality Improvement Division develops outcomes mea-surement and management data and strategies throughout the rehabilitation services field. These goals, like JCAHO's National Patient Safety Goals and those of the International Center for Patient Safety, have moved these accrediting organizations from standards-setting and "inspection" groups to the forefront of overall quality improvement efforts in the larger public health arena.

HEALTH CARE COMPLIANCE PROGRAMS

The federal government's initiative to combat fraud and abuse in health care has become a strong influ-ence on the way hospitals and other health care organizations conduct daily business. Operation Restore Trust was a 2-year project of the Department of Justice and the Office of the Inspector General (OIG) of the U.S. Department of Health and Human Services that targeted the billing practices of home health agencies (HHA), skilled nursing facilities (SNF), hospices, and durable medical equipment (DME) suppliers. The result of that investigation

yielded significant funds returned to the Medicare program in refunds of claims, penalties, and damages. Subsequently, Congress enacted the Health Insur-ance Portability and Accountability Act of 1996 (HIPAA) and the Balanced Budget Act of 1997 (BBA), both of which increased funding for fraud and abuse investigations. The United States Depart-ment of Justice has prosecuted health care organiza-tions under the False Claims Act (FCA), most recently for substandard quality of care. Hence, health care organizations have established corporate compliance programs to promote prevention, detec-tion, and resolution of instances of conduct that do not conform to federal and state law, health care pro-gram requirements of public and private payers, and the organization's ethical and business policies.

A compliance plan defines and describes how the health care organization conducts its business. Laws, regulations, ethical principles, and practice standards provide an infrastructure for clinical prac-tice. The primary categories of compliance activities in health care institutions include:

- Coding, billing, and reimbursement laws and regulations
- Human resources laws and regulations
- Tax and contract laws
- Patient care standards and policies (e.g., informed consent, advance directives, use of restraints)
- Environmental laws and regulations (e.g., infec-tion control, medical waste, radioactive waste)
- Research grants administration (e.g., human subjects review, data management, experimental drugs regulations)
- Ethical standards and codes of conduct

The Department of Health and Human Services Office of the Inspector General's (OIG) recommen-dations for seven elements of a hospital compliance plan are:

1. Written standards of conduct for all employees
2. Development and dissemination of written policies and procedures that promote the organization's commitment to compliance
3. Designation of a chief compliance officer

4. Education and training for all employees regarding legal, regulatory, and ethical issues in health care

5. Auditing and monitoring of billing and other records to detect and resolve identified problems

6. Internal investigation and remediation of systematic and personnel issues

7. Open communication between management and employees about all work practices

Health care compliance programs reduce or prevent risk of civil or criminal liability by ensuring that health professionals and administrators adhere to standards for conducting the business or delivering health care services. Practitioners such as audiologists and speech-language pathologists who provide billable clinical services must do so in accordance with all applicable licensure laws, regulations, and professional standards of care. Practitioners who are ASHA members must also abide by its Code of Ethics. Practitioners must verify competencies to perform procedures according to organizational policies and procedures.

The Centers for Medicare and Medicaid Services (CMS) stipulate Conditions of Participation (CoP) for health care providers and suppliers who participate in the Medicare and Medicaid programs. In addition, specific rules and instructions for providing services are published in Medicare manuals. Information about speech-language pathology services is found in the *Medicare Benefit Policy Manual, Medicare Claims Processing Manual, Medicare State Operations Manual* (survey and certification instructions for inspectors), and intermediary and carrier Local Coverage Determinations (LCD). CMS specifies that speech-language pathology services must be "reasonable and necessary" to the treatment of an individual's illness or injury. Services must be considered under accepted standards of practice to be an effective treatment, and professionals must demonstrate that the services are complex and sophisticated, such that only the qualified speech-language pathologist could safely and effectively perform (or supervise) the service. "Significant, practical improvement" in the patient's condition must be expected within a reasonable period of time. These requirements are specified in the regulations,

and also reflect the federal government's current interest in incorporating quality issues such as appropriateness of care, utilization of resources, and practice standards as compliance issues. Table 13–4 describes basic tenets of compliance related to revenue management, documentation, and billing.

ASHA has long provided guidance to practitioners through programs and publications that address legal, regulatory, and ethical issues. The document "Professional Liability and Risk Management for the Audiology and Speech-Language Pathology Professions" (ASHA, 1994), although over a decade old, is still particularly helpful in delineating ethical practices and risk management strategies. ASHA's "Issues in Ethics" series addresses concerns such as "Conflicts of Professional Interest," "Ethics in Research and Professional Practice," and "Representation of Services for Insurance Reimbursement or Funding." Readers are referred to the ASHA Web site's Online Desk Reference for information on these and other ethical practices issues.

HIPAA—Protecting Confidential Health Information

Health professionals have long been aware of the need to keep information about patients confidential. However, with the advent of electronic health records and databases, a number of intentional and unintentional breaches of health information occurred throughout the country. Consequently, Congress passed the Health Insurance Portability and Accountability Act of 1996 (HIPAA). HIPAA includes three areas of law: insurance portability, antifraud enforcement in public health plans (accountability), and administrative simplification provisions to: protect the confidentiality of health information (PHI), establish standard health care transactions and codes sets, and require health information security safeguards. Although the law was passed in 1996, proposed regulations were not written for the health information provisions until 1999. The compliance dates for these provisions were: April 2003 for the Standards for Privacy of Individually Identifiable Health Information (the Privacy Rule); October 2003 for standard

T A B L E 13–4 Responsibilities of Clinical Staff for Revenue Management and Compliance

Non-physician health professionals must provide billable clinical services in accordance with applicable licensure laws, professional standards of care, and codes of ethics promulgated by professional associations. Clinical staff members must verify their competency to perform services and procedures in compliance with employer competency assessment policies and procedures as well as competency testing requirements established by individual clinical departments or programs. Practitioner eligibility to participate in federally sponsored health care programs must be verified through query of the federal List of Excluded Individuals and Entities (LEIE).

1. Practitioners must also meet other requirements specified by public and private payers regarding:
   - Obtaining physician orders for services and procedures (when required)
   - Establishing medical necessity for services and procedures
   - Documenting physician approval and any required certification and recertification of care plans and services
   - Documenting necessity for skilled levels of care requiring the services of licensed/certified professionals

2. Practitioners must use appropriate diagnosis codes (as directed by the physician, when applicable):
   - Use of correct procedure codes
   - Inclusion of all applicable elements in clinical documentation, at a minimum:
     dates and times of services provided
     types and duration of services provided
     results of services or procedures completed
     identification and signature of professional who provided the service

3. Practitioners must charge only for those services or procedures actually completed.

4. Practitioners should verify, with appropriate signatures, that they either actually performed, or supervised the billable service.

5. Services or procedures performed must match the charge codes (procedure codes) selected by the practitioner for billing. Practitioners should refer to charge descriptions established by clinical departments to match services/-procedures with appropriate charge codes in the hospital's Charge Description Master (CDM) or clinic's master list of charges.

6. Clinical documentation must support charges billed. Services must be documented accurately and completely in the medical or clinical record. Each clinical department must establish documentation guidelines and reporting formats that are consistent with accepted professional standards. Only those claims (bills for services) supported by complete documentation are eligible for payment.

transactions and code sets; and April 2005 for the Security Rule. This chapter section focuses on the privacy rule, although a brief overview of the other provisions is also included.

The Privacy Rule The privacy rule is the first set of standards established by the federal government for the protection of health information. The five basic principles of the rule are:

- Consumer control—patients have new rights to control the release of their medical information.

- *Boundaries*—a patient's health information should be used primarily for health purposes; any other uses must be kept to the minimum

necessary for a specific purpose (e.g., application for life insurance).

- Accountability—specific federal penalties for violating the privacy regulations range from a $100 fine per violation for disclosures made in error, up to $25,000 and 10 years in prison for malicious use of records.

- Public responsibility—specific information is provided about releasing health information for public health, research, fraud and abuse investigations, and quality improvement purposes.

- Security—health care organizations must establish clear procedures to safeguard health information.

The Privacy Rule includes all forms of individually identifiable health information (electronic, written, oral) and applies to the following "covered entities": all health plans, health care clearinghouses, and health providers that conduct financial or other administrative functions electronically. The standards under HIPAA assure that patients have specific rights regarding the use and disclosure of protected health information (PHI). Patients have the right to:

Receive a copy of a covered entity's *Notice of Privacy Practices* **(NPP).** Under HIPAA, a covered entity must provide a patient with a copy of its NPP. The NPP informs the patient of his or her rights with regard to protected health information, gives adequate notice of the uses and disclosures of the individual's PHI a covered entity may make, and informs the patient of the covered entity's legal duties to protect PHI. The NPP must be posted in a prominent area, and a copy offered to each individual. If the organization maintains a Web site, the NPP must be posted electronically. Persons who receive the NPP electronically may request a hard copy. Any member of the public may ask for a copy of the organization's *Notice of Privacy Practices.*

Request restrictions on certain uses and disclosures of PHI. A health care provider must permit an individual to request restrictions on the uses or disclosures of the individual's PHI. The provider is not required to agree to a restriction. However, if the provider agrees, the restriction must be documented and honored, unless the individual rescinds the restriction or an emergency situation warrants waiving the restriction.

Receive communication of PHI at an alternate address or telephone number or in a more private manner ("confidential communications"). A health provider must permit and accommodate reasonable requests by individuals to receive communications of PHI by alternate means. A provider may require that the individual submit a written request.

Inspect and copy his/her own PHI. An individual has the right to inspect and obtain a copy of health information contained in a designated record set. A designated record set is broader than a medical record. The set includes the medical record, billing records, or groups of records that are used by or for the provider or health plan to make decisions about the individual.

Amend the individual's own PHI. An individual has the right to request that a health care provider amend his or her health information or medical record. However, a provider may deny the request for amendment if the record: was not created by the provider, is not part of the designated record set, would not be available for inspection, or is accurate and complete.

Receive an accounting of disclosures of PHI. An individual has the right to receive an accounting (list or log) of certain disclosures of PHI made by the provider for the lesser of either six years prior to the request date or April 14, 2003. The accounting must include: date of the disclosure, name and address (if known) of the person or organization who received the PHI; a brief description of the PHI disclosed; and a brief statement of the purpose of the disclosure that reasonably informs the individual about the basis for the disclosure, or a copy of the actual written request.

File a complaint with the health care provider if the individual feels his/her privacy rights have been violated. In the *Notice of Privacy Practices,* a covered entity must inform an individual about his or her right to file a complaint if the individual feels the covered entity has violated his or her rights or wishes to complain about the organization's privacy policies and procedures. A covered entity may not retaliate against or intimidate an individual for making a complaint. (DHHS, 2003).

The Privacy Rule also contains numerous administrative requirements. Health care organizations must:

- Designate a privacy officer to oversee all activities related to HIPAA implementation and compliance.

- Issue a *Notice of Privacy Practices* to inform patients about how the organization uses and discloses PHI, and make a "good faith effort" to obtain a signed acknowledgement that the patient has received the notice.

- Establish policies and procedures for securing the patient's written authorization to use or disclose a patient's health information for purposes other than treatment, payment, and health care operations, except as permitted by law.

- Develop or revise policies and procedures for ensuring patients' rights under HIPAA.

- Determine what PHI is the "minimum necessary" an employee needs (other than clinicians) to do his or her job (e.g., health care billers, registrars, quality department personnel).

- Revise contracts to include language that assures confidentiality and safeguarding of PHI by business associates (such as third party administrators or information technology vendors) who use and disclose patient information.

- Follow the regulations established for using and disclosing individually identifiable health information for research purposes.

- Establish procedures for ensuring that fund-raising personnel learn only patients' demographic information and dates of service, and that patients can "opt out" or decline to receive fund-raising communications or materials.

Be sure that no marketing materials are sent to patients without first securing a patient's signed authorization (marketing does not include hospital newsletters or other communications regarding a hospital's or clinic's own health-related services or products). Develop a procedure for addressing patient complaints about how organizations use and disclose PHI.

The principal messages regarding the privacy rule for clinicians are:

- Understand patient rights to PHI.

- Safeguard clinical records (use physical and technical controls).

- Provide private areas or take precautions to ensure privacy when discussing matters with or about patients.

- Follow established procedures for disclosing patient information.

- Dispose of records by shredding or using locked bins for later shredding and recycling.

- Take special care when photocopying, printing, and faxing patient information (e.g., don't "mix up" patient information with business records, verify fax numbers).

Table 13–5 lists and defines key terms related to the HIPAA privacy rule.

Electronic Transactions and Code Sets Rule
The electronic data interchange (EDI) provision of HIPAA is intended to improve the efficiency and effectiveness of the health care system by adopting standards for electronic exchange of administrative and financial information in order to eliminate redundant tasks, lower administrative costs associated with paper-based transactions, streamline the flow of information, and improve data quality. Covered entities must conduct certain transactions in a standard format. The transactions covered by the rule include: health care claims, payment and remittance advice, coordination of benefits, claim status request and health plan response, enrollment or disenrollment in a health plan, eligibility for a health plan, health plan premium payments, referral certification and authorization, and first report of injury for state workers' compensation programs. CMS required all providers who file claims electronically to be HIPAA-compliant by October 1, 2005.

Standard code sets are also required to report medical data. Code sets are values used in data fields to identify conditions, procedures, and entities. The following code sets are required to meet HIPAA standards:

International Classification of Diseases, 9th edition, Clinical Modification (ICD-9-CM), Volumes 1 and 2, including the *ICD-9-CM Official Guidelines for Coding and Reporting* for the following conditions: diseases, injuries, impairments, other health-related problems and their manifestations, and causes of injury, disease, impairment, or other health-related problems. The ICD-*9* is updated and distributed by the U.S. Department of Health and Human Services.

T A B L E 13–5 HIPAA Privacy Rule Glossary

Covered entity–a health plan, health care clearinghouse, or health care provider that transmits any health information in electronic form in connection with a standard financial or administrative transaction listed in Section 1173(a)(1) of the act and Section 160.103 of the final rule.

Designated record set–a group of records maintained by or for a covered entity, including the medical records and billing records about individuals maintained by or for a covered health care provider; the enrollment, payment, claims adjudication, and case or medical management record systems maintained by or for a health plan; or data used, in whole or in part, by or for the covered entity to make decisions about individuals.

Disclosure–release, transfer, provision of access to, or divulging in any other manner of information outside the entity holding the information.

Health information–any information, whether oral or recorded in any form or medium, that is created or received by a health care provider, health plan, public health authority, employer, life insurer, school or university, or health care clearinghouse, that relates to the past, present, or future physical or mental health or condition of an individual, the provision of health care to the individual, or the past, present, or future payment for the provision of health care to the individual.

Individually identifiable health information–a subset of health information, including demographic information collected from an individual, that is created or received by a health care provider, health plan, employer, or health care clearinghouse and that relates to the past, present, or future physical or mental health or condition of an individual; the provision of health care to an individual; or the past, present, or future payment for the provision of health care to an individual. There must be a reasonable basis to believe the information can be used to identify the individual.

Protected health information–individually identifiable health information that is transmitted by electronic media; maintained in any medium described in the definition of electronic media; or transmitted or maintained in any other form or medium. Protected health information excludes individually identifiable health information in education records covered by the Family Educational Right and Privacy Act, as amended, 20 U.S.C. 1232g, and Records described at 20 U.S.C. 1232g(a)(4)(B)(iv).

Use–with respect to individually identifiable health information, the sharing, employment, application, examination, or analysis of such information within an entity that maintains such information.

ICD-9-CM Volume 3-Procedures, for procedures or other actions taken for diseases, injuries, and impairments on *hospital inpatients* reported by hospitals related to prevention, diagnosis, treatment, and management. It is anticipated that the ICD-10-PCS will replace the ICD-9 within several years. The November 2003 final draft of the *ICD-10-PCS Coding System and Training Manual* is available at the CMS Web site (http://www.cms.hhs.gov).

Health Care Common Procedure Coding System (HCPCS) contains Level II alphanumeric procedure and modifier codes. These codes are established by the CMS Alphanumeric Editorial Panel and primarily represent items, supplies, and nonphysician services not covered by the American Medical Association's *Current Procedural Terminology* (CPT-4) codes. CPT codes must be purchased from the American Medical Association and are published annually.

The HIPAA Security Rule The Security Rule applies only to *electronic* health information. It requires covered entities to ensure the confidentiality, integrity, and availability of all electronic protected health information (EPHI); to protect against reasonably anticipated threats or hazards to the security or integrity of EPHI; and to prohibit uses and disclosures not permitted or required under the privacy rule. Policies, procedures, and physical and technical safeguards must be established. Examples of policies and procedures include risk analysis, security incident response, data backup and disaster recovery plan, and contingency plans. Physical safeguards refer to facility access, validation procedures, and standards for devices and media controls. Technical safeguards ensure access control on systems that maintain EPHI, security of EPHI transmissions, audit controls, and authentication procedures.

Standard Identifiers Four categories of standard identifiers have been developed to streamline business transactions associated with delivery and payment of health care services:

- National Employer Identifier (NEI)—the Employer Identification Number (EIN) assigned to employers by the Internal Revenue Service (IRS) will be used as the national identifier. Compliance date was July 30, 2004.

- National Health Plan Identifier (PlanID)—the PlanID is issued to each health plan (insured and self-funded group plans, and third-party administrators) and payer. The instructions for applying for PlanID were developed in 2005.

- National Provider Identifier (NPI)—the NPI is a unique 10-digit identifier issued to all health care providers (individuals and organizations), replacing all other identifiers. The official application Web site is: https://nppes.cms.hhs.gov. Compliance date is May 2007.

- Personal Health Identifier—this number would replace the Social Security number for health purposes. Action on this provision has been postponed indefinitely.

The Office of Civil Rights (OCR) in the U.S. Department of Health and Human Services is the HIPAA oversight agency, and its Web site is the official source of information about HIPAA. Readers are also referred to Horner's and Wheeler's article "HIPAA: Impact on Clinical Practice," (2005) and the ASHA Web site for additional information.

PATIENT SAFETY AND QUALITY IMPROVEMENT

Our health care system has received a good deal of bad publicity over the past few years in both the popular and academic press: health care costs too much, hospitals are inefficient, outcomes are often questionable, fraud and abuse associated with government health programs abound, access to care depends upon insurance status, a growing number of persons are uninsured or under-insured, and nonprofit hospitals offer too little charity care. In fact, Dr. Lucian Leape of the Harvard School of Public Health says, "The American health care system is quietly imploding, and it's about time we did something about it" (Stein, 2005, p. 1). This section describes two basic components needed for an effective health care system—patient safety and quality improvement practices.

Patient Safety Initiatives

Patient safety issues have become the foremost concern of health care professionals and organizations across the country since the Institute of Medicine (IOM) published the landmark report *To Err Is Human: Building a Safer Health Care System* (1999). That report was critical of the American health care system, contending that more patients die annually from medical errors and omissions than from motor vehicle accidents, breast cancer, or AIDS. The IOM set a goal of a 50 percent reduction in preventable medical errors within 5 years. Subsequently, both the IOM and the Agency for Health Care Research and Quality (AHRQ) published a series of reports that further defined and described the less-than-optimal state of health care in America. Most notable of these reports was *Crossing the Quality Chasm: A New Health System for the 21st Century* (IOM, 2001). The word *chasm* was used in the report to describe the wide gap between the health care we have versus the health care we could have by establishing a culture of safety across the continuum of care. Six "Aims for Improvement of Health Care Quality" were designated, upon which future safety and quality efforts should be based. The IOM proposed as goals that health care should be:

- **Safe**—avoiding injuries to patients from the care that is intended to help them.

- **Effective**—providing services based on scientific knowledge.

- **Patient-centered**—providing care that is responsive to individual patient preferences, needs, and values and assuring that patient values guide all clinical decisions.

- **Timely**—reducing waits and sometimes harmful delays for those who receive care and those who give care.

- **Efficient**—avoiding waste, including waste of equipment, supplies, ideas, and energy.
- **Equitable**—providing care that does not vary in quality because of personal characteristics such as gender, ethnicity, geographic location, or socioeconomic status.

Concurrently, the Leapfrog Group, a coalition of more than 170 employer-companies, and other organizations who purchase health care plans and services for groups of people developed a set of Leapfrog Safety Practices designed to reduce preventable medical mistakes and improve the quality and affordability of health care; reward physicians and hospitals for instituting safe, effective, and efficient care; and encourage public reporting of quality indicators to help employers, insurers, and consumers to make informed choices about their health care providers. The Leapfrog Safety Practices include: computer physician-order entry; evidence-based hospital referral in which hospitals must meet certain outcome, process, and volume criteria for high-risk surgeries such as coronary artery by pass graft (CABG), abdominal aortic aneurysm repair, and pancreatic resection; intensive care units staffed with specialists in critical care medicine (inten-sivists); and adoption of the National Quality Forum's (2003) *Safe Practices for Better Health Care*. These 30 practices include the three Leapfrog Group standards and 27 other consensus-based practices that have formed the basis for the CMS publicly reported quality measures (which are also the JCAHO's Core Measures) and JCAHO's National Patient Safety Goals.

The JCAHO publishes on its Web site National Patient Safety Goals (NPSG) annually, with subcat-egories and periodic updates, for hospitals and eight other provider types. The 2006 NPSGs for hospitals are:

- Improve the accuracy of patient identification (health professionals must establish the patient's identity prior to providing treatment by using two patient identifiers).
- Improve the effectiveness of communication among caregivers (subgoals include "read-back" of verbal orders and use of approved abbreviations).

- Improve the safety of using medications.
- Reduce the risk of infections associated with health care.
- Accurately and completely reconcile medica-tions across the continuum of care.
- Reduce the risk of patient harm resulting from falls.

JCAHO has also established the International Center for Patient Safety and is developing a set of international patient safety goals.

The Agency for Health Care Research & Quality (AHRQ) is another major player in the pa-tient safety and quality arena. AHRQ is an agency of the U.S. Department of Health and Human Ser-vices whose mission is to improve the quality, safety, efficiency, and effectiveness of health care for all Americans. This research-oriented agency pub-lishes a wide variety of reports, data, and informa-tion for researchers, health care providers, and con-sumers on quality and safety issues. AHRQ's Medical Errors and Patient Safety Web page con-tains extensive resources, ranging from comprehen-sive reports on patient safety issues to fact sheets and "tips." Users can also subscribe to the Patient Safety E-newsletter from this Web page. AHRQ has also established a Patient Safety Network (PSNet). See the Resources section at the end of the chapter for Web addresses.

Among the other important patient safety ini-tiatives is the Institute for Healthcare Improvement's (IHI) "100,000 Lives Campaign." IHI is enlisting hospitals to implement changes that have been proven to prevent avoidable deaths. Six interven-tions are recommended:

- Deploy Rapid Response Teams (RRT) at the first sign of patient decline.
- Deliver reliable, evidence-based care for acute myocardial infarction to prevent deaths from heart attack.
- Prevent adverse drug events by implementing medication reconciliation.
- Prevent central line infections by implement-ing a series of interdependent, scientifically grounded steps called the *Central Line Bundle*.

- Prevent surgical site infections by reliably delivering the correct perioperative antibiotics at the proper time.

- Prevent ventilator-dependent pneumonia by implementing a series of interdependent, scientifically grounded steps called the *Ventilator Bundle.*

IHI hopes to avoid 100,000 deaths over 18 months and every year thereafter by implementing these crucial steps.

In addition to participating in national safety initiatives, most hospitals have established event reporting systems that emphasize the need for each health care practitioner to contribute to the greater good by reporting all errors (including near misses and failures to deliver care) within a "blame-free" environment. Errors, omissions, and near-misses are reviewed by quality and safety committees and action plans are implemented to address infrastructure and process issues that impede practitioners' ability to offer safe, effective health care services. A blame-free environment does not imply that negligence or repeated errors are not addressed through individual disciplinary action, but the traditional culture of blaming individuals for mistakes per se did nothing to improve flawed processes and systems.

Quality and Performance Improvement

We have chosen to separate our discussions of patient safety and quality for purposes of special emphasis, but safety issues are the most basic subset of clinical quality. Quality and performance improvement activities in health care are evolving rapidly. Anything we say within these pages will likely be outdated quickly, as health care purchasers and regulators move rapidly to link quality indicators to payment for services. This linkage is part of a public and private sector initiative called Pay for Performance (PFP). PFP has been defined as "the use of incentives to encourage and reinforce the delivery of evidence-based practices and health care system transformation that promote better outcomes as efficiently as possible" (Johns Hopkins

Outcome Evaluation Program and American Healthways, 2004).

The federal government's pay-for-performance activities began in November 2004 when CMS required hospitals to report their performance on a "starter set" of 10 quality measures. For fiscal years 2005–2007, CMS mandated public reporting of the 10 measures to receive the full annual Medicare "market basket" payment update. Currently, hospitals receive the full payment increase for reporting the measures (subject to a medical record validation audit, which must pass a minimum of 80 percent upper bound reliability). The second phase of PFP will require hospitals (and other health care provider types, including physicians) to meet specific performance thresholds on an expanded set of inpatient and ambulatory quality and efficiency indicators. The second phase is also expected to include emphasis on data collected from a new patient experience-of-care survey that will supplement any existing provider patient satisfaction surveys. Examples of indicators in the inpatient hospital starter set include offering an aspirin to acute myocardial infarction patients at arrival and prescribing an aspirin at discharge; completing a left ventricular function assessment on a heart failure patient; and ensuring that patients with pneumonia receive an initial antibiotic within 4 hours of hospital arrival. At first glance, these items seem too simple to be addressed in the 21st century, but surprisingly, there still is not 100 percent compliance with these basic services.

The hospital quality indicators and pay-for-performance are part of the CMS overall Quality Initiative, which began in November 2002 for skilled nursing facilities (SNF) and expanded to home health agencies and hospitals in 2003. In 2004, the initiative was expanded to kidney dialysis facilities and physician practices (Doctor's Office Quality–Information Technology Project). The initiative is intended to achieve the CMS mission of ensuring "the right care for every patient, every time." Hospital Compare is a new part of the program that joins Nursing Home Compare and Home Health Compare as an online service to give consumers information to help them make informed choices about health care services, while providing stronger rewards and support for high-quality, efficient care. All of the Compare Web pages are found by accessing Medicare's official consumer Web site. Extensive information about specific quality initiatives is found at the CMS Web site.

The private sector is using pay-for-performance as a key strategy to improve quality and control costs. In fact, the private sector was first in establishing various methods of pay-for-performance for hospitals and physicians by basing payment on "report cards" and performance indicators that emphasized utilization controls and efficiency in service delivery. Clinical and service quality indicators have become equally important in more recent private sector initiatives. Management of chronic illnesses, use of prevention tools, emphasis on patient-centered care that requires patient participation and self-management, and use of health information technology are of special private-sector interest and activity. The activities of two organizations are worthy of special mention and study: Bridges to Excellence and California's Integrated Healthcare Association Pay for Performance Program. Readers are referred to the Web sites in the Resources section for specific information.

It is crucial that speech-language pathology and audiology departments, programs, and practitioners develop and implement indicators to evaluate clinical and service quality within the context of the initiatives of the health care community and within their own organization's mission, scope of service, values, goals, and regulatory requirements. ASHA's (2005b) *Quality Indicators for Professional Service Programs in Audiology and Speech-Language Pathology* identifies and describes quality indicators and provides a framework for evaluating programs and services. It is highly recommended reading for all practitioners.

CLINICAL ACCOUNTABILITY: EVIDENCE-BASED PRACTICE

Clinical accountability is not a new concept. The May 1983 issue of *Seminars in Speech and Language* was devoted to the topic. Charles Diggs's article in that issue was titled "Professional Accountability: Present and Future Directions." He predicted the following:

> As a result of continuing economic difficulties nationwide, and consumer demand for quality services at the most reasonable cost possible, practitioners in the future, regardless of setting, will be requested to consider, more and more, both effectiveness and efficiency measures. Effectiveness measures will need to be expressed not only in terms of communication improvement, but also in terms of impact on education and employability. Effectiveness measures will be tempered by increased concern for cost containment, and practitioners will routinely be asked to strike cost/benefit ratios. As a direct result of this emphasis, practitioners will also be called upon to develop innovative assessment and treatment protocols that are designed to yield similar results in shorter periods of time. Of all the predictions for future practitioners, this charge will be the most challenging. (p. 183)

The time has come to fulfill this charge. Gosfield (2005) has referred to the current state of health care as "the era of health care measurement … the ability to evaluate, judge, compare, and pay for performance all depends on some kind of measurement." (p. 1). The CMS Quality Improvement Organizations (QIO) are focusing their efforts on promoting the use of "standardized, effective processes of care" in hospitals across the country as part of the Eighth Scope of Work. These care processes will be used for reporting on clinical and utilization measures linked to pay-for-performance programs. We all know the familiar slogans "what gets measured gets done" and "you cannot manage what you cannot measure." It is imperative for the future of patient care and for the advancement of the professions that clinicians determine systematically what procedures, interventions, and treatments will lead to desired outcomes based on evidence.

Evidence-based practice refers to the application of research data (scientific evidence) to clinical decision making. Clinicians who base their practice on evidence ask themselves:

- How do we use research findings to make clinical decisions?

- How do we use clinical support tools such as guidelines, pathways, and protocols to shape patient care?

- If we choose treatment methods that vary from the guidelines, can we justify those practice variations with other evidence?

- How do we determine if care was delivered in the right setting for the right amount of time?

- Were the services efficient (optimal services delivered at least cost)?

ASHA has developed a number of documents to teach speech-language pathologists and audiologists about evidence-based practice (EBP). Current resources include the position statement *Evidence-Based Practice in Communication Disorders* (ASHA, 2005a); the technical report *Evidence-Based Practice in Communication Disorders: An Introduction* (ASHA, 2004a); and the *Report of the Joint Coordinating Committee on Evidence-Based Practice* (ASHA, 2004c). EBP was an ASHA Focused Initiative in 2005 and an Advisory Committee on Evidence-Based Practice (ACEBP) was established as a standing committee to build upon previous work and expand member knowledge and support in this area. Dollaghan (2004) reminds us that "EBP offers us a framework and a set of tools by which we can systematically improve in our efforts to be better clinicians, colleagues, advocates, and investigators—not by ignoring clinical experience and patient preferences, but by considering these against a background of the highest quality scientific evidence that can be found" (p. 12). See Chapter 28 for a more in-depth discussion of evidence-based practice.

In these times, clinicians are faced with the realization that the value of their services is defined by linking the results of care to cost. Expectations must be established for both clinicians and patients so that appropriate care is provided, but services are not overused. Clinicians should adopt objective criteria for defining necessary services and provide a

consistent clinical and business strategy for decision making. The essence of managing care today is that the use of health care services is controlled to ensure that the right amount and types of care are offered in the appropriate setting. What is new about the concept is that clinicians should not wait for a hospital "utilization review" or "utilization management" department or a payer to tell them that enough is enough; clinicians should be as conscious of cost factors as they are about patient treatment techniques. The clinician's role is not to "fight" the utilization manager but to work with data to determine the most appropriate care within cost parameters. It is imperative to prioritize patient needs, planning and managing care through a continuum approach.

It is important that speech-language pathologists and audiologists participate in the development and implementation of all types of clinical decision support tools. As health care organizations move toward standardizing care and as order sets are automated, only the services of practitioners who have demonstrated the value of their interventions will likely be included in standardized care tools. ASHA has provided many tools to help guide speech-language pathologists and audiologists in offering optimal care. *Preferred Practice Patterns for the Profession of Audiology* (ASHA, 1997) and *Preferred Practice Patterns for the Profession of Speech-Language Pathology* (ASHA, 2004b) are statements that define characteristics of patient care/client activities applicable to all practice settings. The Preferred Practice Patterns are based on a common set of guiding principles and reflect the following fundamental components: professionals and support personnel who perform the procedure, expected outcomes, clinical indications, and clinical process.

Practice guidelines are recommended procedures for specific areas of practice that describe knowledge, skills, and competencies needed for effective practice. Guidelines, knowledge and skills statements, and technical reports are prepared by ASHA task forces and committees and are published in special supplements (and on the ASHA Web site). Clinical decision support tools, with review criteria, are used to place patients within a continuum of care. Audiologists and speech-language pathologists can play important roles within health care organizations by developing continuum-based guidelines and pathways that incorporate principles of utilization management, collaborating with other providers across the continuum, and keeping abreast of trends and opportunities to provide new, different, and more cost-effective services that meet multiple needs. Readers are also referred to the "Health Care Issues" briefs published on the ASHA Web site for detailed information about knowledge, skills, practice parameters, and issues specific to working in acute care, inpatient rehabilitation, home care, and long-term care settings. Audiologists are referred to the ASHA Web site section titled "Resources for Audiologists in Health Care Settings" for extensive practice information.

CLINICAL DOCUMENTATION, CODING, AND PAYMENT FOR SERVICES

Although documentation and coding of services are required for payment, clinicians in all health professions seem to struggle most with these tasks. Instead of viewing documentation as something that reflects pride in what we do, health professionals often think it is a necessary evil or at least a nuisance. The advent of electronic medical records should make the task less onerous. However, the duty will not disappear and may become more exacting. Coding seems to be a great mystery. However, the investment of several hours of basic study of diagnosis and procedure coding, conferring with health information management professionals, and attention to ongoing updates will yield enormous benefit.

Documenting Health Care Services

Accurate and complete documentation is an integral part of every clinician's job. Clinical documentation includes recording every patient encounter (including notation of missed appointments); professional staffing; phone calls, discussions, and correspondence (including e-mail) about or with the patient and/or family/caregiver or other member of the health care

team or referral source. The health care record is first a communication tool among caregivers to facilitate patient care, safety, and clinical and service quality. It is also used to support billing, to provide data for quality improvement and utilization management activities, for research and data repositories, and to protect legal interests of the provider and patient.

Formats for clinical documentation take many forms and depend on work setting. Speech-language pathologists and audiologists who work in acute care hospitals may write on consult forms to report diagnostic procedures and in progress note sections of medical records to describe content and results of individual treatment sessions. Rehabilitation hospitals may use both individual therapy notes and interdisciplinary team reports geared to complement Functional Independence Measure (FIM) reporting (Uniform Data System for Medical Rehabilitation, 1997). Outpatient clinics might use a mix of consultation letters, checklists, typed reports, and treatment logs. Plans of care will likely contain space for physician signatures to meet Medicare requirements for physician certification and recertification of the need for therapy for Medicare beneficiaries. The key to appropriateness of documentation in any setting is determining what one is trying to accomplish and to communicate with others to achieve treatment goals and to facilitate planning for the next level of care.

The trend toward electronic health records (EHR) is increasing. Hurricane Katrina in the late summer of 2005 gave impetus to the initiative to move to an all-EHR system when health professionals discovered in the aftermath that years of paper medical records had been destroyed in flooded hospital basements and in supposedly secure off-site storage locations. The United States Department of Health and Human Services immediately issued proposed regulations and announced other initiatives to accelerate the use of e-prescribing and EHR across the country. Although electronic records will speed the documentation process and enhance communication across settings, the quality and usefulness of records will always depend upon the health professionals who write, type, or speak the information (for voice-activated systems that are being developed for practical use).

There are two parts to the record: the "house-keeping" component and the substantive or content portion. Housekeeping elements include legibility, use of military or 24-hour clock time for hospital records, black-ink only for handwritten records, use of approved abbreviations, no erasures, patient name and record number on every page, and signature and date on every entry.

Elements of required documentation are specified in provider organization policies and procedures, by payers, and by regulatory and accrediting entities such as JCAHO and CARF. CMS requirements are found in the *Medicare Benefit Policy Manual* (at the CMS Web site) and in fiscal intermediary Local Coverage Determinations (LCD). CMS specifies that a therapy plan of care for Medicare beneficiaries include:

- Diagnoses being treated and problem areas identified

- Long-term treatment goals

- Type, amount, duration, and frequency of therapy services

CMS emphasizes the importance of writing functional goals that are objective and measurable. Functional goals reflect the level of communicative independence the patient is expected to achieve outside the therapy environment (at home, in the community, other least restrictive environment), reflecting significant, practical improvement within a reasonable period of time. Progress notes are written for each billing period that describe:

- The initial functional communication level of the patient at this provider setting.

- The current functional level of the patient and progress achieved for this reporting period.

- Assessment and/or treatment techniques, procedures, and methods used.

- The patient's expected rehabilitation potential.

- Changes in the plan of treatment.

Payers and regulators other than Medicare may have additional or different documentation requirements. Format and content of documentation is determined according to practice site, payer source,

and other oversight activities. ASHA updated the 1994 document *Clinical Record Keeping in Speech-Language Pathology for Health Care and Third-Party Payers* (Hasselkus, 2004) to serve as a guide for speech-language pathology programs in establishing, revising, and maintaining accurate and appropriate clinical records. Clinicians must document accurately and completely because it is the right thing to do for the patient and because it achieves a high degree of professional integrity. The application of technology to clinical practice is discussed in depth in Chapter 25.

HEALTH CARE CODING

Health care coding is the "language" of payers. That is, a set of numbers or letters and numbers together represents a health care problem or health care service. The codes link dollars to services. If there is no code to represent a problem or service, payment is usually not forthcoming or is difficult to obtain, The process of acquiring codes is complex and political in our health care system. The following discussion explains the basics of diagnosis and procedure coding.

Diagnosis Coding

Coding links the diagnosis (the illness, injury, or disorder associated with the patient's reason for seeking care) with the health care procedure or service performed by the health care professional(s) treating the patient. *Coding* refers to the numerical (or alphanumerical) representation of a diagnosis or service. The *International Classification of Diseases* (ICD) is the worldwide standard used to classify causes of mortality (death registration) and morbidity statistics (records and surveys, health care claims, and basis for prospective payment). Most of the world uses the new system, the ICD-10 (10th Revision). The official coding scheme for diagnoses used in the United States is the *International Classification of Diseases, Clinical Modification, Ninth Revision* (ICD-9-CM), although the United States does use the ICD-10 for mortality data. The home page of the *Classifications of Diseases, and Functioning & Disability* of the National Center for Health Statistics (part of the Centers for Disease Control) is listed in the Resources section of the chapter. Complete information about the ICD-9-CM, the ICD-10, and the *International Classification of Functioning, Disability, and Health* (ICF) is found there.

The ICD uses three digits followed by decimal points. V-codes are supplemental alphanumeric codes to report reason for visit/encounter and factors influencing health status. Health professionals must code diseases/disorders to the highest degree of specificity possible (to the fifth digit). For example, the code for "late effect of CVA with dysphagia" is 438.82. The code for "late effect of CVA with aphasia" is 438.11. It is important to use the current version of the ICD-9-CM manual (published on CD-ROM and in hardcover). Updated codes are published in the *Federal Register* in April or May of each year as part of the Proposed Changes to the Hospital Inpatient Prospective Payment System (IPPS) and are effective October 1 of that year. CMS places new, revised, and discontinued codes on the MedLearn section of the CMS Web site. Updated codes are also posted at the National Center for Health Statistics site. The *ICD-9-CM Official Guidelines for Coding and Reporting* is used as a companion document to the official ICD-9-CM document. Adherence to the guidelines is required under HIPAA. The diagnosis codes (Volumes 1 and 2) have been adopted under HIPAA for all health care settings. (Note: Volume 3 procedure codes are used only for hospital inpatient settings.) Health care providers and coders, usually employed by health care organizations such as hospitals and physician practices, must work together to achieve accurate and complete documentation, and coding and reporting of diagnoses and procedures. The Official Guidelines are published online at the National Center for Health Statistics Web site.

It is important for speech-language pathologists and audiologists to understand the rules for coding sequences of diagnoses pertinent to the reasons patients seek SLP or audiology services. For example, for patients receiving rehabilitation therapy services in the outpatient setting, the appropriate V-code for the service is listed fist, and the diagnosis or problem for which the service is being performed is listed

second. V-codes in the ICD manual are "aftercare" codes used to cover situations in which the initial treatment of a disease or injury has been performed and the patient requires continued care during the recovery phase, or for the long-term consequences of the disease. For example, the ICD-9 V Code for "encounter for speech-language pathology" is V57.3. The SLP would code V57.3 first, then the problem for which the patient is being seen second (e.g., late effects of CVA, aphasia–438.11). [Note: the other ICD code for aphasia—784.3—refers to the code section 784 "Symptoms Involving Head and Neck" and is meant to be used only when an official diagnosis has not been established or confirmed.] Although lists of diagnosis codes are provided by payers, provider organizations, and a number of sources on the Internet, professionals should not just pick codes from a list without knowing what the code specifies. The section of the ICD manual from which the code is taken is crucial information. Remember to look *first* for correct code assignment in the Alphabetic Index of the ICD-9-CM manual; then search the Tabular List. Initial searches in the Tabular List will lead to coding errors. All documented conditions that coexist at the time of the encounter and require or affect treatment or management of the condition should be coded. Conditions that were previously treated and no longer exist should not be coded (but see exceptions to using history codes in the Official Guidelines document).

The diagnosis, condition, problem, or other reason for encounter should be sequenced first when the patient is receiving diagnostic services only. Other diagnoses (e.g., chronic conditions) may be sequenced as additional diagnoses. If the results of diagnostic testing are normal, code the signs or symptoms to report the reason for the test (many signs and symptoms are listed in Sections 780–799 of the ICD Manual) and explain the normal result in the practitioner's report.

Procedure Coding

Current Procedural Terminology (CPT), published annually and copyrighted by the American Medical Association, is the system used for coding health care services in the United States (except that inpatient hospital procedures are coded by using Volume 3 of the ICD-9-CM). The CPT codes represent specific procedures or services and all are five digits. For example, the code for "evaluation of speech, language, voice, or communication" is 92506. The code for "treatment of speech, language, voice, or communication" is 92507. Although theoretically the codes may be used by any health professional, payers often limit certain codes to specific practitioners. Professionals should know which codes are accepted by individual payers, and it is crucial to code services accurately, regardless of payment. The code must represent the actual service provided. Medicare and other payers have established "edits" that restrict which codes may be billed together. The Medicare edits are called "CCI edits" (Correct Coding Initiative). There are two versions of the CCI Edits—one for physicians and one for hospital acute care services. Medicare Local Coverage Determinations (LCD) also specify which diagnoses and which procedure codes can be billed by different practitioners. Check fiscal intermediary Web sites for additional information.

The Health Care Common Procedural Coding System (HCPCS, pronounced "HickPicks") is maintained and distributed by the Centers for Medicare and Medicaid Services (CMS). The codes are alphanumeric, beginning with a letter followed by four digits. HCPCS Level I codes are the CPT codes. HCPCS Level II codes identify products, supplies, equipment, devices, and services not included in the CPT coding system, such as durable medical equipment, prosthetics and orthotics, and ambulance services. Examples of SLPA codes included in HCPCS are speech generating devices, voice amplifiers, and repair of AAC systems. These codes are required by CMS for claims for covered supplies and devices and by commercial payers. Certain procedure/service codes not described by CPT are also included in HCPCS. The HCPCS is found on the CMS website.

Coding systems provide a standard way to identify and report services and supplies. The systems do not provide a method for determining coverage policy. Therefore, just because a code exists does not mean that payers reimburse health care providers or suppliers for the service or item. However, all services, procedures rendered, and all equipment and supplies provided should be coded. Although all codes may not be payable, for financial tracking and productivity purposes, it is important to account for all aspects of a clinic's or hospital's business.

PAYMENT FOR SERVICES

Payment methodologies for SLP and audiology services vary by employment setting. Medicare prospective payment systems (PPS) dominate health care for acute care inpatient and outpatient services, skilled nursing facilities (SNF), psychiatric hospitals, rehabilitation hospitals and distinct-part units, and home health agencies (HHA). In these settings, Medicare pays on a prospectively determined basis. In the acute-care setting, payment amount depends upon diagnosis-related group category. The SNF PPS payment is per diem (per day) and includes all routine, ancillary, and capital costs related to the services furnished to beneficiaries under Part A of the Medicare program. HHA payments are based on episode of care. Payment in the Outpatient Prospective Payment System (OPPS) is generally based on Ambulatory Patient Classification (APC) groups. PPS applies to hospital outpatient services, certain Medicare Part B services furnished to hospital inpatients who have no Part A coverage, and partial hospitalization services furnished by community mental health centers. Services in each APC are similar clinically, according to resource use. A payment rate is established for each APC. Hospitals may be paid for more than one APC per encounter. However, since CMS issued Program Memorandum AB-00-01 (January 2000), speech-language pathology codes and some audiology codes are paid under the Medicare Physician Fee Schedule (MPFS). The MPFS is considered the prospective payment system for these services under OPPS. In the Inpatient Rehabilitation Facility Prospective Payment System (IRF-PPS), payment is made per discharge, according to certain Case-Mix Groups (CMG). SNF, HHA, and rehabilitation hospitals/units prospective payment systems also require specific patient assessments as part of the conditions of participation (CoP) for that setting and for payment under the system. The patient assessments are:

Home Health Agency	Outcome & Assessment Information Set (OASIS)
Inpatient Rehabilitation Hospital/Unit	Patient Assessment Instrument (IRF-PAI)
Skilled Nursing Facility	Long Term Care Resident Assessment Instrument, Including the Minimum Data Set (MDS), Resident Protocols (RAP), and Utilization Guidelines.

Specific information about the various settings, payment programs, and assessment instruments is found in the Resources section.

Managed care and other commercial payers typically pay per diem, or other specific discounted contract rates for hospital, SNF, and HHA inpatient and outpatient services. Some commercial payers do pay a "percent of actual charges" rate. It is a common misconception that individual charges do not matter in prospective payment system billing. Although payment to facilities or programs does not depend on each individual charge per patient "real-time," *annual determinations of the prospective payment rate calculations is based on actual charges.* All clinicians should account for (or "capture") all services rendered by recording all charges. Recording may be paper-based or electronic. Hospitals and clinics provide charge sheets or charge screens for clinicians that post charges by specific service codes (which may or may not include the actual CPT or HCPCS codes reflected on itemized bills or hospital claims). In community clinic settings, payment is based on fees for service and actual CPT codes are used on bills. A model super-bill is posted on the ASHA Web site under the "Reimbursement" tab. Charges must be supported by accurate and complete clinical documentation that reflects all services, procedures, supplies, and equipment provided. The "Therapy Resources" Web page provided by CMS contains comprehensive information about therapy documentation, coding, billing, medical review, effectiveness, evidence-based practice, and links to other sites.

SUMMARY

The goal of this chapter was to offer context and infrastructure for providing speech-language pathology and audiology services in health care settings. Practice and management concepts were "operationalized" so that clinicians may apply them to everyday clinical practice. The chapter focused on the primary issues and trends in health care. Special emphasis was placed on the realities of public scrutiny of cost, quality indicators, and consumer experience of care.

CRITICAL THINKING

1. Why is it important for clinicians to understand the health care business infrastructure?

2. How can speech-language pathologists and audiologists participate in hospital planning and operations activities?

3. How do pay-for-performance initiatives influence clinical practice?

4. What does evidence-based practice mean in everyday life?

5. What are the implications of public reporting of quality indicators for an organization's quality and performance improvement program?

6. What changes do you foresee in the delivery of health care services in the next 10 years? Why?

7. Why is documentation so important in the health care context? What types of documents might you need to complete as an audiologist or speech-language pathologist? What skills will you need to complete forms and reports in this type of setting?

8. This chapter introduced you to a variety of "codes." Why are these important in the delivery of speech-language pathology and audiology services in health care settings?

9. Make an alphabetical list of all the acronyms and their meanings listed in this chapter for future reference.

REFERENCES

American Speech-Language-Hearing Association. (1994). Professional liability and risk management for the audiology and speech-language pathology professions. *Asha, 36* (Suppl. 12), 25–38.

American Speech-Language-Hearing Association. (1997). *Preferred practice patterns for the profession of audiology.* Rockville, MD: Author.

American Speech-Language-Hearing Association. (2003). Knowledge and skills in business practices needed by speech-language pathologists in health care settings. *ASHA Supplement, 23,* 87–92.

American Speech-Language-Hearing Association. (2004a). *Evidence-based practice in communication disorders: An introduction.* Rockville, MD: Author.

American Speech-Language-Hearing Association. (2004b). *Preferred practice patterns for the profession of speech-language pathology.* Rockville, MD: Author.

American Speech-Language-Hearing Association. (2004c). *Report of the Joint Coordinating Committee on Evidence-Based Practice.* Rockville, MD: Author.

American Speech-Language-Hearing Association. (2005a). *Evidence-based practice in communication disorders.* Rockville, MD: Author.

American Speech-Language-Hearing Association. (2005b). *Quality indicators for professional service programs in audiology and speech-language pathology.* Available at http://www.asha.org/

CARF: The Rehabilitation Accrediation Commission. (2005). About CARF. Available at http://www.carf.org.

Department of Health and Human Services. (2003). Summary of the HIPAA privacy rule. Available at http://www.hhs.gov/ocr

Diggs, C. (1983). Professional accountability: Present and future directions. *Seminars in Speech and Language, 4*(2), 169–185.

Dollaghan, C. (2004, April 13). Evidence-based practice myths and realities. *ASHA Leader, 9,* 12.

Golper, L., & Brown, J. (Eds). (2005). *Business matters: A guide for speech-language pathologists.* Rockville, MD: American Speech-Language-Hearing Association.

Gosfield, A. (2005, September). Performance and efficiency measurement: Implications for provider positioning. *ACG Notes, 17*(2), 1–8. Available at http://www.gosfield.com.

Hasselkus, A. (2004). Clinical record keeping in speech-language pathology for health care and third-party payers. Rockville, MD: American Speech-Language-Hearing Association.

Horner, J., & Wheeler, M. (2005, September 6). HIPAA: Impact on clinical practices. *ASHA Leader, 10*(12), 10–11; 22–23.

Institute of Medicine. (1999). *To err is human: Building a safer health care system.* Washington, DC: National Academy Press.

Institute of Medicine. (2001). *Crossing the quality chasm: A new health system for the 21st century.* Washington, DC: National Academy Press.

Johns Hopkins Outcome Evaluation Program and American Healthways, Inc. (2004). *Outcomes-based compensation: Pay-for-performance design principles.* Available at http://www.rewardingquality.com

Joint Commission on Accreditation of Healthcare Organizations. (2005). About us. Available at http://www.jcaho.org.

National Quality Forum. (2003). *Safe practices for better healthcare.* Washington, DC: Author.

Stein, R. (2005, November 4). For Americans, getting sick has its price. *The Washington Post,* A2. Available at http://www.washingtonpost.com

Uniform Data System for Medical Rehabilitation. (1997). *Guide for the uniform data set for medical rehabilitation* (Version 5.1). Amherst, NY: Author.

RESOURCES

Agency for Healthcare Research & Quality (AHRQ)
http://www.ahrq.gov

American Academy of Audiology (AAA)
http://www.audiology.org

American Hospital Association (AHA)
http://www.aha.org

American Medical Association (AMA)
http://www.ama-assn.org

American Speech-Language-Hearing Association
http://www.asha.org

Bridges to Excellence
http://www.bridgestoexcellence.org

CARF: The Rehabilitation Accreditation Commission
http://www.carf.org

Centers for Medicare & Medicaid Services (CMS)
http://www.cms.hhs.gov

Classification of Diseases & Functioning & Disability
http://www.cdc.gov/hchs/icd9

Health Care Common Procedural Coding System
(HCPCS)
http://www.cms.hhs.gov/medicare/hcpcs

Health Care Compliance Association (HCCA)
http://www.hcca-info.org

Health Insurance Portability & Accountability Act (HIPAA)
http://www.cms.hhs.gov/hipaa/hipaa2
http://www.hhs.gov/ocr/hipaa (Office of Civil
Rights site for HIPAA Privacy Rule)

Healthy People 2010
http://www.healthypeople.gov

Home Health Prospective Payment System
http://www.cms.hhs.gov/providers/hhapps/

Institute for Healthcare Improvement (IHI)
http://www.ihi.org

Institute of Medicine (IOM)
http://www.iom.edu

Integrated Healthcare Association (Pay for Performance)
http://www.iha.org

International Classification of Diseases (ICD-9-CM)
http://www.cdc.gov/nchs/data/icd9/icdguide.pdf

Joint Commission on Accreditation of Healthcare
Organizations (JCAHO)
http://www.jcaho.org

Leapfrog Group
http://www.leapfroggrooup.org

Medical Errors & Patient Safety (AHRQ)
http://www.ahrq.gov/qual/errorsix.htm

Minimum Data Set (MDS)
http://www.cms.hhs.gov/quality/mds30/

National Center for Health Statistics (NCHS)
http://www.cdc.gov/nchs/

National Institutes of Health (NIH)
http://www.nih.gov

National Library of Medicine (NLM)
http://www.nlm.nih.gov

National Provider Identifier (NPI)
http://nppes.cms.hhs.gov

National Quality Forum (NQF)
http://www.qualityforum.org

Outcome & Assessment Information Set (OASIS)
http://www.cms.hhs.gov/oasis

Office of Civil Rights (OCR) (HIPAA Privacy
Rule information)
http://www.hhs.gov/ocr

Office of Human Research Protections (OHRP)
http://www.hhs.gov/ohrp

Office of Inspector General (OIG) (DHHS)
http://www.oig.hhs.gov

Outcome & Assessment Information Set (OASIS)
http://www.cms.hhs.gov/oasis/

Patient Safety Network (PSNet)
http://psnet.ahrq.gov

Prospective Payment Systems (acute-care, inpatient
rehab, inpatient psychiatry)
http://www.cms.hhs.gov/providers/hospital.asp

Skilled Nursing Facility Prospective Payment System
http://www.cms.hhs.gov/providers/snfpps

Therapy Resources–CMS
http://www.cms.hhs.gov/medlearn/therapy/

World Health Organization (WHO)
http://www.who.int

14

Education Policy

DIANE L. EGER, PHD, CCC-A/SPL

SCOPE OF CHAPTER

This chapter answers some key questions about to how education policy has affected speech-language service delivery in the schools. It addresses the federal statutes that have prominently influenced education policy, including the 2004 Reauthorization of IDEA and No Child Left Behind (NCLB). This chapter discusses eligibility, enrollment, dismissal, and paperwork requirements. All speech-language service providers in today's marketplace are burdened with too much paperwork, and school-based speech-language pathologists are no exception. Behind these documentation requirements are (1) key federal statutes influencing education policy for speech and language services in the schools and (2) federal mandates to enroll and dismiss a child into and out of speech therapy. This chapter also discusses the various positive effects on school-based speech and language services that have resulted from federal education policies. These include teaming, integrated services, outcomes measurement, evidence-based practice, and an increased role in literacy. Finally, this chapter briefly notes the impact of key federal laws on audiology in the schools.

FEDERAL LEGISLATION

The federal legislation that has most prominently influenced education policy for school-based speech and language services are Section 504 of the Rehabilitation Act of 1973, the Education for All Handicapped Children Act of 1975 (Part B), the Education for All Handicapped Children Act (Part H), the Individuals with Disabilities Education Act of 1990 (IDEA), the IDEA Amendments of 1997, and the Individuals with Disabilities Education Improvement Act of 2004. As Nelson (1993) notes, "Federal policy in the United States is guided by laws passed by Congress. Other federal influences are based on court interpretations and on position papers, newsletters, and research priorities issued by federal agencies" (p. 153).

Brown v. Board of Education

The American public education system is a major cornerstone of democracy. Our predecessors built a public education system to ensure access to all children. Compulsory education laws have been in every state since 1918. Child labor laws were enacted in 1938. In 1954 the *Brown v. Board of Education* Supreme Court decision "set into motion a new era and struck down the doctrine of segregated education. This decision sparked such issues as women's rights; the right to education and treatment for the handicapped; and the intrinsic rights of individuals" (Neidecker & Blosser, 1993, pp. 8–9).

Further, the democratic process of electing one's leaders necessitates an educated citizenry. The future of the United States depends on public education meeting the challenge of the times. Currently, schools are under increasing pressure to change, and the pressure is from both the payer and the consumer. Businesses want a more educated workforce without having to provide remedial instruction prior to skills training. Local, state, and federal education agencies want each system to be accountable for the outcomes of their students, both those with disabilities and those without. McLaughlin (1997) notes that "Concerns about the post-school outcomes of students with disabilities have been growing for over a decade" (p. 16).

Certainly this issue was part of the motivation for the 2002 No Child Left Behind (NCLB) Act.

Section 504 of the Rehabilitation Act of 1973

Section 504 of the Rehabilitation Act of 1973 (PL 93-112) set the stage for the enactment of PL 94-142 or the Education for All Handicapped Children Act of 1975. Section 504 of the Rehabilitation Act and its later amendments in 1978 were civil rights acts forbidding all recipients of federal assistance from discriminating against persons on the basis of their handicap. This legislation was not specifically aimed at schools but has had great impact on education. It is a broad civil rights law and identifies all school-age children as handicapped who meet the definition of a "qualified handicapped person." All students who qualify for services under IDEA are 504 eligible, but all students who are eligible under 504 are not eligible under IDEA.

PL 94-142 The Education for All Handicapped Children Act of 1975

The Education for All Handicapped Children Act of 1975 was the landmark legislation that changed the face of public education in the United States. PL 94-142 was the response of Congress to the state education systems' failure to meet the needs of children with handicaps across the United States. It was created by Congress to accomplish five main goals:

1. All handicapped children were to have a free, appropriate public education (FAPE).

2. Their rights and those of their parents or guardians were to be protected (due process).

3. States and localities were to be assisted in providing for this education (federal dollars-headcount money).

4. The effectiveness of efforts to educate handicapped children was to be assessed and assured (outcomes).

5. The Individualized Education Program (IEP) was established as the written record of commitment to meet a student's goals as determined by parents and professionals.

This legislation defined special education and mandated a process to include students with handicaps in the regular schools. To receive special education services, the law specified a student must be evaluated and found to have one of the following handicapping conditions:

1. Deaf
2. Deaf-blind
3. Hard of hearing
4. Mentally retarded
5. Multihandicapped
6. Orthopedically impaired
7. Other health impaired
8. Seriously emotionally disturbed
9. Specific learning disability
10. Speech impaired
11. Visually handicapped

The law further specified that this handicapping condition must have a negative impact on academic performance. These requirements have been written into state education regulations and operationalized at the local school building level. Neidecker and Blosser (1993) explain that:

> Public Law 94-142 has had a pervasive and profound effect on public school speech-language and hearing programs. Before the passage of the law, individual states had enacted legislation *permitting* speech and hearing services in the schools, but PL 94-142 *mandated* services for children with speech-language or hearing impairments. In addition, the law established a legal basis for services and provided financial assistance. The scope of speech-language pathology and audiology services are defined in the provisions of the law and mandate the identification and evaluation of communicatively handicapped children as well as the development of an Individualized Education Program (IEP) and its implementation. The regulations also cover the provision of appropriate administrative and supervisory activities necessary for program planning, management, and evaluation. (p. 11)

Revisions of PL 94-142 There have been four major revisions of PL 94-142: PL 99-457, the Education for the Handicapped Act Amendments of 1986; PL 101-476, the Education for the Handicapped Act Amendments of 1990; PL 105-17, the Individuals with Disabilities Education Act Amendments of 1997; and PL 108-446, the Individuals with Disabilities Education Improvement Act of 2004. PL 99-457 extended the rights and protections of PL 94-142 to handicapped children from infancy through age 5. This act initiated program funds for disabled infants and toddlers and increased federal support for preschoolers with handicaps. It also reauthorized discretionary programs of PL 94-142, including personnel training, programs for children with severe disabilities, and research and demonstration projects and materials. PL 101-476 renamed the Education for All Handicapped Children Act as the Individuals with Disabilities Education Act (IDEA). Importantly, it replaced the term *handicapped* with *disabled,* thus expanding services to these children. It also expanded the law to workplace and training centers and added transition plans to the IEP. Significantly, it added the two new categories of "autism" and "traumatic brain injury" to the original 11. There was one relatively minor revision to IDEA. This was PL 102-119 or the Individuals with Disabilities Education Act Amendments of 1991. This act added assistive devices to Part H; stated that preschoolers (3- to 5-year-olds) may have either an Individualized Family Service Plan (IFSP) or an IEP; and changed *case management* to *service coordination.* PL 105-17 imposed new obligations on the states and on schools, established new discipline procedures, revised the funding formula, and added a series of new requirements for IEPs. The latest revision (PL 108-446) reauthorized IDEA to align it with the provisions of NCLB.

PL 99-457 Education for the Handicapped Act Amendments of 1986 Although personnel standards have long been addressed in various federal rules and regulations, they have not been consistently followed in many states. PL 99-457 included provisions requiring state education agencies (SEAs) to use qualified personnel to provide special education and related services as well as early intervention. The regulations for PL 99-457 were finalized in 1989 by the United States Department of Education. The *Technical Assistance Report—Retraining Personnel to Meet the Highest Requirements in the State* (ASHA,1992) noted that the federal law and regulations specified that states must indicate in their state plans for implementing Part B and Part H of IDEA their policies and procedures to ensure that personnel are appropriately and adequately prepared and trained. This "qualified provider" revision has had more impact in the speech and language area than in other areas because, unlike some professions, there are at least four types of certification that directly affect the individual speech-language pathologist (Neidecker & Blosser, 1993). These are certification by ASHA, state certification, state licensure, and state registration. These four types of credentialing are clarified in Table 14–1.

These various types of certification are confusing to new graduates in the field as well as consumers. The 50 states are quite varied in their requirements for employment in the schools. It is critical that a potential school employee for a given state check out the explicit requirements well in advance of seeking employment. In some states, such as Pennsylvania, a separate state exam is required to receive your school certificate and is only given at specified times throughout the year.

PL 101-476 Individuals with Disabilities Education Act (IDEA) The next revision to PL 99-142 occurred in 1990 with the passage of PL 101-476, Education for the Handicapped Act Amendments of 1990, which renamed the act Individuals with Disabilities Education Act (IDEA). IDEA expanded the law to encompass instruction in all settings, including the workplace and training centers and added transition plans to the Individualized Education Program (IEP). Congress not only renamed the law but specified that wherever the word *handicap*

T A B L E 14–1 Certifying and Licensing Agents

Agency	Form	Possible Holder
ASHA	Certificate of Clinical Competence in Speech-Language Pathology and/or Audiology	Person who wishes to be identified by ASHA as a qualified practitioner and/or supervisor in speech-language or audiology. Requires meeting ASHA standards.
State of _____ Department of Education	Certificate to practice in the public school of the State of _____	Person who wishes employment in the State of _____ as SLP and/or audiologist in an educational facility. Requires meeting all state certification standards.
State of_____ Board of SLP and Audiology	License to provide speech, language, and/or audiology Services in State of _____	Person wishing to practice in a voluntary official agency (except specifically named educational facilities) or practice privately in the State of _____ , Requires meeting state board standards and passing examination.
State of _____ Board Of Health or Health Occupations Council	Registration to use title of SLP of Audiologist	Person who wishes to use title of SLP and/or Audiologist in State of _____. Does not bar a person from practicing but does require defined qualifications for registration

SOURCE: From Elizabeth A. Neidecker & Jean L. Blosser. *School Programs in Speech-Language—Organization and Management* (3rd ed). Published by Allyn and Bacon, Boston, MA. Copyright © 1993 by Pearson Education. By permission of the publisher.

appeared in the original law, it should be replaced with *disability*. This is consistent with the international clarification by the World Health Organization definitions of *impairment, disability*, and *handicap*. In addition, this reauthorization expanded the categories of children with disabilities and added children with "autism" and "traumatic brain injury" as new categories. Another major change included in these amendments that has had an impact on students with communication disorders is in the area of transition services. *Transition service* means a coordinated set of activities for a student with a disability 16 years or older, which promotes movement from school to post-school activities. This individualized outcome-oriented plan may include postsecondary education, vocational training, integrated employment (including supported employment), continuing and adult education, independent living, or community participation. The speech-language pathologist is an integral part of these transition plans because the plans are determined to some extent by how effectively the student can communicate. Finally, this law ensures that students who need assistive technology services will receive them from trained personnel.

PL105-17 Reauthorization of IDEA The third revision of PL 94-142 is PL 105-17, known as the Reauthorization of IDEA or IDEA '97. Although this revision preserved the guarantee of a free, appropriate public education (FAPE) to students with disabilities, it imposed new obligations on the SEAs and on schools, established a variety of new discipline procedures, revised the funding formula, and added a series of new requirements for IEPs. The greatest impact on SLPs was in the area of the new IEP requirements. This law aimed to make IEPs more accountable to regular education standards. It also required that students with disabilities participate in statewide or district assessments unless there are legitimate reasons for excluding the child. This change in focus provided tremendous opportunities for the speech-language pathologist to collaborate with regular and special educators to explain the language-learning connection and to assist in developing strategies that account for the linguistic

underpinnings inherent in the regular education curriculum.

The IDEA '97 Final Regulations were released by the United States Department of Education on March 15, 1999, almost 2 years after the passage of PL 105-17. These regulations describe IDEA '97 as retaining the basic rights and protections under IDEA—that is, FAPE for all children with disabilities, including children suspended or expelled from school and procedural safeguards for these children and their parents. It also provides a new and heightened emphasis on improving educational results for children with disabilities through meaningful access to the general education curriculum through IEP improvements and general education reform efforts.

PL 107-110 The No Child Left Behind Act of 2001 The Elementary and Secondary Education Act (ESEA) was reauthorized by PL 107-110 and is known as the No Child Left Behind Act of 2001 (NCLB). It expands the federal role in education. NCLB builds upon the 1965 Elementary and Secondary Education Act (ESEA) by adding specificity and requirements, especially in the areas of standards, assessment, and accountability. At the heart of the law are a number of measures designed to drive significant gains in student achievement and to hold states and schools more accountable for student progress. There are four major components: (1) accountability for results; (2) an emphasis on teaching methods based on scientific research; (3) expanded options for parents of children from disadvantaged backgrounds; and (4) greater flexibility for states and schools in spending federal funds. It asks America's schools to describe their success in terms of what each student accomplishes. Another focus of NCLB is on effective reading instruction. It requires that instructional methods be based upon scientifically based research. ASHA (n.d.) has noted that the issues that significantly impact speech-language pathologists and audiologists in school settings include the following:

- Highly qualified teachers and paraprofessionals
- Use of accommodations, modifications, and alternative assessments for students with disabilities

- Assessment of English language learners
- Sanctions for schools identified as in need of improvement, including the provision of supplemental services
- Accountability and adequate yearly progress

Moore-Brown and Montgomery (2005) note, "Most importantly to speech-language pathologists and other special educators, NCLB now includes requirements for students with disabilities, forging stronger bonds between general and special education" (p. 4). Perhaps the impact of NCLB and the 2004 Reauthorization of IDEA will actually result in one system of education for all students instead of the separate and distinct regular and special education programs that have evolved over the past 30 years. This could be the impetus to successfully integrate the literacy foundation skills into every student's educational experience.

Unfortunately, there are various conflicts between the mandates of NCLB and IDEA. Some of these conflicts have been addressed in the 2004 reauthorization of IDEA. And like many other federal mandates, the law has not provided the funds authorized. Dissatisfaction with the mandates of NCLB has been expressed in lawsuits filed by some states, new state laws that trump federal mandates, and legislation critical of NCLB under consideration in an additional 21 states (Marks, 2005).

PL 108-446 IDEA 2004 The full name of IDEA 2004 is The Individuals with Disabilities Education Improvement Act. The addition of the word *improvement* into the title of this reauthorization of IDEA is significant. The focus of the act is on improving the outcomes for special education and to make IDEA consistent with NCLB. Again it provides a great opportunity for the school-based speech-language pathologist to play an expanded role both in terms of school settings and use of literacy knowledge base in providing services. Since the law now includes homeless children and private school students in Child Find, requires students in charter schools to be served, and allows funds to be spent on eligible students in private schools, SLPs may be assigned to serve the eligible students in these settings. The only

concern is that caseloads are already too high and adding settings could increase these numbers. ASHA (2002a) developed a workload approach rather than the traditional caseload number approach for determining a reasonable caseload size that allows the clinician to meet the needs of individual students and to engage in all of the other professional activities, including mandated paperwork.

The change in the criteria for specific learning disability (SLD) that removes the requirement for a discrepancy between achievement and ability provides an opportunity for the SLP to be involved in the response-to-intervention process in the determination of SLD eligibility. The emphasis of IDEA 2004 on improved "academic achievement and functional performance . . . to the maximum extent possible." Section 1400(c)(5)(E) again provides an opportunity for the SLP to assist the IEP team in the development of curriculum-based goals that consider the impact of the student's communication disorder in successfully accessing the general education curriculum. Another opportunity is the involvement of the SLP in "early intervening services." This term is not to be confused with "early intervention," which deals with services for eligible preschool children. IDEA 2004 allows school districts to use funds to provide support to students who have not been identified as eligible for special education. In addition, changes in IEP procedures and the definition of qualified providers could affect the SLP.

FEDERAL ELIGIBILITY REQUIREMENTS

The major requirements for enrolling and dismissing students into or out of speech and language service was designated in PL 94-142 and modified somewhat in PL 105-17. There were no significant changes made in PL 108-446.

Eligibility for Enrollment

Enrolling a student into speech and language service follows four major steps (1) identification (screening and evaluation), (2) determining eligibility (multidisciplinary team evaluation), (3) developing the IEP/IFSP, and (4) placement into the program. Each state education agency (SEA) and each local education agency (LEA) has developed specific forms, procedures, and documentation steps to enroll a child into special education. Paperwork requirements across states vary, but the steps and order of the IEP process are consistent. Montgomery (1993) lists the steps in the IEP process as follows:

1. Screening, identification, referral
2. Informed consent for evaluation signed by parents
3. Formation of multidisciplinary evaluation team
4. Comprehensive assessment
5. Report of assessment team recommendations
6. IEP meeting and development of IEP
7. Parental consent to program and placement
8. Implementation of IEP
9. Annual review in 1 year
10. Three-year reevaluation

The federal law establishes time lines for each of these steps; however, many SEAs have established their own time lines, which exceed those described in federal statutes. An example of this would be a state education law such as in Pennsylvania, which requires a reevaluation every 2 years instead of every 3 years for students who are mentally retarded.

Identification (Screening and Evaluation) IDEA requires that school districts identify eligible children through a "child find" procedure. Although different SEAs have specific procedures in speech and language, this is generally done by referral from parents, teachers, outside agencies, prereferral teams, or self-referral. If the child fails a screening, then the child proceeds into the formal evaluation process. The federal law requires informed consent for evaluation signed by the parents ("permission to evaluate"). Then the school

district must constitute a multidisciplinary evaluation team (MDT). The team then conducts a comprehensive evaluation. As Neidecker and Blosser (1993) point out, "According to Public Law 94-142, all children with disabilities must be assessed before placement in a special education program or before receiving related services. This assessment cannot be discriminatory based on race, cultural diversity, or disability" (p. 142).

Determining Eligibility The federal law requires that the initial evaluation must determine eligibility for special education and related services and must also determine educational needs. IDEA 2004 requires that the team reviews existing data, including local or state assessments and classroom-based observations for all students. As explained by Neidecker and Blosser (1993), speech and language. "assessment procedures must evaluate the communication behavior and delineate strengths, deficits, contributing factors, and functional implications" (p. 142). In operational terms, this means for initial placement the SLP must conduct a thorough evaluation of the student's communication skills in relation to what is expected in school both socially and within the educational curriculum. This requires formal (norm-referenced tests) and informal (criterion-referenced, curriculum-based, and authentic) components. It also requires input from the student's teacher(s) to verify the impact of any communication concerns on the student's academic performance. This evaluation must determine the child's educational needs, present academic achievement, and related developmental needs. In summary, for a school-age student to be enrolled into a speech-language program, formal tests must verify a disorder, and informal tests and classroom observation must verify the impact of such disorder on academic performance. Both aspects must be present to enroll a student into a speech and language program.

For reevaluations, which are required by federal law at least every 3 years, the focus of the reevaluation by this team of qualified professionals and the child's parents is to determine if the child continues to meet eligibility requirements. The speech and language assessment should be composed of primarily informal measures. IDEA 1997 allowed that, if the team determines that no additional data are needed to determine continued eligibility, it is not required to conduct an assessment unless the parents request one following the notification of their right to do so. IDEA 2004 permits the parent and the LEA to agree that a reevaluation is unnecessary. It is important to consider that each SEA interprets and implements the federal requirements differently. Obviously, each speech-language pathologist must adhere not only to the federal requirements, but also to the SEA and LEA requirements as well.

DEVELOPING THE IEP

One of the most significant concepts in PL 94-142 is the Individualized Education Program. It is developed for all students age 3 or older who qualify for speech and language services. The IDEA Amendments of 1997 added new requirements in the IEP process. The current components of the IEP include the following (Pennsylvania Department of Education, 1998): demographics, IEP team/signatures, special considerations, present levels of educational performance, transition planning, goals and objectives, special education, related services and supplementary aids and services, least restrictive environment, dates (initiation date, anticipated duration date, and the IEP revision date), progress reporting, and exit criteria. The IEP process is at the heart of IDEA and functions as the legal document to describe in writing what has been determined to be the child's program of special education, related services, and supplementary aids and services.

The IEP is developed by the IEP team, which includes the speech-language pathologist, for students with speech and/or language disabilities. The IEP team should write a detailed plan describing the child's educational goals and objectives and the services the school will provide to help the child accomplish them. The IEP team must include

the following: (1) the parents of the child with a disability; (2) at least one regular education teacher of the child; (3) at least one special education teacher or provider; (4) a local education agency representative, who is both qualified to provide or supervise special education services and is knowledgeable about the district's resources; (5) an individual who can interpret the evaluation results; (6) other individuals with special expertise regarding the child; and (7) where appropriate, the child with a disability. The required components of the IEP are outlined in Table 14–2. For a child whose only special education is speech and/or language, all of these components must still be completed. The reauthorization of IDEA designated special considerations that must be addressed by the IEP team. These considerations must be based on valid evaluation data and must be reflected in goals and objectives or services.

A good example of the special considerations now required in the IEP is provided in Table 14–3. This is page 2 of the IEP format developed by the Pennsylvania Department of Education. IDEA 2004 does not require any changes to this format. Obviously, for any student receiving speech and/or language services, question E on Table 14–3 would be answered "yes."

IEP Implementation

Once the IEP has been developed by the IEP team, the parent must formally agree or disagree to the program and placement. After the parent formally designates approval, the IEP must be implemented within the mandated time lines, which differ from state to state. In addition, the team must monitor and report progress toward IEP goal attainment, student growth, and the success of the plan. The IEP must designate how the child's progress toward the annual goals will be measured and the extent to which the progress will enable the child to achieve the goals by year end. The frequency of these reports must be at least as often as the parents of nondisabled children receive progress reports—that is, report cards, parent conferences, and so on.

T A B L E 14–2 Required Components of IEP

Strengths	The strengths of the child and the concerns of the parents for enhancing the education of their child
Evaluation results	The results of the initial evaluation or the most recent evaluation
Present level of educational performance	The effect of the student's disability on the involvement and progress in the general education curriculum (or participation in appropriate preschool activities)
Annual goals and short-term objectives	Measurable goals, benchmarks, or objectives related to meeting general education curriculum or other educational needs that result from the disability
Amount of special education or related services	Projected beginning date, frequency, and duration of service
Supplementary aids and services	Program modification or support services necessary for the student to advance toward attaining annual goals, be involved and progress in the general education curriculum, participate in nonacademic activities, and be educated and participate in activities with other students with and without disabilities
Participation with students without disabilities	Extent of participation with students without disabilities in the general education class and in extracurricular activities
Test modifications	Modifications in the administration of statewide or district assessments of student achievement needed for the student to participate in the assessment (If exempt, the reason the test is not appropriate must be stated.)
Transition service	At age 14, transition services that focus on the student's courses of study; at age 16, transition services that specify interagency responsibilities or needed community links
Notification of transfer of rights	Documentation that the student has been informed of the rights that will transfer to the student upon reaching the age of majority under state law (must notify at least 1 year before the student reaches that age of majority)
Evaluation procedures and method of measurement	Measures of the student's progress (e.g., criterion-referenced test, standardized test, student product, teacher observation, or peer evaluation) and how often the evaluation will take place (e.g., daily, weekly, monthly, each grading period/semester, or annually); progress must be reported as often as progress is reported for general education students.
IEP team members	Signatures of all members of the IEP team that developed the IEP

ORIGINAL SOURCE: Section 614d(3)(A)(i-ii), 614d (1)(A)(i-viii)

SOURCE: From ASHA *Guidelines for the Roles and Responsibilities of the School-Based Speech-Language Pathologist*. © 1999 American Speech-Language-Hearing Association. Reprinted by permission.

DISMISSAL

Dismissal out of therapy is not solely the clinician's decision. The IEP team must identify the levels of performance the student would need to attain to no longer qualify for special education services. This discussion occurs at the initial intake IEP conference and must be revisited at each IEP conference. When the dismissal or exit criteria have been met, the multidisciplinary team must recommend dismissal from therapy, and then the parent must sign the legal document removing the child from service. Because there have been regular progress monitoring reports throughout each school year and because the parent has been aware of the exit criteria from the initial meeting, dismissal should never come as a surprise to the educational team. The speech-language pathologist plays a critical role in providing the educational team with accurate information on the expectancies for the student. For example, if the child's verbal system is characterized by severe oral apraxia,

T A B L E 14–3 Special Considerations the IEP Team Must Address Before Developing the IEP

A. Is the Student Blind or Visually Impaired?

_____ No

_____ Yes—Team must address the need for Braille/Braille instruction based on the student's current and future reading and writing skills and needs and will be included in the development of the IEP.

_____ Yes—Team does not need to address the need for Braille/Braille instruction based on the student's current and future reading and writing skills and needs.

B. Is the Student Deaf or Hearing Impaired?

_____ No

_____ Yes—Team must address the student's language and communication needs, opportunities for direct communication with peers and professionals in the student's language and communication mode, academic level, and full range of needs, including opportunities for direct instruction in the student's language and communication mode in the development of the IEP.

C. Does the Student Exhibit Behaviors That Impede His/Her Learning or That of Others?

_____ No

_____ Yes—Team must develop strategies including positive behavior interventions and supports in the IEP.

D. Does the Student Have Limited English Proficiency?

_____ No

_____ Yes—Team must address the language needs of the student in the development of the IEP.

E. Does the Student Have Communication Needs?

_____ No

_____ Yes—Team must address the communication needs of the student in the development of the IEP.

F. Does the Student Require Assistive Technology Devices and Services?

_____ No

_____ Yes—Team must address the student's assistive technology needs in the development of the IEP.

G. Does the Student Need Transition Services?

1. Will the Student be 14 Years of Age or Older Within the Duration of This IEP?

_____ No—Delete Section III

_____ Yes—Team must address the student's course of study and how it applies to components of the IEP.

Student's Course of Study_____

2. Will the Student be 16 Years of Age or Older Within the Duration of this IEP, or Is the Student Younger and in Need of Transition Services as Determined by the IEP Team?

_____ No—Delete Section III

_____ Yes—Team must address and complete Section III.

H. Is the Student Within Three (3) Years of Graduation?

_____ No—Go to Section II

_____ Yes—Team must address graduation plan below.

Plan for Completion of Necessary Credits for Graduation:

Eligibility for graduation will be based upon: _____

(Continued)

T A B L E 14–3   Special Considerations the IEP Team Must Address Before Developing the IEP (Continued)

Option A—Completion of IEP goals and objectives (Should be linked to planned courses)

or

_____ Option B—Completion of school district Outcomes/Standards

If you selected Option B choose one of the following:

_____ Course requirements (attach a list of courses)

or

_____ Assessment, Independent study, student project, other educational experiences (attach plan).

SOURCE: From the Bureau of Special Education, Pennsylvania Department of Education, 1998. Harrisburg, PA., page 2 of IEP Format.

the clinician must share what this means in terms of prognosis as well as the need for more intensive service. It is incumbent on the speech-language pathologist to set realistic exit criteria on a student-by-student basis. Each student's exit criteria levels should be individualized.

RATIONALE FOR PAPERWORK

One major reason there is so much paperwork for the school speech-language pathologist is because each level of government has its own set of paperwork, and the national caseload monthly average is 50 (ASHA, 2004b). For example, although the federal law is explicit about what must be in each student's IEP, there is great variability in written format and length among SEAs and across school districts even within a given state. Further, some states, such as Pennsylvania, have state education regulations that exceed the federal educational regulations. For example, in Pennsylvania, the multidisciplinary team evaluation for students with mental retardation is mandated every 2 years, not every 3 years as required by IDEA. This one change requires much additional paperwork for a clinician in the Pennsylvania schools with 50 or more students on the caseload. As noted in the ASHA 2004 Schools Survey (ASHA, 2004b), increased paperwork was the most frequently selected response by speech-language pathologists in secondary schools (45%) and in combined school settings (35%) from a list of eight possible effects from NCLB.

Medicaid Reimbursement

Another reason there is so much paperwork for the school-based SLP is the completion of Medicaid forms for all eligible students. Federal provisions incorporated in the Medicare Catastrophic Act of 1988 (PL 100-360) created the opportunity for qualified providers to obtain Medicaid reimbursement for certain health-related services provided to children enrolled in special education programs. According to Achilles and Lewis (1996–1997):

> The intent of the legislation was that, while local school districts are responsible for furnishing education and health-related services to children with disabilities, Medicaid agencies are responsible for reimbursement for health related services provided by schools to Medicaid eligible students to the extent that those services are covered, or included under the state Medicaid plan. (p. 38)

The purpose of Medicaid is to deliver health service to the poor through a federal-state partnership arrangement. A match is established between the federal government and the state government based on a formula related to the economics within a given state. The opportunity to tap federal funds for eligible students provides much needed additional dollars to the schools to assist in financing the high cost of special education services. In locations with many eligible students, this can create a paperwork burden for speech and language staff. In some school districts, funds received from Medicaid reimbursement are used to hire aides to assist in the preparation of the Medicaid paperwork. In many districts, however, this burden is the speech-language pathologist's responsibility.

Currently 47 states allow schools to submit claims to their state Medicaid agency for school-based speech-language and audiology services. The three states that do not allow schools to submit these claims are Hawaii, Tennessee, and Wyoming (ASHA, 2003b). This means it is not uncommon to have additional Medicaid paperwork as a school-based speech-language pathologist. It is critical to follow the ASHA Code of Ethics as well as the state licensure laws when asked to complete these forms. Clinicians must be qualified providers if they sign the form for Medicaid reimbursement. Furthermore if the speech-language pathologist is asked to sign another clinician's forms, that clinician must be "under the direction of" the clinician signing the forms. There is no specific federal guidance on this requirement of "under the direction of" so there is great variability from state to state. ASHA has developed a technical report that addresses the "Under the Direction of" Rule (ASHA, 2004a).

It is also worth remembering that SEAs and LEAs must tap all available resources to survive the ever-increasing costs of special education services. As noted by Achilles and Lewis (1996–1997), in Texas "of the ten approved health related services in SHARS (School Health and Related Services), speech therapy services usually generate the largest single share of the reimbursement amount for the local school district" (p. 41). School-based speech and language services generate a substantial amount of money via Medicaid reimbursement for eligible students. In 1997, Medicaid covered 25 percent of all United States children (ASHA, 2005a). There are school districts that have directed significant dollars that were generated by their speech-language pathologists back into the Speech and Language Programs (Deppe, 2005). Unfortunately, this is not the rule. Because additional paperwork is required to access Medicaid money, school districts should be willing to assist clinicians with this paperwork burden.

Related Service versus Special Education Program

One of the few breaks the school-based speech-language pathologist gets with regard to paperwork is that many of the students on the caseload are receiving speech and language as a related service. For example, in the Allegheny Intermediate Unit (AIU), a large service agency serving the 42 suburban school districts surrounding the city of Pittsburgh, Pennsylvania, in the 1997–1998 school year, 43 percent of the school-age caseloads of district-based clinicians were comprised of students receiving speech and language as a related service (Eger, 1998a). This percentage has continued to increase to almost 50 percent over the past 7 years due to the complexity of students enrolled in regular public schools. In the 2004–2005 school year, 49.7 percent of school-age caseloads of district-based clinicians at the AIU were comprised of students receiving speech and language as a related service (Eger, 2005). IDEA includes "speech-language pathology" as both a related service and as a special education program. IDEA defines "related services" as "developmental, corrective, and other supportive service . . . as may be required to assist a child with a disability to benefit from special education . . . and include the early identification and assessment of disabling conditions in children" [Section 602/22]. Generally, this means that when a student is enrolled in another special education program, such as learning disabilities or hearing, speech and language is considered a related service.

Speech-language pathology is considered "special education" rather than a "related service" when the service consists of specially designed instruction, at no cost to the parent, to meet the unique needs of a child with a disability. As noted in the ASHA (1999) *Guidelines for the Roles and Responsibilities of the School-Based Speech-Language Pathologist,* "state standards may further specify when speech-language pathology services may be considered special education rather than a related service" (p. 5). This means that when a student is only receiving speech therapy for dysfluency or phonology and the rest of the student's education is provided in regular education, speech and language service is considered a special education program. Specifically, this demands that all required steps in the process of placing a child into special education must be followed and completed. The process should be no different than placing the child into a program for autism or learning disabilities.

When our service is considered a "related service" and not a special education program, then the speech-language pathologist's paperwork is minimal. In this instance, the speech-language pathologist usually just provides an insert for the multidisciplinary team report and provides goals and objectives for the IEP. The rest of the written documentation is the responsibility of the special education teacher, with input from the rest of the educational team members. This means that for about 50 percent of the students enrolled on a typical school-age caseload, the clinician has much less paperwork than for the other 50 percent of the caseload. In no way is this meant to suggest that the paperwork is light, but rather that different responsibilities are assigned depending on the type of speech and language service provided. Table 14–4 summarizes the major federal statutes relating to the education of students with disabilities and notes the required paperwork.

IMPACT OF EDUCATIONAL POLICIES ON SLP SERVICES

Although federal laws and policies have increased paperwork, they have had a positive impact on the commitment to educate students with disabilities. Such laws and policies have mandated services and required they be provided by qualified personnel. They have encouraged, both directly and indirectly, that speech and language services be integrated with the rest of the student's educational program. Four distinct outcomes have been noted (1) the requirement for a full continuum of service for students with communication disorders, (2) the use of teaming and the consultative service delivery model, (3) the focus on generating outcome data and applying evidence-based practice in schools, and (4) the increased role of the speech-language pathologist in literacy.

Full Continuum of Service

The full continuum of service for students with disabilities is required by current federal and state rules and regulations and addresses the issues around least restrictive environment (LRE). IDEA 2004 reinforces that students must receive a free appropriate public education (FAPE) in the least restrictive environment to the maximum extent possible. Yell (1998) describes this continuum of placements as follows:

> The purpose of the continuum is to allow school personnel to choose from a number of options when determining a student's placement. The presence of these alternative placements ensures that students with disabilities will not be educated in settings more restrictive than necessary. If a student's individual education program (IEP) planning team determines that the general education placement is not appropriate for a student's individual needs, the student should be moved along the continuum of placements to a setting that offers an appropriate education with the least possible amount of segregation from his or her non-disabled peers. (p. 71)

The determination of placement must be made by each educational team based on the individual needs of each student. For students whose eligibility (disability category) for special education service is designated "speech or language impairment," there should also be a full continuum of service. The full continuum of service in speech and language allows the IEP team to address the LRE issues on an individual basis for students with communication disorders and no other disabilities.

In *The Twenty-Fifth Annual Report to Congress on the Implementation of the Individuals with Disabilities*

T A B L E 14–4 Federal Statutes Relating to Education of Students With Disabilities

Year	Name of Law	Law No.	Highlights	Paperwork Required	Concepts/ Acronyms Created
1973	Section 504 of the Rehabilitation Act of 1973	PL 93-112	Civil rights law to prohibit discrimination on the basis of disability in public or private programs and activities receiving federal financial assistance.	Notice of 504 Eligibility or Noneligibility	504 Coordinator; Self-evaluation; LRE; Related & supplemental aids & services
1975	Education for All Handicapped Children Act of 1975 (EHA) (Part B)	PL 94-142	Mandates a free, appropriate education for all handicapped students between the ages of 3 and 21. Provides for Individualized Education Programs (IEPs), due process, protection in evaluation procedures, and education in the least-restrictive environment.	Permission to Evaluate Multidisciplinary team evaluation report every 3 years Invitation to IEP Provide procedural safeguards document IEP at least annually Parental approval/disapproval of program	FAPE, LRE, PEL, IEP, MDT, LEA, SEA; Due Process Hearings Adversely affects educational performance
1986	Education for All Handicapped Children Act (Part H)	PL 99-457	Extends protections of the EHA to infants and toddlers (birth to age 3) through the establishment of a formula grant program. An important component of early intervention is the comprehensive Individualized Family Service Plan (IFSP).	Same as EHA plus: Multidisciplinary team evaluation report *twice* a year IFSP at least 2 times/year	IFSP; Require Family Involvement; Qualified Provider
1990	Americans with Disabilities Act (ADA)	PL 101-336	A civil rights law to prohibit discrimination solely on the basis of disability by mandating reasonable accommodations across all public and private settings, including private and public schools.	System of Documentation Received to avoid potential liability Public Notice	ADA Coordinator (for school districts with more than 49 employees); Auxiliary aids & services; Undue hardship; Requires new construction to meet regulations
1990	Individuals with Disabilities Education Act of 1990 (IDEA)	PL 101-476	(Includes birth through 21). Expands the discretionary programs, includes the additional categories of autism and traumatic brain injury as separate disability categories. Adds the statutory definitions of assistive technology device and service. Expands transition requirements. Replaced term *handicap* with *disability*.	Transition IEP for 16 yrs and older	AT, TBI, TIEP; Changed the name of the law from EHA to IDEA

(Continued)

T A B L E 14–4 Federal Statutes Relating to Education of Students With Disabilities (Continued)

Year	Name of Law	Law No.	Highlights	Paperwork Required	Concepts/ Acronyms Created
1993	Goals 2000: Educate America Act of 1993	PL 103-85	Describes inclusion of children with disabilities in school reform effort. Develops eight National Education Goals. Ensures that students with disabilities are educated to the maximum extent possible.		
1994	Improving America's Schools Act (IASA)	PL 103-382	Provides for professional development and lists competencies for all persons providing services, including related services and special education.		
1997	IDEA Amendments	PL 105-17	Encourages participation of students with disabilities in the general education curriculum and statewide and district assessments. Encourages parental involvement in the IEP team placement decisions. Ensures that communication and assistive technology needs of students are considered. Encourages use of voluntary mediations rather than attorneys and no cessation of services for disciplinary reasons if related to student's disability.	Additional paperwork required: Permission to Reevaluate Procedural safeguards provided more often Transition Plans start at 14 yrs Progress reports at least as often as regular education Expanded IEP areas to be covered	Progress monitoring; Manifestation determination; Measure progress related to the general education curriculum; All students with disabilities will participate in assessments either with or without accommodations or via alternative assessments.
2002			No Child Left Behind Act of 2001 PL 107-110 Encourages improving academic achievement for all students. Requires students with disabilities be included in statewide assessments that are used to determine whether schools and districts meet state goals. Drives significant gains in student achievement and holds states and schools more accountable for student progress. Focuses on accountability for results, an emphasis on teaching methods based on scientific research, expanded options for parents of children from disadvantaged backgrounds, and greater flexibility for states and schools in spending federal funds. Also focuses on effective reading instruction.	Documentation of statewide assessment results included as part of IEPs and individual evaluations; IEP documentation of appropriate test accommodations on state test for students with disabilities	Adequate Yearly Progress (AYP); statewide accountability system with annual measurable objectives for monitoring and reporting changes in performance among and across student subgroups, schools, and districts; highly qualified teacher; supplemental services; scientific research-based reading programs for children in grades K–3

T A B L E 14–4 (Continued)

Year	Name of Law	Law No.	Highlights	Paperwork Required	Concepts/ Acronyms Created
2003			Individuals with Disabilities Education Improvement Act (IDEA 2004) PL 108-446 Aligns IDEA with provisions of NCLB. Clarifies screening versus evaluation. Prohibits requiring a child to obtain a prescription as a condition for attending school, receiving an evaluation, or receiving service. Expands the "lack of instruction in reading" to include the essential components of reading instruction. Changes criteria for Specific Learning Disabilities so severe discrepancy between achievement and ability not required before receiving special education services. Revises time lines for reevaluation when parent and LEA agree. Eliminates requirement for "short-term objectives and benchmarks" for all children eligible for special education except those who are most severely cognitively disabled.	New data collection on classroom-based observations, educational needs of child, academic achievement & related developmental needs in Evaluation Report LEA must provide summary of student performance when student graduates or "ages out" of special education Documentation of team members whose attendance at IEP the LEA considers "not necessary" Addition of postsecondary IEP goals related to training, education, employment and independent living skills Also reduces Procedural Safeguards Notice to only once a year with exceptions Expedites changes to IEP if parent and LEA agree	Highly Qualified Personnel; Early Intervening Services; "Education needs"; Response to Intervention

SOURCE: ASHA *Guidelines for the Roles and Responsibilities of the School-Based Speech Language Pathologist.* ©1999, American Speech-Language-Hearing Association. (The two right-most columns and all of the information on PL 107-110 and PL 108-446 have been added to the original!) Adapted and reprinted with permission.

Education Act (United States Department of Education, 2003), which represents the data from the 2000–2001 school year, the placement data are as follows:

- Approximately 10 percent of 6- through 21-year-olds were receiving special education under IDEA. Although the percentage is lower than in the 1993–1994 school year, the actual number of students with disabilities being served was higher. There has been a slow increase in the numbers of students served since 1992.

- Around 96 percent of students with disabilities are being educated in regular school buildings. Almost half are in regular classrooms for most of the day.

- Students with speech and language disabilities are most likely to be educated in the regular classroom for longer periods of the day. About 86 percent of these students spend less than 21 percent of their school day being educated outside the regular classroom. Students with the most severe types of disabilities (multiple disabilities, mental retardation, or deaf-blindness) are more likely to be educated outside the regular classroom for longer periods of the day.

- Students with the most severe types of disabilities (deaf-blindness or multiple disabilities) are also more likely to be educated in separate environments.

- Very few students with specific learning disabilities, speech or language impairments, or developmental delay are educated in separate environments.

- Students with speech or language impairments are most likely to be educated with their nondisabled peers. They are also the least likely to be educated in the most restrictive, separate environments.

The prevalence data from this report verify that the speech and language disability category (18.6 percent) is still second only to specific learning disability (49.2 percent) in terms of prevalence across all disability categories. As noted previously, the actual prevalence is significantly higher when speech and language as a related service is considered. In the 1995 ASHA Survey of Speech-Language Pathology Services in School-Based Settings (Peters-Johnson, 1998), about half of the children on clinicians' caseloads had the primary diagnosis of speech-language impairment only, and about half had primary diagnoses other than speech and language. This would suggest that about 42 percent of the children enrolled in special education receive speech and language service. Therefore, it is critical that we provide speech and language services across the continuum of service delivery models if it is to meet the individual needs of the students enrolled.

When we review the ASHA data generated from the national survey of school-based practition-

T A B L E 14–5 Percentage Distribution of Respondents by Service Delivery Models by Age Groups of Children Served

Age Groups	Service Delivery Model				
	TP	SC	CB	CC	RR
Birth to 2 years	24	7	17	52	1
3 to 5 years	50	8	31	10	1
6 to 11 years	78	2	13	5	2
12 to 17 years	65	7	17	7	4
18+ years	48	8	23	16	5

NOTE: TP = traditional pull-out, SC = self-contained classroom, CB = classroom-based, CC = collaborative consultation, and RR = resource room.
SOURCE: From C. Peters-Johnson. LSHSS, 29, page 122. © 1998 American Speech-Language-Hearing Association. Reprinted by permission.

ers (Peters-Johnson, 1998) in terms of service delivery, the overall usage patterns of various models across and within the age groups are apparent. The data presented in Table 14–5 strongly demonstrate that, with the exception of the birth to 2-year age group, the traditional pullout (TP) model is used most frequently. In fact, in the 6- to 11-year age group and in the 12- to 17-year age group it was used 78 percent and 65 percent of the time, respectively. The percentages of respondents using the traditional pull-out model was even higher when data were grouped according to type of communication disorder. These data are presented in Table 14–5.

The overwhelming use of the traditional pull-out model was somewhat surprising since there had been a push for more integrated service for the past 20 years in our professional literature (ASHA, 1991, 1993; Blosser & Kratcoski, 1997; Eger, 1992; Frasinelli, Superior, & Myers, 1983; Nieptupski, Scheutz, & Ockwood, 1980). It was anticipated that the IEP changes enacted in the 1997 reauthorization of IDEA would significantly affect the overwhelming use of the traditional pull-out service delivery models implemented by SLPs in the schools. The changes delineated in IDEA 1997 focused on including regular educators as participants in the IEP meeting and on modifying the content of the IEP by using the general education curriculum as the reference point. All of these changes should have resulted in the greater utilization of more integrated speech and language service delivery models that include curriculum-based assessment and therapy.

However, when we look at the data from ASHA surveys in 2000 (ASHA, 2000) and in 2003 (ASHA, 2003a), ASHA-certified SLPs in school settings are still primarily using the traditional pull-out model of service delivery. The 2000 ASHA Schools Survey reported that a typical school-based SLP spent an average 23 hours per week providing services using the traditional pull-out model, 2 hours using the collaborative consultation model, and only 1 hour using a classroom-based/curriculum-based model. The 2003 ASHA SLP Caseload Report noted that more hours were spent using the traditional pull-out service model than all of the other types of services combined. Clinicians spent 19.9 hours per week on the traditional pull-out model; 3.5 hours on the self-contained classroom; 2.7 hours on the classroom-based/curriculum-based; 1.6 hours on collaborative consultation; 0.5 hours on the resource room; and 0.7 hours on other. Although the overall hours of time spent in models other than the traditional pull-out model are still low, it is worth noting that school-based clinicians are moving in the right direction in terms of accessing more integrated models of service delivery.

In light of our role in literacy learning, it is reasonable to assume that when the pull-out model is deemed most appropriate by the IEP team, it will be an integrated, context-based approach, not the traditional pull-out model. Progress will be measured at regular intervals using curriculum-based assessment. Therefore, there is reason to hope that the language–learning connection will finally be operationalized. All children will have access to the curriculum because the school-based speech-language pathologist will be a working partner with classroom teachers to provide a full continuum of service delivery to students with communication disorders. The ball is in our court, because according to the 2000 ASHA Schools Survey (ASHA, 2000), in most cases (87 percent), the clinician is responsible for determining the type of service delivery model.

Teaming and Consultative Models

For the past 10 years, the experts have talked about the fact that special education should not be a separate system but rather the utilization of effective instructional practices for all learners. Speech-language pathologists understand the critical impact that the language–learning connection has on academic performance. With these two constructs in mind, it is a natural progression to envision a time when school-based speech-language pathologists are a required member of each student's educational planning team. It is clear that teaming facilitates educationally relevant programming to address needs of students in the classroom. An IEP is currently required for each student deemed eligible to receive special education services. However, special education is still a separate system, in that the evaluation procedures, program development, and implementation required by special education rules and regulations (PL 94-142, PL 99-457, PL 101-476, PL 105-17, and PL 108-446) are not afforded to *all* learners. Even with the passage of the No Child Left Behind Act of 2001, it is not common practice to develop individualized student plans for each and every learner. The inclusion movement during the 1990s has certainly demonstrated how powerful school-based teams can be in designing and implementing effective instruction in the regular education setting (Villa & Thousand, 1995).

Speech-language pathologists need to focus more time on developing their teaming skills. Being an effective team member is a set of learned behaviors and should be a required part of the graduate program curriculum at universities. These skills will serve speech-language pathologists well whether in a business, health care, or school environment. According to Schroeder and Collins (1991):

> Team building is certainly not new to organizations today; however, it is becoming increasingly important as the team is replacing the individual as the main focus in innovative organizations. Organizations understand that a team can accomplish more than an individual working alone. Therefore, greater emphasis is being placed on team-building today than in the past. (p. 1)

T A B L E 14-6 Percentage Distribution of Respondents by Various Service Delivery Models and Type of Communication Disorder/Service

Communication Disorder/Service	Service Delivery Model				
	TP	SC	CB	CC	RR
Articulation/phonology	87	3	6	3	1
Fluency	86	2	5	6	1
Voice	79	3	8	9	1
Language	49	8	33	6	4
Dysphagia	61	9	12	16	2
Aural rehabilitation service	58	6	20	15	1
Orofacial myofunctional	78	5	7	8	1
Augmentative/alternative service	29	8	40	21	2
Communication instruction service	32	9	41	15	3
Cognitive communication	42	10	31	11	5
Central auditory processing	51	5	26	14	3
Other	40	19	17	12	12

NOTE: TP = traditional pull-out, SC = self-contained classrooms, CB = classroom-based, CC = collaborative construction, and RR = resource room.

SOURCE: From C. Peters-Johnson. *LSHSS*, *29*, page 123. © 1998 American Speech-Language-Hearing Association, Reprinted by permission.

Public schools are more than educational institutions today. They have become "big business." Hopefully, they are also innovative organizations. Much of the push for innovation has been inspired by the ever-changing school population. To meet the broad range of educational needs of a diverse group of learners, educational teams have been using the consultative service delivery as a viable option. Conner and Welsh (1993) purport that "schools hire speech-language pathologists to facilitate students' communication in the classroom. Thus, speech language pathology services must address not only students' ability to process and use language but also their ability to communicate successfully within the contexts of the total school environment" (p. 35). To do this efficiently and effectively, the consultative or collaborative service delivery model is a natural choice. Both models require excellent teaming skills to be successful.

The collaborative consultative service delivery model for school speech and language services has been described extensively in the literature over the past 15 years (ASHA 1991, 1993, 1996; Cooper, 1991; Coufal, 1993a, 1993b; Dodge & Mallard, 1992;

Ferguson, 1991, 1992; Frassinelli et al., 1983; Magnotta, 1991; Marvin, 1987; Montgomery, 1990, 1992; Moore-Brown, 1991; Russell & Kaderavek, 1993; Simon, 1987). DiMeo, Merritt, and Culatta (1998) described a joint decision-making process used to establish and implement collaborative goals within the classroom setting. This model builds on the mandates of IDEA 1997.

Although the consultative delivery model has been discussed in our literature for years, it is not routinely used by school-based clinicians. In the 1995 ASHA School Survey (Peters-Johnson, 1998), it is clear from the data depicted in Table 14–5 that across age groups, the collaborative consultation (CC) model is used less than 20 percent of the time, except in the birth to 2-years age group. Further, for the 70 percent of the national caseload reflected in the 6- to 17-years age groups, it was used less than 10 percent of the time. This percentage has not changed based on the ASHA 2003 Omnibus Survey results (ASHA, 2003a). It was hoped that the use of the consultative model would increase because of the reauthorization of IDEA and its mandate to measure progress using the general education curriculum and the requirement that the regular education teacher be a member of the IEP team. Federal mandates require the utilization of teams, and the speech-language pathologist must be an effective team player for student's needs to be addressed using the language–learning connection. It is worth noting that burdensome amounts of paperwork, high caseload size, and lack of time for planning, collaboration, and meeting with teachers were reported as the greatest challenges by the majority of school-based ASHA-certified speech-language pathologists in the 2000 Schools Survey (ASHA, 2000).

Outcome Data and Evidence-Based Practice

In the book *Measuring Outcomes in Speech-Language Pathology* (Frattali, 1998), Eger's (1998b) chapter addressing outcome measurement in the schools concludes:

> With education on the public agenda and viewed as the key to economic growth in the twenty-first century, the time has never been more critical for the generation of outcomes data to demonstrate educational results. It has been said that if you don't know where you're going, you won't know when you get there. It is time that we know where we are going in school-based speech and language services, produce the outcomes data to prove when we get there, and use the data to demonstrate that it made a difference. (p.451)

The 1997 reauthorization of IDEA required states to establish performance goals with indicators for children with disabilities that are consistent, to the extent appropriate, with all other goals and standards for children in the state. The focus is on one system, *not* a separate system of special education. These performance indicators will be required to address the performance of children with disabilities on assessment, dropout rates, and graduation rates. In addition, IDEA 1997 mandated that children with disabilities be included in all statewide and district assessment programs with necessary accommodations provided. The state is required to report these data on the number of students with disabilities

participating in regular and alternative assessments as well as their performance on the assessments.

NCLB requires states to adopt challenging academic content and performance standards in reading, math, and science. Each state must establish and specify performance levels of advanced, proficient, or basic in reading, math, and science and then administer academic assessments in these areas annually. By the 2005–2006 school year these state assessments must be aligned with the academic content and performance standards of the state. The focus of accountability has changed from inputs (process) to outcomes. It is no longer acceptable to just measure how many minutes of speech-language intervention a child receives per week; the measure now is what difference such service made in the student's educational performance. Some outcome indicators for students enrolled in speech and language services include IEPs, dismissal criteria, service delivery model effectiveness, and customer surveys. Logemann (1998) notes that we must measure the effects of our interventions and prove what a difference our treatment makes. Gallagher, Swigert, and Baum (1998) summarized ASHA's National Outcomes Measurement System for Speech-Language Pathology and Audiology with specific applications and challenges in the school setting. O'Brien and Huffman (1998) relate managed care to the school setting and highlight what we can expect as judged by the health care arena. The only way to survive the "cost containment fever" that is prevalent in all worksites is to generate outcomes data that verify the cost and value of our services.

In this era of accountability that has been molded by the spiraling costs of health care and special education and the need for improved outcomes in public education, the school-based SLP must apply an evidence-based practice (EBP) approach. The concept of EBP "... emphasizes the systematic and deliberate integration of science and craft, or, alternatively, data and theory" (Justice & Fey, 2004, p. 4). Justice and Fey (2004) explain that the clinician must systematically integrate evidence from scientific investigations with clinical expertise and contextual factors. The concepts of EBP are mandated in NCLB and IDEA 2004 under the term "scientifically based research" (Moore-Brown &

Montgomery, 2005). As succinctly stated by Justice and Fey (2004):

> The emphasis on EBP in school-based speech-language pathology does not place a singular focus on the use of evidence and research when making clinical decisions; rather, it emphasizes the need to consult the best available research to ensure clinical objectivity and currency. In this way, practitioners show greater accountability in their decisions. (p. 5)

Increased Role of the SLP in Literacy

The concept of the language–learning connection and the significant role it plays in learning to read is not new. Perhaps the practical application of this knowledge is more apparent due to the impact of IDEA '97 and NCLB. IDEA '97 required that the IEP goals and objectives allow the student to progress in the regular education curriculum, and NCLB required that states adopt and measure student proficiency in challenging academic standards that apply to *all* students. This impact is reflected in the 2004 ASHA Schools Survey (ASHA, 2004b), where approximately a third of the ASHA-certified respondents noted that they were more involved in literacy activities as a result of NCLB.

In the ASHA Schools 2000 (ASHA, 2000) and 2004 (ASHA, 2004b) surveys, respondents noted that 5 percent of their caseloads were *not impaired*. Although this is not a large percentage, it represents an increase of 25 percent from the 1995 Schools Survey (Peters-Johnson, 1998) findings. Another indicator that the school-based SLP should be involved to a greater extent in literacy learning is reflected by the development of the ASHA guidelines for SLPs with respect to their role in reading and writing (ASHA, 2001). The documents (ASHA, 2001) include an extensive body of research that describes the relationship between oral language learning and reading and states that the position statement was designed to narrow the gap between research and practice. The guidelines also address the National Education Goals (United States Department of Education, America Reads Challenge,

1997) and respond to the national standards movement. They are consistent with the requirements of IDEA 1997. ASHA (2005b) notes:

> Literacy is an essential prerequisite for social well-being, academic achievement and lifetime opportunities. Language problems are both a cause and a consequence of literacy problems in children and adolescents. Because of this, speech-language pathologists play important roles in ensuring that all children gain access to appropriate instruction in reading, writing and spelling—so that no child is left behind. These roles include the following: Early Identification, Intervention, Development of Literacy Programs. (p. 1)

It is noteworthy that IDEA 2004 prohibits eligibility for special education due to a lack of appropriate instruction in reading. The essential components of reading instruction as codified in NCLB and referenced in IDEA 2004 are phonemic awareness, phonics, vocabulary development, reading fluency, and reading comprehension strategies. As stated by Moore-Brown and Montgomery (2005), "The five essential components of reading are familiar to speech-language pathologists, who have the most comprehensive training of any personnel in the school regarding language development and its functional application for activities such as learning and reading" (p. 38).

With the current emphasis of NCLB and IDEA 2004 on post-secondary outcomes, the role of the SLP in literacy with secondary school students has never been more necessary. With this population the clinician must combine relevant treatment with strategies to prepare these students for postsecondary educational and vocational settings (Banotai, 2005). There is reason to be encouraged that with the increased role in literacy of the school-based SLP, more students will be able to succeed in the regular education curriculum. The federal laws and the research suggest that language learning and literacy should be developed and treated within the larger context of school learning and interactions. It should be aligned and integrated with the classroom curriculum and the skills needed to function in the classroom.

IMPACT OF LEGISLATION ON AUDIOLOGY IN SCHOOLS

Four major federal statutes have influenced audiology in the schools. They are Section 504 of the Rehabilitation Act of 1973, PL 94-142 the Education for All Handicapped Children Act, PL 99-457 the Education for the Handicapped Act Amendments of 1986, and PL 101-476 Individuals with Disabilities Education Act. More recent revisions of IDEA in 1997 and 2004 and NCLB may also affect the practice of audiology in the schools. Other federal mandates and provisions, such as universal newborn hearing screening and Medicaid's Early and Periodic Screening Diagnosis and Treatment programs have helped to identify children with hearing loss at earlier and earlier ages and to assist with appropriate referrals and services.

Section 504 of the Rehabilitation Act of 1973

As noted earlier in this chapter, Section 504 of the Rehabilitation Act of 1973 was civil rights legislation and has many similarities to PL 94-192. It provides significant protection to all children whether or not they are identified as eligible under special education laws. Johnson, Benson, and Seaton (1997) suggest that

> We are just beginning to realize the tremendous impact of Section 504 for children having milder, yet still significant, disabilities who may not meet special education "eligibility" requirements. Two groups for which this law has significant implications are children with milder hearing impairments and children having central auditory processing difficulties. For both of these groups, acoustic accessibility is an invisible barrier to their hearing and/or understanding of auditory information. (p. 9)

PL 94-142 The Education for All Handicapped Children Act

This landmark legislation, which changed the face of public education in the United States, clearly specified audiology as a special education "related service." It specified that audiology included the following:

(i) Identification of children with hearing loss;

(ii) Determination of the range, nature, and degree of hearing loss, including referral for medical or other professional attention for the habilitation of hearing;

(iii) Provision of habilitation activities, such as language habilitation, auditory training, speech reading, (lipreading), hearing evaluation, and speech conservation;

(iv) Creation and administration of programs for prevention of hearing loss;

(v) Counseling and guidance of pupils, parents, and teachers regarding hearing loss;

(vi) Determination of the child's need for group and individual amplification, selecting and fitting an appropriate aid, and evaluating the effectiveness of amplification. (34 CFR 300.12[b], pp. 9–10)

This law clearly defined the scope of audiology services that are appropriate for children with hearing impairment in the schools. This definition was essentially unchanged in the 1999 final IDEA Regulations. According to the ASHA *Guidelines for Audiology Service Provision in and for Schools* (ASHA, 2002b), the IDEA regulations clearly delineated the role of the audiologist in the schools. It is important to note, however, that this definition has had limited impact because each state provides its own definitions of services, including audiology services.

Additional regulation was passed in 1976 as a result of a Bureau of Education of the Handicapped study requested by the 1976 House of Representatives Appropriations Committee. This regulation is the Proper Function of Hearing Aids. It states: "Each public agency shall ensure that the hearing aids worn by children with hearing impairment including deafness in the schools are functioning properly" (34 CFR 300.303). This regulation was passed in response to the 1976 study, which found that up to one-third of the hearing aids worn by children in schools were malfunctioning.

PL 99-457 The Education for the Handicapped Act Amendments of 1986

This act extended the provisions of PL 94-142 to preschoolers (3- to 5-year-olds) and authorized early intervention services to handicapped infants and toddlers and their families (birth to age 2). Significantly, audiologists were included as qualified personnel for providing early intervention services.

PL 101-476 Individuals with Disabilities Education Act (IDEA)

The amendments added to PL 94-142 in 1990 renamed the statute IDEA. The most important aspects of these amendments for audiology were the statutory definitions of *assistive technology device* and *assistive technology service*. These definitions in federal law included assistive listening devices and training or assistance to use them so the child can receive a free and appropriate public education.

PL 105-17 1997 IDEA Amendments and PL 108-446 IDEA 2004

IDEA 1997 required service providers, including audiologists, to hold the highest qualifications required by their state for a particular profession. IDEA 2004 may eliminate this provision. It says that the qualifications may match any state-approved licensing, certification, or comparable requirement. IDEA 2004 allows the audiologist to be excluded from the IEP meeting if the parent and the LEA agree, and the new law allows the IEP to be modified without a meeting. These changes could significantly reduce the role of the audiologist at IEP meetings (Banotai, 2005).

IDEA 2004 also includes a change to the definition of *assistive technology device* so that medical devices that are surgically implanted or the replacement of such devices are not considered related services. This clarifies that the surgical implanting of cochlear implants is not included as a related service, but the mapping of the implant is allowed to be part of the related services provided by the audiologist, if the IEP team deems that these services are needed for FAPE.

SUMMARY

It is clear from this review of the key federal statutes that have influenced education policy for speech and language services in the schools that our services are forever changed. Speech and language services have moved from regular education to special education with the advent of PL 94-142 and now back to regular education as well as special education with the passage of NCLB. Significant procedures and paperwork requirements have been mandated for enrolling and dismissing students into and out of therapy. Most of the funding of these services has moved from regular education to special education budgets. Each level of government has established documentation requirements to ensure compliance with state and federal mandates. In general, the impact on speech-language

services in the schools has been positive. The speech-language pathologist is a valuable member of the educational team. Service delivery is more integrated and uses language–learning research to design programs that assist students with success in the educational curriculum. The clinician is measuring student outcomes and reporting progress to parents and the rest of the educational team on a regular basis.

The major influences of federal statutes on audiology services in the schools are: the specification of audiology as a related service; the definition of the scope of audiology services; the inclusion of audiologists as qualified personnel in the provision of early intervention services; and the statutory definitions of assistive technology device and assistive technology service. When audiology services are provided to students with disabilities, they are designated as a "related service." The specific definition of these services is determined at the state level. There is some concern that some of the new provisions of IDEA 2004 could reduce the role of the audiologist at IEP meetings.

CRITICAL THINKING

1. What are the major differences between school-based speech and language services and audiology services as defined in key federal legislation?

2. Why is so much paperwork required for the speech-language pathologist in the schools?

3. Why is "speech and language" designated both a "special education program" and a "related service" in PL 94-142 and its revisions?

4. Have the effects of the key federal statutes been positive or negative on speech and language and audiology services in the schools?

5. Why is it important for the school-based SLP or audiologist to keep abreast of educational legislation at the federal and state levels?

6. What future legislation do you think is needed to provide quality audiology or SLP services in the schools?

7. How can audiologists and speech-language pathologists work more collaboratively in educational settings?

8. What skills do you think a speech-language pathologist or audiologist needs to work effectively in school settings?

REFERENCES

Achilles, J., & Lewis R. C. (1996–1997, Fall). School health and related services (SHARS) program: Medicaid reimbursement. *Texas Journal of Audiology and Speech Pathology, 22*(1), 38–42.

American Speech-Language-Hearing Association. (1991). A model for collaborative service delivery for students with language-learning disorders in the public schools. *Asha, 33* (Suppl. 5), 44–50.

American Speech-Language-Hearing Association, Governmental and Social Policies Coordinating Committee. (1992). *Technical assistance report—Retraining personnel to meet the highest requirements in the state.* Rockville, MD: Author.

American Speech-Language-Hearing Association. (1993). Caseload size and speech-language service delivery in the school. *Asha, 35* (Suppl. 10), 33–39.

American Speech-Language-Hearing Association. (1996). Inclusive practices for children and youths with communication disorders. *Asha, 38* (Suppl. 16), 35–44.

American Speech-Language-Hearing Association. (1999). *Guidelines for the roles and responsibilities of the school-based speech-language pathologist.* Rockville, MD: Author.

American Speech-Language-Hearing Association. (2000). *2000 schools survey, Special report: Service delivery.* Rockville, MD: Author

American Speech-Language-Hearing Association. (2001). *Roles and responsibilities of speech-language pathologists with respect to reading and writing in children and adolescents.* Rockville, MD: Author.

American Speech-Language-Hearing Association. (2002a). *A workload analysis approach for establishing speech-language caseload standards in the schools.* Rockville, MD: Author.

American Speech-Language-Hearing Association. (2002b). *Guidelines for audiology service provision in and for schools.* Rockville, MD: Author.

American Speech-Language-Hearing Association. (2003a). *2003 Omnibus survey caseload report: SLP.* Rockville, MD: Author.

American Speech-Language-Hearing Association. (2003b, June). *Medicaid and third party payments in the schools.* Available at http://www.asha.org/

American Speech-Language-Hearing Association. (2004a). *Medicaid guidance for speech-language pathology services: Addressing the "under the direction of" rule.* Available at http://www.asha.org/

American Speech-Language-Hearing Association. (2004b). *2004 Schools survey report: Caseload characteristics.* Rockville, MD: Author

American Speech-Language-Hearing Association. (2005a, August). *Medicaid payment for school-based services.* Available at http://www.asha.org/

American Speech-Language-Hearing Association. (2005b) *Literacy: Speech-language pathologists play a pivotal role.* Available at http://www.asha.org/

American Speech-Language-Hearing Association. (n.d.) *No Child Left Behind: Fact sheets.* Available at http://www.asha.org/

Banotai, A. (2005, August 15). Strategic instruction: Literacy tools and strategies for secondary school students. *Advance for Speech-Language Pathologists and Audiologists, 15*(33), 7–9, 13.

Blosser, J. L., & Kratcoski, A. (1997, April). PACs: A framework for determining appropriate service delivery options. *Language, Speech and Hearing Services in Schools, 28,* 99–107.

Conner, T. N., & Welsh, R. (1993, June/July). Teams and teamwork—Educational settings. *Asha, 35,* 35–36.

Cooper, C. S. (1991). Using collaborative/consultative service delivery models for fluency intervention and carryover. *Language, Speech and Hearing Services in Schools, 22,* 152–153.

Coufal, K. L. (Ed.). (1993a). Collaborative consultation: A problem-solving process. *Topics in Language Disorders, 14*(1), 1–100.

Coufal, K. L. (1993b, November). Collaborative consultation for speech-language pathologists. *Topics in Language Disorders, 14*(1), 1–14.

Deppe, J. (2005, September 6). Funding answers for school-based members. *ASHA Leader, 4.*

DiMeo, J. H., Merritt, D. D., & Culatta, B. (1998). Collaborative partnerships and decision making. In D. D. Merritt & B. Culatta (Eds.), *Language Intervention in the classroom* (pp. 37–97). San Diego, CA: Singular Publishing Group.

Dodge, E. P., & Mallard, A. R. (1992). Social skills training using a collaboration service delivery model. *Language, Speech and Hearing Service in Schools, 23,* 130–135.

Eger, D. L. (1992). Why now? Changing school speech-language service delivery. *Asha, 34,* 40–41.

Eger, D. L. (1998a). Allegheny Intermediate Unit speech and language program data for the 1997–1998 school year. Unpublished program data. Pittsburgh, PA.

Eger, D. L. (1998b). Outcomes measurement in the schools. In C. Frattali (Ed.), *Measuring outcomes in speech-language pathology* (pp. 438–452). New York: Thieme.

Eger, D. L. (2005). Personal communcation with Vaughn Moreau, Program Director, Speech, Language, Hearing, and Vision Programs, Allegheny Intermediate Unit, Pittsburgh, PA.

Ferguson, M. L. (1991). Clinical forum—Collaborative/consultative service delivery: An introduction. *Language, Speech, and Hearing Services in Schools, 22,* 147.

Ferguson, M. L. (1992). Clinical forum: Implementing collaborative consultation—An introduction. *Language, Speech, and Hearing Services in Schools, 23,* 361–362.

Frasinelli, L., Superior, K., & Myers, J. (1983). A consultation model for speech and language intervention, *Asha, 25,* 25–30.

Frattali, C. M. (Ed.). (1998). *Measuring outcomes in speech-language pathology.* New York: Thieme.

Gallagher, T. M., Swigert, N., & Baum, H. M. (1998). Collecting outcomes data in schools: Needs and challenges. *Language, Speech, and Hearing Services in Schools, 29*(4), 250–256.

Johnson, C. D., Benson, P. V., & Seaton, J. B. (1997). Educational audiology: How did we get here? In *Educational audiology handbook* (pp. 3–15). San Diego, CA: Singular Publishing Group.

Justice, L. M., & Fey, M. E. (2004, Sept. 21). Evidence-based practice in schools: Integrating craft and theory with science and data. *ASHA Leader, 4–5,* 30–32.

Logemann, J. A. (1998). Treatment outcomes and efficacy in the schools. *Language, Speech, and Hearing Services in Schools, 29*(4), 243–244.

Magnotta, O. H. (1991). Looking beyond tradition. *Language, Speech and Hearing Services in Schools, 22,* 150–151.

Marks, A. (2005, August 19). Local discontent with "No Child Left Behind" grows. *The Christian Science Monitor.* Available at http://www.csmonitor.com/

Marvin, C. A. (1987). Consultation services: Changing roles for SLPs. *Journal of Childhood Communication Disorders, 11*(1), 1–15.

McLaughlin, M. (1997). *Special education in an era of school reform—An overview.* Washington, DC: The Federal Resource Center.

Montgomery, J. K. (1990). Consultative collaboration: Making the new model work. *Clinical Connection, 4*(3), 8–9.

Montgomery, J. K. (1992). Perspectives from the field: Language, speech and hearing services in schools. *Language, Speech and Hearing Services in Schools, 23,* 363–364.

Montgomery, J. K. (1993). The law and the school professional. In R. J. Lowe (Ed.), *Speech-language pathology and related professions in the schools* (pp. 67–85). Boston: Allyn and Bacon.

Moore-Brown, B. J. (1991). Moving in the direction of change: Thoughts for administrators and speech-language pathologists. *Language, Speech and Hearing Services in Schools, 22,* 148–149.

Moore-Brown, B. J., & Montgomery, J. K. (2005). *Making a difference in the era of accountability: Update on NCLB and IDEA 2004.* Eau Claire, WI: Thinking Publications.

Neidecker, E. A., & Blosser, J. L. (1993). *School programs in speech-language—Organization and management.* Englewood Cliffs, NJ: Prentice Hall.

Nelson, N. N. (1993). Public policy and service delivery. In *Childhood language disorders in context: Infancy through adolescence* (2nd ed., pp. 115–181). Boston: Allyn and Bacon.

Nieptupski, J., Scheutz, G., & Ockwood, L. (1980). The delivery of communication therapy services to severely handicapped students: A plan for change. *Journal of Association of Severely Handicapped, 45*(1), 13–23.

O'Brien, M. A., & Huffman, N. P. (1998). Impact of managed care in the schools. *Language, Speech and Hearing Services in Schools, 29*(4), 263–269.

Pennsylvania Department of Education, Bureau of Special Education. (1998). *Individuals with Disabilities Education Act Amendments of 1997: Level II implementation training manual.* Harrisburg, PA: Author.

Peters-Johnson, C. (1998, April). Survey of speech-language pathology services in school-based settings-national study final report. *Language, Speech and Hearing Services in Schools, 29,* 120–126.

Russell, S. C., & Kaderavek, J. N. (1993). Alternative models of collaboration. *Language Speech and Hearing Services in Schools, 24,* 76–78.

Schroeder, L., & Collins, A. (1991, March). Team-building in today's business world. *Alternatives in Health and Wellness.* Rockville, MD: Institute for Human Resources.

Simon, C. (1987). Making the collaborative consultative model work: The speech-language pathologist as consultant and teacher in mainstream education. *Journal of Childhood Communication Disorders, 11*(1), 1–234.

U.S. Department of Education. (1996). *Eighteenth annual report to Congress on the implementation of the Individuals with Disabilities Education Act.* Washington, DC: Author.

U.S. Department of Education, America Reads Challenge. (1997). *Read right now.* Washington, DC: Author.

U.S. Department of Education. (2003). *Twenty-fifth annual report to Congress on the implementation of the Individuals with Disabilities Education Act.* Washington, DC: Author.

Villa, R. A., & Thousand, J. S. (Eds.). (1995). *Creating an inclusive school.* Alexandria, VA: Association and Curriculum Development.

Yell, M. L. (1998). The legal basis of inclusion. *Educational Leadership, 56*(2), 70–81.

RESOURCES

American Speech-Language-Hearing Association
10801 Rockville Pike
Rockville, MD 20852-3279

Phone: 800-498-2071, 301-897-5700;
fax: 301-571-0457
Web site: http://www.asha.org

The American Speech-Language-Hearing Association (ASHA) is the professional, scientific, and credentialing association for more than 118,000 members and affiliates who are audiologists, speech-language pathologists, and speech, language, and hearing scientists. Its mission is to promote the interests of and provide the highest quality services for professionals in audiology, speech-language pathology, and speech and hearing science, and to advocate for people with communication disabilities.

The Council for Exceptional Children (CEC)
1110 North Glebe Road, Suite 300
Arlington, VA 22201
Phone: 703-620-3660; TTY: 866-915-5000;
fax: 703-264-9494
Web site: http://www.cec.sped.org
The Council for Exceptional Children (CEC) is the largest international professional organization dedicated to improving educational outcomes for individuals with exceptionalities, students with disabilities, and/or gifted students. CEC advocates for appropriate governmental policies, sets professional standards, provides continual professional development, advocates for newly and historically underserved individuals with exceptionalities, and helps professionals obtain conditions and resources necessary for effective professional practice.

Educational Audiology Association (EAA)
13153 N Dale Mabry Hwy, Suite 105
Tampa, FL 33618
Phone: 800-460-7322
Web site: http://www.edaud.org
The Educational Audiology Association (EAA) is an international organization of audiologists and related professionals who deliver a full spectrum of hearing services to all children, particularly those in educational settings. The Mission of the EAA is to act as the primary resource and active advocate for its members through its publications and products, continuing educational activities, networking opportunities, and other professional endeavors.

The *Special Educator* Newsletter
LRP Publications Dept. 430
747 Dresher Road, P.O. Box 980
Horsham, PA 19044-0980
Phone: 800-341-7874
This bimonthly newsletter provides a look at the trends shaping special education nationwide. It is not specific to speech-language pathology and audiology. The newsletter provides ongoing interpretations of the law and includes cases that involve related services issues.

IDEA Partnership
Web site: http://www.ideapartnership.org
Collaborative work of more than 55 national organizations, technical assistance providers, and state and local organizations and agencies; also includes IDEA and NCLB updates.

U.S. Department of Education
Web site: http://www.ed.gov/offices/OSERS/IDEA/
Updates, IDEA law, technical assistance, regulations, training articles, speeches, *Federal Register* notices, letters, memos.
Web site: http://www.ed.gov/nclb
Overview of NCLB, Updates, A-Z index, information by states, and many other items.

Wrightslaw
Web site: http://www.wrightslaw.com
Up-to-date information about special education law and advocacy for children with disabilities; *The Special Ed Advocate,* a free online newsletter.

15

Service Delivery in Educational Settings

MAUREEN STASKOWSKI, PHD
NICKOLA WOLF NELSON, PHD

SCOPE OF CHAPTER

In this chapter we address the issues of school service delivery from several perspectives. The underlying theme is that speech-language pathologists and audiologists working in school settings have unique potential to work with others to address the communication health of all students. This collaborative consultative role includes direct services to students with speech-language-communication and hearing disorders, but it also includes a wide array of other collaborative services aimed at preventing school failure among children at risk due to language-literacy learning weaknesses, self-regulation problems, and social interaction difficulties.

Meaningful collaborative services cannot be accomplished by SLPs who work in separate rooms, functioning only as the "speech teacher" who slips in and out of the building at odd times, pulling selected children out, playing games or providing activities isolated from the curriculum, and then sending them back to class. Although the job of the school-based SLP brings many challenges, it also has the potential to bring high rewards. SLPs in today's schools have fresh opportunities to change how the position is conceptualized. These are addressed in the first section of the chapter.

The second section addresses SLPs' primary role to help individual students with communication disorders make changes in their communication systems. Individualized service delivery is illustrated with a case study of Sara. As a child with specific speech-language impairment, Sara is a student who can "almost but not quite" fulfill the expectations of the general education curriculum (Nelson, 1998). We describe how speech-language services can assist students like Sara and how service delivery might differ for other students with multiple and severe disabilities.

The third section of the chapter describes varied service delivery models. It ends with a consideration of what it means to shift from a caseload to a workload perspective of what the position of school-based SLP entails. Across the chapter, we indicate how the roles we describe are compatible with mandates of the 2004 version of the Individuals with Disabilities Educational Improvement Act (PL 108-446), known as "IDEA 2004," and the latest version of the Elementary and Secondary School Act, No Child Left Behind, as introduced in Chapter 14. In particular, Sara's case illustrates how the prevention and scientific, research-based practices focus of IDEA 2004 and NCLB influence practice.

SPECIAL OPPORTUNITIES FOR THE SCHOOL-BASED SLP

Between the ages of 5 and 18, children spend the majority of their waking hours in schools using oral and written communication skills to participate academically. They also engage in school-related activities to gain acceptance from peers and experience the affirmation of friends. The ability to participate fully and successfully in academic and extracurricular experiences is limited, for many children with speech, language, and hearing impairments.

Relevance and Continuity

Children with communication disorders experience many advantages from receiving speech-language intervention services in schools. Clinicians have unique opportunities to work with children in the communicative contexts that are critical to their academic success. SLPs and audiologists in schools have direct access to the curriculum. They also have access to classrooms and can observe how students interact with peers in both academic and social contexts. Communication professionals working in schools are well placed to provide services that are relevant to students' most pressing needs and to target improved skills for communicating appropriately in multiple contexts.

Children and adolescents with speech and language impairments face many challenges in school settings. Language impairments, in particular, are associated with difficulties in reading, writing, higher-order thinking, pragmatics, and other aspects of school curriculum (Bashir, Conte, & Heerde, 1998; Catts & Kamhi, 2005; Nelson, 1998; Silliman & Wilkinson, 2004). SLPs and teachers working together can alter the accommodations, treatment strategies, and service frequency to meet students' needs. They can make adjustments when changes in teachers or subjects bring new challenges for students.

SLPs and audiologists in schools often have the opportunity to work with students and their families over a number of years across many developmental and environmental transitions. By virtue of their longitudinal experiences, such professionals can provide effective assessment, therapeutic, and consultative services for students, teachers, and families. This background knowledge also allows school clinicians to take the lead in organizing a network of supports for students with long-term communication difficulties.

Developing Collegial Relationships

Communication professionals in schools who are viewed as full members of the school staff are situated best to make a difference for children. Identification, assessment, and intervention require working closely with other professionals, and the quality of the collaboration makes a difference in the quality of service (Ehren, 2003; Staskowski & Zagaiski, 2003). This has a direct effect on children, as student accomplishments are affected by the "quality of adult relationships within a school" (Barth, 1990, p. 63). The goal is to be considered a member of the school staff and to be included in academic and social activities that will naturally facilitate meaningful service delivery.

Professionals attain collegiality when they engage in dialogue about teaching and learning, observe one another teaching, engage together in activities related to the curriculum, and learn from one another (Barth, 1990). In this way, SLPs benefit from teachers' strategies, knowledge of curriculum, and classroom management. SLPs and audiologists also share information about disabilities, their impact, and strategies for compensating with other professionals, such as occupational and physical therapists, social workers, and psychologists. Trust develops so that professionals feel safe to observe one another in practice, seeking to grow professionally and not fearing criticism.

Working together to address the needs of a population of children or an individual child, collaborative meetings should begin with questions about mutual goals and setting a common purpose (Nelson, 1998). Collaborative climates also are encouraged when communication professionals ask teachers and others to share their own professional advice, articles, books, and resources in areas of common interest. Sharing ideas and resources develops a common frame of reference. This open dialogue gives SLPs and audiologists an opportunity to help teachers, administrators, and parents understand communication disorders while also learning more about what others have to offer.

Becoming part of the school staff requires taking an active role and interest in matters important to the school. Many SLPs have developed relationships with colleagues through participation in school literacy efforts. When coworkers get to know one another, it becomes easier to expose one's doubts and questions, to welcome classroom observations, and to share practices. Even the simple act of eating with teachers in the school lounge or participating in other social events can provide opportunities for coworkers to learn about each other and increase their comfort levels for interacting in other contexts. Other ways that SLPs become part of the schools include participation in staff meetings and on committees, school improvement teams, teams planning initiatives to measure responsiveness to intervention.

One SLP offered to lead the elementary school's application to be considered for a "Blue Ribbon Award." Her hard work paid off when the school adopted a new motto: "All children belong. All children can learn. All children can communicate." Subsequent collaborative efforts were then framed within this common vision. Public relations efforts can intensify during the month of May, which each year this month is designated "Better Hearing and Speech Month." During this time, SLPs promote their services through classroom presentations, school programs, and parent education. ASHA has promotional materials for this purpose, or SLPs may develop their own materials and lessons. For example, one SLP in a middle school offered to do a listening lesson in classrooms during May. The lesson was designed to increase awareness of the importance of good listening and strategies to improve comprehension. Afterward, the teachers made more appropriate referrals for the SLP's service, asked advice, shared materials, and invited the SLP back to the classroom to work together with students on their caseload. Activities such as this promote collegiality and help teachers and SLPs relate services to the curriculum, two vital aspects for services in schools (Staskowski & Zagaiski, 2003).

Bridging Pull-out Services to Classroom Contexts A climate of collegiality facilitates collaborative consultation and coteaching. Many schools already provide a full continuum of speech-language and hearing services, including classroom-based services. When teachers have not worked with communication professionals in this manner, extra effort may be required to introduce them to the possibilities. Table 15–1 summarizes 10 suggestions for gaining invitations from teachers to work with students in their classrooms. All of these strategies can be applied with students of different ages and in a variety of school settings. Although each takes

T A B L E 15–1 Ten Strategies for Being Invited into Classrooms

1. Use curriculum-relevant materials with your student outside the room, then offer a coordinating classroom lesson.

2. Ask advice for working with a student, then suggest working in the classroom to learn more.

3. Demonstrate classroom services during your work with a group of at-risk students.

4. Share observations/suggestions for students that are relevant to teachers' concerns, then offer to come into the classroom to help try the strategies.

5. Offer help during cooperative groups or experiments, then explain goals addressed.

6. Offer to provide a center during center time.

7. Help with an at-risk student or group of students by brainstorming strategies, consulting on implementation, or offering to provide a supplemental intervention.

8. Ask to observe a student to monitor progress and try out strategies for carryover, then offer to return on an ongoing basis.

9. Learn about a teacher's interests, then offer instructional support in that topic, such as a graphic organizer or children's literature selection.

10. Become active on the school improvement committee or other key school activities, then refer back to committee topics when offering to team up with a teacher.

time, efforts to connect with teachers to offer speech and language services in context are rewarded by positive student outcomes. Sharing the load is one way SLPs in schools can reduce the stress of having more to do than is humanly possible.

Roles of SLPs Related to Literacy One of the key factors for SLPs in breaking out of traditional limited roles as a building's "speech teacher" involves conveying what SLPs bring to society's mutual goal to help all students acquire literate communication abilities that will help them succeed in school and in life (ASHA, 2000). SLPs can become important contributors to the school's efforts toward literacy in all areas—prevention,

identification, and intervention for reading and writing difficulties (e.g., Ehren & Nelson, 2005; Staskowski & Zagaiski, 2003; Staskowski & Rivera, 2005; Troia, 2005).

SLPs play an important role planning and implementing early intervention for struggling readers. They help to identify students at-risk for literacy difficulties and are increasingly involved in developing systematic intervention and progress monitoring models for at-risk students (Staskowski & Rivera, 2005). SLPs also help with implementation as they provide ongoing consultation and, in some cases, direct service for small groups of at-risk students. These are important roles in a time when federal initiatives such as No Child Left Behind are placing literacy center stage, especially the early identification and prevention of reading difficulties. SLPs also are becoming more active on district committees that focus on the language arts curriculum. Such work involves designing accommodations, modifications, and differentiated instruction for other subjects.

SLPs and audiologists are playing increasingly collaborative roles in school settings. Although many aspects of the roles make them challenging, the opportunity to work with others to address the communication health of a wide range of students in contexts highly relevant to their needs can make it particularly rewarding. SLPs and audiologists must take deliberate steps to be accepted as full members of the school staff. They must convey to teachers, administrators, parents, and others that their special expertise will help students succeed in school and life.

PROCEDURES FOR SERVING CHILDREN IN SCHOOL SETTINGS

School-based SLPs have core responsibilities in the prevention, identification, assessment, evaluation, and intervention for oral and written communication disorders. They also have other roles related to community partnerships, professional leadership, and advocacy for students, programs, and facilities (ASHA, 1999).

Prevention

Prevention activities are designed to stop or minimize the onset of communication disorders or to reduce the risk of negative impact from a disorder (ASHA, 2004). Activities related to prevention include educating school staff, administrators, and families about communication disorders through awareness activities or in-service presentations. Prevention also includes consulting and collaborating with other educators to improve educational environments and curricula to promote oral and written language. Finally prevention can include consultation, collaboration, or periods of intervention for specific students or groups of students considered at risk for oral or written communication disorders (Moore-Brown, Montgomery, Bielinski, & Shubin, 2005; Staskowski & Rivera, 2005; Troia, 2005).

SLPs have a unique role in assisting school teams for students at risk for speech, language, and learning disabilities (ASHA, 2000). Schools today are challenged by the goal of NCLB to help every child to succeed. This involves tracking the performance of all students and helping struggling students meet expectations. IDEA 2004 allows school teams to use the student's response to scientific, research-based intervention as part of an evaluation for learning disabilities (Sec. 614(b)(6)(a, b)). These efforts are often referred to as responsiveness-to-intervention initiatives.

Responsiveness-to-Intervention: A Prevention Model Responsiveness-to-intervention (RTI) is a framework for preventing and identifying learning disabilities (Graner, Fagella-Luby, & Fritschmann, 2005). This model also may be used for preventing and identifying speech and language disorders (Ehren & Nelson, 2005). Although schools vary in how they execute RTI initiatives, RTI is frequently described as including three tiers of intervention. The first tier includes the provision of research-based instruction in spoken and written language for all students. The progress of all students is monitored. The second tier adds supplemental interventions for students not meeting predetermined criteria on progress measures. Interventions are selected carefully using evidence-based practices, and students' progress is followed more frequently. The third tier involves intensified intervention for students who have not progressed adequately, even with the supplemental interventions in the second tier. In some initiatives, the third tier is the provision of special education. This framework is viewed as an alternative to the use of cognitive referencing, or the discrepancy model, of special education eligibility determination that was used for learning disabilities and frequently for language impairments (Ehren & Nelson, 2005; Troia, 2005). SLPs may offer consultation and classroom-based collaborative services within all three tiers. Sara's case study illustrates how the process begins.

Participation on building teams such as this enables SLPs to become involved with students who are at-risk and to help teachers know which students to refer for formal assessment if they continue to struggle. This is one way in which the SLP's role can expand beyond "speech teacher" to be valued as communication consultant for teachers and students throughout the building. Communication is such a natural phenomenon that many people take it for granted and may not realize that a language disorder or other form of communication impairment may be involved when a student is struggling academically or socially. Comprehension difficulties are particularly likely to be missed. Lack of compliance with teacher directions, for example, may be interpreted as a behavioral issue, when inadequate language skills actually are an important component of the problem. Other children with functional basic communication skills may have higher-level language problems that interfere with their understanding of language of the general education curriculum in both its spoken and written forms. Others may have adequate word-level decoding, spelling abilities, and literal comprehension but may demonstrate difficulties with conversational pragmatics and abstract comprehension and expression.

Small Group Intervention Work and the Classroom   ✳ ✳ ✳

Ms. Brown, a second grade teacher, has been monitoring the progress of all of her students in reading and writing. She meets with the other second grade teachers regularly to analyze class data and talk about students who are struggling. As the SLP, you and the reading specialist (Title I teacher) meet occasionally with the grade level team to discuss students having difficulty and to strategize. You have become familiar with some of the students who are struggling when you have come into the classroom to collaborate with the teacher and to provide intervention for students on your caseload using a writing lab approach (Nelson, Bahr, & Van Meter, 2004). You work with the teacher to revise plans for the upcoming week and decide to begin a new intervention program with a small group of students showing difficulty in reading comprehension. The plan calls for you to work with the group once weekly, including at least one of the students with comprehension problems who is already on your caseload as having a language impairment.

After considering various interventions, you and the team decide to implement the LEARN strategy (Vernon, Schumaker, & Deschler, 1999), a research-validated comprehension strategy for identifying main ideas and learning or remembering the concepts. The plan calls for you to introduce the strategy in small group sessions and consult with the teacher as she supports carryover into general curriculum classroom activities. Additionally, the plan calls for the teacher to work with the small group using the same materials two other times each week. The reading specialist and teacher have begun another intervention program for groups of students whose reading decoding and phonemic awareness problems are more urgent than reading comprehension. The team plans to monitor progress for both groups of students showing learning risks by using periodic read-aloud samples, written story probes, and comprehension checks. Because other students in the same class will be completing the same probes, you plan to use a local comparison group to help the team document whether the students with difficulties are beginning to perform more like their successful peers.

Prevention is enhanced by helping teachers recognize the full range of speech and language difficulties and accommodate students with these problems. Presentations made to educator colleagues on topics such as strategies to support students with listening and reading comprehension difficulties or strategies for children with word retrieval difficulties may have the secondary result of helping teachers know when to request consultation from the SLP about a struggling student or how to incorporate communication goals into the broader curriculum.

Although checklists for speech and language skills can be provided to teachers as an entree to requesting consultation, developing informal relationships with teachers may be the best approach to opening lines of communication. Teachers refer students when their prior experiences lead them to expect that students with better speech, language, and communication will achieve better educational outcomes as well.

Student Assistance Teams When particular students struggle more than others, the next part of the RTI process is to use student assistance or child study teams to intensify services to assist such students with the general education curriculum. Schools vary in their use of procedures for these teams. In some schools, teacher assistance meetings are scheduled on a student-by-student as-needed basis; others have teams that meet regularly. The makeup of child study teams varies for individual students, but members generally include students' parents and main classroom teachers, as well as any additional classroom teachers, special education teachers or teacher consultants, speech-language pathologists, social workers, psychologists, counselors, and principals. After discussing a student's profile of strengths and weaknesses, team members decide on an action plan to address the teacher's concerns and student's needs, but without formal special education referral or assessment.

Sara's Initial Assessment ✳ ✳ ✳

Sara is a second-grade student who is struggling in school. She has been in your small group reading comprehension activities and participates in the collaborative writing lab activities you and the teacher provide twice weekly. Sara is well mannered and soft-spoken. Her teacher, Ms. Brown, describes Sara as a pleasant child but one who frequently does not follow directions during group activities. Ms. Brown has requested help from the school's child study team because Sara is having unusual difficulty in school. At the first meeting, Ms Brown tells the team that in addition to constant difficulty following directions, Sara is below grade level in reading and writing. Her word decoding skills are close to grade level, yet her comprehension skills are below the majority of the class, as shown by her performance in oral reading and retelling tasks during guided reading lessons. Her writing is also primitive. On the fall writing probe (Nelson & Van Meter, 2002), she produced an isolated description, with only 25 words, 10 of which were spelled correctly, while most of her classmates produced longer stories with more fully developed narrative structure. In math, although Sara is

beginning to learn math facts, she has difficulty with mathematical reasoning. The team decides that perhaps the supplemental program was not specific to her needs and a more intensive pre-referral intervention trial would be beneficial.

At the next student study meeting, the team discusses the trial period of intervention. After 8 weeks of intervention, the other students in the group have shown significant improvement in their comprehension and are implementing the LEARN strategy (Vernon et al., 1999) almost independently. Sara, however, has shown only marginal improvement. She attempts the strategy only with a great deal of adult prompting, and her comprehension overall has not shown change. The team decides to intensify the intervention, this time for a 3-week period with more individualized scaffolding. Once again, Sara shows improvement, but she remains heavily dependent on assistance. The team decides Sara should be formally evaluated for eligibility for special education. Her parents sign permission for a formal evaluation with the purpose of determining whether Sara has a disability that makes her eligible for special education services.

COMPREHENSIVE ASSESSMENT LEADING TO ELIGIBILITY

When children are suspected of having speech or language impairments, federal policy requires that comprehensive, culturally appropriate assessments be conducted to determine the existence, nature, and extent of the impairments. As outlined in Chapter 14, eligibility determination is a two-fold process that must assess whether the child has a speech or language impairment and whether the impairment adversely affects a child's educational performance (IDEA 2004 §300.8).

Prior to formal assessment that might qualify a child for special education, parents are asked to give their consent in writing. At this point, the clock starts ticking. That is, the assessment must be completed within a limited number of days following parental consent, such as 45 days or

less, which generally is specified by state regulation. Comprehensive assessments require contributions from more than one source, even in cases in which speech-language is the only area of suspected disability. Teachers contribute observations in classroom contexts; parents share information regarding communicative competence at home; and SLPs provide data from formal and informal assessments, including curriculum-based assessments.

Planning the Assessment

Students who have been followed within a RTI framework are often familiar to the SLP prior to the formal assessment. The SLP can use the information learned through the pre-referral intervention and conversations with the teacher about strengths and weakness to plan the additional assessment needed. This often requires curriculum-based language assessment along with formal or standardized assessments selected to reveal specific areas of speech or language weakness.

Informal Assessment Informal methods play a major role in conducting valid, culturally fair assessments of communication learning needs. When speech-language impairments are suspected, documentation generally includes samples of spoken and written language, data on speech and language performance in curricular tasks, and results of formal standardized assessments.

As noted previously, teacher and parental input are required to document if the condition is a disability. The speech-language impairment must be associated with functional limitations and have a negative effect on daily living needs. According to the requirements of IDEA 2004, the student's assessment must be designed to determine the effect of the communication difficulties on progress within the general education curriculum.

Curriculum-Based Language and Communication Assessment The SLP begins the process of curriculum-based language and communication assessment by conferring with students, parents, and teachers to identify aspects of the curriculum that present the greatest challenges to the student, as well as those that allow the student to demonstrate learning strengths. Curricular contexts include the social, interpersonal "underground" curriculum of developing peer relationships as well as the formal curriculum outlined by school district committees (Nelson, 1998). Once specific areas of the curriculum have been identified as being most in need of attention, the SLP can begin a focused assessment of the student's communication abilities within the targeted context. This form of *curriculum-based language/communication assessment* (CBLA) differs from forms of curriculum-based assessment (CBA) used by general educators to answer the question, "Is the student learning the curriculum?" Rather, it addresses the more specific question, "Does the student have the speech-language-communication skills to learn the curriculum and to participate fully in school?"

T A B L E 15–2 Four Questions for Guiding Curriculum-Based Language Communication Assessment

1. What communication skills are needed for successful participation in this part of the curriculum?

2. What does the student usually do when attempting this task?

3. What communication skills and strategies might the student acquire to become more successful?

4. How should the task be modified?

SOURCE: Adapted from Nelson, N. W. (1989). Curriculum-based language assessment and intervention. *Language, Speech, and Hearing Services in Schools, 20,* 170–184.

Four questions guide the CBLA process (Nelson, 1989, 1998) (Table 15–2). The first question probes communication skills a student needs to participate successfully in problematic curricular activities. To answer this question, the SLP must analyze what it takes, for example, to contribute to oral discussions or to comprehend the language in a social studies textbook and to formulate answers or oral or written questions.

The second question asks what the student usually does when attempting the targeted task. This question may be answered either by observing the student in the classroom or by having the student bring selected curricular materials to the speech-language room. In either case, it is ideal if the SLP can start out as an "onlooker observer" to see what the student does independently, but then shift to a "participant observer" role, asking strategic questions to understand what inner strategies the student may be bringing to the task. For example, after viewing a classroom discussion, the SLP might ask a student what he or she was thinking when the teacher asked for volunteers to answer questions, then probe to find out whether the student knew some answers but did not raise his or her hand. If so, why not?

The third question asks what the student might learn to do differently to perform the activity more successfully. To answer this question, the SLP employs dynamic assessment activities, exploring strategically which cueing, focusing, guiding, or feedback "scaffolds" might assist the student to perform at higher levels of competence. The final question asks whether the task should be modified to make it more accessible. This question can be addressed during the dynamic assessment process, but generally involves more extensive collaborative problem solving with others in the student's educational environment. The goal is to make it possible for the student to be successful in the general curriculum, with an emphasis on keeping the student in that curriculum.

Formal Assessment Formal assessment is required by most state regulations for determining eligibility for special education services. Regulations for IDEA 2004 specify that more than one testing procedure should be used, each validated for the purpose for which it is used. Standardized tests are available to assess articulation and most aspects of language, although informal methods in natural contexts generally are considered more valid for assessing pragmatic aspects of language. For voice and stuttering, validated procedures (in lieu of standardized test scores) are the appropriate means for identifying the disorder.

Determining Eligibility When the assessment is complete, the multidisciplinary evaluation team reviews the results and determines whether a student has an identifiable disability. A student must meet the criteria for a specific disability to be eligible for special services under Part B of IDEA as described in Chapter 14.

The primary challenge facing school-based SLPs is to identify and work with students who need special assistance to progress in the general education curriculum. The charge is to find children with disabilities to provide them with appropriate services from birth to age 21. Students with any of the disabilities listed in the IDEA 2004 definition may need speech-language assessment and intervention services. As described by Eger in Chapter 14, these services may be provided as the student's special education "program" (if the student has a speech-language impairment only), or they may be provided as a "related service" (if the student

has some other disability that is considered primary to the communication disorder). Audiological services are always considered a "related service." Criteria for identifying a disability that involves speech-language or hearing are usually established at the state level, but local agencies may extend those criteria or interpret them differently.

In determining eligibility for service, both informal and formal assessment results are used. Formal assessment results should be interpreted according to the psychometrics of the assessment to determine whether a student's performance differs sufficiently from a particular referent group. The use of a standard cut-off score across test measures (e.g., requiring a score 1.5 standard deviations below the mean) might result in over-identification (i.e., false positive) or under-identification (i.e., false negative) errors depending on the psychometric properties of a particular test (Disney, Plante, Spinello, & Whitmire, 2003). In addition, the range indicated by the test's standard error of measurement (SEM) should be considered. Not all test manuals report SEM, but when available, the high end of the range within which a particular score is predicted to fall, rather than the actual score, should be considered. SLPs also need to be careful to select standardized tests that have demonstrated validity and reliability. The test manual should report the test's *sensitivity,* which is its percent accuracy at identifying children with known disorders as *having* a language disorder, and *specificity,* which is its percent accuracy at identifying children with normal speech and language as *not having* a disability. Both sensitivity and specificity should be at 80 percent or above to be considered valid for identifying disorder (Disney et al., 2003). By using scoring guidelines recommended for the specific test for maximizing specificity and sensitivity ratings, examiners can minimize the chance of making a Type I (false positive) or Type II (false negative) error.

In the not too distant past, many state or local policies required SLPs to compare children's performance to those with the same cognitive or mental age (MA) rather than to peers of the same chronological age (CA). At least partially, such cognitive referencing policies reflected concerns that simply

---

Sara's Assessment Results   ✳ ✳ ✳

For Sara, assessment activities reveal a communication disorder involving language content and form that influences both comprehension and expression in oral and written communication. Sara's need for speech-language intervention services is supported by a language sample and story retelling activity, along with other informal observations and teacher reports that document the adverse effects on Sara's educational performance in several curricular areas. The diagnosis of language impairment is confirmed by the results of two formal tests whose technical manuals provide guidance about scores that maximize the test's sensitivity and specificity.

---

comparing students to others with the same CA would result in huge caseloads. IDEA 2004 states that schools cannot be required to use a discrepancy formula for the identification of learning disabilities. As an alternative, schools may use the student's responsiveness to scientific, research-based intervention (explained previously in this chapter). RTI initiatives are meant to learn first whether students' needs can be met in other ways. They also provide an option for identifying children with language impairment who need speech-language intervention services to develop optimally and benefit fully from their educational experiences (e.g., Ehren & Nelson, 2005).

Planning and Providing Intervention

The essence of a school-based program of service delivery is the design and provision of services to help students acquire the communicative skills for participating in important life contexts. Central features of IDEA 2004 are the provision of a "free appropriate public education" (FAPE) in the "least restrictive environment" (LRE). The exact nature of this service delivery is individually determined. After a student's eligibility is established, a program of intervention is planned by the student's Individualized Education Planning (IEP) team. During this IEP meeting, goals for intervention are written, and the type and frequency of service are planned. The intended outcome is successful participation in the general education curriculum. Modifications and accommodations to that curriculum are also outlined, taking care not to simplify expectations at the sacrifice of students' opportunities to progress and participate with their peers. Families and teachers join in the planning process.

Students' IEPs will include goals and objectives aimed at connecting oral and written language abilities with the increasingly complex communication demands of the general education curriculum. For students with severe disabilities, this may involve efforts to keep them included or active in general curricular activities, but with modified expectations.

Evidenced-Based Practice (EBP)

It is up to practitioners to engage in continuing education and active inquiry that can support them in conducting evidence-based practice (ASHA, 2005). This includes gathering evidence about the effectiveness of their own practice (Hargrove, 2002). In conducting EBP, school teams consider the scientific research base of practices when selecting assessment and intervention practices from pre-referral to assessment and intervention (IDEA, 2004; NCLB, 2001). EBP provides a model and procedures for SLPs and audiologists to determine whether research information applies to a specific student. This includes identifying questions related to the services to the student, searching the literature, critiquing the quality and significance of the evidence, developing a plan, and reevaluating regularly (ASHA, 2005; Hargrove, 2002). Although it is beyond the scope of this chapter to attempt to outline best practice for the wide range of students with communication

Intervention and Follow-up   ✳ ✳ ✳

With Ms. Brown and Sara's parents, you decide to initiate an intervention program that combines classroom-based and pull-out therapy. The pull-out therapy will allow you to work directly with Sara on language comprehension and expression in a small group. In the pull-out sessions, you plan to target a set of grammatical forms and conceptual vocabulary using materials drawn from the classroom curriculum (stories, science textbook, and math problems). For example, you plan to help Sara develop her understanding and use of directional language terms and logical syntactic structures required for classroom direction following. You also plan to help Sara develop self-talk strategies to facilitate listening and reading comprehension. This will guide her through aspects of the classroom routine that are causing particular difficulty. You write these as a set of goals and objectives with measurable benchmarks as part of her IEP. In addition, you plan to continue going into Sara's classroom 1 to 2 days per week to work with

Ms. Brown and the other children on your caseload in the context of the writing lab approach (Nelson et al., 2004).

In providing the intervention, you and Ms. Brown plan activities so that students will have multiple opportunities to work in small groups on their animal reports. You also scaffold Sara's social interaction skills in the small group activities. You and Ms. Brown make ongoing accommodations to the learning environment for Sara and coordinate expectations for Sara to become increasingly independent in listening and reading comprehension. You also help Sara develop competence with more elaborate written language syntax as she prepares her written report. As Ms. Brown becomes increasingly familiar with the grammatical form and language content targets, she begins to emphasize and monitor these structures and vocabulary more frequently in class. She also adopts strategies to check Sara's comprehension and to draw her more actively into classroom discussions.

Working with Sara   ✳ ✳ ✳

You have designed Sara's program to include these features. After your first few sessions with Sara, you and she decide on how to rewrite her therapy goals in her own words. This way, Sara's individualized objectives can be incorporated in her Author Note Book (Nelson et al., 2004). In your pull-out sessions, Sara brings the books she has found that tell about penguins, their habitats, and other facts. You use this reading material to focus on the reading comprehension goals and application of the LEARN strategies (Vernon et al., 1999). She uses the strategy to *Locate* clues that show what is important such as lists in the

text, bold or italicized print, or pictures and tables. Next she *Extracts* key words, and *Assembles* a memory device, *Rehearses*, and *Notes* her score on working with others. You help her to reference her strategy list and to carry out each step. With scaffolding to check whether she understands what she reads, Sara learns to monitor her own comprehension. She goes back and rereads a passage if it does not make sense and is becoming more independent in identifying important information in the text. When you are in the classroom, you keep track of Sara's ability to follow multiple-step directions correctly and independently.

development needs, some features that characterize effective programs in general are student ownership of goals and intervention focused on curriculum-based communication events as well as specific communication skills. See Chapter 28 for more in-depth discussion of EBP.

Reporting on Progress

Requirements for providing special education services that are outlined in IDEA 2004 require that parents receive reports on their children's progress on IEP goals at least as frequently as report cards are

---

Reporting on Sara's Progress   ✳ ✳ ✳

To monitor progress and communicate between school and home, you devise a special page that will be tucked into Sara's classroom homework folder. Weekly, you and Sara confer about which of her goals she worked on that week, and you write a note about one thing that made her feel successful and one thing she wants to work on more. There is space in the folder for Sara and her parents to comment on books they are reading for fun at bedtime.

When report card time arrives for Sara 9 weeks later, you can report that she is making significant progress toward accomplishing her IEP goals. In addition, her scores on a districtwide reading comprehension test have improved. She is now following directions in the classroom with minimal checking by the teacher, and Ms. Brown reports Sara has learned to "chunk" classroom directions into the important

points, keeping track of them on her fingers, rather than trying to repeat them (unsuccessfully) verbatim or simply giving up. She can implement a strategy with moderate assistance that involves drawing the key elements of math story problems with stick figures before attempting to solve them. When she uses this strategy, she can select the correct operation (addition or subtraction) on four out of five story problems, and her parents report that she is now willing to let them help her with her math homework.

Several aspects of school are still difficult for Sara, but with the specialized assistance and team approach her work is manageable and she is making steady progress. She is now frequently sought out as a partner for playground games, and she has stopped telling her mother she has a stomachache each morning before school.

---

sent for all students. This information should be in a language that parents can understand.

SLPs often use percentages to quantify targets in short-term objectives, but it is important that these be real criteria and not just numbers of convenience. For example, what does it mean to set a goal for a student to comprehend 85% of a reading passage? A qualitative description of a student's demonstration of language comprehension when answering questions on classroom tests, or of the student's ability to retell a story with all major narrative elements, might be better measures of improved language comprehension. Broader outcomes, such as fewer questions for repetition of directions in the classroom, are also important to document.

Planning for Children with Multiple Disabilities

The assessment process for students with suspected multiple disabilities should yield information about all areas of concern. This may require input from specialists in several disciplines. In addition to parents and at least one general education teacher,

evaluation and IEP teams for these students might include audiologists, special education teachers, occupational therapists, physical therapists, social workers, psychologists, and school counselors, each of whom may administer formal tests. The evaluation report should represent the team's collective results, as well as input of parents and general educators. At a collaborative meeting, this interdisciplinary group determines the student's category of eligibility.

Determining the most appropriate goals for a student with multiple disabilities requires collaboration with all members of a team, including parents. When goals are written collectively, opportunity exists for all specialists to facilitate the student's growth. For example, the teacher can emphasize communication during classroom interactions using strategies the SLP models. The teacher then can help the SLP identify which strategies are more or less successful so that adjustments can be made in other aspects of intervention. The social worker can emphasize the communicative goals during her social skills group. The occupational therapist facilitates communication during therapy by helping students with hypersensitivities learn how to screen out distracting stimuli. By coming together in this transdisciplinary manner, you can all serve students with diverse needs better and learn from each other how to facilitate students to develop integrated abilities across developmental domains.

Services for individual students encompass a sequence of activities, which sometimes are implemented in recursive cycles more than once across a student's school career. Two guiding principles are individualization and collaboration. In today's schools, SLPs and audiologists might devote a portion of their workload to preventive efforts, helping others implement effective instruction that incorporates principles recognizing interrelationships among hearing, speech, language/literacy, and communication. As part of this work, teams may establish criteria for identifying students who are not improving sufficiently in spite of individualized planning and intensified instructions efforts. Such students must receive the combination of assessment and intervention services specifically tailored to meet their individualized needs.

SERVICE DELIVERY MODELS

Effective intervention helps students with communication disorders participate actively in the curriculum, be more successful in school, and interact appropriately with peers. It works best when an SLP understands a student's communicative needs and strengths, works closely with the student's teachers, knows the curriculum, and knows the child and family's culture. Various intervention models may be used to deliver such services. Regardless of the specific model used, collaboration of SLPs, family members, teachers, and other professionals is essential for effective intervention (ASHA 1999, 2001; Coufal, 1993; Ehren, 2003; Ferguson, 1991; Secord & Wiig, 1990; Simon & Myrold-Gunyuz, 1990). As discussed in detail in Chapter 14, the team is responsible for considering how to keep the student in the least restrictive environment while meeting the student's individualized needs.

In this section we discuss each of the service delivery models that make up a full continuum of speech and language services. Remember that what is "least restrictive" for a particular student is defined relative to that student's needs at any given point in time. The models described here are not discrete and separate but often overlapping and complementary. A combination of models may be best for meeting most students' needs, perhaps including both pull-out and classroom-based components along with consultation, all aimed at developing improved communication skills and generalizing them to natural settings. The ability to provide a combination of models and to provide services that match the student's changing needs improves with flexible scheduling (described later).

Consultative Collaborative Service

In the first section of this chapter, collaboration was emphasized as a feature that characterizes all aspects of an SLP's comprehensive role in today's schools. Consultation services are appropriate whether the student is in pre-referral stages or receiving pull-out or in-class treatment. They are especially important for students in transition from one level to the next, such as the transition from elementary to secondary school, as the student faces more advanced communicative challenges (Bashir, 1989). Consultative services also may be most appropriate for students who have long-term needs that can be addressed best in the natural contexts of daily interactions with other instructional personnel and caregivers. In this model, the SLP consults with the student's teachers and parents as needed, who then provide the direct and ongoing supports for the newly acquired skills. The SLP continues to work with them and the student periodically to monitor independent use of the new skills and to troubleshoot any setbacks.

Family-Centered Service

Family-centered service involves working with families using culturally sensitive practices to foster the communicative development of infants, children, or adolescents. Family-centered practices begin by discovering the communicative needs identified by the family and any concerns the family and student may have for the student's success in the community, school, and home environments. This is crucial for setting appropriate and meaningful goals, using everyone involved with the student to maximize progress toward those goals and to realize changes in communicative functioning across contexts. See Chapter 16 for discussion of early intervention. For students of all ages who use augmentative and alternative communication systems, a family-centered approach to treatment is necessary to choose systems that will be the least intrusive and most beneficial for the student at home and in school. When families are involved in this way over the student's school career, transition planning into settings beyond school into adulthood is greatly enhanced, as required by IDEA 2004.

Classroom-Based Service

Any speech-language intervention that occurs in classrooms may be classified as classroom-based therapy, or it may be called *pull-in* or *push-in* therapy. Classroom-based intervention models and methods vary, but they should be distinguishable from general education classroom instruction (Ehren, 2000). Such models are distinguished by their therapeutic focus and by the explicit intentionality with which SLPs work toward achieving IEP goals. Classroom-based therapy may parallel other programs in language arts and may accompany Tier I and Tier II activities within RTI initiatives. Students without disabilities may benefit by having a communication specialist in the classroom, but the primary focus of the SLP's efforts should be on meeting the needs of one or more students with speech-language impairments.

Classroom-based services have advantages in that ties to a student's curriculum-based needs are immediate, and generalization is enhanced. Students served in the classroom-based model also are less likely to miss important curricular content and are more likely to be viewed by their classmates and teacher as full members of the class (Nelson et al.,

2004). Curricular language demands, both spoken and written, provide the best contexts and content for being relevant to the needs of students with language disorders. Finally, presence in the classroom can provide models of holding higher expectations and scaffolding higher-level communication abilities for students with speech, language/literacy, and communication disorders of all types.

Disadvantages of classroom-based services include giving up full control of session activities. They also require time to plan, and time demands are multiplied when SLPs must meet the needs of students placed in many different general education classrooms. In such cases, it may be possible to group students for certain activities within a grade level. Classroom-based services work best during curricular activities that involve small group activity or individual efforts but with the quiet productive buzz of collaboration. It makes no sense for a SLP to stand at the back of a classroom watching a teacher teach. Nor does it make sense to disrupt other classroom activities by attempting to do traditional speech therapy in the back of a classroom just for the sake of being there. Speech production skills, for example, such as articulation of a difficult phoneme or learning to use easy onset phonation as an alternative to stuttering blocks, are better taught in intensive, frequently scheduled sessions for a short period of time and then moved into the classroom for carryover into everyday communication contexts. Unfortunately, however, research evidence regarding best service delivery models is still rare.

When working within classrooms, different models of collaborative service delivery allow SLPs to address different types of goals. All models require the establishment of a trusting relationship between the SLP and classroom teacher. Examples include team teaching, supplemental teaching, supportive instruction, and small group instruction. The writing lab approach to language instruction and intervention (Nelson et al., 2004) is an example of how several of these methods can be combined using curriculum-based writing projects to address any of the speech, language/literacy, and communication goals that might be on a student's IEP.

Team Teaching

Team teaching has also been called *coteaching* or *complementary instruction* (DiMeo, Merritt, & Culatta, 1998). In a survey of delivery models, team teaching was rated most appropriate by both SLPs and teachers (Beck & Dennis, 1997). When working in this model, the classroom teacher and SLP share responsibility for instructing all students in the classroom, using activities planned jointly to address specialized needs.

Team teaching has many variations. Team members may divide responsibilities or students in different ways, depending on the purposes of the lesson, teaching styles, and nature of the class and students. *Supplemental teaching* (Beck & Dennis, 1997; Elksnin & Capilouto, 1994) involves dividing the class into students who have mastered the material and those who have not, with each team member taking a group. *Supportive instruction* (DiMeo et al., 1998) involves the teacher providing content instruction, with support by the SLP to teach strategies students can use while completing the lesson. The teacher continues to emphasize the use of such strategies in future lessons.

In *coteaching models,* the teacher and SLP share instructional responsibility for some activities by alternating mini-lessons or teaching jointly, with either or both "at the front of the class." For example, in the writing lab approach (Nelson et al., 2004), the SLP might arrange to be in the classroom to coteach a 10-minute mini-lesson at the beginning of a lesson. For example, a mini-lesson might relate to communication processes used in peer editing. The mini-lesson could start with a negative demonstration followed by the class brainstorming the characteristics of good listening and helpful feedback, which the teacher and SLP could model the second time around. Then the teacher and SLP both could move among the peer editing groups as students practice their new skills.

Pull-out Service

Pull-out service refers to pulling a student out of the classroom to receive special services. The student may be grouped with others, as is commonly the case, or seen individually. During these sessions, new communication skills and strategies for addressing curriculum-based communication needs are introduced and practiced. As discussed in the previous chapter, pull-out services have been used predominantly, despite the promotion of classroom-based service delivery models in the literature for the past 2 decades. The current conceptualization of this model is that these services need to be connected with the classroom curriculum, as opposed to traditional pull-out services in which isolated skills or therapy activities were used. Pull-out therapy is especially appropriate for helping students acquire new motor skills for meeting articulation, voice, or fluency needs that require individualized instruction and massed practice trials, especially in the early stages. Pull-out therapy also is appropriate when treatment exercises would be conspicuous or distracting to other children and embarrassing to the student with special needs.

Pull-out therapy may occur on a variety of schedules. When addressing motor skills, more frequent, shorter, sessions may be most beneficial. Students might be seen three or four times per week for 10 minutes of drill rather than for one or two longer sessions. These students also might be seen more intensively for a block of weeks, then put on consult for a block of weeks and then seen again intensively. This type of scheduling allows for more intensive motor skill work. For examples of scheduling speech drill and practice see the Workload Implementation Guide by ASHA (2004).

One disadvantage of pull-out service is that skills developed in isolation may not generalize readily to other contexts. Equally important, missing classroom activities may add to a student's academic risks. These disadvantages may be minimized by using materials from the general curriculum as practice material and by combining pull-out with classroom-based intervention. By doing so, the SLP may gain opportunities to observe the difficulty of the material for the student and may increase the likelihood of generalization of newly acquired skills to classroom contexts. As in other methods, this approach requires ongoing consultation to coordinate the use of curriculum materials by the SLP, to share successful strategies for application in the classroom, and to coordinate with other classroom-based services.

Self-Contained Classrooms

In some states, an SLP with educational credentials may serve as classroom teacher in a self-contained classroom for students with severe primary speech-language impairments. Self-contained special education classrooms may also be provided for students with other primary disabilities, in which cases SLPs provide services using any of the models described previously.

When serving as full-time classroom teacher at the elementary level, SLPs assume responsibility for teaching the general curriculum while providing intensive language therapy throughout the day. The goal is to help students be successful when they reenter general education classes. Self-contained classrooms are usually housed in regular schools, but students may ride buses from other home schools to attend. An SLP may teach a self-contained daily language course for credit at the middle or high school, depending on state and local policy. The student takes the class as a regularly scheduled alternative language arts course, relieving the concern of missing content instruction while receiving language intervention. The emphasis is on spoken and written language, study skills, critical thinking, pragmatics, and other language issues relevant to adolescents (Anderson & Nelson, 1988; Buttrill, Niizawa, Biemer, Takahashi, & Hearn, 1989).

HOW A WORKLOAD APPROACH DIFFERS FROM A CASELOAD APPROACH

SLPs practicing in schools have many responsibilities that stretch beyond direct service to students. It is important that SLPs help administrators and other school staff to understand the breadth of these roles so that they are allowed time to engage activities beyond direct service and can schedule these activities appropriately (Ehren & Whitmire, 2005). In a workload approach SLPs are careful not to fill the available time with direct services, to allow for other vital activities in the daily responsibilities. This improves the quality of services to the students on the caseload and enables the SLP to complete the other important tasks. SLPs' activities can be grouped into a set of "workload clusters" (ASHA, 2002) in the following four categories:

- Indirect services that support student's educational programs
- Indirect activities that support students in the least restrictive environment and general education curriculum
- Activities that support compliance with federal, state, and local mandates
- Direct services to students

Examples of activities in each of these clusters appear in Figure 15–1.

SLPs are working with their schools systems to arrange schedules that accommodate all of these activities in their workday. It is tricky to fit the myriad of services the SLP offers to a caseload of 40–60 or more students into a normal work week. Although demanding at first, a balance of services established in a context of collaborative working relationships can actually streamline the use of the SLP's time. The more SLPs collaborate with general education teachers regarding students on their caseload, the easier it is to consult regarding other children. For example, when providing classroom-based services, SLPs have opportunities to get to know the teaching styles and curriculum, including the "hidden curriculum" of unspoken expectations that are unique to each teacher.

In some places, SLPs have implemented flexible schedules where caseload students are seen in a 3:1 ratio, 3 weeks direct and 1 week indirect for other types of support. Within a flexible schedule, a combination of service delivery types can be used and one can alter the type of service delivery with the changing needs of the students as the curricular demands change. Time to consult and to plan with teachers is built into the schedule, thus acknowledging this activity as essential to a quality program. An example of a 4-week schedule and other workload documentation is available on the ASHA workload Web site.

Direct services to students

- Counsel students
- Evaluate students for eligibility for special education
- Identify students with speech and language impairment
- Implement IEPs and IFSPs
- Provide direct intervention to students using a continuum of service delivery options
- Reevaluate students

Indirect activities that support students in the least restrictive environment and general education curriculum

- Engage in dynamic assessment of students
- Connect standards for the learner to the IEP
- Consult with teachers to match students learning style and teaching style
- Design and engage in pre-referral intervention activities
- Design/recommend adaptations to curriculum and delivery of instruction

- Design/recommend modifications to the curriculum to benefit students with special needs
- Participate in activities designed to help prevent academic and literacy problems
- Observe students in classrooms
- Screen students for suspected problems with communication, learning, and literacy

Indirect services that support students' educational programs

- Analyze and engineer environments to increase opportunities for communication
- Analyze demands of the curriculum and effects on students
- Attend student planning teams to solve specific problems
- Attend teacher/service provider meetings (planning, progress monitoring, modifications to program)

- Communicate and coordinate with outside agencies
- Contribute to the development of IEPs, IFSPs
- Coordinate with private, nonpublic school teachers and staff
- Design service plans
- Design and implement transition evaluations and transition goals
- Design and program high-, medium-, and low-tech augmentative communication systems
- Engage in special preparation to provide services to students (e.g., low incidence populations, research basis for intervention, best practices)

- Interview teachers
- Make referrals to other professionals
- Monitor implementation of IEP modifications
- Observe students in classrooms
- Plan and prepare lessons
- Plan for student transitions
- Provide staff development to school staff, parents, and others
- Program and maintain assistive technology/augmentative communication systems (AT/AC) and equipment
- Train teachers and staff for AT/AC system use

Activities that support compliance with federal, state, and local mandates

- Attend staff/faculty meetings
- Carry out assigned school duties (e.g. hall, lunch, bus, extracurricular)
- Collect and report student performance data
- Complete compliance paperwork
- Complete daily logs of student services
- Complete parent contact logs
- Document services to students and other activities
- Document third-party billing activities
- Participate in parent/teacher conferences
- Participate in professional association activities
- Participate in professional development

- Participate on school improvement teams
- Participate on school or district committees
- Serve multiple schools and sites
- Supervise paraprofessionals, teacher aides, interns, CFYs
- Travel between buildings
- Write funding reports for assistive technology and augmentative communication
- Write periodic student progress reports
- Write student evaluation reports

F I G U R E 15–1 Workload Activity Clusters

SOURCE: From American Speech-Language-Hearing Association (2002). A Workload Analysis Approach for Establishing Speech-Language Caseload Standards in the Schools [Guidelines]. Available at http://www.asha.org/members/deskref-journals/deskref/DRVol3.htm. Reprinted by permission

SUMMARY

This chapter began with an overview of the broad scope of collaborative roles SLPs and audiologists may play in today's schools and the importance of becoming full members of a school's instructional team. Strategies were suggested for

conceptualizing a new view of the school-based SLP as the building's communication consultant, with knowledge and skills that are relevant for addressing the communication health of all students.

The second section presented a sequence of steps for serving the needs of children and adolescents in educationally based settings, consistent with the requirements of IDEA 2004 for using IEPs to provide curriculum-based services to school-age students. Steps for providing services include participation on prevention/intervention teams, conducting interviews, conducting comprehensive assessments, providing intervention, and reporting on progress. Differences for students with multiple disabilities were discussed.

The third section described variations in service delivery models, all set within the goal to help students participate effectively in environments that are least restrictive for them. A continuum of services from less to more restrictive would include consultation/collaboration, family-centered practices, classroom-based intervention, pullout services, and self-contained classrooms. The use of a workload model for addressing the scheduling complexities of conducting SLP practice in today's schools was also discussed. The overriding theme is to encourage readers to think creatively about the goal to be more relevant to students' needs for developing the communication skills that will help them to achieve success within the general education curriculum and in life.

CRITICAL THINKING

1. What strategies might an SLP use for developing collegial relationships and becoming a full member of a school staff? What signs would indicate that an SLP is an accepted member of the faculty? What strategies can an SLP use to develop bridges from pull-out to classroom-based service delivery models? How might you elaborate on the 10 strategies summarized in Table 15–1?

2. Describe a sequence of activities from pre-referral to reporting on progress that would characterize a program of intervention services for a school-age child.

3. Discuss the types of assessment evidence used to show that a student has a disability and that it has an adverse effect on educational performance. How does this coordinate with formal testing results? Why should examiners make sure that test manuals report cut-off scores with regard to maximizing the test's sensitivity and specificity? Describe flaws with the use of cognitive-referenced criteria for identifying language disabilities and how RTI initiatives might be used instead.

4. List and define a continuum of service delivery models for providing school-based services from least to most restrictive. What factors would influence the selection of a model that is "least restrictive" and most appropriate for meeting the needs of a particular child at a particular point in the treatment process?

5. How does a workload model differ from a caseload model for characterizing SLP practice in the schools? What advantages does it bring? List some activities from each cluster in Figure 15.1 that you found surprising or that represent activities you would like to explore.

REFERENCES

Anderson, G. M., & Nelson, N. W. (1988). Integrating language intervention and education in an alternate adolescent language classroom. *Seminars in Speech and Language, 9*(4), 341–353.

American Speech-Language-Hearing Association. (1999). Guidelines for the roles and responsibilities of the school-based speech-language pathologist. Rockville, MD: Author.

American Speech-Language-Hearing Association. (2000). Guidelines for the roles and responsibilities of speech-language pathologist related to reading and writing for children and adolescents. Rockville, MD: Author.

American Speech-Language-Hearing Association. (2002). A workload analysis approach for establishing speech-language caseload standards in the schools. Rockville, MD: Author. Available at: http://www.asha.org/

American Speech-Language-Hearing Association. (2004). Preferred practice patterns for the profession of speech-language pathology. Rockville, MD: Author.

American Speech-Language-Hearing Association. (2005). Evidenced-based practice in communication disorders. Rockville, MD: Author.

Barth, R. (1990). *Improving schools from within*. San Francisco: Jossey-Bass.

Bashir, A. (1989). Language intervention and the curriculum. *Seminars in Speech and Language, 10*(3), 181–191.

Bashir, A., Conte, B. M., & Heerde, S. M. (1998). Language and school success: Collaborative challenges and choices. In D. Merritt & B. Culatta (Eds.), *Language intervention in the classroom* (pp. 1–36). San Diego, CA: Singular Publishing Group.

Beck, A. R., & Dennis, M. (1997). Speech-language pathologists' and teachers' perceptions of classroom-based interventions. *Language Speech, and Hearing Services in Schools, 28,* 146–153.

Buttrill J., Niizawa, J., Biemer, C., Takahashi, C., & Hearn, S. (1989). Servicing the language disabled adolescent: A strategies-based model. *Language Speech, and Hearing Services in Schools, 20,* 185–204.

Catts, H., & Kamhi, A. (2005). *Language and reading disabilities* (2nd ed.). Boston: Pearson Education.

Coufal, K. (Ed.). (1993). Collaborative consultation for speech-language pathologists. *Topics in Language Disorders, 14*(1), 1–14.

DiMeo, J., Merritt, D., & Culatta, B. (1998). Collaborative partnerships and decision making. In D. Merritt & B. Culatta (Eds.), *Language intervention in the classroom* (pp. 37–97). San Diego: Singular Publishing Group.

Disney, S., Plante, E., Spinello, E., & Whitmire, K. (2003). *Educationally relevant assessments*. Rockville, MD: American Speech-Language-Hearing Association.

Ehren, B. (2000). Maintaining a therapeutic focus and sharing responsibility for student success: Keys to in-classroom speech-language services. *Language, Speech, and Hearing Services in Schools, 31,* 219–229.

Ehren, B. (2003). *The pragmatics of teaming*. Rockville, MD: American Speech-Language-Hearing Association.

Ehren, B., & Nelson, N. (2005). The responsiveness to intervention approach and language impairment. *Topics in Language Disorders, 25,* 120–132.

Ehren, T., & Whitmire, K. (2005). Leadership opportunities in the context of responsiveness to intervention activities. *Topics in Language Disorders, 25,* 168–179.

Elksnin, L. K., & Capilouto, G. (1994). Speech-language pathologists' perceptions of integrated service delivery in school settings. *Language, Speech, and Hearing Services in Schools, 25,* 258–267.

Ferguson, M. L. (1991). Collaborative/consultative service delivery: An introduction *Language Speech, and Hearing Services in the Schools, 22,* 147.

Graner, P. S., Faggella-Luby, M. N., & Fritschmann, N. A. (2005). An overview of responsiveness to intervention: What practitioners ought to know. *Topics in Language Disorders, 25*(2), 93–104.

Hargrove, P. (2002). Tutorial: Evidenced-based practices #1 Overview of evidenced-based practice. *Perspectives on Language Learning and Education, 9*(1), 20–22.

Individuals with Disabilities Educational Improvement Act of 2004 (IDEA 2004), Pub. L. No. 108-446 Stat. 2647 (December 3, 2004).

Moore-Brown, B., Montgomery, J., Bielinski, J., & Shubin, J. (2005). Responsiveness to Intervention: Teaching before testing helps avoid labeling. *Topics in Language Disorders, 25,* 148–167.

Nelson, N. W. (1989). Curriculum-based language assessment and intervention. *Language, Speech, and Hearing Services in Schools, 20,* 170–184.

Nelson, N. W. (1998). *Childhood language disorders in context: Infancy through adolescence* (2nd ed.). Boston: Allyn & Bacon.

Nelson, N. W., Bahr, C. & Van Meter, A. (2004). *The writing lab approach to language instruction and intervention*. Baltimore, MD: Brookes.

Nelson, N. W., & Van Meter, A. M. (2002). Assessing reading and writing samples for planning and evaluating change. *Topics in Language Disorders 22*(2), 47–72.

No Child Left Behind Act of 2001 (NCLB), Pub. L. No. 107-110, 115 Stat. 1425 (2001).

Secord, W., & Wiig, E. (Eds.). (1990). *Best practices in school speech-language pathology: Collaborative programs in the schools—Concepts, models, and procedures.* San Antonio, TX: The Psychological Corporation.

Silliman, E.R., & Wilkinson, L.C. (2004). *Language and literacy learning in schools.* New York: Guilford.

Simon, C., & Myrold-Gunyuz, M. (1990). *Into the classroom: The SLP in the collaborative role.* San Antonio, TX: Communication Skill Builders.

Staskowski, M., & Zagaiski, K. (2003). Reaching for the stars: SLPs shine on literacy teams. *Seminars in Speech and Language, 24,* 199–213.

Staskowski, M., & Rivera, E. (2005). Speech-language pathologists' involvement in responsiveness to intervention activities: A complement to curriculum-relevant practice. *Topics in Language Disorders, 25,* 148–167.

Taylor, O. L., & Payne, K. T. (1983). Culturally valid testing: A proactive approach. *Topics in Language Disorders, 3*(3), 8–20.

Troia, G. (2005). Responsiveness to intervention: roles for speech-language pathologists in the prevention and identification of learning disabilities. *Topics in Language Disorders, 25,* 106–119.

Vernon, D. S., Schumaker, J. B., & Deschler, D. D. (1999). *The LEARN strategy.* Lawrence, KS: Edge Enterprises.

16

Service Delivery Issues in Early Intervention

LAURIE NASH KOURY, MA

SCOPE OF CHAPTER

The debate of nature versus nurture began several hundred years ago when Enlightenment philosopher John Locke hypothesized that the infant emerged as a tabula rosa that would be influenced by the environment. Today, society generally believes that children enter the world with innate characteristics that are then influenced by their environment. We see the implementation of this philosophy in the support the federal government has given to establishing and funding early intervention programs. Federal and state legislators have been persuaded that tax dollars should be invested in preventing and remediating early developmental problems. Both immediate and long-term benefits of such intervention are envisioned for the child, parents, and society.

Although early education programs such as preschools, kindergarten, and Head Start have been in existence for some time, what we call *early intervention* in this chapter is a program mandated by Congress in 1997 that ensures that young children are given the best chance for a productive and healthy start to life. Early intervention applies to children, birth to age 3, who are discovered to have or be at risk of developing a handicapping condition or other special need that may affect their development.

In this chapter you will learn the importance of early intervention, its effectiveness, and the legislative context underpinning these programs. You will learn

---

Rosa's Story   ✳ ✳ ✳

My name is Rosa, and I was born two months before I was due. I was so tiny that my mommy could hold me in her hand. I stayed in the hospital for three months before I was strong enough to come home. I get oxygen through a tube in my nose and food through a tube in my stomach. It is hard for mommy and daddy to comfort me, and often we all get frustrated. Sometimes I hear my parents talking in loud voices, or I hear them crying.

When I was in the hospital a woman came to visit from the early intervention program. She told mommy and daddy about the services we could get in our house to help us. She said that I might be able to have

some therapies to help me to learn, to walk, and to talk. She said that she could also help daddy manage the medical bills.

Now two therapists come to visit every week. Sometimes they work together with me. They are helping me to sit up and reach for my toys. I'm learning to taste new foods and say sounds. It can be hard work for me, and sometimes I don't want to do it. But mommy and daddy are happy to see the therapists because they listen and answer their questions. Guess what? I went to the zoo with mommy and daddy in my new wheelchair. Early intervention is helping us. (adapted from Oser & Cohen, 2003)

---

how children are identified for services. Though the early intervention program is federally mandated, individual states set their own guidelines to identify and qualify a child for early intervention services.

Rosa's case, presented in the case study above, illustrates parental feelings of frustration, stress, and helplessness when trying to cope with fragile infants. You will learn how early intervention services include parents and other family members of an exceptional child. The chapter will also introduce the variety of professionals who may constitute an early intervention team and strategies for working effectively as a team member. The development of an Individualized Family Service Plan (IFSP) by the early intervention team will be presented.

Rosa, like the vast majority of children in early intervention programs, received services in her home. Some practical issues, including those related to cultural diversity, for working in the home setting will be addressed. Finally, much progress has been made since the beginning of the early intervention program. As with any service or policy, early intervention will continue to evolve as time passes. The continuing challenges of providing early intervention into the 21st century will be explored.

WHAT IS EARLY INTERVENTION?

According to Oser and Cohen (2003), the first years of life lay the foundation for how babies walk, talk, and learn. Most children grow and develop in predictable ways. For some young children, development proceeds at a slower timetable or in an atypical fashion. The reason(s) for a problem in development may be physical, mental, environmental, or a combination of factors. Oser and Cohen (2003) define *early intervention* as "the process of anticipating, identifying, and responding to child and family concerns in order to minimize their potential adverse effects and maximize the healthy development of babies and toddlers" (p. 3). Agents outside the family are introduced into the home to teach the family how to develop skills and enhance an at-risk child's quality of life. Such intervention may occur from before birth to school entry at kindergarten (Karoly et al., 1998). In this chapter, early intervention is relegated to services provided only from birth to a child's third birthday.

Early intervention may include a wide variety of services, including some combination of public health programs, child care programs, income, and programs to promote early childhood development. Some may also include programs that are of a more general nature such as Medicaid and Food Stamps as part of early intervention. These programs may be general and target the family or may target children with special needs. Early intervention programs can be provided in the home, hospital, center, or a combination of settings. These programs can be funded by some combination of federal, state, local, private, or personal funding. Table 16–1 illustrates examples

T A B L E 16–1 Examples of Range of Early Intervention Programs

Public Health Programs

- Prenatal care
- Home visitation programs for expectant mothers
- Immunizations
- Nutritional supplements

Child Care Programs

- Programs that regulate the quality of child care providers
- Subsidies to families to purchase child care

Income or In-Kind Support Programs

- Medicaid
- Special supplemental Feeding Program for Women, Infants and Children (WIC)

Early and Periodic Screening Diagnosis and Treatment Services

Programs to Promote Early Childhood Development

- Home visitation
- Parenting classes
- Family relationship education
- Family counseling
- Early Head Start
- Head Start
- Healthy Start
- Preschool and Kindergarten
- Part H Infant and Toddler Programs under Individuals with Disabilities Education Act

SOURCES: E. Fish, The Benefits of Early Intervention, *Journal of the HEIA, 10(3)*, pp. 32–34 (2003); L. A. Karoly, P. W. Greenwood, S. S. Everingham, J. Hoube, M. R. Kilburn, C. P. Rydell, M. Sander, & J. Chiesa, *Investing in Our Children: What We Know and Don't Know About the Cost Benefit of Early Childhood Intervention*. Santa Monica, CA: Rand, 1998.

of early intervention programs that may be offered to infants, toddlers, preschool age children, kindergarten children, and their parents.

WHY EARLY INTERVENTION?

There are three main reasons for intervening early with children with special needs (1) to enhance the child's development, (2) to provide support and assistance to the family, and (3) to maximize the child and his/her family's benefit to society (Pathways Awareness Foundation, 2005). Four decades of research in early childhood development indicate that a child's early years provide an important foundation for later development; that early intervention can have a vital influence on how a child will develop to his or her full potential; and that when eligible children do not receive early intervention services, they and their families, as well as society in general, bear the consequences (Oser & Cohen, 2003).

Child Development

It is well established that the pre- and postnatal care is vitally important to eventual child development. Further, we know that children learn and develop most rapidly in their preschool years and that loss of this opportune time will result in later learning difficulties. The brain achieves 90 percent of its total growth by age 3 (Karoly et al., 1998). Thus, early positive and stimulating experience with parents and others affects brain development and consequently physical, cognitive, emotional, communication, and socialization skills. Conversely, negative early experiences may be difficult to overcome (Fish, 2003).

For example, infants with hearing impairment identified after 6 months of age have lower language scores as they age than those who were identified before 6 months of age (Yoshinaga-Itano, Sedy, Coulter, & Mehl, 1998). In general, without formal intervention, research has found a general decline in performance on developmental measures for children with a variety of cognitive disabilities across the first 5 years of life (Shonkoff & Phillips, 2000).

Infants and toddlers who score below the mean of national norms for developmental functioning and do not receive early intervention services often move into the lowest functioning groups as they get older (Mathematica Policy Research, Inc., & Columbia University's Center for Children and Families at Teacher's College, 2002).

Family Support and Assistance

Early intervention services have a significant impact on family members of a child with special needs. The family often feels helplessness, frustration, disappointment, guilt, and social isolation. According to Havens (2005), parents who have a child with a disability may vent their frustrations on each other or the child. Unfortunately, this may result in marital difficulties, sibling rivalry, and child abuse. If a family's overall well-being is compromised, it is likely to have adverse effects on the child's development. Early intervention services can improve parents' attitudes about their child and themselves. These services can improve parenting skills and reduce stress. A reduction in family stress may improve the family's ability to implement the child's program at home (Cooper, 1981; Garland, Stone, Swanson, & Woodruff, 1981; Karnes, 1983; Shonkoff & Hauser-Cram, 1987).

Early intervention programs appear to have many benefits for mothers, in particular. Karoly and colleagues (1998) state that early intervention results in high-risk mothers improving their own quality of life, increasing employment, and reducing drug dependency.

Societal Benefits

Several studies have investigated the effectiveness of early intervention. Karoly and colleagues (1998) of the Rand Corporation evaluated the effects on development, educational achievement, economic well-being, and health for participants versus controls in nine programs across the United States. All programs resulted in some type of gain for the children, and the favorable effects outnumbered the insignificant ones. Specific gains were seen in short-term emotional or cognitive development, improved parent-child relationships, improved educational outcomes for the child, increased economic self-sufficiency for the parent and later the child, lower welfare use, reduced levels of criminal activity, and improvements in health-related indicators such as child abuse, maternal reproductive health, and maternal substance abuse (Rand, 1998).

In general, early intervention has been shown to result in children with special needs requiring fewer special education and other habilitative services later in life, being retained at a grade level less often, and in many cases, being indistinguishable from typical peers years after intervention (Kid-Source Online, 2005). Many studies report that the earlier the intervention, the more effective it is, and the developmental gains are greater (Cooper, 1981; Garland et al., 1981).

Is Early Intervention Cost Effective?

Early intervention services are highly specialized and, often on a short-term basis, more costly than traditional school-aged service delivery models. The Rand Corporation (1998 p. 4), in its evaluation of nine national preschool programs, concluded that "from a statistical point of view, one can be quite confident that the benefits exceed the costs." The researchers also indicated that costs are immediate whereas benefits are realized "only as the years pass and children mature through adolescence to adulthood." Analysts underscore the need to identify who will benefit from programs and how successful demonstration programs can be replicated in the most cost-effective manner at national levels.

YOUNG CHILDREN WITH DISABILITIES

Thus far, we have provided a general description of early intervention for young children. Those youngsters with disabilities are a special subset of those considered at risk.

Legislation

The 1980s saw a growth in national concern for young children with disabilities and their families. A growing body of research, some of it predating PL 94-142, suggested that providing early intervention for children with disabilities yielded important and lasting benefits for both the children and their families. Safer and Hamilton (1993) state that despite the evidence illustrating the benefits of providing early intervention prior to the enactment of PL 94-142, in 1975 Congress, while requiring services for school-age children, included preschool children only on a permissive basis. No support was given for serving infants and toddlers with disabilities, although states were allowed to use some of the federal funds for this purpose. Congress did, however, appropriate funds for the establishment of model programs and research to demonstrate and evaluate the feasibility of providing early intervention to children with disabilities from birth through age 5. By 1985 only 24 states had mandated special education and related services for all children with disabilities beginning at 3 years of age or younger, and only six states had mandated services beginning at birth (Safer & Hamilton, 1993).

In 1984 and 1985 the efficacy of early intervention was framed in cost–benefit terms by the U.S. Department of Education. In addition to efficacy and cost-benefit studies, there was a moral/humanitarian rationale for providing services immediately when a disability was detected, which for many children was at birth or shortly after. Society recognized an imperative or sense of duty to help others in need of assistance. It would be morally objectionable not to provide services when a need was apparent.

In 1985 and 1986, armed with efficacy studies, examples of model programs by states that had mandated services, and arguments made on humanitarian and moral grounds, parents, professionals, and other advocates placed great pressure on Congress to enact comprehensive early intervention legislation for children from birth to age 3 (Safer & Hamilton, 1993). In response, Congress enacted PL 99-457, the Education for the Handicapped Act Amendments (EHA), in 1986. PL 99-457 established the Part H program for infants and toddlers with disabilities and their families.

In 1990, PL 99-457 was further amended to become PL 101-476. The name was changed to Individuals with Disabilities Education Act, or IDEA. IDEA mandated the provision of services for children with disabilities from birth to age 21. Under the law, Congress must periodically review (usually every 5 years) and reauthorize IDEA to ensure the continuation of the programs and services. The first time IDEA was reauthorized was in 1997 (PL 105-17, the IDEA Amendments). The former Part H program for infants and toddlers with disabilities became Part C of IDEA1997. Part B, the section of the legislation that authorizes special education and related services for children ages 3 through 21, was authorized permanently. The most recent reauthorization of Part C was in 2004 (PL 108-446, the Individuals with Disabilities Education Improvement Act of 2004). At present, Part C has not been permanently authorized.

Part C of IDEA authorizes the creation of early intervention programs for infants and toddlers with disabilities and provides federal assistance for states to maintain and implement statewide systems of services for eligible children. Part C is a discretionary program, which means that states have a choice to participate in the program. If they choose to participate, they must fully implement the law's requirements. Currently all 50 states and territories are participating in the Part C program.

Overview to the Part C Program Under IDEA
As stated in IDEA1997 (PL 105-17), Congress established Part C in recognition of "an urgent and substantial need" to:

1. Enhance the development of infants and toddlers with disabilities and to minimize their potential for developmental delay

2. Reduce the educational costs to our society, including our nation's schools, by minimizing the need for special education and related services after infants and toddlers with disabilities reach school age

3. Minimize the likelihood of institutionalization of individuals with disabilities and maximize the potential for their independent living in society

4. Enhance the capacity of families to meet the special needs of their infants and toddlers with disabilities

5. Enhance the capacity of state and local agencies and service providers to identify, evaluate, and meet the needs of historically underrepresented populations, particularly minority, low-income, inner-city, and rural populations. (Sec. 631(a))

In order for a state to participate in the program, it must ensure that early intervention will be available to every eligible child and family. Also, the governor of each state must designate a lead agency to receive the grant and administer the program and appoint an Interagency Coordinating Council (ICC), including parents of young children with disabilities, to advise and assist the lead agency.

The law states that, at a minimum, each state system must include the following 16 key components:

1. A definition of the term *developmental delay*

2. A policy that ensures appropriate early intervention services based on scientifically based research are available to all infants and toddlers with disabilities and their families, including American Indian infants and toddlers and their families residing on a reservation geographically located in the state

3. A timely, comprehensive, multidisciplinary evaluation of each eligible child and a family-directed identification of the needs of each family to appropriately assist in the development of the infant or toddler

4. An individualized family service plan (IFSP), including service coordination, for each eligible child and family

5. A comprehensive child find and referral system, consistent with Part B of IDEA

6. A public awareness program focusing on early identification of infants and toddlers with disabilities, including the preparation and dissemination of information to parents

7. A central directory of services and other resources, including research and demonstration projects

8. A comprehensive system of personnel development

9. Policies and procedures to ensure that personnel are appropriately and adequately prepared and trained

10. Designation of a single line of responsibility in the lead agency

11. A policy pertaining to contracting with local service providers

12. A procedure for timely reimbursement of funds

13. Procedural safeguards

14. A system for compiling data

15. A state interagency coordinating council

16. Policies and procedures to ensure, to the maximum extent appropriate, early intervention services are provided in natural environments (Sec. 635(a))

Early Intervention Eligibility/Developmental Delay

A major challenge to state policy makers in implementing the Early Intervention Program for Infants and Toddlers with Disabilities, Part C under IDEA, is defining developmental delay and criteria of eligibility. The federal law defines an infant or toddler with a disability as an

individual under 3 years of age who needs early intervention services because the individual is experiencing developmental delays in one or more of the domains of cognitive development, physical development, communication development, social or emotional development and adaptive development; or has a diagnosed physical or mental condition which has a high probability of resulting in developmental delay. (Sec. 632(5)(A))

States are required to define the term *developmental delay* and establish procedures to determine when such a condition is present. Brown and Brown (1993) state that "procedures to determine the presence of delays include the use of tests, informed clinical opinion, and multidisciplinary team decision making" (p. 27). When states use quantitative standardized procedures to determine the presence of developmental delay, levels of functioning may include standard deviation, percentage of delay, number of months of delay, and developmental quotients.

There is currently a great variation from state to state in the procedures that have been established to define developmental delay and eligibility (Shackelford, 2004). While states and jurisdictions have flexibility in determining developmental delay, 13 rely only on test-based criteria, and 38 use a combination of test-based and non-test-based criteria. Three states use only professional judgment and/or documentation of atypical development. Depending on the state, the percentage of delay for eligibility ranges from a 25 percent to 50 percent delay in one developmental domain or a 25 percent delay in two developmental domains. Some states rely on standardized scores ranging from 1.5 to 2.0 standard deviations below the mean in one developmental domain or 1.0 to 1.5 standard deviations below the mean in two developmental domains (Shackelford, 2004). The reader is referred to Shackelford (2004) for information comparing individual state and jurisdictional eligibility definitions under Part C of IDEA.

According to Benn (1991) and Shonkoff & Meisels (1991), there is an insufficient number of reliable and valid instruments for the birth to 2 age group; thus, determining delay by traditional assessment can be problematic. For that reason states are required to ensure that informed clinical opinion/judgment is included to determine eligibility. Shackelford (2004) states that informed

clinical opinion can be based on the observation of discrepancies in developments, without specifying a particular level of delay. Informed clinical opinion is typically derived from the consensus of a multidisciplinary team that includes parents and information from multiple sources (Harbin, Gallagher, & Terry, 1991; Benn, 1991; Shackelford, 2002).

Diagnosed Physical or Mental Condition Diagnosed physical or mental conditions can establish a child's eligibility based on the high probability of the occurrence of developmental delay associated with the condition (Sec. 632(5)(A)(ii)). The federal law does not specify which conditions are to be included; however, examples are provided to the states for guidance. Examples include Down Syndrome and other chromosomal abnormalities; sensory disorders (i.e., hearing and vision loss); inborn abnormalities in metabolism; neurological disorders; congenital malformations; severe attachment disorders, including failure to thrive; seizure disorders; and fetal alcohol syndrome (Shackelford, 2004).

On a state-by-state basis there are differences of professional opinion on which conditions should be included under established conditions eligibility; however, having an established condition constitutes *presumptive eligibility*. This means that the child is eligible for early intervention services regardless of whether the delay is present at the time of the identification. An example would be children diagnosed with Down syndrome who might not be developmentally delayed at birth; however, it is universally held that children with a diagnosis of Down syndrome should receive early intervention services to help minimize future delay (Brown & Brown, 1993).

At Risk After the creation of the early intervention program under IDEA, many states were interested in serving children at risk, but fears of highly increased numbers of eligible children and highly increased costs reduced the number of states that included children at risk in their definitions of eligibility. Brown and Brown (1993) state that "the term *at risk* refers to children who are in danger of having substantial developmental delays if early intervention services are not provided" (p. 30). These children may not demonstrate an abnormality in development but have biological or environmental factors in their medical history or home life that may increase the risk of delay in the future.

According to Shackelford (2004), examples of biological/medical risk conditions include low birth weight, intraventricular hemorrhage at birth, chronic lung disease, and failure to thrive. Children at environmental risk are those individuals whose current care-giving situation places them at greater risk for delay than the general population. Shackelford goes on to say that examples of environmental risk include family substance abuse, family social disorganization, poverty, parental age, parental educational attainment, and child abuse or neglect. Some states that choose to serve at-risk children use a multiple risk model with a range of three to five risk factors required for eligibility of services. A few states require less delay for eligibility when biological/medical and/or environmental risk factors are present. Currently nine states include children at risk under their eligibility definition. Several states that are not serving children at risk have indicated that they will monitor the development of these children and refer them for early intervention services as delays are manifested (Shackelford, 2004).

Screening, Evaluation, and Assessment

According to the National Early Childhood Technical Assistance Center (2005a), screening, evaluation, and assessment are distinct processes with different purposes under Part C of IDEA. Screening, which includes developmental and health screening, is a procedure designed to identify children who should receive more intensive evaluation to determine the existence of a delay in development or a particular disability. Evaluation is used to determine the existence of a delay or disability. Assessment is used to determine the individual child's present level of performance and early intervention or educational needs.

Developmental Screening Many children with behavioral or developmental disorders are not being identified early in the United States (Oser & Cohen, 2003). Part C requires that each state's child find system must include the policies and procedures that the state will follow to ensure that all infants and toddlers in the state who are eligible for services under Part C are identified, located, and evaluated. Developmental screening can allow for earlier detection of delays and improve child health and well-being for identified children. According to the National Center of Birth Defects and Developmental Disabilities (2005), developmental screening can be done by various professionals in community, school, or health care settings. The role of health professionals has become important to developmental screening. Health professionals have regular contact with children birth to age 3, which allows them an opportunity to monitor development through periodic developmental screening. The American Academy of Pediatrics (AAP) and the American Academy of Neurology recommend that all infants and toddlers be screened for developmental delays as part of office-based primary care.

Role of Audiologists and Speech-Language Pathologists in Screening Hearing plays a vital role in the acquisition of speech and language, social-emotional, and cognitive skills. Over the past 10 years, the emphasis on universal early detection of hearing loss in infants has grown considerably. The passage of the Newborn and Infant Hearing and Intervention Act of 1999 had important implications for audiologists and speech-language pathologists. Research findings and improvements in screening technology have influenced and resulted in updates of hearing screening guidelines ASHA, 1997a). In *Guidelines for the Audiologic Assessment of Children From Birth to 5 Years of Age* (2004a), ASHA advocates the use of portions of developmental screening tools, such as the *Early Language Milestone Scale* (Coplan & Gleason, 1993), to screen prelinguistic communicative behavior in children from birth to 4 months and to screen receptive and expressive language skills in children 5 through 24 months of age.

The Joint Committee on Infant Hearing (JCIH) (2000) states that hospital-based screening is the first step in a comprehensive program of detection and intervention of hearing loss. The JCIH position statement provides a comprehensive program with a suggested time line for detection and intervention that also includes diagnosis, integration with the baby's medical care, provision of family support services, and data management/tracking procedures.

With rising numbers of infants born prematurely with resulting neurodevelopmental sequelae, speech-language pathologists also play a significant role in screening, evaluation, and intervention in neonatal intensive care units. ASHA (2004b, 2004c) developed two position statements to address the roles and knowledge/skills needed by speech-language pathologists to provide services in neonatal intensive care units (NICU). Speech-language pathologists provide a continuum of services for infants and families in the NICU to identify infants at risk for communication, cognition, and feeding/swallowing problems.

According to the First Words Project (2005), a delay in language development may be the first evidence of a developmental delay when serious health or physical impairments are not present. Research has identified a group of "language predictors" that are indicators of later language development and promise earlier and more accurate identification (McCathren, Warren, & Yoder, 1996; Wetherby & Prizant, 1993, 1996). Wetherby and Prizant (2001) have developed a screening *Infant-Toddler Checklist* as one component of their *Communication and Symbolic Behavior Scales-Developmental Profile*. The purpose of this profile is for early identification of children who are at risk of developing a communication impairment and to monitor changes in the child over time. Information on this checklist can be found on the First Words Project Web site (see Resources at the end of this chapter).

Rescorla and Alley (2001) conducted two studies demonstrating the reliability, validity, and clinical utility of the *Language Development Survey* (LDS) (Rescorla, 1989) as a screening tool for the identification of expressive language delay in toddlers. The LDS can be used by health care providers, early childhood teachers and caregivers, speech-language pathologists, and child find agencies to screen children for possible language delays at around 24 months of age.

Evaluation

Part C of IDEA requires that each state system include provisions for a timely, comprehensive, and multidisciplinary evaluation. Evaluation is defined as the procedures used by qualified personnel to determine a child's initial and continuing eligibility, consistent with each state's definition of infants and toddlers with disabilities. Part C states that there should be a family-directed evaluation "of the resources, priorities, and concerns of the family and the identification of the supports and services necessary to enhance the family's capacity to meet the developmental needs of the infant or toddler" (Sec. 636(a)(2)).

Part C further states that the early intervention evaluation must include (1) a review of pertinent records related to the child's current health status and medical history and (2) an evaluation of the child's level of functioning in each of five developmental domains: cognitive development, physical development, communication development, social-emotional development, and adaptive development.

The Evaluation Process A strategy for beginning the evaluation process is preassessment planning (Johnson, McGonigel, & Kaufman, 1989). Preassessment planning involves two steps (Kjerland & Kovach, 1989). According to Johnson, McGonigel, and Kaufman (1990), "the service coordinator, who serves as the facilitator for the evaluation process, obtains information from the family on the concerns they have about their child and on their needs concerning the time, location, and extent of their participation in the evaluation process" (p. 55). The service coordinator reviews this information with the evaluation team who then decides which assessments should be used and plans the evaluation to fit the family's needs.

The evaluation process is facilitated through an integrated team approach, often called an *arena assessment*, where members of a team of professionals from a variety of disciplines collect information on the five developmental domains defined by IDEA Part C (Foley, 1990). According to Foley (1990), "the members of the team, lead by the family, plan in advance what questions they will be attempting to answer, which assessment instruments will be used, and what time and location would best facilitate child performance" (p. 56). Procedures may vary from one jurisdiction to another, but typically, one team member will be designated the facilitator for the evaluation. The facilitator and parent will directly engage the child in activities during the evaluation. Usually, at least one other team member will be present and be engaged in completing individual assessment tools. The other team member(s) may or may not interact directly with the child.

Areas of Evaluation

IDEA Part C requires that the child's current level of functioning be determined in each of these five developmental domains:

Cognitive development—assessing a child's visual pursuit and object permanence, means ends abilities, operational causality, spatial relationships, schemes for relating to objects, verbal imitation, and gestural imitation.

Communication development—assessing a child's prelinguistic communication behavior, expressive language abilities, receptive language abilities, pragmatic language abilities, speech acquisition skills, and oral-motor development related to feeding and prespeech development.

Physical development—assessing a child's fine and gross motor development, including reflexes, balance, nonlocomotor, locomotor, receipt, and propulsion in the gross motor area and grasping, hand use, eye-hand coordination, and manual dexterity in the fine motor area.

Social-emotional development—assessing a child's temperament, expression of emotions and feelings, self-concept, peer interaction, adult interaction, coping, and play skills.

Adaptive skills development—assessing a child's independent feeding skills, dressing skills, grooming and hygiene skills, toileting, sleep patterns, and household independence/responsibility.

Assessment of Results

Once it is clear through the evaluation process that an infant or toddler is eligible for early intervention services based on each state's criteria for eligibility, IDEA Part C states that assessment activities will be conducted to identify the child's unique strengths and needs and the appropriate services to meet those needs. In addition, "a family-directed assessment of the resources, priorities, and concerns of the family and the supports and services necessary to enhance the family's capacity to meet the developmental needs of their infant or toddler with a disability" will be conducted (Sec. 636(a)(2)). An early intervention assessment should be a flexible, collaborative decision-making process where teams of parents and professionals repeatedly revise their judgments and reach consensus about the changing needs of young children and their families (Bagnato & Neisworth, 1991). Assessment is ongoing throughout the period of a child's eligibility.

THE INDIVIDUALIZED FAMILY SERVICE PLAN (IFSP)

The purpose of assessment under Part C is to determine the content of the Individualized Family Service Plan. The outcome of the assessment will be goals and objectives for the child and the family, determination of related services to be provided, and "baseline" measurement of the child's level of functioning, which will serve as a point of comparison for measuring progress (McLean & McCormick, 1993). The IFSP is the "vehicle through which effective early intervention is implemented in accordance with Part C of the Individuals with Disabilities Education Act" (Bruder, 2000). Each plan is tailored to the individual child and his or her family. Part C acknowledges the family as the central focus of early intervention policies and practices. Through the IFSP process, team members plan, implement, and evaluate services tailored to the family's unique concerns. According to Part C, the IFSP (Sec. 636(d)) shall be in writing and contain statements comprising the following eight components:

1. The child's present levels of physical development, cognitive development, communication development, social or emotional development, and adaptive development

2. The family's resources, priorities, and concerns relating to enhancing the development of the child with a disability

3. The major outcomes to be achieved for the child and the family; the criteria, procedures, and timelines used to determine progress; and whether modifications or revisions of the outcomes or services are necessary

4. Specific early intervention services necessary to meet the unique needs of the child and the family, including frequency, intensity, and method of delivery

5. The natural environments in which services will be provided, including justification of the extent, if any, to which the services will not be provided in a natural environment

6. The projected dates for initiation of services and their anticipated duration

7. The identification of the service coordinator who will be responsible for implementing the plan and coordinating with other agencies and persons 8 Steps to support the child's transition to preschool or other appropriate services.

The United States Department of Education's Division for Early Childhood (DEC) established rules (1993) requiring non–Part C services needed by a child, including medical and other services, be described in the IFSP, along with funding sources for those services. Part C requires that the IFSP be evaluated and revised annually and that periodic reviews be conducted at least every 6 months or sooner, if requested by the family.

Principles to Guide the IFSP Process

According to Sandall (1993), "the extent to which the process of developing and implementing a family service plan is positive and supportive is determined largely by the attitudes and skills of the early intervention professionals" (p. 130). McGonigel (1991) developed a set of principles that are necessary for professionals to understand in order to develop effective family service plans. In order for professionals to develop an effective family service plan, several principles need to be taken into account. According to McGonigel (1991), respect for and acceptance of diversity is a hallmark of family-centered intervention. The services must be flexible and matched to the needs of individual families taking into account each family's racial, ethnic, cultural, and socioeconomic diversity. McGonigel (1991) further indicates that services should be provided in as normal an environment as possible to best integrate the child and his or her family into the community. To accomplish this, family and provider partnerships or collaboration are critical.

SERVICE COORDINATION

Under Part C, service coordination is defined as an active, ongoing process that assists and enables families to access services and assures their rights and procedural safeguards. Each family of an infant or toddler that receives services under Part C is assigned a service coordinator who:

1. Coordinates the necessary evaluations and assessments,

2. Facilitates the initial IFSP meeting and subsequent reviews,

3. Assists the family in receiving the services and supports described on the IFSP

4. Assures their rights and safeguards

States have different approaches or models of service coordination and service coordination caseloads vary according to the different models. In practice, at least four different service coordination models have been identified (Hurth, 1998): dedicated service coordination, early interventionist service coordination, interagency service coordination, and intake service coordination. Table 16–2 illustrates different models of service coordination.

T A B L E 16–2 Service Coordination

Dedicated Service Coordination

- Service coordination is primary job focus
- Service coordinators may be employed by early intervention programs or independent or program

Early Interventionist and Service Coordination

- Service coordinator is also a service provider

Interagency Service Coordination

- The service coordinator that is the most appropriate match to a family's needs may be selected from a choice of several different agencies

Interim or Intake Service Coordination

- Interim or intake coordinator facilitates the first 45 days of a family's entry into the early intervention system
- At first IFSP meeting a permanent service coordinator is selected

SOURCE: J. Hurth, *Service Coordination Caseloads in State Early Intervention Systems.* Chapel Hill, NC: National Early Childhood Technical Assistance System, 1998.

Service Delivery Collaboration: Teaming

After the IFSP has been developed, Part C requires an integrated team approach to intervention. The types of teams that typically function in early intervention have been identified as multidisciplinary, interdisciplinary, and transdisciplinary. Bruder and Bologna (1993) state that the "components that differentiate the types of teams have been identified, including the role of the family, the mode of communication between team members, the role-clarification process, and the mode of intervention" (p. 117).

In the *multidisciplinary* team approach, which is usually associated with the medical model, professionals maintain their respective discipline boundaries with only minimal, if any, coordination, collaboration, or communication with other team members. Bruder and Bologna (1993) report that the parent is invited to share information, and the professionals, in turn, share information with the family through an "informing" conference. There is

little integration across disciplines, and the family is a passive recipient of information about the child. Therapy and assessment are conducted in isolation.

The *interdisciplinary* team approach was developed as a response to dissatisfaction with the multidisciplinary model. This model is based on a commitment to coordination, collaboration, and communication. According to Bruder and Bologna (1993), "parents may be active members of the team, but their input is generally considered secondary in importance to material collected by the professionals" (p. 117). There usually is an exchange of information among the service providers prior to intervention or at team meetings, but it generally ends at that point. Therapy and assessment conform to the same isolation tenets as the multidisciplinary approach.

The *transdisciplinary* team approach addresses the problems of the multidisciplinary and interdisciplinary approaches. Bruder and Bologna (1993) state that "on a transdisciplinary team the members share roles and purposefully cross discipline boundaries" (p. 117). All team members, including the family, work together to accomplish mutually agreed-upon intervention outcomes. The professionals' roles are defined by the needs of the situation rather than by the function of a specific discipline (Bruder, 2002). A critical component of effective transdisciplinary teams is a continuous need for communication among all members of the team. This concept is often difficult to implement. According to McWilliam (2000), "team members must be open with each other, be willing to share their knowledge, and be open to acquiring new skills." In addition, "each team member must develop skills in problem solving, conflict resolution, and team consensus-building" (p. 2).

In reality, maintaining a transdisciplinary approach can be challenging. State and national licensing issues may impede the concept of "role release." Many clinicians come from training backgrounds where the interdisciplinary approach is the norm. In some instances, a child may receive services from multiple disciplines where very different philosophies of intervention are implemented. For example, a team working with a child diagnosed with autistic spectrum disorder could possibly be comprised of a speech language pathologist delivering service based on a developmental model and a special education teacher delivering service based on a behavioral model such as Applied Behavioral Analysis (ABA). Open communication between team members in such a scenario may be problematic.

One interaction strategy that has come to be identified closely with the transdisciplinary team approach is consultation. *Consultation* can be defined as a process of interaction between two professionals concerning a current work problem. Typically the consultee is having some difficulty and has decided to seek guidance via a consultant whose area of specialized competence the consultee seeks (Caplan, 1970).

A second interaction strategy that has come to be identified with the transdisciplinary team approach is *integrated therapy*. Part C states that to the maximum extent appropriate services are to be provided "in natural environments, including the home and community settings in which children without disabilities participate" (Sec. 632(4)(G)). Integrated therapy helps to meet the federal mandate and can be defined as training in environments where the skill is to be performed (Nietupski, Scheutz & Ockwood, 1980). Orelove and Sobsey (1991) provide four assumptions that should govern the transdisciplinary team approach to integrated therapy:

1. Natural environments are the best place to assess and develop a child's abilities.

2. A child should be taught skills he or she needs for everyday living. These skills are best taught through daily routines and activities.

3. Discipline-specific objectives should be implemented in all settings in which a child functions.

4. Skills should be taught and reinforced in natural settings.

Transdisciplinary teamwork makes integrated therapy possible. As an example, Kilgo and colleagues (2003) state that during snack time in an inclusive early childhood program for toddlers, the speech-language pathologist works with a child on communication goals such as requesting snack items as well as socialization with peers. The physical therapist works with the child on his ambulation skills to the table, and the occupational therapist provides the proper positioning of the child at the table while eating. The child participates in the regular routines of the classroom and is not removed from the classroom for isolated therapies. The classroom teacher can then implement the therapists' goals during other activities in the room, and the caregivers can do the same at home. Integrated activities provide the child with many opportunities to practice and generalize new skills in natural settings.

PERSONNEL AND DISCIPLINES IN EARLY INTERVENTION

Part C of IDEA states that early intervention services should be provided by "qualified personnel" and include: special educators, speech-language pathologists, audiologists, occupational therapists, physical therapists, psychologists, social workers, nurses, nutritionists, family therapists, orientation and mobility specialists, and pediatricians and other physicians.

Professional requirements for providing early intervention are based on the highest requirements in the state applicable to the professions. According to Brown and Rule (1993), "a qualified service provider is one who has met state-approved or state-recognized certification, licensing, registration, or other comparable requirements that apply to the area in which the person is providing early intervention services" (p. 256).

Many professional organizations have recognized the need to define and teach competencies to members of their discipline who serve infants and toddlers with disabilities. ASHA has described services and roles of speech-language pathologists and audiologists who provide early intervention services (1989, 1990, 2004a). In addition, ASHA has sponsored training for early intervention personnel through meetings and conferences.

Not all states have developed early intervention standards that are applicable across disciplines, but many have adopted a common core of standards. Fenichel and Eggbeer (1991) identify three content-independent issues pertinent to all personnel preparing to work in early intervention. (1) observation and interacting with young children and families, (2) individualized supervision, and (3) support from colleagues from various disciplines. In addition, all personnel training for jobs in early intervention need instruction in the areas of family theory, teaming, typical and atypical infant development, service coordination, and cultural diversity (Brown & Rule, 1993).

WORKING WITH CULTURALLY AND LINGUISTICALLY DIVERSE FAMILIES

Given that the United States is one of the most culturally, ethnically, racially, and linguistically diverse countries in the world, there is an immediate need for speech-language pathologists and audiologists working with the birth to age 3 population to upgrade their levels of multicultural knowledge and skills to better address the needs of these children and families. According to McLean (1997), "service providers' lack of experience with and knowledge of diverse families make the development of relationships with them difficult and often contributes to families' under utilization of services" (p. 1).

Different Cultural Views on Health and Disorders

Western health practice is largely based on "fixing" diseases or medical maladies. Treatment is designed to repair the physical malfunction. Speech therapy is ordered to "fix" communication disorders or improve communication functionality.

Traditional non-Western cultures usually believe in the connection between illness and an external force. It is believed that health is a result of physical and spiritual harmony with nature and physical maladies are states of disharmony. If a child exhibits a speech disorder, the family may exhibit guilt or shame. They may respond by covering up or hiding the problem and not seek intervention. Speech-language pathologists and audiologists providing early intervention must be aware of how parents perceive their child's communication disorder and are willing to accept treatment for it (Cole, 1989; ASHA, 1991).

Different Service Delivery Preferences Among Minority Language Groups

Speech-language pathologists and audiologists, as a Western cultural group, believe they are "experts" in the treatment of children with communication disorders due to their academic training. As a group, SLPs and audiologists are often frustrated when family members do not appear willing to participate in therapy activities.

Clinicians must be aware that strong cultural influences often determine the amount of family participation in the treatment of their child or even the refusal of treatment (ASHA, 1985). For additional information, a variety of resources are available from the Early Childhood Research Institute on Culturally and Linguistically Appropriate Services (ASHA, 2003). Also, see Chapter 23 on multicultural issues for more discussion of this topic and communication disorders.

TRANSITION FROM EARLY INTERVENTION TO PRESCHOOL SPECIAL EDUCATION

Many children will continue to need the services provided to them under the Early Intervention program after their third birthday. Preschool special education services are designed for children with special needs ages 3 through 5 and are provided free of charge through the public school system. This program is mandated through Part B of IDEA, which, unlike Part C, has been permanently authorized. The transition from early intervention services to preschool special education services requires that the child be evaluated to determine if he or she has a disability as defined by IDEA Part B and to determine if that disability is considered educationally handicapping. If the child is found eligible, the family will meet with school district personnel to write an Individualized Education Program designed to meet that child's individualized needs. Children transitioning from early intervention to preschool special education programs usually begin the transition process sometime between the ages of 2 years 6 months and 2 years 9 months. A bibliography of reference materials on the transition from early intervention programs to preschool special education programs designed for parents and professionals can be found through the NECTAC Clearinghouse on Early Intervention and Early Childhood Special Education (2005).

PRACTICAL ISSUES FOR SPEECH-LANGUAGE PATHOLOGISTS AND AUDIOLOGISTS

This chapter has dealt with the legislative context and the policies and procedures of implementing Part C of IDEA. The remainder of this chapter will provide clinicians with information describing the practical issues facing speech-language pathologists and audiologists as early intervention service providers.

Employment Opportunities

Speech-language pathologists and audiologists working in early intervention programs may be employed in salaried positions (full time and part time) or as independent contractors working for specific counties, hospitals, clinics, or private service provider agencies. Speech-language pathologists and audiologists provide services to children in homes, daycare/preschool facilities, center-based programs, and outpatient clinics. In 1999, 6,054 speech language pathologists and 577 audiologists were employed and contracted to provide early intervention services to infants and toddlers with disabilities and their families in the United States

and outlying areas (United States Department of Education, 2002).

Credentials Many states require that speech-language pathologists and audiologists have state licensure and ASHA's Certificate of Clinical Competency (CCC) to provide early intervention services.

IDEA 2004 eliminated the "highest qualified provider" requirement that had previously been included in the law due to concerns about personnel shortages. Now qualifications for speech-language pathologists must be consistent with any state-approved or state-recognized certification, licensing, or other comparable requirement applicable to their professional discipline.

Home Care Services

Of all the different early intervention settings covered under Part C, the home setting is where the vast majority of early intervention services are provided. In 1999, 68 percent of infants and toddlers who received early intervention received it in their own home (United States Department of Education, 2002). For most children, the home is the least restrictive, natural environment for learning. Having family members/caregivers present during treatment sessions provides the clinician with opportunities to teach family members therapy techniques and to provide carryover activities for the family to engage their child. Often older siblings can be enlisted to "work with" the child. Direct family education increases the number of opportunities a child will have for learning speech and language. A clinician may only spend 1–2 hours per week with a child, whereas the family is usually with the child 24 hours a day, 7 days a week. Providing services in the child's home also provides opportunities for understanding and assessing the emotional impact of a young child with special needs on the family unit. Thus, more authentic counseling and education can be customized to meet these needs.

Infection Control

Clinicians should follow their provider agency's infection control procedures to protect children, family members, caregivers, and themselves from infection or potential infection. Provider agencies generally have infection control policies and procedures in place. Most employees and contractors are required to be oriented to the Occupational Safety and Health Administration infection control plan on an annual basis.

Often clinicians feel awkward asking to wash their hands after a session has been completed as they feel it might be insulting to the family. A simple solution is to tell the family at the initial treatment session, "It is the agency's policy that we wash our hands before and after working with each child. Where would you like me to do this?" Clinicians should wash their hands with pump-bottle soap and dry their hands with paper towels. If these are not available, the clinicians should check with their provider agency on the use of alcohol-based hand cleaners.

The policy of bringing a clinician's personal toys, books, and games into the child's home varies by jurisdiction. Some areas prohibit this practice, and clinicians (therapists and evaluators) must use whatever is found in the child's home. Some homes will have few or no age-appropriate toys. In such cases, some clinicians purchase inexpensive items and leave them at the child's house. For those jurisdictions that allow personal toys to be used, clinicians will need to follow their provider agency's infection control procedures to clean and store the items after use. See Chapter 21 for more discussion of infection prevention.

Physical Environment

As a clinician doing home care, you must be prepared to work in homes in various degrees of maintenance and cleanliness that may conflict with your own lifestyle. You may want to carry with you an extra pair of socks, a blanket, and a small plastic tablecloth. Families may want clinicians to remove their shoes. When removing sandals, you should put on a pair of socks so as not to go barefoot. If you are uncomfortable with the level of cleanliness in the designated area where services are to be delivered, spread a blanket on the floor and provide services on the blanket. When engaging the child in art activities, cover the table or other work area with a plastic tablecloth to prevent damage to the family's furniture. Clinicians should also be aware of their own nonverbal communication that may signal disapproval of the environment or cultural differences reflected in the home.

You may also find that the child's home is noisy and that there are family members, including siblings and visitors, in the home during a treatment session. In some cases, it is appropriate to include siblings in the treatment session. If, however, the environment is not conducive to your goals, you will need to discuss this tactfully with the parent or caregiver before the next session. You should also be sensitive to cultural differences in the home as some parents may be more comfortable having family members present for the visit.

Safety

It is unlikely that anything will happen to you when providing early intervention services in a home setting, but some suggestions are in order. A rule of thumb when providing home care is to act as though you know exactly what you are doing and where you are going. As the old saying goes, "attitude is everything." Always be alert to your surroundings. If visiting a home in a high crime area, try to schedule a visit in the morning, and if necessary, ask for a security escort or buddy up with another team member for the visit. If you feel unsafe about entering a home, do not enter. Clinicians should use a cell phone or find a public phone and call a supervisor for instructions. Program your cell phone with "911" or another emergency number. Try to park where your car can be seen from the family's door. Remove your car keys before leaving a family's house, have the keys ready to unlock a car door, and check the back seat for any intruders. If possible, do not carry a purse in plain view. Keep valuables locked in the car trunk or hidden from view in the car. Report all safety concerns to a supervisor. If the environment inside the house appears to be unsafe or unfit for the child, a call to a supervisor is indicated to discuss reporting the safety issues to your local child protection agency.

CONTINUING CHALLENGES OF PROVIDING EARLY INTERVENTION

With reauthorization of IDEA in 2004, early intervention has come of age. PL 99–457 was amended in 1986 to support states to serve infants and toddlers with disabilities. Much progress has been made; however, as with any service or policy, early intervention will continue to evolve as time passes. Issues and challenges continue to face early intervention providers.

Definitions and Eligibility

The criteria for defining, identifying, and declaring infants and toddlers and their families eligible for early intervention services vary widely from state to state. Eligibility continues to be a major issue because economic and human resources are limited. Only a limited number of states provide services to children and their families at risk for serious developmental problems. The Zero to Three Policy Center recommends that the existing category of "diagnosed physical or mental conditions" includes "family conditions that have a high probability of resulting in a developmental delay, such as significant parental mental illness, parental substance abuse, and significant family violence" (Oser & Cohen, 2003, p. 10).

Family Centeredness

Many early intervention services focus on the target child and involve the family only in limited ways. For programs to be family-centered, professionals must view their roles as much more than just providing parents with information and training and being present to sign forms at IFSP meetings. According to Thurman (1993), professionals can only be truly family-centered if they accept the family, along with the child, as the focus of services. Services must be designed to meet the needs and desire of the family, and professionals must accept each family's unique social, moral, and cultural values.

Personnel Preparation

Several challenges are associated with the development and maintenance of family-centered professionals. The first is developing graduate programs that prepare clinicians for this type of employment. Thurman and colleagues (1990) state that while many college faculty members have extensive experience in preparing special education and related services personnel generally, some faculty have limited experience preparing personnel for the birth to age 3 population. In addition, university training programs may lack the necessary expertise for preparing such personnel. The United States Department of Education Office of Special Education Programs has been funding projects at various universities and colleges for preparing early intervention professionals since the establishment of Part C; however, much more work needs to be done to develop widespread training programs throughout the United States.

In addition, Thurman (1993) states "for any field that is changing as quickly as early intervention, ongoing staff development and in-service training will continue to present challenges" (p. 313). It is important that in-service training be easily accessible and cost effective. Many provider agencies require annual continuing education in the field of early intervention. Models of in-service training need to be responsive to developing trends and practices and address the needs identified by staff and administrators.

Early Intervention and Advocacy

Since the concept of early intervention was created at the federal level, the number of infants and toddlers with disabilities receiving services has increased more than sixfold. It becomes easy to be complacent and assume that all children and families who need services will receive them; yet, many children with disabilities still are not receiving needed services. According to the General Accounting Office (GAO, 2001) data collected suggested that many children do not receive early and periodic screening, diagnostic, and treatment services (EPSDT) for which they are eligible. A major reason cited for not all eligible children receiving EPSDT is a lack of awareness among parents regarding the service availability. The challenge of advocating the necessary levels of funding to ensure that early intervention services are provided continues.

More than 4 decades of knowledge regarding early childhood development and the benefits of early childhood intervention have been compiled into a report from the National Research Council and Institute of Medicine, *From Neurons to Neighborhoods: The Science of Early Childhood Development* (Shonkoff & Phillips, 2000). Continued research into early childhood development and benefits of early intervention such as that cited in this comprehensive report is needed to support policy recommendations.

It would be easy to blame the lack of services for eligible children on inadequate funding.

Thurman (1993) states "It is often easy to advocate the position that the source of any problem and especially the lack of services, lies in inadequate funding. Beginning from this premise, it would be quite logical to always advocate for more money, although more money does not necessarily mean more or better programs." (p. 314). Effective advocacy must be based on program evaluation and evidence-based practice. Early intervention is competing for a piece of the public funding pie, and therefore, the challenge is to develop cost-effective, evidence-based programs that meet the needs of infants, toddlers, and their families.

Early intervention professionals must also advocate for their families and teach their families to advocate for themselves. Such advocacy is the basis of service coordination and transdisciplinary teaming, the backbone of family-centered early intervention.

SUMMARY

Early intervention is a program federally mandated since 1997 that helps infants and toddlers obtain a productive and healthy start to life. Ample evidence supports the benefits for the child, family, and society from intervention during the early years. In this chapter the legislative context for the Individuals with Disabilities Education Act (IDEA) Part C—Infants and Toddlers with Disabilities was presented. Early intervention was defined by IDEA. Rules and regulations for identifying, qualifying, and treating

children in early intervention programs were discussed. Transdisciplinary teaming and family-centered intervention were defined. Practical issues for the delivery of SLP and audiological services to infants and toddlers in the home setting were addressed. The need to continue research to develop cost-effective, evidence-based programs that meet the needs of infants, toddlers, and their families and the continuing challenges of providing early intervention services into the 21st century were explored.

CRITICAL THINKING

1. Why is early intervention important to child development, families, and society? Is early intervention cost effective? Cite examples from the literature in your discussion.

2. IDEA (PL 101-476) was landmark legislation in terms of the promise it held for children birth to age 3 and their families. Discuss the legislative history of early intervention. How did the laws evolve to serve this age group

   from the 1970s to present day? In establishing Part C, what did Congress recognize an "urgent and substantial need" to do?

3. How are children found eligible for the early intervention program? Is there a universal definition for *developmental delay*? What areas of development are required to be evaluated? Discuss the difference between screening, evaluation, and assessment.

4. Define an IFSP and sequence the IFSP process. What principles are necessary for professionals to understand to facilitate an effective IFSP process?

5. Discuss the importance of teaming in the delivery of early intervention services. Define the three types of teams and discuss the challenge of family-centered service delivery with each. What are the advantages and disadvantages of working on a team in an early intervention program?

6. What practical principles should you keep in mind as you provide early intervention services in a child's home? Consider what you would do if you had to provide services in a variety of types of homes that differ from your personal home experiences.

7. Critique your own clinical and interpersonal skills. Are you ready to provide early intervention services?

REFERENCES

American Speech-Language-Hearing Association. (1985). Clinical management of communicatively handicapped minority language populations. *Asha, 27*(6), 29–32.

American Speech-Language-Hearing Association. (1989). *Communication-based services for infants, toddlers, and their families.* Rockville, MD; Author.

American Speech-Language-Hearing Association. (1990). The roles of speech-language pathologists in service delivery to infants, toddlers, and their families. *Asha Supplement, 32*(4).

American Speech-Language-Hearing Association. (1991). Multicultural action agenda 2000. *Asha, 33*(5), 39–41.

American Speech-Language-Hearing Association. (1997a). *Guidelines for audiologic screening.* Rockville, MD: Author.

American Speech-Language-Hearing Association. (2003). Serving children who are culturally and linguistically diverse. Available at http://www.asha.org/

American Speech-Language-Hearing Association. (2004a). *Guidelines for the audiologic assessment of children from birth to 5 years of age.* Rockville, MD: Author.

American Speech-Language-Hearing Association. (2004b). Roles of speech-language pathologists in the neonatal intensive care unit: Position statement. *Asha Supplement, 24,* 60–61.

American Speech-Language-Hearing Association. (2004c). Knowledge and skills needed by speech-language pathologists providing service to infants and families in the NICU environment. *Asha Supplement, 24,* 159–165.

Bagnato, S. J., & Neisworth, J. T. (1991). *Assessment for early intervention: Best practices for professionals.* New York: Guilford.

Benn, R. (1991). *A state wide definition of eligibility under PL 99-457, Part H: A final research report.* Detroit, MI: Merrill-Palmer Institute.

Brown, W., & Brown, C. (1993). Defining eligibility for early intervention. In W. Brown, S. K. Thurman, & L. Pearl (Eds.), *Family-centered early intervention with infants & toddlers: Innovative cross-disciplinary approaches* (pp. 21–42). Baltimore, MD: Paul H. Brookes.

Brown, W., & Rule, S. (1993). Personnel and disciplines in early intervention. In W. Brown, S. K. Thurman, & L. Pearl (Eds.), *Family-centered early intervention with infants & toddlers: Innovative cross-disciplinary approaches* (pp. 245–268). Baltimore: Paul H. Brookes.

Bruder, M. (2000). *The individual family service plan (IFSP).* Available at http://ericec.org/digests/e605.html

Bruder, M. (2002). *Early intervention for children with disabilities.* Available at http://www.bridges4kids.org/

Bruder, M., & Bologna, T. (1993). Collaboration and service coordination for effective early intervention. In W. Brown, S. K. Thurman, & L. Pearl (Eds.), *Family-centered early intervention with infants & toddlers: Innovative cross-disciplinary approaches* (pp. 103–128). Baltimore: Paul H. Brookes.

Caplan, G. (1970). *The theory and practice of mental health consultation.* New York: Basic Books.

Cole, L. (1989). E pluribus pluribus: Multi-cultural imperatives for the 1990s and beyond. *Asha, 31*(9), 65–70.

Cooper, J. (1981). *An early childhood special education primer.* Chapel Hill, NC: Technical Assistance Development System.

Coplan, J., & Gleason, J. (1993). Test-retest and inter-observer reliability of the Early Language Milestone Scale, Second Edition. *Journal of Pediatric Health Care, 7*(5), 212–219.

Division for Early Childhood. (1993). *DEC recommended practices: Indicators of quality in programs for infants and young children with special needs and their families.* Reston, VA: Council for Exceptional Children.

Fenichel E., & Eggbear, Z. (1991). Preparing practitioners to work with infants, toddlers, and their families: Four essential elements of training. *Infants and Young Children, 4*(2), 56–62.

First Words Project. (2005). *First Words Project home page.* Available at http://firstwords.fsu.edu/

Fish, E. (2003). The benefits of early intervention. *Journal of the HEIA, 10*(3), 32–34.

Foley, G. (1990). Portrait of the arena evaluation: Assessment in the transdisciplinary approach. In E. D. Gibbs & D. M. Teti (Eds.), *Interdisciplinary assessment of infants: A guide for early intervention professionals* (pp. 271–286). Baltimore, MD: Paul H. Brookes.

Garland, C., Stone, N. W., Swanson, J., & Woodruff G. (Eds.). (1981). *Early intervention for children with special needs and their families: Findings and recommendations.* Westar Series Paper No. 11. Seattle, WA: University of Washington.

General Accounting Office. (2001). GAO-01-749 Medicaid: Stronger efforts needed to ensure children's access to health screening services July 2001. Available at http://www.gao.gov/

Harbin, G. L., Gallagher, J. J., & Terry, D. V. (1991). Defining the eligible population: Policy issues and challenges. *Journal of Early Intervention, 15*(1), 13–20.

Havens, C. A. (2005). Becoming a resilient family: Child disability and the family system. Available at http://www.ncaonline.org/

Hurth, J. (1998). *Service coordination caseloads in state early intervention systems.* Chapel Hill, NC: National Early Childhood Technical Assistance System.

Johnson, B., McGonigel, M., & Kaufman, R. (1989). *Guidelines and recommended practices for the individualized family service plan.* Washington, DC: National Early Childhood Technical Assistance System and Association for the Care of Children's Health.

Joint Committee on Infant Hearing. (2000). Year 2000 position statement: Principles and guidelines for early hearing detection and intervention programs. Available at http://www.jcih.org/

Karnes, M. B. (Ed.). (1983). *The underserved: Our young gifted children.* Reston, VA: Council for Exceptional Children.

Karoly, L. A., Greenwood, P. W., Everingham, S. S., Hoube, J., Kilburn, M. R., Rydell, C. P., Sander, M., & Chiesa, J. (1998). *Investing in our children: What we know and don't know about the cost benefit of early childhood interventions.* Santa Monica, CA: Rand.

KidSource Online. (2005). What is early intervention? Available at http://www.kidsource.com/

Kilgo, J. L., Aldridge, J., Denton, B. l., Vogtel, L., Vincent, J., Burke, C., & Unanue, R. (2003). *Transdisciplinary teaming: A vital component of inclusive services.* Available at http://www.acei.org/

Kjerland, L., & Kovach, J. (1990). Family-staff collaboration for tailored infant assessment. In E. D. Gibbs & D. M. Teti (Eds.), *Interdisciplinary assessment of infants: A guide for early intervention professionals* (pp. 287–298). Baltimore, MD: Paul H. Brookes.

Mathematica Policy Research, Inc., & Columbia University's Center for Children and Families at Teacher's College. (2002). *Making a difference in the lives of infants and toddlers and their families: The impacts of Early Head Start.* Available at http://www.acf.hhs.gov/programs/opre/ehs/ehs_resrch/reports/impacts_vol1/impacts_vol1_title.html

McCathren, R. E., Warren, S. F., & Yoder, P. J. (1996). Prelinguistic predictors of later language development. In K. Cole, P. l. Dale, & D. Thal (Eds.), *Assessment of communication/language* (pp. 57–75). Baltimore, MD: Paul H. Brookes.

McGonigel, M. J. (1991). Philosophy and conceptual framework. In M. J. McGonigel, R. K. Kaufmann, & B. H. Johnson (Eds.), *Guidelines and recommended practices for the individualized family service plan* (2nd ed., pp. 7–14). Bethesda, MD: Association for the Care of Children's Health.

McLean, M. M. (1997). *Family/professional relationship: Service utilization.* Unpublished manuscript, CLAS Early Childhood Research Institute, Champaign, IL.

McLean, M. M., & McCormick, K. (1993). Assessment and evaluation in early intervention. In W. Brown, S. K. Thurman, & L. Pearl (Eds.), *Family-centered early intervention with infants & toddlers: Innovative cross-disciplinary approaches* (pp. 43–79). Baltimore, MD: Paul H. Brookes.

McWilliam, R. A. (2000). Recommended practices in interdisciplinary models. In S. Sandall, M. McLean, & B. Smith (Eds.), *DEC recommended practices for early intervention/early childhood special education* (pp. 47–54). Longmont, CO: Sopris West.

National Center on Birth Defects and Developmental Disabilities. (2005). Developmental screening. Available at http://www.cdc.gov/ncbddd/child/devtool.html

National Early Childhood Technical Assistance Center. (2005a). *Screening, evaluation and assessment.* Available at http://www.nectac.org/

National Early Childhood Technical Assistance Center. (2005b). Minibibliography. Transitions from infant toddler services to preschool education. Available at http://www.nectac.org/

Nietupski, J. l., Scheutz, G., & Ockwood, L. (1980). The delivery of communication therapy services to severely handicapped student: A plan for change. *Journal of the Association for the Severely Handicapped, 5*(1), 13–23.

Orelove, F. P., & Sobsey, D. (1991). *Educating children with multiple disabilities: A transdisciplinary approach* (2nd ed.). Baltimore, MD: Paul H. Brookes.

Oser, C., & Cohen, J. (2003). *Improving early intervention: Using what we know about infants and toddlers with disabilities to reauthorize Part C of IDEA.* Washington, DC: Zero to Three Policy Center.

Pathways Awareness Foundation. (2005). *Where can I turn? I need more answers.* Available at http://www.pathwasawareness.org/

PL 105-117. (1997, June). Individuals with Disabilities Education Act Amendments of 1997 (IDEA 1997). *Federal Register.*

Rand. (1998). *Early childhood interventions: Benefits, costs and savings.* Available at http://www.rand.org/

Rescorla, L. (1989). The Language Development Survey: A screening tool for delayed language in toddlers. *Journal of Speech ad Hearing Disorders, 54,* 587–599.

Rescorla, L., & Alley, A. (2001). Validation of the Language Development Survey (LDS): A parent report tool for identifying language delay in toddlers. *Journal of Speech, Language and Hearing Research, 44,* 434–445.

Safer, N. D., & Hamilton, J. L. (1993). Legislative context for early intervention services. In W. Brown, S. K. Thurman, & L. Pearl (Eds.), *Family-centered early intervention with infants & toddlers: Innovative cross-disciplinary approaches* (pp. 1–20). Baltimore, MD: Paul H. Brookes.

Sandall, S. R. (1993). Curricula for early intervention. In W. Brown, S. K. Thurman, & L. Pearl (Eds.), *Family-centered early intervention with infants & toddlers: Innovative cross-disciplinary approaches* (pp. 129–172). Baltimore, MD: Paul H. Brookes.

Shackelford, J. (2002). *State and jurisdictional eligibility definitions for infants and toddlers with disabilities under IDEA.* NECTAC Notes (11). Chapel Hill: The University of North Carolina, FPG Child Development Institute, National Early Childhood Technical Assistance Center.

Shackelford, J. (2004). *State and jurisdictional eligibility definitions for infants and toddlers with disabilities under IDEA.* NECTAC Notes (16). Available at http://www.nectac.org/

Shonkoff, J. P., & Hauser-Cram, P. (1987). Early intervention for disabled infants and their families: A quantitative analysis. *Pediatrics, 80,* 650–658.

Shonkoff, J. P., & Meisels, S. J. (1991). Early childhood intervention: The evolution of a concept. In S. J. Meisels & J. P. Shonkoff (Eds.), *Handbook of early childhood intervention* (pp. 3–31). New York: Cambridge University Press.

Shonkoff, J. P., & Phillips, D. (Eds.). (2000). *National Research Council and Institute of Medicine: From neurons to neighborhoods: The science of early childhood development.* Washington, DC: National Academy Press.

Thurman, S.K. (1993). Some perspectives on the continuing challenges in early intervention. In W. Brown, S. K. Thurman, & L. Pearl (Eds.), *Family-centered early intervention with infants & toddlers: Innovative cross-disciplinary approaches* (pp. 303–316). Baltimore, MD: Paul H. Brookes.

Thurman, S. K., Brown, C., Bryan, M., Henderson, A. l., Klein, M. D., Sainato, D. M., & Wiley, T. (1990). Some perspectives on preparing personnel to work with at risk children birth to five. In L. M. Bullock & R. L. Simpson (Eds.), *Monograph on critical issues in special education: Implications for personnel preparation* (pp. 97–101). Denton, TX: University of North Texas, Programs in Special Education.

U.S. Department of Education. (2002). *Twenty-fourth annual report to Congress on the implementation of the Individuals with Disabilities Education Act.* Available at http://www.ed-gov/about/reports/annual/osep/2002/index.html

Wetherby, A., & Prizant, B. (1993). *Communication and Symbolic Behavior Scales-Normed Edition.* Chicago: Applied Symbolix.

Wetherby, A., & Prizant, B. (1996). Toward earlier identification of communication and language problems in infants and young children. In S. J. Meisels & E. Fenichel (Eds.), *New visions for the developmental assessment of infants and young children* (pp. 289–312). Washington, DC: Zero to Three/National Center for Infants, Toddlers, & Families.

Wetherby, A., & Prizant, B. (2001). *Comunication and Symbolic Behavior Scales Developmental Profile-Preliminary Normed Edition.* Baltimore, MD: Paul H. Brookes.

Yoshinaga-Itano, C., Sedy, A., Coulter, D., & Mehl, A. (1998). Language of early and later- identified children with hearing loss. *Pediatrics, 102*(5), 1161–1171.

RESOURCES

ASHA Resources and Activities Related to Early Intervention in Speech-Language Pathology (Birth to 5 Years) http://www.asha.org/

Family Village School Early Intervention Resources http://www.familyvillage.wisc.edu/education/ei.html

First Words Project http://firstwords.fsu.edu

Global Early Intervention Network http://www.atsweb.neu.edu/cp/ei

Zero to Three: National Center for Infants, Toddler and Families http://www.zerotothree.org

17

Service Delivery Issues
in Private Practice

KENNETH E. WOLF, PHD

SCOPE OF CHAPTER

Private practice, regardless of the profession or discipline, at one time was fairly easy to understand, namely working independently for oneself in one's own office. That simple definition has been broadened over the past 10–20 years. Currently, private practice describes those who work for themselves, work full or part time for others and then for themselves after hours, contract with other professionals and work in a variety of locations, have a single business location, supply professional staff to other agencies and corporations that require services, and serve as consultants. And the list goes on. Just about any type of service offered by a speech-language pathologist or audiologist may fall within the realm of private practice. The common denominator is the person(s) who owns the business and is ultimately responsible for all of its aspects, including business, professional, practice standards, and obligations.

Private practice appeals to many who desire employment autonomy—being one's own boss and taking the ultimate risk and responsibility for economic and professional success. Private practice has often been associated with the health care environment, as that was the primary focus of the service delivery base. Today, however, private practice goes beyond health care, extending into the educational arena as well. Therefore, many of the service delivery issues described in the health care and education settings need to be fully understood and may have significant implications for the private practitioner. (The reader is referred to other chapters in this text for additional information regarding other work settings.)

A recent ASHA survey (2004d) revealed that 17.8 percent of its members were engaged in private practice in 2004 (7.3 percent full time and 10.5 percent part time). Those who are employed in such settings will likely face issues similar to other health care and education employees. Owners of private practices, although confronted with comparable issues, have even greater responsibility, with prosperity and survival the overriding concerns.

This chapter cannot address all aspects of private practice. ASHA (1991a, 1991b, 2005e, 2005f, 2005g) and the American Academy of Private Practice in Speech-Language Pathology and Audiology provide valuable information about initiating and working in a private practice (see the Resources section). Rather, this chapter provides an overview of key issues to be considered by those who work in private practice environments. Included is a discussion of the practitioner confronting business and professional issues and how these issues may differ from those in other work settings. The chapter concludes with consideration of issues that have emerged or are about to emerge that will influence speech–language pathologists and audiologists in private practice.

T A B L E 17–1 Basic Questions Before Starting a Private Practice

Questions to Ask Yourself

- Do I enjoy working alone?
- Do I have the knowledge and skills to work independently?
- Do I have the skills to manage the stress of owning my own practice?
- Do I understand the people and community in which I have my practice?

Business Questions to Ask

- Do I know the need for private practice in the community in which I will work?
- Do I know the financial climate in the community in which I will work?
- Are there small business support groups in the community that I can turn to for advice?
- What are the financial requirements for starting and maintaining a private practice?
- What types of payments and reimbursement schedules are available and needed to support the practice?
- What are my long-term financial needs?

SOURCE: Adapted from P.S. Currie, *Starting a Private Practice* (2004). Available at http://www.audiology online.com/

SERVICE DELIVERY ISSUES IN PRIVATE PRACTICE

Although private practice offers many alluring features, it also holds some obvious and hidden pitfalls (Currie, 2004). Entering private practice requires speech-language pathologists and audiologists to actively and honestly self-evaluate their personal skills, talents, likes and dislikes, and knowledge of business and the business climate, all in addition to addressing the challenges of their profession (Currie, 2004; Goffinet, 2005). Table 17–1 offers some basic questions about oneself and business in general that should be approached honestly before the audiologist or speech-language pathologist commits to starting a private practice. Then the speech-language pathologist or audiologist who decides to enter private practice will understand

that he or she immediately assumes a role greater than that of service provider. He or she must think and perform as a business person, an administrator, a clinician, probably a supervisor, and possibly a teacher and/or researcher as well. As such, establishing a private practice requires advanced thinking and questioning.

Private Practice Options

One of the first decisions a professional must make is whether to enter private practice on a full-time or part-time basis. The percentage of speech-language pathologists and audiologists working in full-time private practice has been relatively stable for nearly 20 years; 6–8 percent of the speech-language pathologists and 20–30 percent of the audiologists. During the same period (1986–2003), there has been a slight downward trend in the percentages engaged in part-time private practice; 10–22 percent of the speech-language pathologists and 7–16 percent of the audiologists (Zingeser, 2005). Unfortunately, the data that identify those who limit their work activity to part time versus those engaged in part-time private practice as a supplement to their primary or other employment are not available. The important issue is that private practice may offer greater flexibility for the individual who cannot work full time. Some professionals may want or need flexible scheduling, and others may wish to "moonlight" to generate additional income. Regardless of full- or part-time status, those who enter private practice must treat such a venture with the same dedication and commitment as they would any business venture. Such commitment is critical to the individual's success and to the way one is viewed by peers and professional colleagues. Respect will only come from high-quality professional behavior and exhibiting the highest level of professionalism. The remainder of this chapter addresses issues from the perspective of the full-time practitioner-owner; however, the information may easily be applied to those who engage in part-time private practice.

Private practice offers professional and business autonomy, without the requisite accountability to a boss or supervisor. However, accountability of performance may be even greater than that of an employee. As a private practitioner, the final responsibility for all decisions and performances rests with the practitioner. Income is dependent on services being delivered in a timely and appropriate manner, and thus all absences (e.g., illness, vacation, or other emergency) must be covered, just as they would in any other employment setting. Financial obligations (e.g., monthly bills, salaries, other expenditures) associated with the practice must be honored. This often means additional work for the private practitioner beyond his or her clinical service delivery hours or hiring employees to perform these functions. In short, numerous nonbillable activities are encumbered in a successful private practice.

Solo or Affiliated Practice A private practice assumes one of three legal organizational structures: solo proprietorship, partnership, or corporation (ASHA, 2005e; United States Small Business Administration, 2005). *Solo proprietorship* is a business run by one individual for his or her own benefit. *Partnership* is a business owned by two or more persons and may be either general or limited. *General partnership* is an agreement between two or more persons to join together to carry on a business venture for profit, with each partner contributing money, property, labor, or skill and receiving equal shares of profit or loss and unlimited personal liability for the debts of the business. *Limited partnerships* limit personal liability for the debt of the business to the amount invested by the partner. *Corporation* is a legal entity whose scope of activity and its name are restricted by its charter and must be granted permission to operate under the laws of that state. The corporation is liable for the debts and taxes, not the owners and the managers. The advantages and disadvantages of each entity are summarized in Table 17–2; for more detail, ASHA (2005e) offers a discussion of business practices on its Web site.

One of the first issues to be considered is the decision between solo practice or affiliation with another professional(s) either as a partnership or other working agreement. Such an affiliation may be with another speech-language pathologist, audiologist, physician, health care provider, or educator, assuming the affiliation does not violate any legal statutes of a particular state. Such a decision is based, at least in part, on other factors that are described in this chapter, but also on one's own goals, objectives, personality, and answers to the basic questions posed in Table 17–1. Zingeser (2005) reported that 60 percent of speech-language pathologists in private practice were solo, and those in group practices were nearly equally divided between group practices that were exclusively communicative disorders professionals or other disciplines. Audiologists were less likely to be in solo practices (48 percent), but those in group practices tended to be with other audiologists or speech-language pathologists. Solo versus affiliated practice must be considered fully in business terms and based on legal and professional advantages and disadvantages.

T A B L E 17–2 Primary Advantages and Disadvantages of Three Types of Business Entities

Solo Proprietorship	Partnership–General and Limited	Corporations
Advantages:	**Advantages:**	**Advantages:**
▪ Simple	▪ Greater availability of capital	▪ Limited liability to stockholders
▪ Minimum legal restrictions	▪ Greater resources for decision making, support, and creative activity	▪ Perpetual life of the corporation
▪ Ease of discontinuance		▪ Ease of transferring ownership
▪ Owner is truly the boss		▪ Ease of expansion of the corporation
Disadvantages:	**Disadvantages:**	**Disadvantages:**
▪ Difficult to raise capital	▪ Unlimited liability in general partnership	▪ Government regulations
▪ Limited life of the business	▪ Divided authority among the partners	▪ Higher costs to organize
▪ Unlimited liability		▪ Corporation is limited to operate in state chartered unless permission granted from other states
		▪ Double taxation (corporate and personal)

SOURCE: Adapted from American Speech-Language-Hearing Association, Frequently Asked Questions About Business Practices (2005). Available at http://www.asha.org/

Location The location of the practice is important. Will it be a free-standing independent practice or located within another practice site? If an independent practice, should it be in a specific type of building with potential referral sources as tenants, or might the goals and objectives of the practice be equally or better accomplished in another location that offers a greater degree of traffic (self-referral), easier patient/client access, or lower rent? For example, if the primary objective is to sell hearing aids, the practice should be located in an accessible area, preferably on the first floor, with appropriate signage and visibility for walk-up traffic to maximize opportunities for self-referrals. Lower rents at a strip-mall may be more advantageous than a more expensive medical building. Conversely, if the practice is expected to focus more on diagnostic audiology, then a location in a medical building in reasonable proximity to referring physicians may be necessary. Zingeser (2005) reported that speech-language pathologists in private practice were most likely to provide services in their clients' homes (59 percent) or in a free-standing clinic or office (34 percent). On the other hand, audiologists in private practice overwhelmingly provided services in a free-standing clinic or office (75 percent) or in a health care setting (25 percent).

If the practice is to be located within another practice, additional considerations are warranted. Will this practice function autonomously within that larger practice, simply renting space or perhaps equipment and/or staff? This is often a way of establishing a practice, building it to a level for eventual relocation or merger with the preexisting practice. The advantage of such an agreement is that some assistance is usually offered, if no more than the affiliation with an ongoing successful practice.

Other private practitioners have no physical office space of their own for serving patients/clients, but work as independent contractors providing a service in another's facility for them and their patients/clients. In this case, the work activities and responsibilities must be distinct from that of an employee. As an independent contractor, the practitioner must at least minimally set his or her own working hours; have an established rent agreement and/or fee schedule that is charged to the existing practice; carry his or her own insurances; and meet all other local, state, and federal requirements. Responsibility for equipment ownership and maintenance, supplies, and staff must be agreed on by the independent contractor and the owner of the practice site. These agreements are found between audiologists or speech-language pathologists, other health care professionals, or educational facilities.

Business Plan A business plan that details the *whats* and the *hows* must be established during the initial development of a private practice. This plan will tell the story of the business (Goffinet, 2005), describing the practice and how it will be financed, marketed, and managed. In other words, the plan will drive what the practice is intended to do and how those intentions will be accomplished. The major elements of a business plan are outlined in Table 17–3. The plan typically delineates such areas as physical, personnel, and financial needs, resources, and strategies. It describes the space, equipment (professional and office), supply needs, and personnel requirements, if any, in addition to the practitioner-owner. Each item in the plan has some financial implication (cost) that needs to be identified. *Pro forma* income projections will be needed. Revenue streams and access to patients should also be identified in the plan along with strategies for attracting and building a solid referral base. Without a continuous source of patients/clients, the practice cannot be maintained. This plan should be used in each phase of practice development and should be revisited periodically, at least annually to assure progress is being achieved in a measurable way. The United States Small Business Administration (2005)

T A B L E 17–3 Core Elements of a Business Plan

Introduction
- Description
- Ownership and legal structure
- Skills and experience you bring to the business
- Advantages over competitors

Marketing
- Services to be offered
- Customer demand
- Market
- Planned advertising and marketing
- Pricing strategy

Financial Management
- Source and amount of equity capital
- Monthly operating budget for first year
- Expected return on investment
- Monthly cash flow for first year
- Projected income statements for first year
- Break-even point
- Methods of compensation
- Maintaining accounting records

Operations
- Day-to-day management
- Personnel
- Insurances and agreements
- Equipment

Concluding Statement
- Summarize goals and objectives
- Review with colleague or consultant
- Approach a lender

SOURCE: Adapted from U.S. Small Business Administration, *Small Business Start-up Basics* (2005). Available at http://www.sba.gov/startings_business/index.html

provides an excellent and comprehensive overview and tutorial for preparing a business plan and how to get started.

Most businesses require start-up capital to launch. That capital is usually achieved through financing and loans. Private practices are indeed businesses, and as such, there is a degree of risk. Commercial lenders, therefore, rarely capitalize 100 percent of a new business. At one time, private practices in the health care environment (including medical practices) were considered relatively low risk. However, at least in some markets, health care practices have been viewed as a greater risk to lenders than in the past. As a result, lenders expect to review and analyze the business plan and, where applicable, other documents such as affiliation agreements and/or partnership agreements. Most importantly, lenders demand evidence of financial commitment and risk sharing on the part of the practitioner. In other words, is the practitioner placing any of his or her finances into the project? Typically, commercial lenders prefer that the practitioner enter such a venture with at least 10 percent of the up-front capital needed to launch the practice.

Licenses, Certification, and Insurances It is understood that the practitioner, and those who provide services on his or her behalf, will hold valid and current licenses to practice his or her profession as required by the laws of the state(s) in which they are performing services. At the time of this writing, 50 states regulate audiologists and 47 states regulate speech-language pathologists (Colorado, Michigan, and South Dakota do not) (Diggs, personal communication, 2005). In states where there is no licensure, ASHA certification is the only national credential available. Additionally, ASHA certification is recognized by the Centers for Medicare and Medicaid Services as the credential for the provision of speech-language pathology and audiology services. In states with licensure, ASHA certification may not be required. However, the private practitioner is always in competition with other providers to gain access to patients/clients and referral sources. The more credentials one has, the more attractive his or her practice may be to potential and actual patients/clients and/or referral sources. Thus, even if ASHA certification is not required, it may be viewed as just one more characteristic that positively differentiates between practitioners. Additional licenses may be required to own, name, and/or operate a business. These licenses may vary depending on the exact nature, structure, and location of the practice and on municipal and/or state regulations.

Insurances are also required. Professional liability insurance is needed not only for the practitioner-owner but also for each clinical service provider in his or her employment. Many provider contracts also proscribe the minimum limits of insurance. Typically, liability insurance in the range of $1 million per occurrence, and $3 million to $5 million aggregate are common minimum limits of liability. Proof that liability insurance is currently in effect is a common requirement. Worker's compensation and unemployment insurances are required for all employees. Health and disability insurance will be available only if the practitioner purchases them. Independent contractors are often required to show proof of their own worker's compensation as part of their contractual agreement. Additional insurances are also advisable to protect the practice and its contents from loss due to fire, theft, accident, or other liability.

Specialization It is difficult for one practitioner to be an expert in all aspects of his or her profession. Therefore, many elect to limit their practice to a specific area such as dysphagia, aphasia, voice, or stuttering or to a specific age group such as geriatrics or neonatal assessment. Those who limit their practices within these narrowly defined areas often maintain that only those with specialized training and experience may provide the best and most competent services, and such an argument may be valid. Currently, three areas have established Specialty Recognition Boards: Child Language, Fluency, and Swallowing and Swallowing Disorders. Specialty Board recognition is beyond ASHA certification. Holders of such recognition may identify themselves as a *Board Recognized Specialist in that specialty* if they so desire, and such individuals often believe that it provides a potential marketing advantage over those who are not so recognized (ASHA, 2005h). However, specialty recognition is a voluntary program within ASHA and is not required for practice in any area or with any specific population group. Other specialty groups outside of ASHA (i.e., the Academy of Neurologic Communication Disorders and Sciences) have established their own requirements and offer specialty certification. Nevertheless, the ASHA Code of Ethics (Principle of Ethics II, B) requires that all clinicians be trained, competent, and experienced in any area of clinical service they perform (ASHA, 2003c). See Chapter 2 for more information on certification and licensure.

Specialization may be desirable for some, but it may also have some disadvantages, particularly in the managed health care arena. Managed care organizations (MCOs) often want to provide services to the greatest number of patients with the least amount of administrative support and complications (i.e., cost). If an individual or group practice is capable of providing quality and competent services to a broader and more diverse population than those competing for the same contract, the generalists may be viewed more favorably. The advantage to the MCO is a single contract covering all of its needs in a given service area, as opposed to multiple smaller contracts that in the aggregate provide the same total coverage as the single larger contract. The more contracts the MCO must manage, the greater its administrative costs. In other words, restricting specialization too severely may limit access to contracts, patients/clients, and referrals, depending on the market served. If a narrowly defined service area is desirable, specialization definitely should be considered. However, early in the development of a private practice, general practice may be required to facilitate its growth.

Referral Base Practice sites cannot exist without patients/clients who require services. Publicly funded programs, such as public schools and public hospitals, may have greater access to patients/clients, especially for those individuals who cannot or elect not to pay for services out of pocket. Private practices, however, are totally dependent on those who can and will pay for services or who have someone else (e.g., a third party) pay all or the majority of the expenses associated with that service. Thus, the private practice is in competition with the publicly funded service providers and other private group and individual practices. The successful practice must have a mechanism for sustaining patient/client referrals, which includes access to such populations, providing quality, and marketing.

The changes in funding of health care services have resulted in access to patients becoming a much larger issue than it once was, especially in markets with high managed care penetration. When indemnity insurance was the predominate health care coverage mechanism, patients were able to seek services from almost any licensed provider, and their insurance company would reimburse at a reasonable rate. Under the current system, patients may be obligated to seek services only from paneled or approved providers if they want to receive the maximum coverage benefit. If services are provided by other than a paneled provider, the patient's financial responsibility for that service increases, sometimes dramatically. However, most MCOs do not allow for any willing provider and limit the number of providers per profession as a way of maintaining efficient management of their group. The fewer number of providers they have to deal with in terms of record keeping and payments, the less expensive their administrative costs. Thus, there is competition among providers to be paneled, and without such status, access to patients may be severely compromised (Griffin, 1995; Klontz, Napp, White, & Wolf, 1997; Kreb, 1997; Wolf, 1995).

Private practitioners typically join provider networks to maintain or increase their access to patients/clients. Sometimes, there is a fee associated with being a network provider. Some network affiliations (paid for or not) actually mean little more than being listed in a larger book of acceptable providers. None of these affiliations guarantee referrals, only access and possible referrals. One strategy for maintaining access to patients/clients that some private practices have used is to form their own provider networks and offer the network to the MCO as a single provider (e.g., Kreb et al., 1995; Napp, 1997). The network maintains its own administrative structure, making referrals, collecting payments, and distributing payments to the providers. A provider network may also offer broader geographic coverage for that profession or specialty, a greater range of subspecialties, faster service, increased ease, and greater flexibility to the patients/clients. These advantages are often reflected in patient/client satisfaction. Additionally, the MCO may still maintain cost containment, having multiple service providers from the network, but only having to maintain and manage a single account to the network. In other words, a significant segment of the administrative overhead is shifted to the network. One disadvantage to the providers within the network is the cost of its maintenance. These costs may require significant monthly fees to the network or still greater reduction in the net reimbursement to the provider. Regardless of the type of network affiliation, without it, access to patients, and possibly the viability of the practice, may be compromised in the current health care environment (ASHA, 2005e; Griffin, 1995).

Staff and Consultants Maintaining a smooth functioning practice requires good business practices and performance. As stated earlier, this often means additional work for the private practitioner beyond his or her clinical service delivery hours (work that is not billable to patients or MCOs) or hiring employees to perform those functions. If the practitioner-owner is devoting most of the working day to direct patient services, no one is available to answer telephones, schedule patients, greet the public, and provide nonpatient-related services. Today's society is dependent on technology, and voice mail is one of the most common technologic applications. However, a high proportion of the public, particularly patients in need of service, prefer to talk to a real person, especially if they are contacting a small business. And patient/client satisfaction is critical to continued patient/client access. Remember, the front door to the practice for the rest of the world is that initial telephone contact, and it provides a lasting impression. Thus, one staff position that should be considered is an office receptionist.

Depending on the size and needs of the practice, other full- or part-time employees may be needed such as a billing clerk or service and/or office manager. A trustworthy and knowledgeable accountant and attorney, at least on a part-time or as-needed consulting basis, are also necessary. A banker who works specifically with that particular practice is also valuable. Other consultants to be considered might include a general business manager, marketing professionals, and investment consultants.

As the practice expands, the professional obligations to provide services may exceed the abilities of a single practitioner-owner. At that time, additional professional colleagues must be considered. Assuming there are neither plans nor desire for an additional partner, then the only other options are to consider professionals who are employees or independent contractors. Both have advantages and disadvantages in terms of costs and responsibility to the practice. Employees may be slightly less costly in terms of salary, but may expect benefits and have other associated costs such as health, worker's compensation and professional liability insurances; taxes; and holiday, sick leave, and vacation time. Independent contractors may be more expensive for the services they render, but have none of the other associated costs. In addition, the practice only pays contractors when there is enough work to generate income.

Whether the additional personnel are employees or independent contractors, the practitioner-owner must determine if the additional services are cost-effective. If the additional caseload is to be handled by existing personnel, and there are ample existing resources to do so through excess capacity, then the additional caseload is sound. If the cost of expansion will not cover the additional expenses associated with it and/or be reasonably justified indirectly, it would seem prudent to forestall such activities and possibly reconsider in the future. If the additional patient/client services produce enough revenue to just meet the additional expenses associated with the expansion, then it becomes a decision for the practitioner-owner to determine if the additional work and responsibility are justified for little or no immediate net economic gain. One factor to consider is the potential gain in terms of goodwill with referral sources and probability of economic gain in the future. Finally, if the expansion is revenue positive and a sound business and professional move, it should be implemented (Wolf, Cohen, & Arnst, 1994). However, growth simply for the sake of growth or undertaken too rapidly has been catastrophic and sometimes fatal to small businesses, and private practices are no exception.

Productivity Productivity standards have not been developed for speech-language pathologists and audiologists. However, the ASHA Omnibus Survey indicated that speech-language pathologists across health care settings average about 5.8 hours (out of 8 hours) per day in patient/client services (ASHA, 2003a). Audiologists average slightly more time: 6.6 hours (out of 8 hours) per day in patient care (ASHA, 2003b). Although these are only averages, they provide an indication of the amount of work expected to maintain practice. These figures indicate how hours of the workday are allocated, but may not be a true indication of productivity.

Another aspect of productivity that is almost never mentioned in relation to speech-language pathology and audiology is the ratio of revenue generated to cost to provide that service. In some businesses, this ratio is the major, if not the only, indicator of productivity. The impact of a negative ratio is obvious; no business can survive if it costs more to provide a service than can be generated from providing it. But how large must that ratio be for the service (or employee) to be worthwhile to the practitioner-owner? In some financial businesses and professions, it is not unrealistic to expect and demand employees to generate revenues that are four to eight times their annual salary (i.e., 4:1 or 8:1). An informal survey of some speech-language pathology practice sites, including private practices, indicates that such revenue generated to cost expenditures is more likely to be less than 2:1. Those types of productivity ratios are critically important to the financial viability of a small business such as a private practice. Another type of productivity indicator will be discussed later in the chapter under the discussion of evidence-based practice and benchmarks.

Other Issues

Other issues that will affect your ability to run an effective, efficient, and productive private practice include payment for services, the evidence-based practice approach, information technology, the creation of value for clients, cultural competence, ethical values, research and education, and volunteerism.

Payment for Services The structure of the health care payment landscape has changed drastically over the past two decades. The traditional system was based on a retrospective payment model,

whereby services were provided and the practitioner received payment for those services *after* the fact—thus, the term *retrospective fee-for-service reimbursement*. The financial risks for health care fell mainly on the payer in a retrospective fee-for-service model, even with significant preestablished discounts. Although it began earlier, the 1990s witnessed a strong movement toward a prospective payment or capitated system. Under capitation, the provider agrees to accept a flat or fixed per-member, per-month premium (PMPM), paid in advance, for a guaranteed number of covered lives or enrollees, usually for several thousand lives. The provider also agrees that any member of that covered population group who needs such services, regardless of the actual cost to the provider, will receive such services in a timely manner. In other words, there is a shift in the financial risk. Under the prospective capitated system, more of the risk is shared between the payer and the provider. (For a more detailed discussion of prospective payment system see Wolf (2001)).

Most providers remain under a retrospective reimbursement system, whereas networks and some Medicare and Medicaid programs may contract with the MCOs under capitated agreements. The providers within the network bill the network retrospectively for services rendered. Often those services require prior authorization from the network for payments to be made in a timely manner. Further, since the capitation that the network receives is usually discounted from full fee-for-service, the reimbursement rates to the providers are further discounted, sometimes severely. Private practitioners must know their costs and required reimbursement rates before affiliating with any provider network, if at all (Wolf & Kreb, 1996).

Understanding his or her own price structure, diagnostic and procedural coding, and payer fee schedules is imperative for the practitioner-owner. Private practitioners must also know the reimbursement sources for their profession. For example, Zingeser (2005) reported that private pay (out-of-pocket) was the largest source of payment for both audiologists (49%) and speech-language pathologists (41%) in private practice, followed by private insurance (25% for audiologists; 15% for speech-language pathologists) and Medicare/Medicaid (21% and 20% for audiologists and speech-language pathologists, respectively). Understanding and adjusting the payer mix for the practice is important for sustenance and sustainability of the practice.

Evidence-Based Practice The concept of evidence-based medicine began to emerge in the United Kingdom and Canada throughout the 1990s. The process quickly became applicable to all aspects of health care delivery, evolving into evidence-based health care (EBHC) (McKibbon, Eady, & Marks, 1999) and today referred to as *evidence-based practice* (EBP). Evidence-based practice is used to establish practice guidelines, clinical pathways, and benchmarks for quality of care (Wolf, 1999). An evidence-based approach to care communicates to the professions, consumers, and payers that best practices are rooted in data with the expectation of accuracy (diagnostics) and benefit (therapy) (Plante, 2004).

The transition to an evidence-based approach to clinical decision making is not without challenges (Dollaghan, 2004; Sackett, Straus, Richardson, Rosenberg, & Haynes, 2000). EBP de-emphasizes practitioner intuition, opinion, and unsystematic clinical experience. Instead, EBP requires that decisions are reached through the systematic examination of evidence from clinical research. It is dependent on the scientific method (Evidence-Based Medicine Working Group, 1992; Sackett et al., 2000). EBP does not ignore clinical experience, but instead considers it in context against high-quality evidence that meets a priori standards (McKibbon et al., 1999; Sackett et al., 2000). As such, EBP demands that practitioners be efficient and effective searchers of the literature. Once that literature is identified, it must be critically appraised, not only for its scientific and clinical merit, but also for its applicability to the target patient or population.

The need for clinical trials in communication sciences and disorders has emerged within the past decade (Logemann, 2004). However, evidence garnered from other types of studies (e.g., meta-analyses or case studies) or from publications in non-peer reviewed journals, may be helpful (Kent, 2004).

Therefore, it is critical that clinicians not only learn about EBP, but also how to use and interpret it. A more extensive discussion of EBP is beyond the scope of this chapter. ASHA has embraced the concepts of EBP and issued a technical paper and position statement (ASHA, 2004c, 2005d), as well as an extensive array of Web-based tutorials (ASHA, 2005a) on the topic.

Benchmarks may be useful in terms of productivity standards. Instead of measuring productivity based on hours of service, as has been used in the old paradigm, comparisons with established benchmarks may be a more meaningful standard (Wolf, 1999). In other words, standards and rewards are based on achieving outcomes rather than number of hours worked. Productivity standards also are valuable when competing for a contract with a managed care organization. The private practice that can demonstrate outcomes data and benchmarks has an advantage over those that cannot and is likely to be more appealing to MCOs and other contractors. In fact, at the time of this writing, Congress is considering federal legislation that will amend Medicare reimbursement to require providers to report quality measures and indicators. Those that do not report such measures may receive lower reimbursements compared to those that do.

What do payers want? Payers want the best possible outcome. They do not want a test score. They want to know if a patient can be discharged, go home, recover, and get back to work. Payers want that outcome for the least amount of money and in the least amount of time. Practitioners who can provide data related to outcomes, time, and cost are in the best position to succeed. In other words, providers need to keep costs down and quality high, achieve maximum patient satisfaction, and be able to measure it and prove it (Wolf, 1999). Health care delivery has become a process that balances cost and risk and that also affords an acceptable outcome and level of quality (Wolf et al., 1994). See Chapter 27 for further discussion of this topic.

Information Technology The use of information technology has become a mainstay in health care delivery. Computers are used not only to facilitate a smooth functioning office by integrating scheduling, billing, inventory, and payroll, but also for scientific and clinical purposes. Access to the information superhighway via the Internet has become an integral aspect of practice. Some practices have developed Web sites to describe their practice, schedule appointments, provide access to patients for their questions, and serve as a source of information and educational materials about communication disorders. Patients are turning to the Internet to gather information about diagnosis and treatment and bringing that information to their health care providers. Providers must know what the patients are reading and whether that information is or is not a viable option. Additionally, providers are turning to the Internet for literature searches and information applicable to their practices and to receive their professional literature via electronic publishing. Clinically, electronic medical records have become common, but are still undergoing refinement. Many practices and MCOs are requiring that patient data be used to build databases, leading to internal benchmarks.

Creating Value Speech-language pathology and audiology services are beneficial to those who receive them, but if those services are to be paid for, the consumer (and the payer) must perceive a value from those services. In other words, patients/clients must perceive that services are worth reaching into one's own pocket and paying for them, if they are not covered by insurance, the schools, the government, or some other third party payer (Kreb & Wolf, 1997). Marketing speech-language and hearing services to those who receive them and pay for them has been a frequent topic and objective for many professionals and organizations. The real and perceived value of those services, however, must be constructed before there is any chance of generating a successful marketing program. The creation of value begins at the level of the individual provider-to-patient/client relationship.

To illustrate the creation of value, Kreb (personal communication, 1998) uses the example of orthodontia. Huge numbers of children and young adolescents receive orthodontia annually in the United States. How many of them truly require such services for functional purposes? How many believe they need such services because of cosmetic reasons? At costs typically over $3,000 per child, how many parents are willing to pay for these services themselves, as insurance companies rarely, if ever, cover orthodontia? The answer is simple. In almost all cases, orthodontia is paid for by the consumer, actually the parents, because they perceive a value in those services, whether functional or cosmetic. When there is perceived value, it is much easier to market services.

On the other hand, Cohen (1993) described an example of an elderly couple he observed dining in a restaurant. Coffee and dessert were desirable, if included in the price. However, when they learned that dessert and coffee were a la carte, they declined. In other words, if there is no additional out-of-pocket expense, they want it, but if it means added cost, there is question of the desire and value of the additional items.

Are speech-language pathology and hearing services perceived by the education and health care consuming public like orthodontia or like dessert and coffee at a restaurant? Are the services desired and perceived to hold value only if someone else is paying for the services, or are consumers willing to forego other valued services and products to pay for speech-language or hearing services? The professions need to be viewed in such positive light that individuals are willing to undergo some financial sacrifice to receive services, creating a high degree of value. Until that perceived value is achieved, marketing efforts are at risk of being compromised and falling short of their objective.

The burden of creating value and marketing cannot be placed solely on the professions and their professional associations. Each practitioner must be actively involved in the process by marketing his or her own practice and establishing its value. These activities include marketing, advocacy, and educating individuals at all levels of health care, education, government, politics, and the corporate worlds (Nelson, La Puma, & Wolf, 1998). Time, energy, and resources need to be planned for and dedicated to these efforts. ASHA has developed many such tools and offered workshops that may be a vital stepping stone for the practitioner (see the ASHA Web site for the most current information).

Cultural Competence The United States has become increasingly diverse. Racial and ethnic minorities are 28 percent of the current population and are expected to comprise more than 40 percent by 2030 (United States Census Bureau, 2000). The 2000 U.S. Census found that about 18 percent of people over the age of 5 years spoke a language other than English at home (Moxley, Madhendra, & Vega-Barachowitz, 2004). Some communities are changing more rapidly than others, but all are undergoing shifts in demographic composition. Diversity is reflected in attitudes, customs, and expectations about health care, illness, disease and healing, and presents challenges to the health-care system (Wolf & Calderon, 1999); further, education parallels health care (Medrano, 2003). Thus, clinicians and educators need to be competent to offer services that are responsive to and effective for a myriad of populations (ASHA, 2004b). To abide by the Code of Ethics, speech-language pathologists and audiologists may need additional or continuing education. Therefore, maintaining or developing new knowledge and skills to be culturally competent is a requirement of not only good, but also ethical practice (ASHA, 2005b; Crowley, 2004). Success as a practitioner-owner in the 21st century may depend on the ability to develop cultural competence as well as clinical competence, to ensure that any cultural differences that may exist between the practitioner and the patient/client do not bias or affect clinical outcomes (Wolf, 2004; Wolf & Calmes, 2004). ASHA has developed guidelines (ASHA, 2004b) as well as ethical statements (ASHA, 2005b) for delivering culturally competent services. The reader is encouraged to visit the ASHA Web site for access to many additional tools and references.

Ethical Practices Every day, the practitioner-owner will be faced with clinical, business, and personal decisions that are likely to have competing values and interests. Ethical considerations guide that decision-making process (Chabon & Morris,

2005). The ASHA Code of Ethics clearly and succinctly delineates appropriate behaviors for its members (ASHA, 2003c), and all members are bound by this code. The Principles of Ethics and the Rules of Ethics describe the fundamental aspects of ethical conduct as related to service delivery, research, scholarly activity, and those who are served by speech-language pathologists and audiologists. The Principles of Ethics form the underlying moral basis, whereas the Rules of Ethics are statements of minimally acceptable behaviors. The Code of Ethics clearly delineates members' responsibilities to hold paramount the welfare of the persons they serve, responsibility to the achieve and maintain the highest level of professional competence, responsibility to the public, and responsibility to the professions and to colleagues, students, and members of other professions. ASHA maintains an active ethics education program, including publication of articles and periodic development of *Issues in Ethics Statements* (ASHA, 2005c). An Ethical Practices Board processes and adjudicates formal ethics complaints from members or the general public.

Research and Academic Affiliations Individuals in private practice are as dependent on research and the acquisition of new knowledge as any other professional. In fact, a great deal of the data used to generate databases, practice guidelines, and benchmarks will have to emerge from the private practice environment to be meaningful and representative. This need creates an extraordinary opportunity for collaboration with researchers and university training programs. Additionally, university training programs often seek a broader range of practicum sites in which to train their students, and the private practice site offers a rich teaching environment that may not be paralleled in other clinical speech-language pathology or audiology venues. Further, academic and teaching responsibilities provide another mechanism for the practitioner to remain current. Finally, an academic affiliation, even as an adjunct instructor, often adds market value to the practitioner in the eyes of the public and/or other professional colleagues. For these reasons, like colleagues in medicine, some private practitioners are carving out a segment of their time for teaching and affiliating with academic institutions.

Continuing Education Mandatory continuing professional development for maintaining ASHA certification began in 2003 for audiologists and in 2005 for speech-language pathologists. The new requirements were based on trends in client demographics, emerging issues, changes in practice patterns, skills validation studies, independent research on consumer advocacy, and extensive internal peer review comments. Some states also require participation in mandatory continuing education programs to maintain licensure. Additionally, many hospital credentialing committees require annual evidence of continuing professional development to maintain hospital privileges. Continuing education is necessary regardless of the mandatory status. The ASHA Code of Ethics, Principle of Ethics II (C) (ASHA, 2003c), states that practitioners will remain current in their practice and knowledge base. Maintaining a continuing education transcript demonstrates that these professionals have a commitment to lifelong learning, without the need to do so by mandate. Regardless of

mandate or voluntary participation, the individual who is engaged in private practice needs to dedicate time and resources to maintaining currency through continuing education.

Volunteerism Volunteerism is the backbone of any professional organization. However, individuals in the later part of the 1990s were volunteering less than any previous generation (Blanken & Liff, 1998; Ellis, 2005). Unfortunately, speech-language pathologists and audiologists are no different than the rest of society, and there is greater competition for their volunteer time to ASHA and other groups. As a result, decisions, regulations, practice guidelines, advocacy and position papers are being drafted and approved by those willing to volunteer their time to do so. The voice of the private practice community needs to be heard if it is to influence any such actions. That means practitioners need to be involved and participate, giving more of their time for which they cannot be reimbursed. However, this investment of time and effort may have significant rewards, personally and professionally.

SUMMARY

This chapter presented some of the issues facing the individual who elects to enter the private practice environment. Although some who enter private practice are employees and/or part-time practitioners, the information was presented from the perspective of the practitioner-owner. Options and advantages of private practice were discussed, along with the business considerations unique to a practitioner-owner. Included were topics such as development and maintenance of a business plan, funding and loans, licenses and insurances needed to practice, referral bases and networks, and the use of staff and consultants. Additional topics not unique to the private practitioner, but that affect the delivery of speech-language pathology and audiology services in the private practice arena, were also discussed. Those issues include retrospective versus prospective payments systems, treatment outcomes,

accountability, evidence-based practice, the use of information technology, the need to create value for speech-language pathology and audiology services, the need to participate in education and advocacy activities, the need for cultural competence, the potential to participate in research and affiliate with an academic institution, a commitment to lifelong learning and continuing education, ethical practice, and finally a call for increased volunteerism. Some issues are shared with other delivery environments such as health care and education, and readers are referred to those chapters for more information.

ASHA has recently published a useful resource for speech-language pathologists who want to know more about business practices (Golper & Brown, 2005). That text was written by an ad hoc committee that included individuals coming from private practice. Two policy documents are also available, based on the work of that committee (ASHA, 2003d, 2004a). However, no single article, chapter, or book will adequately provide all of the information to describe the service delivery issues in private practice. Individuals who elect the world of private practice will need to network with colleagues, participate in professional development, and dedicate themselves to a commitment that goes beyond serving patients/clients. Private practice requires involvement in the business, practice, and professional issues of speech-language pathology and audiology service delivery.

CRITICAL THINKING

1. You have been working in the public schools for the past 4 years and occasionally providing evening, weekend, and vacation coverage for some colleagues in hospitals. Now that you have experienced work in both the education and health care environments, you think you would like start you own practice. Describe the process you will undertake to help you decide if private practice is appropriate for you.

2. Your business is competing with two others of about the same size and scope of services for a contract to provide services. Discuss how evidence-based practice might be used to help you win that contract.

3. Describe how you as a private practitioner will participate in the creation of value for our services and why it is important.

4. Owner-practitioners must participate in several activities that are nonbillable and may actually detract from their profit. Therefore, explain why it is important for private practitioners to participate in ASHA, AAA, and other state and national professional organizations.

5. How might you as a private practitioner benefit from an affiliation with a research and academic facility?

6. What are the disadvantages of establishing a private practice in either speech-language pathology or audiology?

REFERENCES

American Speech-Language-Hearing Association. (1991a). Considerations for establishing a private practice in audiology and/or speech-language pathology. *ASHA, 33* (Suppl. 3), 10–21.

American Speech-Language-Hearing Association. (1991b). Report on private practice. *ASHA, 33* (Suppl. 6), 1–4.

American Speech-Language-Hearing Association. (2003a). *2003 omnibus survey: Caseload report: SLP*. Rockville, MD: Author.

American Speech-Language-Hearing Association. (2003b). *2003 omnibus survey: Practice trends in audiology*. Rockville, MD: Author.

American Speech-Language-Hearing Association. (2003c). Code of ethics (revised). *ASHA Supplement, 23,* 13–15.

American Speech-Language-Hearing Association. (2003d). Knowledge and skills in business practices needed by speech-language pathologists in health care settings. *ASHA Supplement, 23,* 87–92.

American Speech-Language-Hearing Association. (2004a). Knowledge and skills in business practices for speech-language pathologists who are managers and leaders in health care organizations. *ASHA Supplement, 24,* 146–151.

American Speech-Language-Hearing Association. (2004b). Knowledge and skills needed by speech-language pathologists and audiologists to provide culturally and linguistically appropriate services. *ASHA Supplement, 24,* 152–158.

American Speech-Language-Hearing Association. (2004c). *Evidence-based practice in communication disorders: An introduction.* Rockville, MD: Author.

American Speech-Language-Hearing Association. (2004d). *Highlights and trends: ASHA counts for 2004.* Available at http://www.asha.org/

American Speech-Language-Hearing Association. (2005a). *Web-based Tutorials.* Available at http://www.asha.org/

American Speech-Language-Hearing Association. (2005b). Cultural competence. *ASHA Supplement, 25,* 1–2.

American Speech-Language-Hearing Association. (2005c). *Ethics.* Available at http://www.asha.org/

American Speech-Language-Hearing Association. (2005d). *Evidence-based practice in communication disorders.* Rockville, MD: Author.

American Speech-Language-Hearing Association. (2005e). *Frequently asked questions about business practices.* Available at http://www.asha.org/

American Speech-Language-Hearing Association. (2005f). *Private practice in speech-language-pathology.* Available at http://www.asha.org/

American Speech-Language-Hearing Association. (2005g). *Resource guide for audiologists in private practice.* Available at http://www.asha.org/

American Speech-Language-Hearing Association. (2005h). *Specialty recognition: FAQs.* Available at http://www.asha.org/

Blanken, R. L., & Liff, A. (1998). *Facing the future: Preparing your association to thrive.* Washington, DC: Foundation of the American Society of Association Executives.

Chabon, S. S., & Morris, J. (2005). Raising ethical awareness in the practice of speech language pathology and audiology: A 24/7 endeavor. *CSHA, 35*(1), 6–8.

Cohen, M. (1993). Planes, trains, and speech therapy. *CSHA, 20*(2), 12–13, 16.

Crowley, C. J. (2004). The ethics of assessment with culturally and linguistically diverse populations. *ASHA Leader, 9*(5), 6–7.

Currie, P. S. (2004). *Starting a private practice.* Available at http://www.audiologyonline.com/

Dollaghan, C. A. (2004). Evidence-based practice in communication disorders: What do we know, and when do we know it? *Journal of Communication Disorders, 37*(5), 391–400.

Ellis, S. J. (2005). Tracking volunteer trends. *Association Management, 57*(1), 72–74.

Evidence-Based Medicine Working Group. (1992). Evidence-based medicine: A new approach to teaching the practice of medicine. *Journal of the American Medical Association, 268*(17), 2420–2425.

Goffinet, M. (2005). Private practice: Where do you begin? *Access Audiology, 4*(4). Available at http://www.asha.org/

Golper, L., & Brown, J. (Eds.). (2005). *Business matters: A guide for speech-language pathologists.* Rockville, MD: American Speech-Language-Hearing Association.

Griffin, K. (1995). Managed care and the professions. In S. Holzberger (Ed.), *Meeting the managed care challenge: Strategies for professionals and the professions.* Rockville, MD: American Speech-Language-Hearing Association.

Kent, R. D. (2004). Science in the courtroom and the clinic. *ASHA Leader, 9*(16), 33.

Klontz, H. A., Napp, A. C., White, S. C., & Wolf, K. E. (1997). *The competitive edge for audiologists negotiating with managed Care.* Rockville, MD: American Speech-Language-Hearing Association.

Kreb, R. A. (Ed.). (1997). *A practical guide to applying treatment outcomes & efficacy resources.* Rockville, MD: American Speech-Language-Hearing Association.

Kreb, R. A., Swigert, N. B., Conoway, J., Markus, G., von Unwerth, F. H., & White, S. C. (1995). PPOs: Are they good for ASHA members? *ASHA, 37,* 39–41.

Kreb, R. A., & Wolf, K. E. (1997). *Successful operations in the treatment outcomes driven world of managed care.* Rockville, MD: National Student Speech-Language-Hearing Association.

Logemann, J. A. (2004). Clinical trials: CSDRG overview. *Journal of Communication Disorders, 37*(5), 419–423.

McKibbon, A., Eady, A., & Marks, S. (1999). *PDQ: Evidence-based principles and practice.* Saint Louis, MO: B.C. Decker.

Medrano, M. A. (2003). *Affirmative action: Challenges and opportunities in creating a diverse health care workforce.* Paper presented at the Association of American Medical Colleges, Washington, DC.

Moxley, A., Madhendra, N., & Vega-Barachowitz, C. (2004). Cultural competence in health care. *ASHA Leader, 9*(7), 6–7, 20–22.

Napp, A. (1997). Developing networks at state and regional level for negotiating empowerment. In H. A. Klontz, A. C. Napp, S. C. White, & K. E. Wolf (Eds.), *The competitive edge for audiologists and speech-language pathologists*. Rockville, MD: American Speech-Language-Hearing Association.

Nelson, J. A., La Puma, J., & Wolf, K. E. (1998). When the patient's health plan limits care: An ethics roundtable. *ASHA, 40,* 48.

Plante, E. (2004). Evidence-based practice in communication sciences and disorders. *Journal of Communication Disorders, 37*(5), 389–390.

Sackett, D. L., Straus, S. E., Richardson, W. S., Rosenberg, W., & Haynes, R. B. (2000). *Evidence-based medicine: How to practice and teach EBM* (2nd ed.). New York: Churchill Livingstone.

U.S. Census Bureau. (2000). *U.S. Census 2000.* Available at http://www.census.gov/

U.S. Small Business Administration. (2005). *Small business startup basics.* Available at http://www.sba.gov/starting_business/index.html

Wolf, K. E. (1995). What audiologists need to know about managed care. In S. Holzberger (Ed.), *Meeting the managed care challenge: Strategies for professionals and the professions*. Rockville, MD: American Speech-Language-Hearing Association.

Wolf, K. E. (1999). Preparing for evidence-based speech-language pathology and audiology. *Texas Journal of Audiology and Speech Pathology, 23,* 69–74.

Wolf, K. E. (2001). Service delivery issues in private practice. In R. Lubinski & C. M. Friattali (Eds.), *Professional issues in speech-language pathology and audiology* (2nd ed., pp. 301–315). San Diego, CA: Singular.

Wolf, K. E. (2004). Cultural competence in audiology. *ASHA Leader, 9*(7), 8–9.

Wolf, K. E., & Calderon, J. L. (1999). Cultural competence: The underpinning of quality health care and education services. *ASHA, 28*(2), 4–6.

Wolf, K. E., & Calmes, D. (2004). Cultural competence in the emergency department. *Topics in Emergency Medicine, 26*(1), 9–13.

Wolf, K. E., Cohen, M. S., & Arnst, D. J. (1994). Managed care: Costs and risks. In B. S. Cornett (Ed.), *Managing managed care: A practical guide for audiologists and speech-language pathologists*. Rockville, MD: American Speech-Language-Hearing Association.

Wolf, K. E., & Kreb, R. A. (1996). Actuary data: what's in it for you? *ASHA, 38*(2), 33–36.

Zingeser, L. (2005). Trends in private practice among ASHA constituents, 1986–2003. *ASHA Leader,* 10–11, 14.

RESOURCES

American Academy of Audiology
8300 Greensboro Drive, Suite 750
McLean, VA 22102
Phone: 702-790-8466; 800-AAA-2336
Web site: http://www.audiology.org

American Academy of Private Practice in Speech-Language Pathology and Audiology
Web site: http://www.aappspa.org

American Speech-Language-Hearing Association
10801 Rockville Pike
Rockville, Maryland 20852
Phone: 301-897-5700
Web site: http:// www.asha.org

For ASHA's overview of state associations, regulatory agencies, state laws and other relevant information see: http://www.asha.org/about/legislation-advocacy/state/info/

Marsh Affinity Group Services, a Service of Seabury and Smith
1440 Renaissance Drive
Park Ridge, IL 60068-1400
Phone: 800-503-9230
Web site: http://seaburychicago.com/default.asp

U.S. Small Business Administration
See local white pages for address and telephone number Web site: http://www.sba.gov

18

Strategically Promoting Access to Speech-Language Pathology and Audiology Services

BROOKE HALLOWELL, PHD

BERNARD P. HENRI, PHD

SCOPE OF CHAPTER

It is ironic that the provision of quality speech-language pathology and audiology services to persons who need them is most threatened at a time when the number of persons throughout the entire age range needing such services is increasing steadily. Before we can strategically counteract the forces that threaten access to speech-language pathology and audiology services, we must have both a clear understanding of what the barriers to access are and a sound rationale for the need for our services. In this chapter, we discuss the factors that impede access despite a growing need for services. We will then discuss strategic means of enhancing access through: optimizing reimbursement for clinical services, finding alternative ways to fund clinical services, pursuing legislative channels to enhance access, engaging in advocacy, using care extenders, taking advantage of technology, educating the public, and modifying our service-providing environments.

BARRIERS TO ACCESS

Reimbursement and funding problems constitute the greatest barriers for access to audiology and speech-language pathology services. An emphasis on cost containment in all areas of health care delivery is at the root of many of those problems (Henri & Hallowell, 1999b). Children and adults with disabilities face unique difficulties as they attempt to obtain services through our progressively more unwieldy health care system (Mitchell & Gaskin, 2004; Ronder, Kastner, Parker, & Walsh, 1999; White, 2002). Overall, access to our services is being reduced by the coverage and reimbursement limitations imposed by managed care and health maintenance organizations (MC/HMOs), Medicare's Prospective Payment System (PPS), Medicare's on-again off-again reimbursement caps, and the ongoing efforts in many states to relinquish control of public education to local school boards (ASHA, 2006; Frymark & Mullen, 2005; Hiller & Lewis, 1995; Rodwin, 1995).

Physician referrals are decreasing, authorizations for evaluations and treatment are slow in coming, reimbursement rates are being reduced, denials are increasing, and the appeals process is cumbersome and lengthy. As a result, some health care employers are eliminating positions or are placing clinicians on as-needed schedules, actions that further reduce access to services. Primary care physicians are guarding more aggressively scarcer financial resources to ensure the availability of basic health care for their patients. Many physicians see audiology and speech-language pathology services as a low priority or a service that should be paid for by other entities, such as school districts, public service organizations, or clients themselves. Insurance companies are following suit.

THE NEED FOR SERVICE

Why is it critical that an individual obtain services for communication disorders? What are the consequences to a child or adult of diminished communicative effectiveness when services are inaccessible or otherwise unavailable? The answers to these questions must be addressed and elaborated upon continuously by members of our professions if we are to substantiate the need for our services to consumers, third party payers, legislators, and other professionals in health care and education. Likewise, the effectiveness of our interventions must be documented and promoted continuously.

The need for health care services, including those provided by audiologists and speech-language pathologists, is expected to increase up to 35 percent by the year 2012 (United States Department of Labor, 2004). There are several reasons for this growing need:

- There is a greater emphasis on health promotion and disease prevention (Marge, 1993).

- The elderly population is growing, with corresponding increases in hearing loss and neurologically based speech-language problems (United States Department of Labor, 2004).

- Advances in medical technology are saving lives and increasing the life span (United States Department of Labor, 2004).

- The bilingual/multilingual population, which has a proportionately greater need for speech and language diagnostic and intervention services, is expanding (Uffen, 1998).

- There is a greater emphasis on early identification and diagnosis, as well as increased referrals of students to professionals (Marge, 1993; United States Department of Labor, 2004).

- There are increased enrollments in elementary and secondary schools, including enrollments in special education (United States Department of Labor, 2004).

Another factor affecting the need for services to persons with communication disorders is the accelerating speed with which our world is moving into and through the "Information Age" (Toffler,

1980), requiring persons to have progressively more effective communication abilities. On a daily basis, we are required to manage greater amounts of complex language-based information. Those who have untreated communication challenges risk becoming marginal participants in our society, observers standing on the sidelines. Reading abilities, particularly in the country's large urban school districts, are plummeting. In some districts, up to 75 percent of fourth graders are failing basic reading proficiency tests (Marrison, 1999). Recent research demonstrates that children who are poor readers, particularly those raised in poverty, often experience careers of academic failure and may eventually become trapped in lives of generational poverty, accompanied sometimes by teenage parenthood and criminal behavior (Jesuit & Smeeding, 2002). The prevalence of language learning disabilities and illiteracy in state prisons provides dramatic evidence of the cost of not providing speech-language pathology and audiology services. Up to 75 percent of individuals remanded to adult correctional facilities have significant communication disorders, which are vitally linked to literacy (Voinovich, 1996). Likewise, teenage mothers raised in poverty have a high prevalence of speech-language and literacy problems. Such problems may affect not only their own economic and social futures but also those of their children, who may not benefit from literate environments or from competent speech-language models (Hock & Deschler, 2003). Additionally, in high-technology industries, employers report difficulty recruiting candidates with even minimal literacy and mathematical abilities (Gage, 1995). For many individuals, access to our services is crucial for establishing the communication skills necessary for success in school, employment, and social interaction.

Despite worldwide efforts to improve the ways individuals with disabilities are treated and regarded, the social consequences of communication disorders remain fundamentally challenging. Many individuals with communication disorders face "attitudinal barriers, marginal social status, rejection, distrust, stigmatization and loss of esteem" (Chapey & Hallowell, 2001, p. 12).

OPTIMIZING REIMBURSEMENT FOR CLINICAL SERVICES

Unless the financial viability of service providers and their institutions is ensured, there will be limited or no access to speech-language pathology and audiology services (Henri & Hallowell, 1996). A primary means by which financial viability can be maintained is through the enhancement of clinical revenues. In today's managed care environment, multiple sources of reimbursement for evaluations, treatment, and consultation must be identified and developed. Contractual agreements with managed care organizations can be carefully negotiated to ensure clinical revenues and minimize financial risk (Breakey, 1994). One must know in detail the policies and procedures of multiple payers and stay abreast of changes in policies and procedures of each payer. This requires an unprecedented amount of communication with payers.

One especially effective approach to optimizing an organization's payer reimbursements is to identify the five most common reasons for authorization and/or treatment denials an organization experiences and then develop action plans to address each reason. Generally, the most common reasons for denials include:

- An appropriate physician referral was not obtained.

- The service provided was not covered by the client's benefit plan.

- The service was determined to be "not medically necessary."

- The authorization period had lapsed.

- The patient was no longer improving.

Given that these causes typically make up 80 percent to 90 percent of the reasons for denial, clinical professionals and administrators may best use their time and resources by proactively attending to the sources of each of these problems. By implementing careful documentation strategies, along with ongoing verification procedures to ensure attention to each of these potential pitfalls, service providers may greatly reduce the proportion of reimbursement claims denied. Many service-providing agencies have implemented automated denial management systems for a systematic approach for analyzing claim problems, tracking of denials and appeals, and prevention of future denials (c.f., Danbe, 2002).

Also essential to solid clinical revenue is a sound understanding of the diagnosis and treatment classification coding systems that are the basis for reimbursement—that is, the International Classification of Diseases (ICD-9) and Common Procedural Terminology (CPT) codes, as they relate to speech-language pathology and audiology services. Still, a failure to stay abreast of variations in coding and billing procedures from one insurance carrier to another can be costly. Fortunately, implementation of the Health Insurance Portability and Accountability Act (HIPAA) is helping reduce problems of inconsistency in billing codes used by various payers through required use of uniform coding processes. Educating administrators and payers about projected health care cost savings associated with speech, language, swallowing, and hearing services is an additional means of enhancing access to these services. Consider an important example provided by Johnson (1997). In efforts to reduce payments for treatment under its own health maintenance organization, representatives at Henry Ford Hospital in Detroit proposed to eliminate reimbursement for several speech-language pathology services that had long been covered. Johnson, who was overseeing those services at the time, reports that he was able to demonstrate that eliminating the coverage for these services would conservatively cost the hospital approximately $1.6 million in revenue. As a result, the proposal to restrict coverage was withdrawn.

An additional means of clinical revenue enhancement is offering services for which clients or their employers pay directly. Direct payment is the usual form of reimbursement for some services, such as accent modification programs and individualized coaching programs for professional speakers. Patients and clients may also pay out-of-pocket for most clinical services. Emphasizing the possibility of direct payment to those who can afford it may be an alternative route to access care that is not dependent on insurance coverage and may also help enhance providers' clinical revenues.

Rebutting Denials Based on "Medical Necessity"

As managed care and health maintenance organizations attempt to rein in health care costs, the loosely defined and broadly applied concept of medical necessity is frequently being used to deny authorizations or reauthorizations for care (Brown, 1999; Ireys, Wehr, & Cooke, 2000). Strictly defined, medical necessity relates to treating conditions proceeding from illness or injury. First-level claims reviewers, whose purpose it is to protect health insurance company funds, typically apply this restricted definition.

In most instances, these reviewers have little to no understanding of speech-language pathology or audiology services and, thus, are poorly prepared to render informed decisions concerning the medical necessity of these services. Because of their limited experience with the services provided by our professions, third party payers are often more easily convinced of the necessity for the treatment of physical disabilities than they are of the need to treat problems associated with cognitive and communication disorders. Professionals in audiology and speech-language pathology must be able to provide substantive arguments demonstrating how most of our services do, in fact, meet definitions of medical necessity.

The following perspectives, drawn from the medical literature, offer guidance concerning the rebuttal of denials based on an apparent lack of demonstrated medical necessity. Berman (1997) states that, because medical necessity has no standardized definition, its inclusion in contract language gives the health plan considerable discretion determining the use, scope, and duration of covered benefits. Writing on behalf of the American Academy of Pediatrics (AAP), he recommends the following criteria be used to guide decisions concerning medical necessity:

- Is the service appropriate for the age and health status of the individual?

- Will the service prevent or ameliorate the effects of a condition, illness, injury, or disorder?

- Will the service aid the overall physical and mental growth and development of the individual?

- Will the service assist in achieving or maintaining functional capacity? (p. 858)

The AAP (2005) has expanded the scope of the definition to address health problems, evidence of effectiveness, and value for children. Perkins and Olson (1998), writing on behalf of the National Health Law Program, propose a model definition of medical necessity for physical care contracts. They state that medically necessary care is the care that, in the opinion of the treating physician, is reasonably needed:

- To prevent the onset or worsening of an illness, condition, or disability;

- To establish a diagnosis;

- To provide palliative, curative or restorative treatment for physical and/or mental health conditions; and/or

- To assist the individual to achieve or maintain maximum functional capacity in performing daily activities, taking into account both the functional capacity of the individual and those functional capacities that are appropriate for individuals of the same age. (p. 1)

Kahan and colleagues (1994) declare that a procedure is medically necessary if the following criteria are met:

- The procedure is appropriate,

- It would be improper care not to recommend this service,

- There is sufficient likelihood that the procedure will benefit the patient, especially in light of associated risks, and

- The benefit to the patient is not "minor." (p. 359)

Finally, ASHA (2005d) has published *Medical Necessity for Speech-Language Pathology and Audiology Services,* a comprehensive document providing additional information supporting why our services meet the definition of medical necessity.

Evidence-Based Practice

Evidence-based practice (EBP) is a concept being applied increasingly by many payers to further restrict access and reduce care and, thus, their payments. This topic is discussed in depth in Chapter 28. EBP represents an approach to clinical care wherein decision making is based on an analysis of the data from clinical research (Ellrodt, Cho, & Cush, 1997). As defined by Sackett et al., 1996 (in Dollaghan, 2004), evidence-based practice is ". . . the conscientious, explicit, and judicious use of current best evidence in making decisions about the care of individual patients . . . [by] integrating individual clinical expertise with the best available external clinical evidence from systematic research" (pp. 71–72). Simply stated, health insurance companies (HICs) are now proposing that authorizations and reimbursements will occur only for those interventions for which efficacy and effectiveness are supported by well-controlled studies. While laudable in principle, implementation of strict EBP rules has the potential to significantly reduce access to all health care disciplines for minorities and underrepresented groups (women, children and adolescents, people of color, and the elderly) who generally have not been included in studies of clinical effectiveness (Newacheck, Stoddard, Hughes, & Pearl, 1998; Perkins & Olson, 1998; Weinick, Weigers, & Cohen, 1998). As a result, Perkins and Olson (1998) emphasize that these groups suffer disproportionately when a HIC's coverage is dependent on proof of a treatment's effectiveness.

Despite recent concerted efforts to address treatment efficacy and outcomes research in communication sciences and disorders, work to develop a solid foundation in EBP through our own disciplines lags behind the implementation of EBP requirements imposed by the insurance industry and by state and federal policymakers (Lerner, Gesek, & Adams, 2003). ASHA has prepared extensive bibliographies summarizing treatment efficacy in various clinical areas such as stuttering, cognitive and communicative problems associated with traumatic brain injury, feeding and swallowing disorders, hearing loss, hearing aids, audiological rehabilitation, aphasia, child language disorders, autistic spectrum disorders, phonological disorders, and dysphagia. This information has been developed to help support claims of effectiveness and to reverse denials based on the concepts of medical necessity and evidence-based medical necessity. It may also be used advantageously when negotiating contracts with HICs. These resources can be accessed online through ASHA. The Preferred Patterns for the Profession of Audiology (ASHA, 2005e) and the Preferred Practice Patterns for the Profession of Speech-Language Pathology (ASHA, 2005f) offer especially helpful guidance to support clinicians' assertions that services are medically necessary and appropriate.

ALTERNATIVE FUNDING APPROACHES

Agencies may enhance access to services by systematically developing program funding alternatives that supplement clinical revenues. Alternative funding sources help to ensure the fiscal stability of a service-providing agency (Greenfield, 1994; Rosso & Associates, 1991). These alternatives have long been central to the operation of most not-for-profit agencies, which are commonly required to provide services to clients regardless of their ability to pay. In the midst of grave reductions in clinical revenues in the current service delivery arena, alternative funding sources are now more critical than ever (Henri & Hallowell, 1999a, 1999b). Even for-profit agencies are developing their own not-for-profit foundations or are partnering with extant foundations that will help support the provision of services to clients whose access might otherwise be curtailed.

Service-providing agencies can best support their nonclinical revenue base by strategically developing a funding plan consisting of several possible revenue sources. Henri and Hallowell (1999a) describe the means for developing such a strategic plan. Essential steps include:

1. Creating a resource development, or fund-raising team, including members of the organization's Board of Directors, the chief executive officer or executive director, an experienced development professional, staff, volunteers, and any additional "friends" of the organization.

2. Composing a case statement that describes the agency's purpose and details why donors should invest their resources in its programs and services.

3. Establishing a donor base of individuals, patients/clients, foundations, and corporations that support the concerns of persons with communication disorders. The donor base may include, but should not rely solely on, aggregated donor bases, such as United Way or Easter Seals Society.

4. Engaging in specific fund-raising activities. These may include:

   ■ An annual fund campaign. This is typically conducted during the last quarter of a calendar year to take advantage of contributions that individuals and corporations make to reduce their income tax liability.

   ■ Special events. Examples are benefit concerts, special recognition dinners, golf outings, fashion shows, marathons, and evenings at the theater. In addition to raising operating revenue for the organization, these events generate publicity, media attention, and community goodwill. They also introduce potential donors to the agency and its purpose.

   ■ Planned and deferred giving programs. These long-range funding programs yield benefits in an average of 5 to 7 years. They include bequests, gift annuities, charitable remainder annuity trusts, charitable remainder unitrusts, pooled income funds, charitable life insurance, and gifts of real estate and goods (e.g., works of art). Guidance from professionals with expertise in planned giving, estate planning, law, and accounting are essential to successful planned and deferred giving programs.

- Corporate partnerships. Partnerships between corporations and agencies serving persons with communication disorders may help to improve client access through agencies' improved fiscal stability. Corporations are most likely to "adopt" an agency or one of its programs in communities where corporations have a significant presence (e.g., in areas where their corporate headquarters are located).

- Fraternal organizations. Community fraternal organizations such as the Rotary, Junior League, Kiwanis, Lions, Elks, and Eagles are all sources of usually client- or program-specific funding. SERTOMA and Scottish Rite, though present in only certain regions of the United States, are also fraternal organizations with long-standing histories of support for audiology and speech-language pathology services. All entertain proposals to fund services, equipment, or instrumentation needed by individuals unable to afford these.

- Research funding to support clinical services. Clinical research funding from local, regional, state, and federal agencies may strengthen a service-providing agency's fiscal stability. Often, research materials purchased through grant funds (e.g., diagnostic equipment, published tests, treatment materials, computers, and software) enrich not only the research environment but the organization's clinical environment as well. Also, indirect cost or "overhead" monies allotted by funding agencies can be used to support an agency's general operational costs, thus enhancing clinical access.

Agencies that do not have resident development expertise can contract with fund-raising consultants for specific resource development projects and/or long-range planning. In many instances, these arrangements are more cost-effective and further allow the organization's staff to concentrate upon more profitable activities, such as acquiring major gifts.

LEGISLATION IMPROVING ACCESS

Several pieces of federal and state legislation have been passed to ensure that children and adults with special conditions have access to adequate and appropriate levels of service (Barlow, 1997). Knowledge of federal laws, their state equivalents, and the rules and regulations that guarantee access to special services, including speech-language pathology and audiology, is essential. The Social Security Act, for example, contains several "titles"—that is chapters or subsections that ensure reimbursement for speech-language pathology and audiology services, including:

- Title 5, the Crippled Children's Act, the funding base for states' Bureaus for Children with Medical Handicaps

- Title 18, Medicare, which provides for speech-language pathology and audiology coverage (Medicare coverage is also available for persons under the age of 65 who have disabilities lasting longer than 2 years, such as chronic neurological conditions.)

- Title 19, Medicaid, which also includes Aid to Aged, Blind and Disabled; Early Periodic Screening Diagnosis and Treatment, EPSDT; and state-contracted Medicaid HMOs

- Title 20, the Social Services Subsidy, that in some instances supports social work services, which, in turn, can help families access speech-language pathology and audiology services

- Title 21, Children's Health Insurance Program (CHIP), a new funding source for speech-language pathology and audiology services, usually administered by a state's Department of Human Services, Medicaid Division

- The Disabilities Education Act, the primary funding vehicle for states' special education programs

- The Rehabilitation Act, which funds rehabilitation services, including audiology and speech-language pathology, for persons ranging in age from 16 to 64

Many of these reimbursement mechanisms have mixed histories in terms of their effectiveness in supporting services for populations with special chronic or degenerative conditions (Smith & Ashbaugh, 1995). Several other pieces of federal legislation indirectly support our services. The Americans with Disabilities Act (ADA), for example, does not ensure funding per se, but may require employers to make available certain resources in cases where communication disorders have a demonstrated impact on an individual's ability to perform their job duties. Likewise, the Rehabilitation Act is a national law that prohibits discrimination against qualified people with disabilities for employment in the federal sector. Additionally, the No Child Left Behind Act (NCLB) is intended to support education of all children, including those with disabilities, in the public schools, through high standards, an emphasis on school and teacher accountability, and selective funding programs. However, the effectiveness and legitimacy of many of the principles guiding NCLB remain areas of concern for many as varied aspects of this law are implemented (e.g., Hock & Deshler, 2003).

ADVOCACY AND PROFESSIONAL ASSERTIVENESS

The goals of improved access and quality of care of most current HICs are often in direct conflict with their goals of cost containment (Carlson, 1995; Engelhard & Childress, 1995; Henri & Hallowell, 1999a; Hiller & Lewis, 1995; Rodwin, 1995).

Improving access for speech-language pathology and audiology services requires that action plans for advocacy be thoughtfully developed and executed at various levels of governmental bureaucracies, in the public and private reimbursement arenas (Henri & Hallowell, 1996; Henri, Hallowell, & Johnson, 1997).

The child, teenager, or adult coping with a communication disorder is often at a disadvantage when the need for personal advocacy concerning access or reimbursement arises. Many individuals with communication disorders find it difficult to advocate vigorously for their own needs. This problem may be further compounded by difficulties related to communication infrastructure, travel, and distance from legislators in rural areas. Furthermore, individuals who would benefit from our services often do not have the knowledge necessary to confront a complex bureaucratic system to obtain coverage for needed services. Audiologists and speech-language pathologists thus have numerous opportunities to initiate or support consumers' advocacy efforts. These opportunities require that we professionals be knowledgeable about the content and the process required for an effective advocacy effort (Barlow, 1997).

Historically, most audiologists and speech-language pathologists have had little experience, and often little inclination, to participate in the arena of public policy development, political advocacy, and lobbying. Given the ongoing dramatic challenges to consumer access and the consequent fiscal instability of service-providing agencies, though, it is no longer possible for clinicians, administrators, educators, and consumers to remain passive, adopting a "let someone else do it" attitude. Together, professionals and consumers must participate in coordinated efforts aimed at educating and influencing decision makers about the value of audiology and speech-language pathology services and especially about the societal consequences of not providing these services. Information related to access issues must be disseminated and used as a basis for action. Specific actions for advocacy are described here and are outlined in Table 18–1.

T A B L E 18–1 Actions for Advocacy and Professional Assertiveness

Advocacy Among Clinicians and Clinical Administrators
- Continuing education
- Consumer education and mobilization
- Marketing to and education of referral sources
- Appealing denials of treatment authorization and reimbursement
- Financial support
- Active writing to legislators
- Inviting legislators to work settings
- Visiting legislators in their local offices or on Capitol Hill
- Engaging in quality assurance

Advocacy Among Consumers and Their Significant Others
- Active pursuit of coverage for speech-language pathology and audiology services
- Reporting of health care policy coverage inconsistencies
- Education of employers
- Mobilization of consumer groups

Advocacy Among Educators and Students
- Continuing education concerning modes of service delivery and health policy and about the effects on persons with communication and swallowing disorders
- Curricular revision
- Engagement in concerted legislative advocacy

Advocacy Among Clinicians and Clinical Administrators

Specific action steps in which clinicians and clinical administrators may make solid contributions to advocacy efforts to improve consumer access are summarized here.

- *Continuing education.* Clinicians who consistently and attentively read current publications and participate in seminars and workshops to improve their knowledge concerning managed care and its impact upon our services will be most effective as advocates.

- *Consumer education and mobilization.* Clinicians must take advantage of the direct access they have to consumers to provide counseling and education that will motivate consumers and their families to appreciate:

  - the complex relationships between an individual's communication abilities and the success one experiences in other life arenas, such as progress in school or independent living;

  - any restrictions consumers' MCOs place on the treatment of communication and/or swallowing disorders; and

  - specific means by which consumers may become more involved in advocacy.

- *Education of and marketing to third party payers.* Providers must convince managed care representatives of the need to include speech-language pathology and audiology services in health care plans (Henri et al., 1997).

- *Marketing to and education of referral sources.* Many of the decision makers who have the greatest potential for making an impact on patient access are often unaware of the issues faced by persons with communication and swallowing problems and of the vital role that SLPs and audiologists play. It is important that decision makers such as physicians, discharge planners, and directors of student services and special education programs be educated about the link between communication abilities and one's success in life.

■ *Appealing denials of treatment authorization and reimbursement.* Providers must work with their clients to vigorously appeal all decisions denying coverage of services. A concerted appeals process in a service-providing agency helps improve access to services in that agency, as success rates for concerted appeals are high (Henri, Hallowell, & Johnson, 1997). To support these efforts, ASHA published in 2002 a helpful document, *Appealing Health Plan Denials.* This resource provides model letters that can be sent to HICs to reverse authorization and reimbursement denials as well as treatment efficacy statements that can be appended to an appeal letter as a supporting document.

■ *Financial support.* Contributions to ASHA's Political Action Committee (ASHA-PAC) help to advance concerted professional advocacy efforts at state and federal levels. The purpose of the PAC is to provide financial support to "incumbents, challengers and open seat candidates for the U.S. House and Senate who recognize the importance of speech-language pathology and audiology services and who demonstrate concern for the rights of all citizens to receive these services" (ASHA, 2005a).

■ *Writing to legislators.* As they want to remain in office and be re-elected, legislators have a vested interest in knowing their constituents' concerns. Without the strong voice of professionals who understand the impact of policy decisions on consumers, legislators are unlikely to be sensitive to and knowledgeable about critical issues important to informed decision making. Professionals do not need to be sophisticated about legislative processes to join in legislative campaigns to address the numerous challenges to patient access. National, state, and local organizations offer ample guidance.

Joining one or both of ASHA's grassroots advocacy networks, HealthNet (for health care professionals) and EdNet (for professionals working in schools), both free of charge, allow professionals to receive occasional electronic mailings of "Action Alerts" from ASHA. These include concise descriptions of issues that need to be addressed and specific actions professionals may take. These actions almost always involve calling, writing, or e-mailing legislators. At each annual ASHA convention, ASHA's Congressional Affairs staff offers hands-on help with letter writing and model letters. Further assistance is available through the "Professionals" segments of ASHA's Web site, and additional guidance can be found in an ASHA publication edited by Golper and Brown (2004), where advocacy processes are analyzed and discussed as critical to business practices within the profession.

■ *Inviting legislators to work settings.* Hosting a member of Congress in the clinical environment allows clinicians to directly discuss and demonstrate problems of access, the need for access, and the ways in which speech-language pathology and audiology services improve the quality of life of legislators' constituents.

■ *Visiting legislators in their local offices or on Capitol Hill.* The Governmental Affairs staff of ASHA arranges appointments for professionals visiting Washington, DC, and provides in-person briefings and other materials. Because legislators have temporary terms, it is a good idea to visit and write to elected officials on a yearly basis to keep them informed about critical access and service delivery issues confronting children and adults in their districts.

■ *Participating in clinical research.* Given the dire need for empirical research to support EBP, clinicians' roles in research are more important than ever. For those not having skills, time, training, or resources to initiate or oversee research programs, there are ample possibilities for collaboration with university-based researchers.

■ *Engaging in quality improvement.* By maintaining ongoing quality improvement programs, providers continue to demonstrate cost-effective, functional treatment outcomes, which are essential to local, state, and national advocacy efforts. Again, ASHA has developed a number of resources to assist its membership in developing and maintaining quality improvement programs.

Advocacy Among Consumers and Their Significant Others

Consumers and their significant others are among the most powerful and credible advocates in improving access to audiology and speech-language pathology services. As there are often limitations due to consumers' communication disorders, support from family and from clinicians in encouraging consumer advocacy is essential. Specific ways in which consumers and their significant others may make solid contributions to advocacy efforts to improve access to services include active writing to legislators and visiting legislators in their local or Capitol Hill offices, as described previously under "Advocacy Among Clinicians and Clinical Administrators." Additional steps are described briefly here. Backing by the SLP or audiologist in each of these efforts may be helpful, as may be the support of the consumer's primary care physician.

■ *Active pursuit of coverage for speech-language pathology and audiology services.* It is important that consumers pursue adequate coverage by HICs. Consumers often are unaware of the coverage provided by their health care policies and restrictions that many place on speech-language pathology and audiology services. Careful study of a health plan's coverage and policies is the first step toward proactively seeking greater access to services. For those covered by employer-sponsored plans, staff members of the employer's human resources department may offer assistance in checking on specific coverage issues. Referring an insurance case (or "utilization") reviewer to a particular policy document may easily resolve some coverage issues. In cases in which needed services are not covered, consumer appeals to third party payers regarding the need for services to enhance independence, educational status, medical management, and/or overall quality of life may help to shape future policy modifications.

■ *Reporting of health care policy coverage inconsistencies.* When there are discrepancies between what an insurance company purports to cover, through its promotional materials and policy documentation, and its actual practice in terms of authorizing and/or reimbursing for services, appeals brought about by consumers are critical. Discrepancies can be reported at a variety of levels. Working through a hierarchy of contacts is recommended, beginning with HIC case reviewers, thereon to consumer liaisons, and up to CEOs. If necessary, state insurance commissioners may be contacted. If reporting at each of these levels fails, contacting your United States congressman or senator representative often helps. Other avenues for advocacy in the face of restricted services include letters to the editor in newspapers and professional journals, and carefully constructed press releases that may lead to newspaper, radio, and/or television coverage of access problems. If aired constructively, such media coverage may help to foster public education about access issues while exerting due pressure on HICs, the success of which depends upon public credibility.

■ *Education of employers.* Organizations that pay for insurance coverage for their employees should be urged to reconsider contracts with companies that have a pattern of limiting or violating their coverage policies or of not covering critically needed services. Consumer feedback to employers' human resources departments helps raise awareness of a plan's effectiveness and worth and has been found to be especially effective.

■ *Mobilization of consumer groups.* The advocacy power of individual consumers may be compounded exponentially through consumer groups. Personal and political advocacy efforts among members of local, state, and national organizations for persons with specific communication disorders may be especially effective in the retention and expansion of access to services.

Advocacy Among Educators and Students

Before they enter the clinical workforce, it is important that students gain awareness and knowledge of professional practice issues and how they may work to foster positive changes within their profession. Such preparation is especially essential in medical, rehabilitation, and skilled nursing contexts, where supervisors and other experienced practitioners are increasingly called to engage in billable clinical service as opposed to training and supervisory activity related to issues of insurance coverage (i.e., coding, authorizations, documentation, billing, appeals, and marketing). Graduates who are savvy about these issues and about productive actions for advocacy will have a distinct advantage over others in the job market and in their initial stages of clinical practice.

An additional advantage to having students get involved in professional practice issues is that students are capable of achieving significant advocacy work while they are still in school.

Specific actions in which faculty members and students may engage to advance advocacy for clinical access are addressed here.

■ *Continuing education concerning modes of service delivery and health policy and about the effects on persons with communication and swallowing disorders.* Because of the recency of the gravest challenges accompanying the expansion of managed care and major federal health care policy changes, few university faculty members have practiced in environments in which there have been significant threats to consumer access. Still, it is essential that all faculty members obtain an understanding of managed care principles and their ramifications for the practice of speech-language pathology and audiology. Such an understanding, in turn, helps foster students' potential for strategic advocacy as well as effective future professional practice (Hallowell & Henri, 1996; Vekovius, 1995). Continuing education is available through current publications, Internet resources, conferences, seminars, and workshops. Two methods of advocacy by educators and students are curricular revision and engagement in concerted legislative advocacy.

■ *Curricular revision.* Course work emphasizing the interconnections among functional clinical outcomes, cost-effectiveness of intervention, reimbursement, and consumer access will help to foster professional advocacy for years to come. Infusing such concepts throughout the curriculum will help students to see the import of such concepts in their current and future professional roles (Hallowell & Henri, 1996; Vekovius, 1995).

■ *Engagement in concerted legislative advocacy.* Students and faculty have clout as political constituents whose voice may have an impact on legislators. It is important that faculty and students be encouraged to participate in advocacy efforts sponsored by ASHA, the National Student Speech-Language-Hearing Association, and by state and local student and consumer groups. Academic classes or student groups may organize letter-writing campaigns involving significant numbers of participants.

CARE EXTENDERS

One way to cope with limitations in access to professional specialized care that many persons with communication and swallowing disorders are facing is to expand the reservoir of individuals who may provide needed care. "Care extenders" consist of individuals who are not certified or licensed SLPs or audiologists, but who nevertheless are involved in helping to further the development or rehabilitation of communication and swallowing skills. Ideally, they are trained and monitored by a fully certified clinician. They may be "support personnel" (aides, technicians, or assistants), clinicians in training, family members, or community volunteers.

Support Personnel

Many SLPs and audiologists find the use of professional aides, technicians, and assistants to be essential for ensuring clients' access to care (Kimbarow, 1997;

Paul-Brown & Goldberg, 2001). Support personnel may help in the handling of large caseloads, such that more clients are treated and/or more treatment time per client is offered than would otherwise be possible. Support personnel may also allow fully credentialed clinicians more time to treat individuals with severe and complex communication disorders, thus improving overall quality of care. An additional advantage is that the level of care needed by an individual may be more closely matched with the level of training and experience of an aide or assistant.

Services once thought to be within the sole domain of the speech-language pathologist or audiologist, but that do not require the skills and expertise of professionals with all the training and experience required for clinical certification, may now be offered by persons whose services are far less costly. Support personnel vary widely in their level of academic and on-the-job training. Speech-language pathology aides, for example, generally have training in specific areas of practice and have more limited responsibilities than assistants. Within the United States, states vary in the use of terms used to refer to the various levels of training and/or licensure required of support personnel. State laws also vary in terms of the tasks in which support personnel are permitted to engage. Some states do not permit the use of support personnel. Of the 47 states that regulate audiology, 18 have licensure laws that regulate support personnel in audiology. Of the 44 states that regulate speech-language pathology, 29 have licensure laws that regulate support personnel in speech-language pathology (ASHA, 2005b).

Examples of tasks that speech-language pathology assistants may perform under the supervision of an SLP, according to ASHA's *Guidelines for the Training, Use, and Supervision of Speech-Language Pathology Assistants* (ASHA, 2005c), include conducting speech-language screenings and participating in treatment plans or protocols that have been established by a certified speech-language pathologist. Examples of tasks that audiology technicians may perform under the supervision of an audiologist include conducting

hearing screenings, application of electrodes for electronystagmography testing, and calibration checks for audiological equipment. Support personnel may perform clerical duties; document test results and patient/client progress; prepare diagnostic and treatment materials; schedule diagnostic and treatment activities; and participate in research projects, in-service training, and public relations programs. Examples of tasks that support personnel are generally not permitted to perform include diagnostic testing or interpretation of test results, hearing aid fitting, patient/client or family counseling, development or modification of a patient/client's individualized treatment plan, and discharging a patient/client from services.

Despite the advantages mentioned, the use of support personnel remains controversial in the field of communication and swallowing disorders. Clinicians opposing support personnel maintain that the quality of care rendered to patients is diminished and that the job security of licensed professionals is threatened. There is also concern that cost-minded health care and educational administrators will abuse the use of support personnel by compelling them to provide services outside their scope of practice and by implementing cost-saving hiring practices wherein ideal supervisor-to-support staff ratios are exceeded (Henri & Hallowell, 1999b). An additional disadvantage is that many HICs still do not recognize support personnel as qualified service providers and therefore do not pay for treatment delivered by these persons. See Chapter 10 for more discussion of this topic.

Graduate Students

The provision of supervised evaluation and treatment services by graduate students in speech-language pathology and audiology has long been a source for extending care to clients/patients. In many university clinics, ample free and low-cost services are made available to surrounding communities while providing diverse clinical learning opportunities to student clinicians. Additionally, networks of student volunteers may be helpful in extending services beyond clinical and diagnostic treatment sessions. Examples are students serving as communication partners (Lyon, 1992), inhome respite caregivers (Hallowell, 2000), or as volunteers in a wide array of clinical educational contexts.

Trained Volunteers

Trained volunteers can be effective care extenders. As no compensation is involved, and as these individuals are clearly identified to clients/patients as volunteers, there are fewer legal and licensure-related problems than in the use of multiskilled professionals. Volunteers provide additional opportunities to practice and maintain developing communication skills (Kagan, Black, Duchan, Simmons-Mackie, & Square, 2001; Lyon, 1992). Before their direct involvement with patients or clients, volunteers may be required to observe treatment sessions and then may be guided by the clinician in the provision of treatment-reinforcing activities such as repetitive drills. Volunteers may also be trained to handle other tasks, such as clerical work, scheduling, and equipment maintenance, allowing skilled clinicians more time to spend with clients/patients.

Family Members and Other Caregivers

Given the current health care service delivery climate, family members are now often required to assume greater responsibilities in caring for their significant others (Teng et al., 2003). As with trained volunteers, coaching and training by the skilled clinician is essential. Treatment-complementing activities provided by a properly guided caregiver can be highly effective (Des Rosier, Cantanzaro, & Piller, 1992; Evans, Bishop, & Haselkorn, 1991; Landi et al., 2004). With increased family member involvement, it will become necessary to identify the unique variables that minimize or prevent successful caregiver follow-through at home or elsewhere (Jorgensen et al., 1999; Thomas et al., 2002).

Multiskilling of Professionals

Multiskilling is the cross training of professionals to enable them to perform functions that have been exclusively within the scope of practice of a profession other than his or her own (ASHA, 1996). Multiskilling is one more means by which patients' access to care may be enhanced, because it ideally enables more professionals to provide needed services. Multiskilling also has cost-saving implications in that it is less expensive to hire one individual to perform a series of tasks that traditionally have required multiple professionals.

Consider a home health patient recovering from a stroke. The patient may have a speech-language pathologist visit three times per week to work on compensatory swallowing strategies for dysphagia, an occupational therapist visit five times per week to work on activities of daily living, a physical therapist visit five times per week to work on mobility and strength, and a nurse visit once per week to obtain a blood sample and record vital signs. Under a multiskilling model, a home health agency may have each of those specialized professionals conduct initial diagnostic evaluations and develop care plans based on contact with the patient. Then, rather than each professional repeatedly visiting the patient, one multiskilled professional would carry out the multiple plans of care specified by the group of specialists.

The cost-saving implications for multiskilling are evident. Likewise, it is clear that multiskilling may increase patient/client access to services through the sheer number of professionals trained to offer a service. Still, if not implemented carefully, with respect to the training needed to perform skilled services, multiskilling poses a serious threat to the integrity of the specialized health care professions. Also, job security of some certified clinical professionals may be threatened. In some contexts, the responsibilities and required skills of multiskilled professionals are unclear (ASHA, 1996; Pietranton & Lynch, 1995). The regulations for the training, experience, licensure, and certification required for each specialty may be breached in many contexts where multiskilled personnel perform in areas beyond their scope of practice.

ASHA's position statement on multiskilling (ASHA, 1997) indicates that it is acceptable for multiskilled providers to perform basic activities that do not require professional-level skills, such as taking blood pressures or assisting with bed-to-wheelchair transfers. It is unacceptable to provide cross-training of clinical skills.

TECHNOLOGICAL ACCESS

Advances in technology improve and augment the clinical services of speech-language pathologists and audiologists. For many individuals, these advances improve access to services, particularly those with limited physical accessibility to evaluations or therapy. Technology also may aid clinicians in accessing current information that will improve their clinical skills. See Chapter 25 for continued discussion of technology as a professional issue.

Telehealth

Telehealth is the use of electronic information and communications technologies to provide and support health care services when there is a distance between participants (Craig & Patterson, 2005; Field, 1996). The term *telehealth* is sometimes used interchangeably with *telemedicine,* although many authors and practitioners in health professions prefer the connotation of the former term, as it is more inclusive of professions outside of primary medical practice. Audio, visual, and text media are generally combined in telehealth applications. From its inception, one of the most promising aspects of telehealth has been the improvement of access to care in remote areas where skilled service providers are scarce or absent (Berman & Fenaughty, 2005). In addition to the lack of geographic access to service providers, other barriers to care might be alleviated by telehealth. As aptly summarized by Field (1996), these barriers include:

- Distance from primary, secondary and tertiary medical services;

- Poor transportation (e.g., lack of automobile, limited or nonexistent bus service), even for relatively short distances;

- Inadequate financial resources, particularly insurance coverage or directly subsidized services;

- Family, educational, and cultural factors (e.g., illiteracy, distrust of technology);

- Delivery system characteristics, including poor coordination of care, long waiting times for appointments, inadequate numbers or kinds of specialists, and bureaucratic obstacles to services; and

- Gaps in our knowledge about how these factors interact to affect the use of services and what can be done to overcome or eliminate barriers to access. (p. 174)

In addition to expanding access for disadvantaged populations and patients in rural areas, opportunities are emerging for expansion of home health services through technology (Baer, Williams, Vickers, & Kvedar, 2005; Martinez, Villarroel, Seoane, & Pozo, 2004; Ogasawara et al., 2003; Woo, Hui, & Chan, 2004). As home health care is one of the most rapidly expanding forms of service delivery, it is essential that professionals in our disciplines stay abreast of telehealth mechanisms that may allow replacing some home visits with video visits, checking up on carryover of treatment activities, and furthering patient and family education (cf. Warner, 1997). An additional advantage of providing care through distance technology is that it may expand clinicians' availability to persons who live in areas that are considered unsafe, such as some urban neighborhoods and even within active international war zones (Doolittle, Otto, & Clemens, 1998; Khazei, Jarvis-Sellinger, Ho, & Lee, 2005).

In conjunction with the expansion of digital technology, enabling image capturing, compression, transmission and interpretation, interest in telehealth is expanding rapidly across a vast array of health care professions. High-speed, high-bandwidth telecommunication systems are expanding globally (Long, 1998). In addition to improved access, advantages reported by evaluators of some rural telemedicine programs include reduction of duplicative diagnostic services, improved consumer confidence in local medical personnel and facilities, reduced need for referral to service providers outside the local area, improved recruitment and retention of health care personnel, and improved continuing education for service providers (Brown, 2005; Hickman & Dyer, 1998). Clinical applications in telehealth are found in virtually every health specialty (Myers, Luecke, Longan, & Revell, 1998; Ridenour & Komoroski, 1998; Thrall & Boland, 1998; Wakefield, Holman, Ray, Morse, & Kienzle, 2004). Much of what we know about possibilities for remote service delivery for diagnosis and treatment in communication and swallowing disorders is derived from research and applications from other disciplines (cf. Burtt, 1997). For example, research in long-distance interpretation of radiographic imaging (e.g., Pauly, 1993) may have important implications for diagnostic interpretation of videofluoroscopic studies of swallowing. On a regulatory level, cases in which state regulations have been developed to control the delivery of services from medical practitioners between states (Scott, 2004) may also be applied to SLPs and audiologists.

Few published empirical studies directly address the effectiveness of telehealth delivery in audiology and speech-language pathology. Studies involving comparisons of face-to-face and telehealth assessments support the feasibility, reliability, and acceptability of telehealth evaluations of acquired speech and language disorders (Duffy, Werven, & Aronson, 1997; Glykas & Chytas, 2004; Mashima et al., 2003; Sicotte, Lehoux, Fortier-Blanc, & Leblanc, 2003; Wertz et al., 1992; Wilson & Onslow, 2004).

New developments in technological access to care will be shaped by ongoing developments in health policy as it affects telehealth (Gaffney, 1997; Milio, 1996). The factors that will be most influential in continuing efforts to expand service delivery options for professionals in our disciplines include:

- Licensure issues, especially for services provided between states

- Training in use of telehealth technology

- Establishment of standards

- Reimbursement issues

- Patient confidentiality issues

- Attitudes of providers and patients

- Means of ensuring quality of clinician-patient relationships

- Potential cost savings

- Demonstration of clinical outcomes

- Telecommunications infrastructure and cost (Hibbert et al., 2004; Hill & Theodoros, 2002; Long, 1998; Ostbye & Hurlen, 1997; Thrall & Boland, 1998; Yoo et al., 2004).

Information Technology

Given that access to care involves more than direct contact with a skilled clinician, the notion of technological access also includes the use of telecommunications and information technology to improve access to information that may allow consumers and potential consumers to learn about communication problems, diagnostic and treatment options, and prevention strategies (Kuster, 1997). For those who remain without computers and connection to the Internet and/or telephones, access to information resources is tenuous. Funding for technology through regional clinics and public facilities, such as libraries, is highly variable across the country, and is often subject to changes in tax or grant allocations and annual budgets. Deficits in language and literacy skills may impose further obstacles to care for disadvantaged populations. Gaps in access may actually widen if information services are improved only for those with the means, education, and skills to pursue those services (Field, 1996).

EDUCATING THE PUBLIC

Most individuals take communication for granted and are frequently unaware of the link between one's communication abilities and one's success in life. To improve access to speech-language pathology, audiology, and swallowing services, it is increasingly more critical to improve the general public's and consumers' awareness and knowledge about speech-language pathology and audiology services.

We are reminded of the scene in the movie of a few years ago, *Regarding Henry*, starring Harrison Ford, in which his character suffers a brain injury resulting in aphasia. In this movie, Mr. Ford's speech and language treatment is provided by the physical therapist! Clearly, at least in Hollywood, we have a long way to go to educate our communities concerning the roles and responsibilities of SLPs and audiologists.

ADJUSTMENTS IN SERVICE-PROVIDING ENVIRONMENTS

Certain environmental and operational adjustments must be made to improve client access to speech-language pathology and audiology services. Flextime and compressed workweeks are rapidly becoming the norm. Recognizing the value of schedules that are more convenient for their customers, organizations are expanding their daily work hours and, as a result, improving their revenues. Speech-language pathology and audiology providers must follow suit. In environments where traditional appointment schedule models create significant client/patient hardships, creative, nontraditional scheduling approaches have been found helpful. Some settings, for example, are currently experimenting with "fluid" appointment schedules wherein a child's treatment appointment can occur anytime between 9 a.m. and 12 p.m. or 1 p.m. and 4 p.m. As clients arrive during these time periods, they are integrated into the ongoing 3-hour session to receive their treatment, whether it be 30, 45, or 60 minutes. They leave when their time period ends. These models have, additionally, been found to improve attendance.

Another tactic being used to improve access and attendance is the development of interagency collaborations in which several agencies contribute to fund a minibus or to bring clients to their locations. Other environmental adjustments must be explored to ensure maximum access to our services. To improve geographic access, satellite offices (leased, shared, or donated space) should be considered. Finally, while expensive, home visits have been useful as one avenue for improving access for persons with limited resources and mobility challenges.

SUMMARY

In this chapter, we identified significant barriers that influence access to audiology and speech-language pathology services and stressed the broad and serious consequences of current service delivery trends on our field. We also emphasized the growing need for our services along the age continuum. Access to audiology and speech-language pathology services can be significantly enhanced through comprehensive, focused strategies that remove or minimize barriers and maximize the use and impact of health care and educational resources, both financial and human. With this in mind, we described effective strategies to improve revenues, decrease costs, and increase clinical outcomes. To subsidize diminishing reimbursements, strategies to create alternative funding sources were presented. More than ever, it is today the responsibility of all audiologists and speech-language pathologists to ensure that barriers are eliminated and resources are maximized. To accomplish these goals, our roles in educating the public and in advocacy were described in detail.

CRITICAL THINKING

1. What are the key factors that have led to a growing need for services in speech-language pathology? What are the key factors that have led to decreased access to those services?

2. Imagine that you are the CEO of a not-for-profit center for the treatment of communication disorders. What are the key steps that you would take to maximize your center's (a) clinical revenues and (b) nonclinical revenues?

3. When justifying your services to a managed
    care organization, how you would defend the
    treatment for each of the conditions listed
    below as "medically necessary"?

    - adult dysphagia
    - adult aphasia
    - child language delay
    - child articulation disorder
    - child hearing impairment
    - adult hearing impairment
    - child central auditory processing disorder

    In addition to your own descriptions of med-
    ical necessity, what other information and
    references might you include in your docu-
    mentation to third party payers regarding the
    medical necessity of your services?

4. In what specific actions for advocacy might
    you engage in your current educational or
    work context to enhance access to service in
    speech-language pathology and audiology for
    persons who need them? Write an action
    plan for achieving one or two of those
    actions within the next month, either alone
    or with students or professional colleagues.
    Include specific dates for each activity in
    which you would need to engage to achieve
    that action.

5. What is the role of local, state, and national
    professional organizations in improving access
    to audiology or speech-language pathology
    services?

6. Suppose you have a client who needs a
    hearing aid but has no health insurance or
    financial means to purchase the device. Do
    you have a responsibility to help the client
    find financial aid? What sources might help in
    this situation?

REFERENCES

American Academy of Pediatrics. (2005). Policy statement: Model contractual language for medical
necessity for children. *Pediatrics, 116* (1), 261–262.

American Speech-Language-Hearing Association.
(1996). Technical report of the ad hoc committee
on multiskilling. *Asha, 38* (Suppl. 16), 1–9.

American Speech-Language-Hearing Association.
(1997). Position statement: Multiskilled personnel.
Asha, 39 (Suppl. 17), 13.

American Speech-Language-Hearing Association.
(2002). *Appealing health plan denials.* Prepared by the
Health Care Economics & Advocacy Team.
Rockville, MD: Author.

American Speech-Language-Hearing Association.
(2005a). Congressional relations. Available at
http://www.asha.org/

American Speech-Language-Hearing Association.
(2005b). Frequently asked questions about speech-
language pathology assistants. Available at
http://www.asha.org/

American Speech-Language-Hearing Association.
(2005c). *Guidelines for the training, use, and supervision
of speech-language pathology assistants.* Available at
http://www.asha.org/

American Speech-Language-Hearing Association.
(2005d). Medical necessity for speech-language
pathology and audiology services. Available at
http://www.asha.org/

American Speech-Language-Hearing Association.
(2005e). Preferred practice patterns for the profession of audiology. Available at http://
www.asha.org/

American Speech-Language-Hearing Association.
(2005f). Preferred practice patterns for the profession of speech-language pathology. Available at
http://www.asha.org/

American Speech-Language-Hearing Association
(2006). Medicare caps back & fees cut, pending
Congressional action. Available at http://
www.asha.org/

Baer, C. A., Williams, C. M., Vickers, L., & Kvedar, J. C.
(2005). A pilot study of specialized nursing care for
home health patients. *Journal of Telemedicine and Telecare, 10,* 342–345.

Barlow, T. (1997). *Managed care for children with disabilities and the interface of legislative policies. (#PB9711).* Honolulu, HI: Pacific Resources for Education and Learning.

Berman, S. (1997). A pediatric perspective on medical necessity. *Archives of Pediatric Adolescent Medicine, 151,* 858.

Berman, M., & Fenaughty, A. (2005). Technology and managed care: Patient benefits of telemedicine in a rural health care network. *Health Economics, 14,* 559–573.

Breakey, L. K. (1994). *Negotiating managed care contracts. Managing managed care: A practical guide for audiologists and speech-language pathologists,* Ad Hoc Committee on Managed Care. Rockville, MD: American Speech-Language-Hearing Association.

Brown, E. (1999) Medically necessary? *Physician Executive, 25* (2), 74–77.

Brown, N. A. (2005). Information on telemedicine. *Journal of Telemedicine and Telecare, 11,* 117–126.

Burtt, K. (1997). Nurses use telehealth to address rural health care needs, prevent hospitalizations. *American Nurse, 29,* 21.

Carlson, R. (1995). Managed care creates conflicts of interest. *Indiana Medicine,* 248–254.

Chapey, R., & Hallowell, B. (2001). Introduction to language intervention strategies in adult aphasia. In R. Chapey (Ed.), *Language intervention strategies in adult aphasia* (4th ed., pp. 3–17). Baltimore, MD: Williams & Wilkins.

Craig, J., & Patterson, V. (2005). Introduction to the practice of telemedicine. *Journal of Telemedicine and Telecare, 11,* 3–9.

Danbe, L. (2002). Too many delayed or denied claims? A system for denial management may be in order. *Getting paid in behavioral healthcare, Journal* V. 7, pp. 5–6.

Des Rosier, M., Cantanzaro, M., & Piller, J. (1992). Living with chronic illness: Social support and the well spouse perspective. *Rehabilitation Nursing, 17,* 87–91.

Dollaghan, C. A. (2004). Evidence-based practice in communication disorders: What do we know, and when do we know it? *Journal of Communication Disorders, 37,* 391–400.

Doolittle, G. C., Otto, F., & Clemens, C. (1998). Hospice care using home-based telemedicine systems. *Journal of Telemedicine and Telecare, 4,* 58–59.

Duffy, J. R., Werven, G. W., & Aronson, A. E. (1997). Telemedicine and the diagnosis of speech and language disorders. *Mayo Clinic Proceedings, 72,* 1116–1122.

Ellrodt, A. G., Cho, M., & Cush, J. J. (1997). An evidence-based medicine approach to the diagnosis and management of musculoskeletal complaints. *The American Journal of Medicine, 103,* 3S–6S.

Engelhard, C. J., & Childress, J. F. (1995). Caveat emptor: The cost of managed care. *Trends in Health Care, Law & Ethics, 10,* 11–14.

Evans, R., Bishop, D., & Haselkorn, J. (1991). Factors predicting satisfactory home care after stroke. *Archives of Physical and Medical Rehabilitation, 72,* 144–147.

Field, M. J. (Ed.). (1996). *Telemedicine: A guide to assessing telecommunications in health care.* Washington, DC: National Academy Press.

Frymark, T. B., & Mullen, C. (2005). Influence of the prospective payment system on speech-language pathology services. *American Journal of Physical Medicine & Rehabilitation, 84*(1), 12–21.

Gaffney, T. (1997). State legislatures increasingly addressing telehealth/telemedicine, *American Nurse, 29,* 7.

Gage, S. (1995, June 12). Workforce crisis won't disappear without effort. *Crain's Cleveland Business, 16,* 11.

Glykas, M., & Chytas, P. (2004). Technology assisted speech and language therapy. *International Journal of Medical Informatics, 73,* 529–541.

Golper, L., & Brown, J. (Eds.). (2004). Business matters: A guide for speech-language pathologists. Rockville, MD: American Speech-Language-Hearing Association.

Greenfield, J. M. (1994). *Fund raising fundamentals: A guide to annual giving for professionals and volunteers.* New York: John Wiley & Sons.

Hallowell, B. (2000). A student-run respite network for caregivers of persons with dementing illness. *Communication Connection, 14*(1), 10.

Hallowell, B., & Henri, B. P. (1996). Preparing students for the realities of health care changes: Incorporating concepts of managed care and health care financing into clinical training programs. *HEARSAY: Journal of the Ohio Speech and Hearing Association, 11,* 40–42.

Henri, B. P., & Hallowell, B. (1996). Action planning for advocacy: Issues for speech-language pathologists and audiologists in the face of the expansion of managed care. *HEARSAY: Journal of the Ohio Speech and Hearing Association, 11,* 61–64.

Henri, B. P., & Hallowell, B. (1999a). Funding alternatives to offset the reimbursement impacts of managed care. Newsletter of Special Interest Division 2, Neurophysiology and Neurogenic Speech and Language Disorders. Rockville, MD: American Speech-Language-Hearing Association.

Henri, B. P., & Hallowell, B. (1999b). Relating managed care to managing care. In B. S. Cornett (Ed.), *Clinical practice management in speech-language pathology: Principles and practicalities.* Gaithersburg, MD: Aspen Publishers.

Henri, B. P., Hallowell, B., & Johnson, C. (1997). Advocacy and marketing to support clinical services. In R. Kreb (Ed.), *A practical guide to treatment outcomes and cost effectiveness* (pp. 39–48). Rockville, MD: American Speech-Language-Hearing Association Task Force on Treatment Outcomes and Cost Effectiveness.

Hetherington, L. T. (1998). High tech meets high touch: Telemedicine's contribution to patient wellness. *Nursing Administration Quarterly, 22,* 75–86.

Hibbert, D., Mair, F. S., May, C. R., Boland, A., O'Connor, J., Capewell, S., & Angus, R. M. (2004). Health professionals' responses to the introduction of a home telehealth service. *Journal of Telemedicine and Telecare, 10,* 226–230.

Hickman, C. S., & Dyer, W. M. (1998). Improving telemedicine consultation with TeleDoc and the emergent technologies. In M. L. Armstrong (Ed.), *Telecommunications for health professionals* (pp. 204–214). New York: Springer Publishing.

Hill, A., & Theodoros, D. (2002). Research into telehealth applications in speech-language pathology. *Journal of Telemedicine and Telecare, 8,* 187–196.

Hiller, M. D., & Lewis, J. B. (1995). Managed health care benefit plans: What are the ethical issues? *Trends in Health Care, Law & Ethics, 10,* 109–112, 118.

Hock, M. F., & Deshler, D. D. (2003) "No Child" leaves behind teen reading proficiency. *The Education Digest,* 27–35.

Ireys, H. T., Wehr, E., & Cooke, R. E. (2000). Defining medical necessity. *The Exceptional Parent, 30*(3), 37–39.

Jesuit, D., & Smeeding, T. (2002). *Poverty and Income Distribution.* Syracuse, NY: Maxwell School of Citizenship and Public Affairs, Syracuse University.

Johnson, A. (1997, March). *Managed care 101.* Seminar presented at the Ohio Speech-Language Hearing Association Annual Convention, Columbus, OH.

Jorgensen, H. S., Reith, J., Nakayama, H., Kammersgaard, L. P., Raaschou, H. O., & Olsen, T. S. (1999). What determines good recovery in patients with the most severe strokes? The Copenhagen stroke study. *Stroke, 30,* 2008–2012.

Justice, L. M., Chow, S. M., Michel, C., Flanigan, K., & Colton, S. (2003). Emergent literacy intervention for vulnerable preschoolers: Relative effects of two approaches. *American Journal of Speech-Language Pathology, 12,* 320–332.

Kagan, A., Black, S. E., Duchan, J. F., Simmons-Mackie, N., & Square, P. (2001). Training volunteers as conversation partners using "supported conversation for adults with aphasia" (SCA): A controlled trial. *Journal of Speech, Language, and Hearing Research, 44,* 624–638.

Kahan, J. P., Bernstein, S. J., Leape, L. L., Hilborne, L. H., Park, R. E., Parker, L., Kamberg, C. J., & Brook, R. H. (1994). Measuring the necessity of medical procedures. *Medical Care, 32,* 357–365.

Khazei, A., Jarvis-Selinger, S., Ho, K., & Lee, A. (2005). An assessment of the telehealth needs and healthcare priorities of Tanna Island: a remote, underserved and vulnerable population. *Journal of Telemedicine and Telecare, 11,* 35–40.

Kimbarow, M. L. (1997, Fall). Ahead of the curve: Improving service with speech-language pathology assistants. *Asha, 39,* 41–44.

Kuster, J. M. (1997, Fall). Telehealth and the Internet. *Asha, 39,* 55.

Lai, J. C. K., Woo, J., Hui, E., & Chan, W. M. (2004). Telerehabilitation—a new model for community-based stroke rehabilitation. *Journal of Telemedicine and Telecare, 10*(4), pp. 199–205.

Landi, F., Onder, G., Cesari, M., Barillaro, C., Lattanzio, F., Carbonin, P. U., & Bernabei, R. (2004). Comorbidity and social factors predicted hospitalization in frail elderly patients. *Journal of Clinical Epidemiology, 57,* 832–836.

Lerner, J. C., Gesek, J., Adams, S. (2003). Will using evidence-based approaches to a standards development process improve Medicaid policy making? Report on a promising effort. *Journal of Ambulatory Care Management, 26*(4), 322–333.

Long, J. D. (1998). TeleHealth and direct health care delivery: An introduction. In M. L. Armstrong (Ed.), *Telecommunications for health professionals* (pp. 187–203). New York: Springer Publishing.

Lyon, J. G. (1992). Communication use and participation for adults with aphasia in natural settings: The scope of the problem. *American Journal of Speech-Language Pathology, 1,* 7–14.

Marge, M. (1993). Disability prevention: Are we ready for the challenge? *Asha, 35,* 42–44.

Marrison, B. (1999, January 9). Fourth graders flunking state reading test at an alarming rate. *Cleveland Plain Dealer,* A1, A11.

Martinez, A., Villarroel, V., Seoane, J. & Del Pozo, F. (2004). A study of a rural telemedicine system in the Amazon region of Peru. *Journal of Telemedicine and Telecare, 10,* 219–225.

Mashima, P. A., Birkmire-Peters, D. P., Syms, M. J., Holtel, M. R., Burgess, L. P. A., & Peters, L. J. (2003). Telehealth: Voice therapy using telecommunications technology. *American Journal of Speech-Language Pathology, 12,* 432–439.

Milio, N. (1996). U.S. policy support for telehealth: Organizational response to a new policy environment. *Journal of Telemedicine and Telecare, 2*(2), 87–92.

Mitchell, J. M., & Gaskin, D. J. (2004). Do children receiving Supplemental Security Income who are enrolled in Medicaid fare better under a fee-for-service or comprehensive capitation model? *Pediatrics, 114* (1), 196–204.

Myers, M. K. S., Luecke, J., Longan, D., & Revell, T. (1998). Practical aspects of telemedicine from the user's perspective: Neonatology, general medicine, and inmate health care. In M. L. Armstrong (Ed.), *Telecommunications for health professionals* (pp. 215–229). New York: Springer Publishing.

Newacheck, P. W., Stoddard, J. J., Hughes, D. C., & Pearl, M. (1998, February). Health insurance and access to primary care for children. *New England Journal of Medicine, 338,* 513–519.

Ogasawara, K., Ito, K., Jiang, G., Endoh, A., Sakurai, T., Sato, H., Okuhara, Y., Adachi, T., & Hori, K. (2003). Preliminary clinical evaluation of a video transmission system for home visits. *Journal of Telemedicine and Telecare, 9,* 292–295.

Ostbye, T., & Hurlen, P. (1997). The electronic house call: Consequences of telemedicine consultations for physicians, patients, and society. *Archives of Family Medicine, 6,* 266–271.

Paul-Brown, D., & Goldberg, L. R. (2001). Current policies and new directions for speech-language pathology assistants. *Language, Speech, and Hearing Services in the Schools, 32*(1), 4–17.

Pauly, A. (1993). Telemedicine permits long-distance diagnosis. *Diagnostic Imaging, 15,* 57–59.

Perkins, J., & Olson, K. (1998). The threat of evidence-based definitions of medical necessity. *Health advocate.* Los Angeles: National Health Law Program.

Pietranton, A. A., & Lynch, C. (1995). Multiskilling: A renaissance or a dark age? *Asha, 36,* 37–40.

Ridenour, N., & Komoroski, K. S. (1998). Multidisciplinary collaboration in telehealth and telenursing. In M. L. Armstrong (Ed.), *Telecommunications for health professionals* (pp. 230–241). New York: Springer Publishing.

Rodwin, M. A. (1995). Conflicts in managed care. *The New England Journal of Medicine, 332,* 604–607.

Ronder, R. W., Kastner, T., Parker, S. J., & Walsh, K. (1999). Serving people with developmental disabilities in Medicaid managed care. *Managed Care Quarterly, 7* (2), 23–30.

Rosso, H. A., & Associates. (1991). *Achieving excellence in fund raising: A comprehensive guide to principles, strategies, and methods.* San Francisco: Jossey-Bass.

Scott, R. (2004). Investigating e-health policy—tools for the trade. *Journal of Telemedicine and Telecare, 10,* 246–248.

Sicotte, C., Lehoux, P., Fortier-Blanc, J., & Leblanc, Y. (2003). Feasibility and outcome evaluation of a telemedicine application in speech-language pathology. *Journal of Telemedicine and Telecare, 9,* 253–258.

Smith, G., & Ashbaugh, J. (1995). *Managed care and people with developmental disabilities: A guidebook.* Alexandria, VA: National Association of State Directors of Developmental Disabilities Services, Inc.

Teng, J., Mayo, N. E., Latimer, E., Hanley, J., Wood-Dauphinee, S., Cote, R., & Scott, S. (2003). Costs and caregiver consequences of early supported discharge for stroke patients. *Stroke, 34,* 528–536.

Thomas, P., Chantoin-Merlet, S., Hazif-Thomas, C., Belmin, J., Montagne, B., Clement, J., Lebruchec, M., & Billon, R. (2002). Complaints of informal caregivers providing home care for dementia patients: The Pixel study. *International Journal of Geriatric Psychiatry, 17,* 1034–1047.

Thrall, H. H., & Boland, G. (1998). Telemedicine in practice. *Seminars in Nuclear Medicine, 28*(2), 145–157.

Toffler, A. (1980). *The third wave.* New York: Bantam Books.

Uffen, E. (1998). Where the jobs are: Keeping an eye on the future. *Asha, 40,* 25–28.

U.S. Department of Labor, Bureau of Labor Statistics. (2004). *Occupational Outlook Handbook,* 14–18.

Vekovius, G. T. (1995). Managed care 101: Introducing managed care into the curriculum. *ASHA, 37,* 44–47.

Voinovich, G. V. (1996, February). *1996 state of the state address.* Address presented to the Ohio General Assembly, Columbus, OH.

Wakefield, B. J., Holman, J. E., Ray, A., Morse, J., & Kienzle, M. G. (2004). Nurse and patient communication via low- and high-bandwidth home telecare systems. *Journal of Telemedicine and Telecare, 10,* 156–159.

Warner, I. (1997). Telemedicine applications for home health care. *Journal of Telemedicine and Telecare, 3*(1), 65–66.

Weinick, R. M., Weigers, M. E., & Cohen, J. W. (1998). Children's health insurance, access to care, and health status: New findings. *Health Affairs 17,* 127–136.

Wertz, R. T., Dronkers, N. F., Bernstein- Ellis, E., Sterling, L. K., Shubitkowski, Y., & Elman, R. (1992). Potential of telephonic and television technology for appraising and diagnosing neurogenic communication disorders in remote settings. *Aphasiology, 6,* 195–202.

White, P. H. (2002). Access to health care: Health insurance considerations for young adults with special health care needs/disabilities. *Pediatrics, 110* (6), 1328–1335.

Wilson, L., & Onslow, M. (2004). Telehealth adaptation of the Lidcombe program of early stuttering intervention: five case studies. *American Journal of Speech-Language Pathology, 13,* 81–93.

Yoo, S. K., Kim, D. K., Jung, S. M., Kim, E., Lim, J. S., & Kim, J. H. (2004). Performance of a web-based, realtime, tele-ultrasound consultation system over high-speed commercial telecommunication lines. *Journal of Telemedicine and Telecare, 10,* 175–179.

RESOURCES

See the reference list for specific guidelines from ASHA pertaining to clinical practice issues discussed in this chapter. ASHA's Web site at http://www.asha.org includes numerous resources for those wishing to learn more about access, funding, and legislative and advocacy issues. The "Professionals" section in particular contains vast amounts of information regarding the access issues discussed in this chapter. For hands-on help with letter writing to legislators, contact the governmental affairs section of ASHA's Web site or call ASHA's Action Center at 800-498-2071.

Internet links for learning about and contacting consumer groups related to a wide variety of communication and swallowing disorders may be easily accessed through Dr. Judith Kuster's Web site "Net Connections for Communication Disorders and Sciences" at http://www.communicationdisorders.com. Also available through this site are additional resources related to technology.

Providing Quality Care

19

Policies and Procedures

PAUL RAO, PHD

SCOPE OF CHAPTER

Fourteen years ago I interviewed 28 graduate students on the topic of policies and procedures (Rao, 1992). Each student was unfamiliar with the existence or location of the university clinic's P&P manual. There was also a general lack of familiarity with the need for a P&P manual, what might be covered in a P&P, and what difference a P&P makes in a clinic's operation. To follow up on that survey, I (Rao, 2005) conducted another informal survey in a local graduate school class of prospective audiologists and speech-language pathologists (N=30). The "good news" is that more than 90 percent of the respondents were able to explain why P&Ps were necessary and where in the clinic they could find the manual. In a follow-up interview with the instructor in the Professional Practices class and with several of the graduate students, it was increasingly clear that there was significantly greater awareness of the legal mandates and institutional accountability that affected their current training and future practice. Students had come a long way in their understanding of this important professional practice.

This chapter familiarizes you with what commonly constitutes a P&P manual and answers the following questions: What is a policy and procedure? What should be included in a P&P manual? When, why, how, and by whom are P&Ps written? After reading this chapter, you will have a clearer idea of what is entailed in "managing by the book" in a variety of speech-language pathology and audiology employment settings. According to Rizzo and Trudeau (1994), in establishing an Audiology and Speech-Language Pathology Department, the development of clear policies and procedures can serve a vital function by defining expectations and standards of performance. As my expertise is in the area of hospital-based speech-language pathology, many illustrations will be derived from that area of clinical practice. However, much of the rationale, principles, and operational procedures discussed here may be applied to audiology as well, and to universities, schools, private practices, and other settings.

DEFINING TERMINOLOGY

Before we can discuss the topic of P&Ps, we need to lay the groundwork for delving into this multifaceted topic. Each of us comes to the topic with a seemingly high degree of familiarity. All of us are required to follow P&Ps in our workplace. As parents, we likely have undocumented P&Ps in the home to maintain order. Clearly one must differentiate between a policy, a procedure, a plan, and a guideline.

What Is a Policy?

According to CARF, The Rehabilitation Accreditation Commission (2005), a policy is a "written course of action or guidelines adopted by leadership" (p. 222). Organizations seeking CARF accreditation may consult the CARF Glossary when determining their conformance with standards that require a policy. The key word in the CARF definition is *leadership* and its inferred responsibility and overall accountability. According to the Society of Human Resources Management (SHRM) (1998), a policy is a "broad statement that reflects an organization's philosophy, objectives, or standards concerning a particular set of management or employee activities" (p. 7). For example, a policy may describe what an employee is entitled to in terms of vacation days and how many days may be retained in one's leave bank from year to year. The policy statement provides a basis for management practices, and a framework within these practices is established.

The human resources function of an organization should review organizational policies periodically and revise those that are obsolete so that they

no longer influence decision making. A policy is thus an organization's "guide" to be followed under a given set of circumstances. A good policy will not force a manager into narrow or rigid decision making. Rather, it will provide guidance for handling a wide range of organizational issues and will establish a framework for both management and staff decision making. For example, a P&P on documentation in a medical setting may state, "It is the policy of the Speech-Language Pathology Department to document a comprehensive evaluation in the medical record within 48 hours of the first patient contact." This statement is an explicit and measurable guide to policy, and all clinical staff members should be cognizant of what the policy is. An example of a policy from a university setting might be a statement of the quality point average that must be maintained to continue graduate study.

The Bureau of Business Practice (BBP) (1988) describes good policies as "broad, current, comprehensive, inviolate, written to specify responsibility for action, and used frequently" (p. 11). These attributes are essential ingredients of P&Ps if they are to be user-friendly and convey the mission, philosophy, and goals of a given program, department, or organization. Kaluzny, Warner, Warren, and Zelman (1982) stress that P&Ps are an organization's written rules and regulations that describe the values of the organization, defining specific directions, goals, and expectations. Rao (1991) notes that a P&P manual can also be used as a management tool and a training aid for employees to avoid misunderstanding and errors. If you were to "Google" the words *policies* and *procedures,* you would obtain more than 28 pages of references on the Web in a variety of industries that provide timely illustrations of P&Ps.

What Is a Procedure?

According to CARF (2005), a procedure is a "how to description of actions to be taken . . . need not be written unless specified by CARF" (p. 223). Here again, the organization may wish to determine if a given procedure needs to be formally documented based on CARF's specification in the relevant standards. According to SHRM (1998), a procedure "is a detailed, step-by-step description of the customary methods of handling activities" (p. 8). Using an example mentioned previously, a procedure for vacation pay may establish necessary actions for a planned absence. The employee must request the absence at least one week in advance of the vacation, and no more than a specific number of employees can be off at the same time. A procedure may outline the manner in which a particular policy is to be implemented, but it cannot take the place of that policy. According to Rizzo and Trudeau (1994), procedures should be written to reflect the most efficient method for carrying out a task. They should reflect current regulations and standards of relevant accreditation programs. Recall that a good policy is inviolate. Policies change slowly and infrequently. Procedures, on the other hand, change often, as dictated by any number of factors, such as funding, staffing, equipment, space, accreditation standards, and technology. The steps necessary for a graduate student to be advanced to candidacy, for example, constitute an academic procedure.

What Are Institutional, Departmental, and Programmatic P&Ps?

All organizations should have an *institutional* P&P manual that applies to all employees. Such a manual includes a host of P&Ps that need not necessarily be restated in a departmental manual (e.g., the institution's policy on sexual harassment or dress code). Many institutions are organized by *departments* (e.g., Dietary or Medicine in a health care setting; Early Childhood Education or Speech-Language Pathology and Audiology in a university setting). Each department is required to have its own P&P manual, including those P&Ps specific to the department. For example, in a hospital setting, only Audiology and Otorhinolaryngology may have a P&P on cerumen removal, whereas *all* patient care policies have a P&P on documentation and infection control. Other agencies and institutions may be organized along *programmatic* or product lines. In a rehabilitation facility, for instance, product lines such as a stroke program or a brain-injury program commonly exist. The persons served with a given diagnosis (e.g., stroke) are admitted to a special geographic area in the facility (e.g., stroke unit). A number of professional disciplines, including nursing, physical therapy, occupational therapy, and speech-language pathology, form an interdisciplinary team to treat persons with stroke. The services the stroke team provides constitute the stroke *program.* CARF (2005) requires the various rehabilitation programs within an institution to have P&Ps, such as admission criteria (how a person served enters a given program), continued stay criteria (how long a person served remains in the program), discharge criteria (when and how a patient leaves the program), and exit criteria (when a person served is no longer followed by the program). Thus, each program must also have a P&P manual to guide the interdisciplinary team in delivering the desired programmatic care.

What Is a P&P Manual?

For ease of access and use, all P&Ps for a given institution, department, or program should be kept together in a central manual either in hard copy or on an electronic database or disc. Frequently, this manual takes the form of a large three-ring binder, from which outdated P&Ps can be removed readily and into which new or revised ones can be inserted easily. In this millennium, a manual copy is likely to be necessary for persons in an organization without easy computer access or who may not be computer literate. Increasingly, organizations are supporting "dummy computer terminals" throughout a given environment where all employees can access company policies as well as any other need to know employee resource (e.g., the employee handbook).

In addition to the P&Ps themselves, several manual components facilitate consistent, efficient, and effective use. The first of these, according to the BBP *Personnel Policy Manual* (BBP, 1988), is a complete and detailed table of contents that lists major areas of policy and, under each major heading, the specific P&Ps in that area. In conjunction with a table of contents, the BBP suggests the use of a simple numbering system, whereby each major heading is assigned a corresponding section number (e.g., Clinical Policies = Section #200), and each subordinate P&P within that section has an individual subsection number (e.g., Client Referral and Assignment = #200.01). This system enhances an employee's or manager's ability to identify and locate the necessary P&P at a glance. As a CARF surveyor, the author has had an opportunity to examine and review literally hundreds of P&Ps, and most use a numbering format as just described. However, many institutions also organize their P&Ps alphabetically under macro categories. Other P&P manual components recommended by the BBP (1988) include a written explanation of the relationship between the P&P manual and other manuals, handbooks, and printed material in existence within the organization; a statement of the purpose of the P&P manual; and a statement of the organization's practice with regard to ensuring compliance with its policies and procedures. For example, at my place of employment, I chair the institutional P&P Committee and report that *plans* have been separated from P&Ps. Thus, the Plan Manual includes the organization's required plans such as performance improvement, information management, safety, and infection control. Organizations may also publish rules and guidelines that are separate from the P&Ps but have managerial approval. The SHRM (1998) states that rules "reflect management decisions that actions be taken—or avoided—in a given situation" (p. 6). For instance, most companies want to ensure that alcoholic beverages are not consumed during work hours. Management may therefore establish a rule that alcoholic beverages cannot be brought onto or consumed on company property.

NECESSITY AND VALUE OF POLICIES AND PROCEDURES

As a manager, you need show up in court only once to defend a personnel action to fully appreciate and then embrace the potent and prerequisite nature of P&Ps in any organization. The P&P Manual can be a manager's "best friend."

Accrediting and Regulatory Requirements

A P&P manual is required by accrediting, certifying, licensing, and regulatory bodies such as the Joint Commission on the Accreditation of Healthcare Organizations (JCAHO), CARF, state licensing boards, state education agencies, and the American Speech-Language-Hearing Association's Council on Academic Accreditation in Audiology and Speech-Language Pathology. These organizations establish and promote minimal standards that must be met by an institution seeking accreditation. Many of these standards must be translated into P&Ps for dissemination and implementation throughout the institution or practice setting. For example, JCAHO (2005) requires that all institutional policies be reviewed and approved at least every 3 years except the Human Resources P&P, which must be updated annually. Without a P&P manual, it is likely that the responsible program would be cited by CAA, JCAHO, CARF, or other accrediting or licensing agencies for noncompliance with a standard.

For example, when reviewing the CARF 2005 standards, the reader is cognizant of what is required for each standard. In Section #1, Criterion B, Accessibility #2 of CARF's 2005 Standards Manual dealing with Business Practices in Medical Rehabilitation notes that the organization "must have an accessibility *plan* that addresses barriers in the following areas:
a) Architectural;
b) Environmental;
c) Attitudinal;
d) Financial;
e) Employment;
f) Communication;
g) Transportation; and
h) Any other barrier identified by the:
   1) person served;
   2) personnel;
   3) other stakeholders" (p.13).
However, in Section #1, Criterion D, Rights of Persons Served, #3, the standard states that "the organization implements policies promoting the following rights of the person served:
a) Confidentiality of information;
b) Privacy;
c) Freedom from the following:
   1) abuse;
   2) financial or other exploitation;
   3) retaliation;
   4) humiliation; and or
   5) neglect" (p. 21).

Finally in the same Section and Criterion #4, CARF requires the organization to "implement a policy and written procedure by which the person served may make a formal complaint, file a grievance, or appeal a decision made by the organization's personnel or team members" (p. 22). Although the presence of a P&P manual is no guarantee of quality, without it an organization cannot become accredited (Rao, 1991).

According to Golper and Brown (2004), "while accrediting standards address a broad range of areas (e.g., provision of care, ethics, leadership, human resources, information management, environment of care), individual clinicians will be most affected by the organization's policies and procedures, the requirements for 'qualified providers,' and the need to maintain competencies to practice with the population with which they are working (e.g., age range and disorder types)" (p. 64). Golper and Brown (2004) present a sample of a department-specific policy and procedure on staffing.

Legal Considerations

We live in a litigious society in which nearly every decision can be called into legal question. In addition, government oversight of Medicare and Medicaid waste that began in 1993 with new money and power granted by Congress has empowered the Office of Inspector General in the United States Department of Health and Human Services (2005) to require every health care provider to establish a corporate compliance plan to prevent, detect, and correct any violations of federal and state fraud and abuse laws. In audiology and speech-language pathology, there is no shortage of potential litigants: clients, payers, and professionals. The P&P manual is a prerequisite for documenting compliance with existing laws. According to Applegate (1991),

> You want your policy manual to be as clear as possible because it often plays a key role in court if any employee sues you for wrongful termination or any other labor dispute. Many courts around the country have ruled that a policy handbook often serves as a contract between employees and employer. (p. C8)

The legal and regulatory climate alone has changed so rapidly during the past decade that a host of new policy areas have emerged. The Family and Medical Leave Act, which is intended to provide employees equal opportunity to take time off from work to care for a child or parent, has resulted in a number of new legal requirements for employers and service providers. The law thus mandates a number of changes in the Human Resource function of the P&P manuals of many organizations.

HIPAA is the most significant recent federal law that compels organizations to have in place a host of new, explicit policies and procedures. The Health Insurance Portability and Accountability Act (2003) encompasses three major rules and regulations (1) privacy, (2) transactions, and (3) security. HIPAA was designed specifically to ensure that health care providers make every effort to ensure that protected health information (PHI), or a patient's medical records, are kept private. The final rule applies to all information, whether electronic, written, or oral. Today when you enter a heath care institution, you will receive a privacy notice, and you may observe new procedures that reflect a culture of confidentiality. Providers are now required to train all staff in the specifics of the HIPAA Rules and Regulations. Provisions of the HIPAA statute generally carry significant penalties. Civil penalties range up to $100 per person, per violation, up to $25,000 per year. Criminal penalties apply as well— up to $50,000 in fines and a year in prison for knowingly disclosing PHI; up to $100,000 in fines and 5 years in prison if the disclosure is under false pretenses; and finally up to $250,000 in fines and 10 years in prison if the disclosure is for commercial advantage. Thus it is imperative that providers have in place the P&Ps to address all three components of HIPAA and have evidence of training all staff on relevant policies and procedures.

Identification and Definition of Relevant Rules and Regulations

The P&P manual is a comprehensive compendium of all relevant rules and regulations with which an organization must comply. Accreditation standards aside, a manager cannot operate effectively without written P&Ps. Although control of all management decisions may not be possible, a framework for managerial and clinical decision making is necessary. The P&P manual should not be designed to establish a rigid set of rules but should enable managers to (1) appreciate how far the impact of their decisions might reach, (2) encourage logical and consistent thinking, and (3) provide an opportunity for all employees to operate in a cohesive manner (Rao, 1991). Many P&Ps are management protocols designed for the smooth and efficient operation of a department. The P&P manual should be the last word on what is required of an employee. It is designed to equip both employer and employee with a means to ensure compliance with all relevant rules and regulations.

WHAT TO INCLUDE IN A POLICY AND PROCEDURE MANUAL

A variety of administrative, clinical, and professional policies and operational procedures for audiology and speech-language pathology must be considered when gathering, expanding, or revising a policy and procedure manual. Standards set forth by accrediting bodies, as well as legal requirements at the federal, state, and local levels, also serve as guidelines for many of the items to be incorporated as standard components of a P&P manual. Beyond these standards, requirements, and general areas of consideration, the content of a P&P manual is determined by the individual needs of a given program or department and by those of the institution in which it operates.

Accrediting Body Requirements

Anyone in healthcare realizes that there is increasing attention being paid to safety and quality and a host of federal compliance initiatives. When one "opens shop," usually the very first order of business is to document all the policies required by accreditation bodies. If you wish to admit patients and be paid,

usually the ticket that must first be punched to enter the health care arena is meeting the various stringent accreditation requirements. Schools and universities must first ensure that they have the correct policies and procedures in place prior to any admissions.

ASHA Council on Academic Accreditation (CAA) in Audiology and Speech-Language Pathology The core standards considered essential by ASHA CAA (ASHA, 2005) for the provision of quality services and instruction in the university setting are:

- Standard 1.0 Administrative Structure and Governance
- Standard 2.0 Faculty/Instructional Staff
- Standard 3.0 Curriculum
- Standard 4.0 Students
- Standard 5.0 Program Resources

Specifically, ASHA CAA standards include the need for a written mission statement that describes the department's purpose and scope of practice and that remains up-to-date in relation to changing needs by means of periodic and systematic review. ASHA's CAA requires that the administration of an audiology and speech-language pathology university department be based on established P&Ps that are consistent with the department's stated mission and goals. ASHA maintains that any policies related to clinical decision making in the field must be established in consultation with persons holding a current ASHA Certificate of Clinical Competence (CCC) in the respective profession.

Sample Mission Statement This following mission statement, as well as corresponding measurable and attainable goals and objectives, is located in the first section of our department's P&P manual and may drive a number of core policies such as admission and discharge criteria. The National Rehabilitation Hospital's (NRH) Speech-Language Pathology Service mission statement (National Rehabilitation Hospital, 1998) is:

The mission of the Speech-Language Pathology (SLP) Service of National Rehabilitation

Hospital's Medical Rehabilitation Network is to apply state-of-the-art theory and knowledge in the realm of communication sciences and disorders to the quality of care of persons with communication/swallowing disorders in order for them to achieve maximum independence and optimum functioning within the community. The SLP Service is committed to the assessment and treatment of individuals exhibiting communication/swallowing disorders; to educating and counseling patients and their families regarding the nature, cause, treatment, and prevention of conditions which may result in a communication &/or swallowing disturbance; to educating the NRH network and community at large regarding current concepts in the application of communication sciences to the communicatively impaired population; to expanding the knowledge base of the communication sciences through clinical research; and to serving as an advocate for persons with communication impairments. A continuous performance improvement and outcomes management program is the foundation of the SLP Service's efforts to render the highest quality of care in an effective and efficient manner. All activities of the SLP Service will be in accordance with the Scope of Practice and Code of Ethics of the American Speech-Language-Hearing Association and with legal and professional standards established for certification, licensure, accreditation, and protection of patient and staff rights. (p. 1)

Joint Commission on Accreditation of Healthcare Organizations (JCAHO) JCAHO (2005) requires that certain P&Ps be established for specific functions such as patient rights and organizational ethics, assessment and care of patients, special procedures, performance improvement, leadership, environment of care, human resources, infection control, medical affairs, and nursing leadership within health care organizations seeking JCAHO accreditation. These include P&Ps regarding documentation in the medical record, fire and safety, infection control, equipment inspection and preventative maintenance, and special procedures (e.g., the P&P for responding to a medical emergency) Other JCAHO requirements of particular import to the SLP manager/supervisor include a policy on the following: orientation of new employees; age-based competencies; evidence of a performance improvement plan with appropriate indicators addressing important aspects of care; a comprehensive staffing model and plan that assures one level of care; the presence of an organizational chart and explanation of the relationship of the SLP department to other hospital departments; and a statement of the scope of services/plan of care provided.

CARF: The Rehabilitation Accreditation Commission CARF has developed its own set of standards for rehabilitation organizations that wish to obtain CARF accreditation. Evidence that these standards are met must be present at the organizational level and also at the individual program level (e.g., brain-injury program), if the organization seeks specialty program accreditation. To the extent that audiology and speech-language pathology departmental policies and procedures may complement or reinforce organizational or specialty program P&Ps in meeting the standards of this and other accrediting bodies, you should consider them for inclusion in a departmental P&P manual. CARF standards (2005) in their "requested survey resource documents" that may have relevance for the audiology and speech-language pathology departmental P&P manual include, but are not limited to:

- Documentation of the program's or department's role in the continuum of care
- Measurable criteria for the initiation and termination of specific treatments
- Policies and procedures that promote safety and security
- Procedures for filing grievances and appealing decisions
- Policies for advance directives and resuscitation orders

- Admission, continued stay, discharge, and exit criteria per department and program

- Policies that address confidentiality of records, release of records, records retention, records storage, and protection of records from fire and water damage

- Policies for electronic records that address protection of records, privacy of records, and security of records

- Policies concerning ethical conduct

- Policies and procedures related to taking and reporting disciplinary actions against practitioners

- Procedures for handling vehicle accidents and road emergencies

- Administrative policies and procedures

- P&Ps that identify the functions and the responsibilities of rehabilitation physicians providing treatment

Federal, State, and Local Requirements In addition to the components of a P&P manual required by accrediting bodies, laws and regulations at the federal, state, and local levels may also dictate organizational and departmental P&Ps. The presence of and compliance with these P&Ps are not always regularly monitored through formal site visits or surveys. However, when compliance with the law is called into question in the form of litigation or other civil action, your ability to demonstrate the presence of and adherence to federal, state, and local regulations is of paramount importance. With the advent of corporate compliance to combat fraud and abuse, it is imperative that your staff is familiar with and compliant with your organization's plan, policies, and procedures that ensure compliance with all federal, state, and local laws.

Federal Requirements In the last decade, a relevant example of a federal law that has been enacted and that has significant impact on P&P requirements is HIPAA (2003), previously described in detail. In the early 1990s another landmark federal law

that has had dramatic impact on the American scene is the Americans with Disabilities Act (ADA) (PL 101-336) (1990). This law prohibits discrimination on the basis of disability in employment, public services and transportation, privately operated public accommodations and services, and telecommunication services. P&Ps regarding recruitment, employment, promotion, and termination of employees; job descriptions, performance standards, and performance appraisals for staff; access to job training and continuing education opportunities; access to services provided; physical accommodations; and telecommunications, to name a few, must reflect compliance with the law by removing barriers to persons with disabilities through the provision of reasonable accommodations.

State and Local Requirements Local requirements obviously vary among jurisdictions but frequently have significant impact on P&Ps involving such areas as fire safety, infection control, and/or the parameters of employees' entitlement to family/medical leave. State licensure requirements for audiology and speech-language pathology have been adopted in 47 states, although specific exemptions to these requirements sometimes exist. For example, school speech-language pathologists in Maryland are exempt from state licensure requirements but are bound by the state's Department of Education standards. Many states are also enacting laws to deal with speech-language pathology assistants. All such state and local requirements must be incorporated into the P&P manual.

Other Necessary Policies and Procedures

Beyond the P&Ps dictated by accrediting bodies and federal, state, and local licensing agencies, P&Ps should be documented for a variety of administrative and mission-driven rationales.

Administrative Issues Administrative issues for which you may want to develop and maintain P&Ps include staff vacation, sick, and administrative leave; dress code for the workplace; access to secretarial support; staff productivity levels; staff meetings; and

T A B L E 19–1 Sample Performance Standards for Staff Speech-Language Pathologists

A. Quality of Work

1. Accurately evaluates communication abilities of assigned patients and plans and organizes treatment to achieve functional outcomes.

   Outstanding: Consistently and independently reaches projected functional outcomes as a result of providing superior evaluation and treatment.

   Commendable: Consistently and independently reaches functional outcomes as a result of providing appropriate evaluation and treatment.

   Competent: Consistently reaches projected functional outcomes with supervisory input.

2. Accurately documents diagnostic and treatment services in a timely fashion in accordance with SLP and Program policies and guidelines.

   Outstanding: Consistently and independently.

   Commendable: Consistently with occasional supervisory input.

   Competent: Consistently with more than occasional supervisory input.

SOURCE: From "National Rehabilitation Hospital Performance Standards for Staff Speech-Language Pathologists, by P. Rao and T. Goldsmith, 1998 *National Rehabilitation Hospital Speech-Language Pathology Service Policies and Procedures Manual*, p.220.04-0. Copyright 1998 by the National Rehabilitation Hospital. Reprinted by permission.

management reports. One essential element is the establishment and annual review of *job descriptions* that delineate the duties and responsibilities; requisite language and mathematical skills; reasoning ability; physical demands; lines of authority; work environment; any equipment, aids, tools, materials, or vehicles used; certificates, licenses, and registrations; and required education and experience. Likewise, you should consider establishing the department's P&P regarding development and utilization of *performance standards* to be used to objectively measure performance within the critical components established for each job title. Sample performance standards for a staff speech-language pathologist are illustrated in Table 19–1 and for audiologists in Table 19–2.

Clinical Issues As stipulated by JCAHO, CARF, and ASHA CAA, another essential P&P should provide for a program of continuous evaluation and improvement of the quality of clinical care rendered to consumers. This particular P&P defines the parameters within which a performance improvement (PI) program can be developed to support the PI plan outlined by the leadership of the organization. Other clinical issues for which you may consider developing a P&P include

patient referral and assignment; general and/or specific evaluation and treatment protocols; treatment planning, implementation, and discontinuation; department-specific medical record documentation standards (for a concise review of this topic, refer to Paul-Brown, 1994); education and counseling of those who are served and their families; and maintenance of standards of ethical practice. Perhaps more than any other area of practice, additional P&Ps related to clinical issues may be largely determined by the individual needs of a particular clinical setting. For example, with prospective payment in place in all post-acute settings since 2002, a P&P addressing the Minimum Data Set (Briggs Corporation, 1995), the outcome system designed for long-term care, or a P&P regarding completion of the Inpatient Rehab Facility- Patient Assessment Instrument (IRF-PAI) would appear to be an obvious priority.

Professional Issues Beyond strictly administrative or clinical issues, examples of other areas for which you may develop written P&Ps include continuing professional education, student training, research activity, and professional presentations and publications. When issues arise requiring an administrative decision about these activities, or when questions of

T A B L E 19–2 Sample Performance Standards for Staff Audiologists

A. **Quality of Work**

1. Accurately provides assessment and (re)habilitation of auditory and/or vestibular function of assigned patients to enhance communication and functional competence.

  Outstanding: Consistently and independently evaluates and enhances abilities as a result of providing superior evaluation and treatment.

  Commendable: Consistently and independently evaluates and enhances abilities as a result of providing appropriate evaluation and treatment.

  Competent: Consistently evaluates and enhances abilities with supervisory input.

2. Accurately documents diagnostic and treatment services in a timely fashion in accordance with Audiology and Departmental policies and procedures.

  Outstanding: Consistently and independently.

  Commendable: Consistently with occasional supervisory input.

  Competent: Consistently with more than occasional supervisory input.

3. Appropriately incorporates age, cognitive level, and communication skills into evaluation, treatment, and patient education.

  Outstanding: Consistently and independently.

  Commendable: Consistently with occasional supervisory input.

  Competent: Consistently with more than occasional supervisory input.

SOURCE: From "Washington Hospital Center Competency Standards for staff audiologists" by T. Wilson-Bridges and C. Surowicz, 2005 Washington Hospital Center Hearing & Speech Center Clinical Procedures & Protocols Manual, 200.30.

appropriateness, equity, or protocol are raised, it is extremely helpful to have ready and consistent access to clearly articulated P&Ps with regard to these areas of professional practice.

HOW TO WRITE POLICIES AND PROCEDURES

Now for the mechanics of drafting and approving P&Ps. It takes nearly a village to get consensus on many of your draft policies. However, many P&Ps are so transparently obvious and required that authors frequently "borrow" standard P&Ps. For example, many CARF surveyors whose organizations are eventually surveyed have a penchant for finding "best practices" in a given facility and asking for permission to copy same back at their facility. The dictum seems to be for the more obvious P&Ps, "do not recreate the wheel."

Components and Format

Specific P&P components and format will vary from organization to organization, but within an organization or department, each P&P should reflect consistent documentation and presentation of policies, practices, and procedures. A sample format, as well as component definitions, utilized at National Rehabilitation Hospital (NRH) in Washington, DC, follows:

Title/Section/Department/Effective Date;

  Section 1.0 Purpose: A positive statement of the intention or aim of the policy conveyed to the reader in as few words as possible.

  Section 2.0 Policy: A brief descriptive statement articulating the policy.

  Section 3.0 Procedure: A sequence of prescribed steps for implementing the policy.

Section 4.0 Responsibilities: An explanation of the policy and expectations of personnel implementing it.

Section 5.0 Applicability: A statement of those personnel to whom the policy and procedure apply.

Section 6.0 Signature Approval: Evidence of approval by the designated authority.

Section 6.0 References: Other existing documents or policies and procedures which are cited in, or related to, the policy and procedure. (NRH, 1998, #213.3)

The original effective date and latest revision date should be documented and clearly visible on each P&P within a department or organization. At NRH, revised P&Ps are disseminated to staff with an attached memo via e-mail. This e-mail draws the reader's attention to the specific revisions made to the P&P. A computerized format is becoming increasingly necessary with efforts of organizations to become paperless. The computerized format was adapted from the Windows version of Policies Now (Knowledge Point, 1996), which permits the author to write customized personnel policies in minutes. The Society of Human Resources Management (2005) has established a policy handbook from a variety of sources on its Web page, wherein the person who accesses the Web page can click to view and download any one of the following P&P related materials:

- A complete handbook
- At-will employment policies
- EEO/Affirmative Action
- Exempt/nonexempt
- Overtime
- Drug/alcohol policies
- Sexual harassment
- Electronic communication
- Voluntary/involuntary separation

A number of proprietary companies are also in the P&P business (see Resources). Medical Consultants Network, Inc. (1999) customizes P&Ps for client organizations and provides them in a three-ring binder and an electronic version. The available 43 manuals cover all of the key JCAHO functions and other health care policy needs. Its marketing mantra is "Why reinvent the wheel?" A similar venue can be found in Hospital and Physician Publishing, Inc. (1999), which provides updated manuals on a quarterly basis to subscribers. This publisher offers more than 250 P&P manuals in both paper and electronic form and highlights its currency with JCAHO standards and breadth of topics. A manager starting from scratch in a new facility might be well served to investigate these off-the-shelf, state-of-the-art options.

NRH has attempted to reduce its reliance on a paper manual and to take advantage of computer technology. Besides the hard copy of the "heavy" P&P manual, which is centralized in administration, NRH had also automated its P&Ps in 1998 on Lotus Notes and disseminated them on a local area network (LAN). Consistent with the goal of performance improvement, the NRH P&P Committee elected to simplify the process and eliminate redundancy. As NRH has expanded to more than 40 sites over a 20-year institutional history, the organization needed to arrive at a network policy on policies and procedures that provided the required P&Ps for each site, program, and department. However, the former organization policies that were applicable under one roof, such as the fire and safety policy, were no longer applicable at the outpatient sites that had no inpatients and were under the rules and regulations of local jurisdictions and the fire code of the particular building in which the site was housed.

NRH P&Ps are organized under the following categories: Patient Care, Care Coordination, Pharmacy, Dietary, Medical Affairs, Admissions, Infection Control, Quality Improvement, Administration Communications and Development, Human Resources/Employee Health, Accounting/Budget and Reimbursement, Patient Financial Services, Materials Management, Medical Records, and Safety Policies. The header for the automated NRH P&Ps is shown in the following box.

The search is made easy via a keyword approach. For example, if you are interested in the policy on restraints, the computer will call up all policies that deal with restraints. If you are interested only in site-specific policies, the computer will organize only those P&Ps dealing with outpatient sites. There are specific security protocols for "read only" versus "contributing editor" versus "author only." Anyone who has access to the NRH LAN can connect to the P&P pages then read, and if desired, print.

Title	Title of P&P	Number	P&P#
Policy Statement	Statement	Policy Type	Type e.g., department
Forms/Attachments		Scope staff	Scope e.g., all
Initial Effective Date	e.g., 11/01/04	Revision Date	e.g., 11/01/05

Style P&Ps should be written in clear, concise language that can be easily and quickly understood by all employees to whom the P&Ps apply. Technical or professional jargon and ambiguous statements should be avoided to minimize the possibility of misinterpretation. The BBP (1988) recommends use of active voice when possible and suggests that exclusive passive voice use makes P&Ps sound "dull and pompous." The BBP also suggests that short, but not choppy, sentences enhance P&P readability.

WHO SHOULD WRITE POLICIES AND PROCEDURES

Normally, there is not a long line of employees wishing to be responsible for P&Ps in a given department and organization. The want ad would suggest that the prospective individual is computer literate with excellent organizational and detail-oriented skills. In addition, the "czar" or "czarina" of your P&Ps must be skilled in grammar, patience, and persistence.

Primary Responsibility

In most cases, the department director has primary responsibility for drafting and revising departmental P&Ps. This task may be delegated to subordinate staff in some instances, but the responsibility for final review remains with the director. Other director-level responsibilities include assuring appropriate dissemination of and ready access to all applicable P&Ps as well as assuring compliance with and enforcement of both department-specific and organizational P&Ps.

Solicitation of Input

In many organizations, employees are encouraged to recommend new P&Ps and to suggest revisions to existing P&Ps. A recent example in the author's experience involved staff suggestions regarding the employee dress code. In 1999, NRH embarked on a cultural transformation entitled "New Value" (Rao, 2002) that was modeled after the Disney corporation. Disney has an extremely strict dress code and a "zero tolerance" policy for noncompliance with the dress code policy. When NRH implemented its revised dress code (2002) with an accompanying "style book," NRH Team Members felt dictated to and controlled with little to no input on the policy and apparently nil degrees of freedom with complying with the strict dress code policy. The SLP Service opted to be creative in its advocacy for a less stringent dress code policy. During one of the senior management staff meetings, the SLP Service provided an impromptu breakfast of home-made pastries with each serving topped with a toothpick and a flag like "'jean" fabric. The obvious message was that employees would really appreciate senior management's approval of a trial "jean therapy day." After little discussion, an exemption to the strict dress code was approved with an allowance of a monthly "dress down/jean therapy" day that could be thematic and fun (e.g., Halloween/Freaky Friday Dress Down Day). A regular practice of soliciting staff input on a P&P manual's usefulness and on suggestions for additions or changes to the manual is one grassroots mechanism of assuring that your manual is the current, accurate, relevant, and authoritative resource it is intended to be. NRH hosts an annual town hall for staff to provide input on current and proposed policies, practices, and guidelines.

Administrative Review and Approval

Although generally developed and/or approved at the department director level, department-specific P&Ps also frequently require review and approval by a member of an organization's senior management staff before dissemination and implementation. For P&Ps that involve or have an impact on departments other than the one initiating the policy, review and approval by other affected department directors are also needed. Interdisciplinary clinical procedures, such as modified barium swallow studies, provide such opportunities for interdepartmental collaboration. The originating department director is responsible for obtaining all necessary authorizations and signatures in accordance with the organization's policy.

WHEN SHOULD POLICIES AND PROCEDURES BE WRITTEN?

The need for P&Ps may be prompted by a number of factors. Updates in the standards manuals of JCAHO, CARF, and ASHA CAA may include new or additional requirements that prompt P&Ps. P&Ps may also be dictated by federal, state, or local regulations.

New Policies and Procedures

For all of the previously cited reasons, new policies may be required of an organization as well. In 1991, the Department of Labor required health care organizations to offer the hepatitis B vaccine to all employees. This federal regulation eventually was added to the NRH policy on "Employee Health." Installation of new technology and equip-

ment also may require a P&P to clearly specify indications for application, responsibilities, and procedures.

For example, NRH recently had a ventilation system installed in a "TB room," and staff training and policies and procedures were required before patients could reside in the high technology room. Development of an entirely new program or service within the department may be further grounds for development of a new P&P. If your department, which formerly treated only adolescents and adults, embarks on the management of children, for instance, the department would clearly require new P&Ps regarding a number of critical areas that are unique to children (e.g., age-based competencies, revised and adapted testing and treatment protocols, and manner of obtaining informed consent). In 2002, NRH was licensed to operate 12 pediatric rehabilitation beds. A number of new policies had to be developed and approved before pediatric patients could be admitted to the newly built unit. Obviously issues such as "medical emergency" in a 6-year-old differ from those of an adult in terms of equipment, protocol, and practice. Finally, evolving societal standards may prompt a P&P. One example in this area is a preemployment drug screening, which has become an increasingly common employment prerequisite because of the prevalence of drug use in society. If a drug screening practice is adopted, a corresponding P&P must be in place.

Policy and Procedure Review and Revision

Most organizations establish a schedule of P&P review, which is at least as frequent as the minimum P&P review schedules mandated by accrediting and licensing bodies. JCAHO, for example, requires P&P review every 3 years. CARF requires an annual review of all job descriptions in the organization. Such review schedules are designed to assure that necessary and appropriate revisions to P&Ps are reflected in an organization's current manual. Factors that might prompt the revision of a given policy are the same factors one would consider when drafting a new policy. For example, the NRH SLP Service recently revised its policy on documentation of progress notes. Originally, SLPs were responsible for writing inpatient progress notes every 2 weeks. However, because of a national trend toward shortened lengths of stay (LOS) for rehabilitation patients, along with a change in local standards (managed care companies were requiring more frequent notes), the SLP Service revised the policy from documenting progress every 2 weeks to documenting a daily "log" note and a weekly progress note. The SLP Service has modified a number of other policies for a variety of reasons. Table 19–3 details that process, stating the nature of the policy, the nature of the change, and the primary reasons for revision of sample P&Ps.

P&P revision may also result from the performance improvement data of the institution, program, or department. These PI data may have identified a problem in the structure or process of a given P&P. For example, a PI team reviewing the NRH system for scheduling patients for therapy determined that canceled therapy time was excessive and that the scheduling system was

not "Y2K compliant." Once barriers to patient flow were identified and removed, improved patient care was obtained with a new and compliant scheduling system. When the revised scheduling structure and process were fine-tuned and clinical and scheduling staff were trained, the revised P&P was documented and disseminated hospital-wide.

ACCESS TO POLICIES AND PROCEDURES

It should be clear from this chapter that the P&P manual is intended to be a dynamic management tool—consulted often, revised periodically, and available to all staff. Familiarity with the P&P manuals of an institution, program, and department can be accomplished by following several steps:

■ **Orientation.** All new employees should be provided an opportunity to read the P&P manual and to ask questions about its contents during the

T A B L E 19–3 Original Policy, Revised Policy, and Reason for Revisions in NRH SLP'S 1998 P&P Manual

Original Policy	Policy Revision	Reason for Revision
Biweekly inpatient progress summaries	Weekly inpatient progress summaries and daily logs	Shortened length of stay (LOS)
Discharge Summary within 48 hours of discharge	Discharge Summary within 24 hours of discharge	Referring institutions request more timely data. Physicians request data for medical discharge summaries. Case Managers request more timely reports to enhance continuity of care.
Written Evaluation Report within 5 working days of initial contact	Written Evaluation Report within 2 working days of initial contact	Shortened LOS & External Case Managers' request
Uniform staff working hours from 8:00 a.m. to 4:30 p.m.	Establishment of flexible schedule options	Staff retention & expand tour of duty to reach patients' families
Modified Barium Swallow studies conducted off-site	Modified Barium Swallow studies conducted on-site	New equipment at NRH precluded the need to go off-site

SOURCE: From *The National Rehabilitation Hospital Speech-Language Pathology Service Policies and Procedures Manual* by P. Rao and T. Goldsmith, 1998, pp. 220.01–220.40. Copyright 1998 by the National Rehabilitation Hospital. Reprinted by permission.

probationary period of employment (typically the first 3 or 4 months of employment). Written verification by the employee that he or she has read the P&Ps and agrees to abide by them is standard practice in many organizations. In addition to this initial orientation to existing P&Ps, new or revised P&Ps must be circulated through all current staff, and written verification of an awareness and understanding of the new and/or revised P&P should be obtained.

■ **Location.** The hard copy of the P&P manual must be located where all staff within a given program, site, or department have free and easy access. It is suggested that a sign-out sheet for the P&P manual be maintained in a central location so that the manual can be readily located if it is in use. Clearly, access to the P&Ps on the LAN is dependent on available computers and the individual's authorization to read versus edit the P&P.

■ **Promulgation.** In addition to orienting new employees to the entire P&P manual, and current employees to new and revised P&Ps, the department, program, or site manager is strongly encouraged to regularly highlight or note important policy issues in staff meetings. If the manager has observed confusion about a given P&P, an informational review and discussion is a necessary first step in promulgating the policy. Another method of updating employees on P&Ps is to write a "Did You Know?" column as a regular feature in your institution's newsletter. Such a column can highlight certain P&Ps and clarify any common problems of misinterpretations. Managing *by* the book is easier if staff know what is *in* the book. Finally, if the institution holds regular all-staff meetings, this is a perfect forum for stressing a compliance issue with a given P&P.

SUMMARY

A policy and procedure manual is perhaps the single most important tool a manager can have, to the extent that it:

1. Clearly articulates the department's and the organization's mission, philosophy, and goals
2. Documents compliance with all applicable laws, rules, regulations, and standards
3. Provides a sound framework for logical and consistent decision making

This chapter defined the terms, policy, and procedure; argued for the necessity and value of P&Ps; and offered suggestions regarding what to include in a hard copy and computerized version of a P&P manual. Because a P&P manual is *useful* only to the degree that it is *used,* recommendations were also made for the regular review and revision of P&P manuals, as well as the promulgation of P&Ps to all applicable staff.

CRITICAL THINKING

1. Why establish a P&P manual rather than simply maintain a notebook of memoranda and guidelines?

2. You have been hired to establish a new audiology and speech-language pathology clinic. What P&Ps would you develop first and why?

3. What commercial resources are available to help you construct policies that conform with national accrediting groups?

4. In your current academic and/or clinical setting, is there a new P&P that needs to be established and a current one that needs to be revised? Why does it need revision? Practice formulating a new one.

5. Recall one instance in your practice when a disagreement or debate ensued over a particular institutional practice. Was the P&P instrumental in resolving this conflict? How could the conflict be avoided?

6. Why and how should staff be involved in creating new policies and procedures? What are the advantages to seeking staff input?

7. What four media forms could you use to disseminate information

regarding new or revised P&Ps in your organization?

8. Why is it important for a private practitioner to have a policy and procedures manual if there is only one clinician?

REFERENCES

Americans with Disabilities Act, (1990) Public Law (101-336), Federal Register. Available at http://www.hhs.gov/ocr/ada/finalreg.html

American Speech-Language-Hearing Association. (2005), *Standards manual for CAA Accreditation*. Rockville, MD: Author.

Applegate, J. (1991, September 23). Succeeding in small business. *Baltimore Evening Sun*, p. C-8.

Briggs Corporation. (1995). *Minimum data set*. Version 2.0. Des Moines, IA: Author.

Bureau of Business Practice. (1988). *Personnel policy manual*. Englewood Cliffs, NJ: Prentice Hall.

Commission on Accreditation of Rehabilitation Facilities (CARF). (2005). *Standards manual for CARF accreditation*. Tucson, AZ: Author.

Department of Labor, Occupational Safety and Health Administration. (1991). Occupational exposure to blood-borne pathogens: Final rule. *Federal Register, 56,* 235.

Golper, L. A., & Brown, J. E. (2004) *Business matters: A guide for speech-language pathologists*. Rockville, MD: American Speech-Language-Hearing Association.

Health Insurance Portability and Accountability Act (August 2003) Complete Privacy, Security, and Enforcement (Procedural) Regulation Text (45 CFR Parts 160 and 164), December 28, 2000 as amended May 31, 2002, August 14, 2002, February 2003, and April 17, 2003. Available at http://www.hhs.gov/ocr/hipaa/finalreg.html

Hospital and Physician Publishing, Inc. (1999). *Policy and procedures manual*. Marion, IL: Author.

Inpatient Rehabilitation Facility Prospective Payment System (August 15, 2005) Final Rule (42 CFR Part 42). Available at http://www.hhs.cms.gov/irfpai/finalreg.html

Joint Commission on Accreditation of Health Care Organizations. (2005). *Comprehensive accreditation manual for hospitals*. Oakbrook Terrace, IL: Author.

Kaluzny, A. D., Warner, D. M., Warren, D.G., & Zelman, W. N. (1982). *Management of health services*. Englewood Cliffs, NJ: Prentice Hall.

Knowledge Point. (1996). *Policies now!* Petaluma, CA: Author.

Medical Consultants Network, Inc. (1999). *Policy and procedure manual*. Englewood, CO: Author.

National Rehabilitation Hospital. (1998, August). *Speech-language pathology policy and procedure manual*. Washington, DC: Author.

National Rehabilitation Hospital. (1998, September). Policy and procedure on policy and procedures, #700.00. Washington, DC: Author.

National Rehabilitation Hospital. (2005, November). Hand hygiene. *The National Rehabilitation Hospital policy and procedures manual*. Washington D.C: Author.

Office of the Inspector General, Department of Health and Human Services. (2005). *Work plan: Fiscal year 2005*. Washington, DC: U.S. Government Printing Office.

Paul-Brown, D. (1994). Clinical record keeping in audiology and speech-language pathology. *Asha, 36,* 40–43.

Rao, P. (1991). The policy and procedure manual: Managing by the book. In C. Frattali (Ed.), *Quality improvement digest*. Rockville, MD: American Speech-Language-Hearing Association.

Rao, P. (1992, November). *Interview with graduate students on policies and procedures*. Baltimore, MD: Loyola College.

Rao, P. (2002, May). Cultural shift happens: A new value framework. Course presented to the Maryland & D.C. Health Information Management Association.

Rao, P. (2005, September). *Interview with graduate students on policies and procedures*. Baltimore, MD: Towson University.

Rizzo, S. R., & Trudeau, M. D. (1994). *Clinical administration in audiology and speech-language pathology*. San Diego, CA: Singular Publishing Group.

Society for Human Resources Management. (1998). Policy handbook on the Web. Alexandria, VA: Author. Available at http://www.shrm.org

RESOURCES

CAA Accreditation Manual, Standards Manual for CAA
accreditation. American Speech-Language-Hearing
Association
10801 Rockville Pike
Rockville, MD. 20852-3279
Phone: 888-498-6699
Web site: http://www.asha.org/

Commission on Accreditation of Rehabilitation
Facilities (CARF), Standards manual for CARF
accreditation. 4891 East Grant Road
Tucson, AZ 85712
Phone: 800-444-8991
Web site: http://www.carf.org

Hospital and Physician Publishing, Inc.
P.O. Box 158, Ordill Area #7, Bldg 2-1
Marion, IL 62959
Phone: 618-997-9375

Joint Commission on Accreditation of Health Care
Organizations. (JACHO) One Rennaissance Blvd.

Oakbrook Terrace, IL 60181
Phone: 630-792-5000
Web site: http://www.jcaho.org

Knowledge Point
1129 Industrial Ave
Petaluma, CA 94952
Phone: 707-762-0333
E-mail: kp@knowledgepoint.com

Medical Consultants Network, Inc.
3191 South Broadway
Englewood, CO 80110-2423
Phone: 800-538-6264
Web site: http://www.medconnetwork.com

Society for Human Resources Management
606 North Washington Street
Alexandria, VA 22314-1997
Phone: 703-548-3440
E-mail: shrm@shrm.org

APPENDIX 19–1

Sample P&P

NRH POLICIES & PROCEDURES

Title: **Hand Hygiene**   **Section:**

Purpose: This policy outlines the procedure for maintaining   **Scope:**
                   hand hygiene, which is the most effective way to   **Number:**
                   prevent transmission of disease.

Forms: **Effective Date of**
                                                                  This Version:

1. **Policy:** All team members must follow the guidelines for hand hygiene

2. **Procedure:**

    A. To reduce the number of organisms on the hands, use the following guidelines:
       1. When hands are visibly soiled or contaminated, wash with soap and water.
       2. If hands are not visibly soiled, use an alcohol based hand-rub.

    B. Decontamination of hands is required for, but not limited to the following:
       1. Before having direct contact with patients
       2. Before performing procedures such as catheter insertion, peripheral vascular catheter, or other invasive devices that do not require a surgical procedure
       3. After contact with patient's intact skin (e.g. when taking pulse or blood pressure and lifting patients)
       4. After contact with body fluids or excretions, mucous membranes or dressings
       5. After removing gloves
       6. When moving from a contaminated body site to a clean body site during patient care
       7. After eating, drinking or using the bathroom

    C. Dispensers
       1. Liquid soap dispensers are replaced or cleaned and filled with fresh product. Liquids are not added to a partially filled dispenser.
       2. Alcohol-based hand rub containers are replaced as needed.
       3. Dispensers are located in every patient room and in patient care areas or close proximity.

    D. Soap and water handwashing steps
       1. Apply soap to wet hands.
       2. Lather and briskly rub hands together over all surfaces of hands, fingers, and fingernails for at least 15 seconds.
       3. Rinse thoroughly under a stream of warm water.
       4. Dry completely with a paper towel.
       5. Turn off water with paper towel.

E. Alcohol-based hand rub steps for decontamination
   1. Ensure hands are free of visible debris prior to using the alcohol-based hand rub.
   2. Dispense product into palm of one hand and place fingernails of other hand into the foam and rotate. Repeat procedure for opposite hand. Then rub product over both hands.
   3. Rub until the alcohol has evaporated.
   4. Wash hands with soap and water after 7–8 alcohol uses, and/or when there is a build up of the emollients on the hands.
   5. Alcohol-based hand-rub is flammable. Do not use near electrical outlets or oxygen.

F. Gloves
   1. Wear gloves when in contact with blood or other potentially infectious materials, mucous membranes and non -intact skin.
   2. Change gloves during patient care when moving from a contaminated body site to a clean one.
   3. Remove gloves after having contact with a patient. Do not wear the same pair of gloves for the care of more than one patient.

G. Nails
   1. Nails must be clean, short and natural.
   2. Artificial nails, extenders, nail wraps or other nail applications may not be worn by staff providing direct patient care.
   3. Polish, if worn, will not be chipped.

Reference: Guidelines for Hand Hygiene in Health-care settings: Recommendations of the Healthcare Infection Control Practices Advisory committee and the HICPAC/SHEA/APIC/IDSA
Hand Hygiene Task Force (2002)
CDC: Guidelines for Hand Hygiene

Approved By:

_____

Edward A Eckenhoff President/CEO

Additional Signature Information:

20

Leadership and Communication Skills

ANN W. KUMMER, PHD

SCOPE OF CHAPTER

In the professions of audiology and speech-language pathology, most of us consider ourselves as clinicians, not as leaders. We evaluate and treat individuals for a variety of communication and swallowing disorders. We counsel families, and we work with physicians and other professionals. Most of us are not in what would be classified as a traditional leadership position. Leadership skills are important, however, for clinicians who must advocate for their clients, students, and patients, interact with other professionals on teams and at conferences, communicate persuasively with caregivers, and serve on professional committees, boards, and associations at local, state, and national levels. In addition, many of you will assume traditional management or administration positions in your individual settings.

In addition to leadership skills, good communication skills are critical to the success of audiologists and speech pathologists in all positions. Certainly it can be said that communication is our business. We are experts at it! Even so, we are not all experts in business communication. Although we are acutely aware of the physical prerequisites and the necessary cognitive and functional skills that are required to communicate, we ourselves must demonstrate effective workplace communication with management, peers, clients, and families.

The purpose of this chapter, therefore, is to discuss the necessary leadership and communication skills for success in the workplace. How these skills relate to the activities of both managers and clinicians will be particularly stressed.

LEADERSHIP

A *leader* is a person who *influences* others to act in a certain way to achieve certain goals. *Leadership*, therefore, is the process of influencing or directing others to follow (Yukl, 1981).

Follow the Leader

We usually think of leaders as those who are in positions of power or authority. In fact, those individuals who are at the top of an organizational chart should all be good leaders. However, anyone can be a leader in certain situations. Leadership is not job-specific; instead it is situation-specific. We all serve as both leaders and followers, depending on the situation, the group, and the environment. For example, in one day an individual can be a department director (leader), a committee member (follower), a middle manager (leader and follower), a parent (leader), an advocate for legislative change (leader), a clinician (leader), a student supervisor (leader), and a member of a patient care team (leader and follower).

Effective leadership depends as much on the follower accepting direction as it does on the leader giving it. "Followers" include employees, committee members, students, and clients. Because followers must consent to being influenced by the leader, the leader must obtain the trust and loyalty of the followers to influence them to follow a certain path. How the leader obtains this trust and loyalty often depends on the leader's relationship with others and ability to communicate effectively with the followers.

Leader versus Manager: What Is the Difference?

In general, leaders are the ones to develop a plan or course of action, and managers are the ones who see that the plan is implemented (Zaleznik, 2004). A *manager*, therefore, is an individual who oversees the operations of a business or organization and controls the day-to-day operations, resources, and expenditures (Mintzberg, 1998). In contrast to a leader, a manager usually has a particular position of authority that does not change with the situation.

TABLE 20–1 Differences Between a Manager and a Leader

Leader	Manager
Originates ideas	Follows directions
Asks what and why	Asks how and when
Has global perspective	Has a day-to-day perspective
Looks toward the future	Focuses on the present
Watches the horizon	Watches the bottom line
Develops	Implements
Makes the rules	Plays the game
Promotes change	Maintains a steady course
Plans	Does
Takes initiative and risks	Follows a predetermined course
Deals with people	Deals with things
Looks at the forest	Looks at the trees

Reprinted from L. A. C. Golper and J. Brown, *Business matters: A guide for speech-language pathologists*. Rockville, MD: American Speech-Language-Hearing Association, 2004. Reprinted with permission.

The roles that the leader and manager play in an organization are very different, although they are not mutually exclusive and often overlap (Kotter, 1998). Table 20–1 shows the contrasting roles of the leader and manager. Since the roles are different, the skills that are required to fulfill these roles are also different. As a result, some individuals are better suited for one role versus the other.

It has been said that most companies are overmanaged and underled. If true, these organizations will remain static and have difficulty dealing with a culture of rapid change. For an organization to be truly successful, it is important to have both effective leaders and effective managers. Having a balance between the two is particularly important for service and health care organizations that have to compete in an increasingly complex and ever-changing environment.

Leadership in Audiology and Speech-Language Pathology

Opportunities for leadership are not reserved for the "boss" or those who are in administrative positions.

In fact, there are many opportunities for leadership roles at our individual workplaces, in our communities, or through professional associations, such as ASHA, state associations, and other professional organizations. These opportunities may include serving on or even chairing committees, initiating an advocacy effort, or leading a parent or family training group. Even in the purely clinical arena, each staff audiologist or speech-language pathologist (SLP) serves as a leader every day. For example, the SLP is the leader of his or her client's treatment "team." In this role, the SLP influences the patient, family members, and other treating professionals to do certain things in order to achieve certain goals. The SLP has the ability to influence others with the professional degree, the demonstration of professional knowledge, and skill. This builds the trust and confidence in the SLP's ability, which is required for others on the treatment team to follow the SLP's direction. The SLP must have the ability to effectively communicate the plan with good interpersonal skills. Therefore, even if they do not hold a formal position of authority, clinicians must have good leadership and communication skills to be effective in the workplace.

The Leader's Source of Influence is Power

Influence is the ability, or the *power*, to convince others to believe or act in a certain way. All leaders need to have power or influence to achieve their goals through others (Maxwell, 2002). Although power often has a negative connotation, use of the right type of power can be positive and is necessary for effective leadership.

Many authors have described five basic sources of power in a work setting (Yukl, 1981; Hellriegel, Slocum, & Woodman, 1983). Although they are sometimes labeled differently, the meanings behind the labels for these sources of power are the same.

The most obvious source of power is called *legitimate* (or *position*) *power*. This is the power that is given to the boss, supervisor, or chairperson by virtue of a particular leadership position. The boss is the designated leader of a group and has *legitimate* authority to tell his or her staff what to do, when to do it, and how to do it. This source of power is solely based on the level of authority inherent in the position and is not based on any personal or professional attributes of this leader.

The second source of power is *reward power*. Reward power is the leader's ability to give the followers something of value in return for their work. If the leader is the boss, then the ability to offer salary, benefits, and promotion is the basis of this type of power. The reward or incentive does not need to be monetary, however. The leader may have the ability to reward with special privileges or assignments. Even the ability to publicly recognize and thank the follower gives the leader reward power.

Punishment (or *coercive*) *power* is the opposite of reward power. Punishment power is the ability to take something away from a noncompliant follower. The things that might be taken away are also things that serve as effective rewards for the employee (e.g., salary, benefits, promotion, job security). The employee may also be coerced to comply with the demands of the leader due to a fear of reprisal, lack of respect, or embarrassment if there is noncompliance with the leader's demands. Although this type of power is effective in the short term, it leads to employee dissatisfaction in the long run. When employees are unhappy, this can cause poor performance and reduced productivity and ultimately lead to turnover, all of which are costly to the organization. Therefore, effective leaders use punishment power sparingly, if at all.

Expert power is unrelated to the leader's position or legitimate authority. Instead, a leader has expert power when employees or others recognize his or her special knowledge, skill, and expertise, particularly in difficult situations. An effective leader must have sufficient, maybe even extensive, knowledge in appropriate areas for expert power. With this source of power, the employees or followers have confidence in the leader's ability to understand the issues and to lead them competently. In this case, the employees or followers respect the leader and feel that they are in good hands. The greater the expertise, the more authority and power the leader will have.

Personal (or *referent*) *power* is a source of influence that depends on the leader's personality and charisma. For this type of power, the leader's personal characteristics are more important than his or her position or level of authority. Personal power results in the type of influence that a best friend or admired colleague would have on an individual. To have personal power, the leader must be high in *emotional intelligence,* which is the ability to manage relationships effectively and work well with others (Goleman, 1995, 2002, 2004; Heifetz, 2004). Leaders with personal power tend to have excellent communication skills, since effective communication enhances interpersonal relationships. Personal power is also gained when the leader shows a great deal of respect and encouragement for others and displays characteristics of honesty, integrity, and trustworthiness. As a result of these characteristics, followers have a strong personal identification with the leader and want to please the leader with compliance.

Considering these five sources of power, which is most effective in influencing others? Although the first three sources of power are typically associated with being the "boss," most leaders would agree that a more effective source of influence is expert power and the *most* effective source of influence is personal power (Yukl, 1981; Hellriegel, Slocum, & Woodman, 1983). Therefore, a person with authority, but lacking expert or personal power, will have great difficulty influencing others in the long run, especially in situations where the followers do not see personal value in following the request.

Mutual Dependency of the Leader and Follower

In addition to understanding sources of power, the leader should understand the mutual dependency inherent in the leader-follower relationship. Both parties have need for something from the other. As such, there must be a balance in the relationship whereby the leader and follower both receive what they value in exchange for what they give. In the work setting, the boss or supervisor is dependent on the employee for a certain amount and type of work. The chairperson of a committee is dependent on the members to complete their tasks in order to accomplish committee goals. The followers (e.g., employees, committee members) expect certain rewards from the leader in exchange for their efforts. These rewards may be material (such as pay) or

psychological (such as recognition). The leader must continually satisfy the needs of the follower to retain the position of leadership and power.

Successful organizations have one thing in common: They realize that employees are the organization's most valuable resource. Leaders who understand the importance of employee satisfaction through appropriate rewards are likely to find that the employees reciprocate with improved job performance (quality and quantity) and with loyalty to the organization.

Given the concept of mutual dependency and the need for balance in the relationship, the role of the "boss" should be reconsidered. Contrary to popular belief, the employee does not work "for" the boss. Instead, they both work for each other. In fact, an effective boss or leader should realize that his or her job is to make the employee or follower happy, because a happy employee is an effective employee. This is done by acting as a "servant leader." If employees are happy with the rewards received in exchange for their work and the employees have all the necessary resources for the job, they are likely to provide quality services, be productive, and stay in the position. Since the costs of poor quality, low productivity, and turnover are significant, making the employee happy is an important responsibility for the boss.

Development of Leadership Skills: Nature versus Nurture

Are good leaders born that way, or are they the result of training and experience? The answer to this question is that it is probably a combination of both. Leadership skills can be learned and constantly improved, particularly in a model environment (Heller, 1999). Good role models and mentoring relationships are crucial in the development of leadership skills. In addition, an entrepreneurial culture can help the individual learn to take on the responsibilities that are typically given to leaders. In fact, the best way to develop leaders in an organization is to create challenging opportunities for young or inexperienced employees to "step up" and take responsibility and then to provide coaches for mentoring. Successful businesses encourage and reward employees who help to develop leaders within their ranks.

T A B L E 20–2 Common Characteristics of Effective Leaders

Character: demonstrates integrity, honesty, and trustworthiness; admits mistakes and apologizes; has extreme humility and modesty; ambition is for the institution rather than for self; tells the truth; has a personal and organizational code of ethics; is fair to all; doesn't use power for selfish purposes; is a role model of behavior; is genuine and candid; is inspiring; respects others; has self-awareness, self-regulation, and self-discipline; and is diplomatic and tactful.

Relationship Orientation: listens to others and communicates effectively; shows respect; takes time for people; has strong interpersonal skills; is concerned about the welfare of employees; recognizes others; appreciates the contributions of others; shows confidence in the ability of others; works cooperatively; gives frequent positive feedback; smiles and is courteous; shows compassion; is positive in dealings with others; is emotionally mature; is empathetic and supportive; is respectful, trustworthy, and fair-minded; doesn't take advantage of others; empowers others and delegates; and supports and celebrates others' successes.

Competence and Drive: shows the knowledge and skills to get the job done; is ambitious and achievement oriented; assertive and decisive; a problem-solver; is a visionary and is forward-thinking; doesn't get discouraged about setbacks or failures; is tolerant of stress; has strong need to produce results; takes initiative and risks; focuses on results; benchmarks and networks with others; demonstrates a desire to make a difference; is committed; engages in continuous performance and quality improvement; is passionate about the mission and vision.

Adapted from L. A. C. Golper and J. Brown, *Business matters: A guide for speech-language pathologist.* Rockville, MD: American Speech-Language-Hearing Association, 2004.

Although many leadership skills can be learned and developed, some individuals have more "leadership potential" than others. This potential has a great deal to do with personality traits and communication abilities. In this way, nature has a role in the making of a good leader. Certainly, great leaders are not all alike, and they accomplish their goals through many different methods and approaches. However, research shows that they share certain personality and behavioral characteristics.

Leadership Characteristics

Many authors list personality and behavioral characteristics that are typical of great leaders. Great leaders are not always the most visible or most vocal people. In fact, great leaders blend personal humility with strong ambition for the organization (Collins, 2001). These leaders take pride in the accomplishment of others (Maxwell, 1999). They channel their ambition to work for the good of the organization rather than for the good of themselves and their personal egos.

A compilation of common of leadership characteristics can be found on Table 20–2. Covey (2000) surveyed 54,000 people about characteristics of effective leaders. In his survey, the most frequent characteristics named, in order of frequency, were related to integrity, communication, a people orientation, vision, and caring.

It should be noted that the characteristics on Table 20–2 have a common theme and, therefore, are categorized under three main headings: character, relationship orientation, and competence and drive. It soon becomes apparent that the first two categories (character and relationship orientation) are related to the leader's personal power. The final category (competence and drive) is what establishes the leader's expert power. To determine if you have these qualities, see the Assessment of Leadership Qualities in Appendix 20–1.

The three categories of common leadership characteristics support the concept that personal power and expert power are strong sources of influence. They are necessary for effective leadership, yet they are unrelated to the leader's formal position in an organization.

The Roles of a Leader

Leadership roles can be divided into two basic categories: the visionary role and the motivational role (Golper & Brown, 2004). The combination of these roles requires the leader to engage in high levels of both task-oriented (visionary) and relationship-centered (motivational) activities. These activities are all done for the primary purpose of accomplishing certain goals through the entire team members (leader and followers).

T A B L E 20–3 Leadership as Applied in the Role of a Clinician

Mission: To work with patients with feeding and swallowing disorders.

Vision: To significantly improve or correct all disorders treated and make a positive impact on the life of every patient who is treated.

Values: To conduct therapy with honesty and integrity; to give the best effort possible for each session; to include the family in the therapeutic process; to respect the wishes and goals of the patient and family; to treat patients and families with respect and dignity.

Strategy: To learn as much as possible about each patient; to develop comprehensive, individualized treatment plans; to seek advice and feedback from others as needed; to coordinate treatment with other caregivers; to train the family to understand the problem and how to work with the patient at home; to provide a home program of therapy and update after each treatment session; to attend at least one continuing education course on dysphagia this year.

The *visionary role* encompasses the way in which leaders define, envision, strategize, and plan to set a path for others to follow. An effective visionary leader attends to four aspects of this role: mission, vision, values, and strategy. The aspects of this role can be done for an entire organization, for a department, for a program, or even for clinical activities. Table 20–3 shows an example of how this can be applied to the role of a clinician.

In the visionary role, the leader must first define the mission of the organization or group and be sure that this is clear to all within the organization. The *mission* is the organization's primary purpose or function. Even when chairing a small committee, the leader should make the mission of the committee clear so that the members know what is expected and what is outside the realm of responsibility for the committee. A clear mission statement helps to determine and direct the activities of the members of the organization toward a common focus. Examples of mission statements include the following:

- Hospital X will improve health care of our patients and transform the delivery of care through fully integrated, globally recognized research, education, and innovation.

- Hospital Y will provide a high standard of patient care, research, and education to improve the health care of infants, children, and adolescents in the community, nation, and world.

- The dysphagia team will improve the quality of services by increasing the skills of our members and providing more education to our patients and their families.

- The mission of Special Interest Division X is to promote the development of knowledge and skills among affiliates through research and the exchange of information in our specialty areas.

Once the mission is clear, the leader must develop a vision. A *vision* is the long-term goal and reflects what the organization should be like in the future. Using information at hand, leaders must be able to plan prospectively, process many different kinds of information, and use their perceptions as a basis for judging environmental forces. The vision should always be developed with input from a variety of stakeholders (e.g., patients and families, senior management, referring physicians, third party payers, and staff). It should be developed with both an analytical and objective perspective, as well as an emotional and subjective view.

Examples of vision statements include the following:

- To be a leading resource for the community of scientists and clinicians specializing in XYZ disorders.

- To be the leader in improving the outcomes for at-risk infants.

The next aspect of the visionary role is defining values. *Values* have to do with the principles that are important while trying to carry out the mission and achieve the vision. Values provide the followers with a guideline of acceptable and expected performance and behavior (Dye, 2000). It also lets them know what is not acceptable. Knowingly or not, leaders always set the tone for standards of behavior in the group. If the leader allows goals to be accomplished through inappropriate behavior, the followers will either do the same, or leave. So that everyone knows the "rules of the game," it is important for the leader to determine the values of the organization or group. The following are examples of typical value statements:

- We will treat patients and families as partners and members of the health care team.

- We recognize the value and worth of all individuals, regardless of racial, cultural, or personal differences.

- We will provide service to our customers with respect for their time.

- We will treat our coworkers with respect and dignity.

- We will work cooperatively with all team members and acknowledge their contributions to the goals of the team.

The last aspect of the visionary role involves developing a strategic plan. The *strategic plan* is a detailed document that serves as guide or roadmap for achieving the goals of the vision. It usually has specific steps with timelines for accomplishment. Just like the vision, the strategic plan must take into account the interest of all stakeholders. When developing a strategic plan, the leader must also consider what resources will be needed (money, people, time, materials, equipment, space, training, and technology) to accomplish the goals. Once completed, the strategic plan should serve to focus and guide the activities of the organization toward accomplishment of certain predefined goals.

To implement the strategic plan and work toward the vision, the leader is dependent on other people to carry out the plan. A leader may have a great strategy, but all will fail unless he or she has the "power" to get others to follow the plan. Therefore, once planning is complete, the leader takes on the motivational role.

In the *motivational role,* the leader must be able to clearly communicate the plan and demonstrate the need to implement the plan. After the followers are convinced of the need to implement the plan, the leader must then continually encourage,

energize, and empower them to follow the strategic plan to accomplish the determined goals. In order to do that, the leader must be involved in constant communication, training, and coaching. Once followers have the knowledge and skills to do the job, it is important to motivate them to do the job on their own. Great leaders delegate and empower followers to take responsibility, be creative, and be successful. In fact, John Quincy Adams said: "If your actions inspire others to dream more, learn more, do more and become more, you are a leader."

Although pay in the form of salary and benefits is a primary motivation for taking a job, it is not the only motivation. Motivation alone may not be enough to keep an employee in the job. It is the leader's responsibility to be sure that the employee has the resources necessary to do the job and that the employee has a positive and supportive work environment.

BUSINESS COMMUNICATION

Business communication refers to the method in which we exchange information in the workplace in order to communicate a plan and influence others to follow. When the people (leaders and staff) in an organization fail to communicate effectively with each other, accomplishment of goals is difficult and the organization is at great risk.

Communication in the Profession of Communication Disorders

As audiologists and speech-language pathologists, we are aware of the importance of communication skills in interpersonal relationships. We are experts in communication disorders, and we know what to do to remediate communication disorders. However, we often forget that effective communication is more than just hearing clearly, understanding a message, and speaking intelligibly. Effective communication requires us to listen carefully to understand and speak effectively to convey our thoughts. The ability to communicate in this way is actually a high level "metaskill" that is necessary to exchange information and intent effectively with other individuals.

In our own professional business, we need to communicate effectively with our "customers," including patients or clients, families, physicians, teachers, colleagues, other health care providers, administrators, and third party payers. It is clear that without effective interpersonal communication skills, quality and productivity will suffer due to the lack of ability to influence, persuade, and negotiate—all necessities for workplace success.

Communication in Leadership Roles

Although most of us can hear and convey our ideas effectively, we are often ineffective when it comes to truly listening to others. The visionary role is dependent on the leader's ability to understand the environment and the needs of the organization in order to craft a plan. This means the leader must listen carefully to others to obtain the necessary information.

The leader's success in performing the motivational role depends on his or her ability to communicate the plan and to engage others to embrace the plan and follow direction. Effective communication is the crux of motivating employees, and employee motivation is critically important to the job's success. Employees are motivated when managers communicate clear expectations, instructions, and time frames. This fosters within the employees a sense of security, respect, power, and control in their jobs. On the other hand, employees are demotivated when they are unsure of the leader's direction, expectations, and priorities. Furthermore, leaders need to communicate constant encouragement and support, as well as acknowledgement and appreciation for achievement of outcomes. Toward this end, the leader must understand what motivates the followers so that there is a balance in the relationship between what is received by the leader and what is received by the followers.

We have also discussed the mutual dependency between a leader and follower. Because of this mutual dependency, the lines of communication must be open between the individuals who rely on one another. Considering all of these points, effective leaders must demonstrate excellent communication skills to be effective. Leaders must be able to clearly communicate goals and expectations, and followers must be able to listen attentively to perform to expectations. This helps to avoid conflicts and misunderstandings, and it allows leader-follower teams to succeed in any arena.

Use of Communication in Leadership Roles

Leaders depend on their communication skills for a variety of purposes. Let's consider some common examples.

Communication of Mission, Vision, Values, and Strategies The leader must be able to grasp the "big picture" to determine the organization's mission, vision, values, and strategies. The leader should be knowledgeable about inside and outside forces and activities that have the potential to affect the organization. In addition, the leader must consider and analyze the organization's strengths, weaknesses, opportunities, and threats (SWOT) to determine the strategic plan. To accomplish these tasks, the leader must communicate with all stakeholders. This would include *external customers* (i.e., patients/clients, families, physicians, other professionals, and insurance companies) and *internal customers* (i.e., senior management and staff). The leader must be able to listen carefully to others, gather information, analyze the information, and then determine the plan with input and constant feedback from others. The leader then needs to be able to share the plan with the followers. Throughout all of these activities, the leader must be able to listen carefully to, and communicate effectively with, others.

Communicating Expectations The leader cannot realistically expect followers to perform in a certain way if the followers do not know the expectations of performance. The ability to read minds is a rare talent. Unclear expectations cannot only result in failure but can also cause the follower to feel insecure and unhappy. The leader will encounter additional problems when it is time to provide feedback of behavior or performance, especially if there are issues with performance or accomplishment.

Therefore, it is incumbent upon the leader to communicate clear expectations of performance. A discussion about the expectations is important to ensure a clear understanding of what is expected and when. This should be done verbally in person and also documented in writing for further reference.

Coaching (Mentoring) A *coach* (or *mentor*) is someone who trains, teaches, encourages, and provides constant feedback to improve the performance of others. Coaching is an important leadership role because the leader is always dependent on others to accomplish tasks. Therefore, the leader must make sure others have the knowledge, skills, resources, and information to get the job done. The more knowledgeable and trained the follower is, the better the ultimate outcome will be. The followers must also be continually encouraged and supported so that they have confidence, a positive attitude, and the desire to do the job well.

A truly successful leader takes pride in the success and accomplishments of those under his or her leadership. The leader in an organization should foster a culture of continuous learning through coaching and mentoring at all levels. When coaching and continuous learning are part of the culture, the services continue to improve and job satisfaction remains high.

In audiology and speech-language pathology, we have training and experience in "teaching" and helping others change behaviors. These coaching and teaching skills should not be limited to our clients; instead they should be transferred to other leadership activities with employees, committee members, coworkers, and graduate students.

Constructive Feedback The term *constructive feedback* tends to have a negative connotation. In fact, constructive feedback can be both positive and negative. Positive feedback is news or input to an employee about a good effort or result. Negative feedback is news to an employee about inadequate performance, areas of weakness, areas that need improvement, and opportunities for growth. Unfortunately, the word *negative* can develop defensiveness and resistance. Therefore, this word should be avoided. Instead, the focus of this type of feedback should be on change, improvement, and professional growth.

Whenever possible, constructive feedback should be information-specific, issue-focused, and based on observations rather than subjective impressions. Successful leaders develop a routine that includes frequent, in-depth discussions about performance with employees or followers. The boss should let the employee know that the purpose of the feedback is to help him or her to be successful.

Giving positive feedback is easy, but giving negative feedback is hard for most leaders. As a result, leaders sometimes soften the feedback to avoid confrontation or hard feelings. This may hurt the employee in the long run, however, especially if he or she did not get a clear message of what to do differently. A strong leader is one who can give both positive and negative feedback. Open and honest feedback helps employees by giving them guidance as to how to perform, what is expected in the future, and how to succeed. Honest feedback of this type is also good for the ultimate goals of the organization because it helps the employee to contribute appropriately to team goals.

Asking the employee specific questions is a useful tool in the feedback process. Such questions might include: What have you accomplished this year? Why was this successful? What were your challenges or disappointments? What could you have done differently or better in retrospect? What would you like to learn to do this year? How can I help? Asking questions is a great way to start a meaningful discussion and unveil unclear expectations that affect performance. It also helps employees to self-evaluate and encourages them to take responsibility for learning and developing skills.

Reward and Recognition Although recognition in the form of salary and benefits is a primary motivation for taking a job, it is not the only motivation. It may not be enough to keep an employee in the job. Effective leaders understand that recognition, praise, and thanks for doing a good job are highly motivating to employees. This may be especially true for those in professional positions, such as audiologist and speech-language pathologist. Recognition signifies that someone noticed the individual's hard work and appreciated it. At the same time, recognition communicates what the organization values—that is, what great performance looks like. It is positive reinforcement for expected performance. Recognition and praise become particularly important in situations where pay is restricted by regulations, policies, or the organization's budget.

Recognition is easy to give and inexpensive (usually free). Yet for some leaders, giving praise and recognition is difficult or simply forgotten. Given the studies that indicate the power of recognition in the workplace, it should be a priority for leaders in all positions of leadership!

Recognition does not need to be formal. Employees value personalized, spur-of-the-moment recognition for their contributions. They also appreciate public recognition (in a meeting, for example) that is timely and addresses the unique contributions of the individual. Note that frequent recognition of others enhances the leader's personal power.

Sharing Relevant Information The leader should keep employees informed of anything that has the potential to affect themselves, the work unit, or the organization. When the leader is not proactive in communicating with employees, the employees must rely on rumors and the "grapevine." At the very least, this form of communication is inefficient and usually inaccurate. In addition, it is often destructive in that it undermines the leader's effectiveness and can force the leader to constantly correct misinformation and misperceptions. Communicating information well means not "hoarding" the truth (Bartolome, 1999).

Actually, sharing information, whether it is good news or bad news, has a positive effect on others' performance because it helps to foster a positive atmosphere of honesty and trust. Withholding information can have a negative effect because it can cause fear, insecurity, and distrust (Golper & Brown, 2004). Therefore, an effective leader recognizes the importance of frequent communication with followers and communicates good and bad news openly and honestly. In some organizations, this open environment with honest communication of both the good and the bad is called *transparency*.

Managing Conflict Most leaders know that conflict over issues is natural and often necessary. Conflict helps individuals to consider different options and ultimately to make better choices. By avoiding conflict, some leaders do more harm to the organization. Ignoring conflict and ducking tough issues can ultimately lead to a culture that cannot tolerate honesty and straight talk (Argyris, 1999). Therefore, the leader must encourage team members to argue and challenge each other without destroying their ability to work together in the future. The leader's challenge is to be sure that disagreements do not become personal.

When conflict does become personal, the leader must deal with this directly and swiftly to maintain a positive work environment. The leader should meet with those in conflict individually or in small groups to allow people the opportunity to vent anger. It is important, however, that everyone knows in advance why these meetings are being held and that they understand that personal attacks and blame are not appropriate in these meetings. The challenge for the leader is to listen carefully to all sides and then arbitrate a resolution. This situation can truly test the leader's communication skills.

Developing Relationships, Trust, and Loyalty Establishing effective working relationships with others takes time and effort. However, the best leaders make certain that each person in the group feels connected and valued. When leaders communicate individually with others, clarify expectations, coach and mentor, give employees the opportunity to do their best, recognize and praise them, and encourage individuals to develop their skills, they help develop good working relationships and loyalty. This builds the leader's personal power to keep the followers productive and task-oriented.

Advocacy Advocacy involves taking responsibility to influence others to do certain things. It is a process of marshalling resources and information to bring about a change (Golper & Brown, 2004) Audiology and speech-language pathology present many opportunities to be involved in advocacy efforts for our clients and the profession as a whole.

Advocacy requires that the leader is knowledgeable (and therefore has expert power) and has good communication skills to persuade others. In our professions, advocacy can include working with legislators on issues such as mandating that health care plans offer a benefit option for audiology and speech-language pathology coverage, repealing the $1,500 therapy cap under Medicare, determining requirements for state licensure, and requiring schools districts to hire only master's level speech-language pathologists.

Although we typically think of advocacy as involving the legislative process, it is actually much more extensive and is something leaders must do frequently. For example, a department director may advocate for increased salaries, more space, or additional equipment based on a strong argument using relevant information. A committee leader may advocate for a change in a procedure based on the information that has been gathered and analyzed by the committee. A clinician may advocate for a change in the frequency of therapy based on information gathered regarding the patient's needs, previous response to therapy, and prognosis.

Again, advocacy is influencing others through the dissemination of information. The effectiveness of advocacy efforts clearly relies on the power of the leader (expert power and even personal power) and the ability to effectively communicate information to convince others of the need for the change.

Barriers to Effective Communication

Although there is little argument that effective communication is extremely important in interpersonal relationships and in organizations, it seems to be difficult to achieve. There are many barriers to effective communication, especially in the area of listening (Nichols & Stevens, 1999).

Hearing is passive and takes no effort. Listening, on the other hand, is active. It requires that we focus on the speaker, maintain attention, and seek to understand. Since listening requires effort, it is no surprise that when we hear others speak, we typically only remember a small portion of what we have heard.

The problem is that we listen and attend to other things at the same time. Since only a part of our mind is paying attention, it is easy to drift and think about other things while listening to the speaker (like what we will have for dinner). We can become impatient and even lazy about trying to understand. We are also distracted by competing issues for our attention (like the conversation at the next table). In some cases, we are busy thinking about a response instead of listening to the other person. Our emotions and interpersonal relationship with the speaker also affect our ability to listen and understand. Finally, personal filters, assumptions, judgments, biases, culture, and beliefs can distort what we hear.

Because listening is so difficult and we listen with a personal bias, what we think we heard and understood can be very different than what the speaker actually intended to communicate! To counter these barriers, effective leaders participate in a process called *active listening*.

Active Listening

Active listening is a structured form of listening and responding that focuses the attention on the speaker. The goal of active listening is to improve the mutual understanding of both parties through specific techniques. Some of the principles of active listening include the following:

- *Focus on the speaker.* You already know your thoughts. Therefore, spend more time trying to understand the other person's thoughts. Listen about 80 percent of the time and talk about 20 percent of the time.

- *Empathize.* Try to "walk in the other person's shoes" and see the other person's perspective. Empathizing does not mean you need to agree with the speaker. It just means that you must ignore your own thoughts and perceptions for the moment and see the issue from the other person's perspective.

- *Acknowledge.* Show that you are listening and trying to understand through verbal and nonverbal confirmation. Use nonverbal communication and body position (e.g., leaning forward) to encourage the speaker and signal interest.

- *Don't interrupt.* Let the speaker complete the point without interruption and without rushing him or her.

- *Ask questions.* Ask sincere and relevant questions to clarify a statement or gather more information. A question that begins with "why" puts people on the defensive (e.g., "Why did you do that?"). Therefore, "why" questions should be avoided. However, more effective types of questions may include:

- What are your ideas for the committee?
- What should be done next?
- How do you want to do that?
- What are your challenges?
- What can I do to help?

- *Paraphrase to confirm understanding.* Paraphrasing is a technique that good active listeners use frequently. It is a way to confirm understanding by restating the information that was received. The speaker confirms, clarifies, or explains further based on the listener's restatement. Some common ways to paraphrase or confirm understanding may start with the following:

  - What I hear you saying is. . . . Is that what you meant?
  - It seems that you are frustrated when. . . . Is that correct?"

Methods of Communication

In past generations, communication was accomplished by phone or mail or in person. In addition, workers in the majority of professions had predictable work hours, often 9 to 5. Today, many people check e-mail messages (or voice mail) before leaving home in the morning and before going to bed at night. Late-night e-mails from workaholics, insomniacs, and others are now common. Although this form of communication is convenient, it does not replace the need for individual or group face-to-face meetings. In fact, any communication that involves emotion, problem solving, or differences of opinion is best done with a traditional face-to-face meeting.

Meetings are important because they can make people feel part of the group. Participative meetings help people to feel that their opinion is heard and that it matters. It gives them an opportunity to ask questions and clarify misunderstandings. In addition, meetings allow the individuals to communicate more effectively with tone, posture, eye contact, and body language. Thus, an effective leader must determine the most important mode of communication (fast *versus* personal) for each type of situation.

SUMMARY

There is general agreement that a leader must have power to be effective. Although five sources of power were discussed, most authors agree that expert power and personal power are the most effective in influencing others for maximum performance. These sources of power are important as the leader fulfills the major roles discussed in this chapter. For the visionary role, the leader needs knowledge and competence. Therefore, expert power is important. For the motivational role the leader must interact with the followers. Therefore, personal power is needed.

Communication skills are also extremely important in these leadership roles. For the visionary role the leader must be able to listen carefully to obtain information to develop the plan. For the motivational role, the leader must then communicate the plan clearly to influence others to act. In summary, effective leaders require excellent communication skills, expertise, and strong interpersonal skills. It may be a cliché, but in leadership positions, it pays to be nice!

CRITICAL THINKING

1. Think of influential people and people of authority in your work setting and in you personal life. Consider each person's primary source of influence or power. Which of these people are most influential, and why?

2. What situations that occur in the work setting require leadership skills?

3. What are some ways that audiologists and speech-language pathologists can assume leadership roles in the profession?

4. What is meant by "servant leader"? Why is it important for followers to be satisfied with the leadership?

5. Why do effective leaders require effective communication skills?

6. Describe some techniques for active listening. How can these techniques help a leader in

performing the visionary or motivational roles?

7. Evaluate your own leadership and communication skills. What are your assets and what skills could be improved? Why would it be important to improve your leadership and communication skills?

REFERENCES

American Speech-Language-Hearing Association. (2005). How ASHA works with you. Rockville, MD: Author.

Argyris, C. (1999). Skilled incompetence. In *Harvard Business Review on effective communication* (pp. 101–118). Boston: Harvard Business School Publishing.

Bartolome, F. (1999). Nobody trusts the boss completely—Now What? In *Harvard Business Review on effective communication* (pp. 79–100). Boston: Harvard Business School Publishing.

Collins, J. (2001). *Good to great.* New York: Harper Business.

Covey, S. (2000). Leadership is a choice. In *Lessons in leadership program guide* (p. 4). Lexington, KY: Wyncom.

Dye, C. F. (2000). *Leadership in healthcare: Values at the top.* Chicago: Health Administration Press.

Goleman, D. (1995). *Emotional intelligence.* New York: Bantam Books.

Goleman, D. (2002). *Primal leadership: Realizing the power of emotional intelligence.* Boston: Harvard Business School Publishing.

Goleman, D. (2004). What makes a leader? *Harvard Business Review, 82*(1), 82–91.

Golper, L. & Brown, J. (2004). *Business matters: A guide for speech-language pathologists.* Rockville, MD: American Speech-Language-Hearing Association.

Heifetz, R. A. (2004). Question authority. In S. Clarke (Ed.), Voices: Leading by feel. *Harvard Business Review, 82*(1), 27–37.

Heller, R. (1999). *Learning to lead.* New York: DK Publishing.

Hellriegel, D., Slocum, Jr., J. W. & Woodman, R. W. (1983). *Organizational behavior* (3rd ed.). St. Paul, MN: West Publishing.

Kotter, J. P. (1998). What leaders really do. In *Harvard Business Review on leadership* (pp. 37–60). Boston: Harvard Business School Publishing.

Maxwell, J. C. (1999). *The 21 indispensable qualities of a leader: Becoming the person others want to follow.* Nashville, TN: Maxwell Motivation.

Maxwell, J. C. (2002). *Leadership 101: What every leader needs to know.* Nashville, TN: Maxwell Motivation.

Mintzberg, H. (1998). The manager's job: Folklore and fact. In *Harvard business review on leadership* (pp. 1–36). Boston: Harvard Business School Publishing.

Nichols, R. G., & Stevens, L. A. (1999). Listening to people. In *Harvard Business Review on effective communication* (pp. 1–24). Boston: Harvard Business School Publishing.

Tannen, D. (1995). The power of talk: Who gets heard and why. *Harvard Business Review, 73*(5), 138–148.

Yukl, G. A. (1981). *Leadership in organizations.* Englewood Cliffs, NJ: Prentice Hall.

Zaleznik, A. (2004). Managers and leaders: Are they different? *Harvard Business Review, 82*(1), 74–81.

RESOURCES

Business Communication Quarterly http:// bcq. theabc.org/

Harvard Business Review Online http:// harvardbusinessonline.hbsp.harvard.edu

Making the Most of Your Membership: How ASHA Works With You http://www.asha.org/about/ leadership-projects/involvement.htm

Tannen, D. (1995). *Talking from 9 to 5: Women and men at work.* London: Virago Press.

Tannen, D. (2001). *You just don't understand: Women and men in conversation.* New York: Quill.

APPENDIX 20–1

Assessment of Leadership Qualities

ANN W. KUMMER, PHD

Instructions: Rate your leadership qualities the way you think others would rate you based on their perception. Then ask others to rate you anonymously and compare your perception with theirs. Any rating under 3 is an important area for development.

	1	2	3	4
Character:				
Has integrity, honesty, trustworthiness, code of ethics				
Admits mistakes and apologizes; has humility and modesty				
Has ambition for organization, not just for self				
Doesn't use power for selfish purposes				
Is fair to all				
Is a role model of behavior; is inspiring to others				
Has self-awareness, self-regulation, and self-discipline				
Is diplomatic and tactful, respectful, genuine, caring				
Relationship Orientation:				
Has strong interpersonal skills				
Is concerned about the welfare of employees				
Listens to others and communicates effectively				
Recognizes and appreciates the contributions of others				
Is empathetic, supportive, respectful, compassionate, and positive				
Gives frequent positive feedback; smiles and is courteous				
Doesn't take advantage of others				
Shows confidence in the ability of others; empowers others				
Supports and celebrates the successes of others				
Competence and Drive:				
Shows the knowledge and skills to get the job done				
Is achievement-oriented with a strong need to produce results				
Is assertive, decisive, committed, a problem-solver				
Takes initiative and risks				
Is a visionary and forward-thinker				
Doesn't get discouraged about failures or setbacks				
Is tolerant of stress				
Benchmarks and networks with others				
Engages in continuous performance and quality improvement				
Is passionate about the mission and vision of the organization				

Key:
1- Never
2- Sometimes
3- Usually
4- Always

21

Infection Prevention

ROSEMARY LUBINSKI, EDD

SCOPE OF CHAPTER

Little did you know on entering the professions of audiology or speech-language pathology that, in addition to your professional knowledge base and clinical skills, you would need to know about such topics as communicable diseases and universal precautions. Whether you practice in a health care institution, educational setting, private practice, or community speech, language, or hearing clinic, it is essential to know procedures to protect yourself, your family, and your clients from the spread of infectious diseases. Although infectious diseases are not new or unique to the populations with whom we work, changing demographics of our society, mainstreaming into educational settings, increased service to high-risk populations, and increase in certain communicable diseases are a few of the factors that prompt serious attention to risk management. Therefore, this chapter provides a rationale for protecting yourself and others, presents a basic discussion of infection pathways and types, and outlines ways of incorporating a hygiene plan into your clinical practice with all clients. Finally, we discuss some special situations related to the topic of infection prevention. This chapter encourages you to use a commonsense approach to creating a hygienic environment that minimizes the potential of infection transmission.

IMPORTANCE OF INFECTION PREVENTION TO SPEECH-LANGUAGE PATHOLOGISTS AND AUDIOLOGISTS

Although those of you who practice in health care facilities are likely to be aware of clean practices or risk management, this subject is often "ignored" by professionals working in other settings such as schools or private practice (McMillan & Willette, 1988). This is most unfortunate because clients with infectious diseases can range from toddlers in early intervention programs to elderly persons seeking a hearing aid from a dispensing audiologist. The reasons for an increase in infections are complex but include changing and increased population growth, poverty, expansion of populations into remote areas, improved transportation providing easier spread of disease, and inadequate public health infrastructure (Engender Health, 2005). Changing demographics of our client population suggest that you are likely to work with individuals who may be at high risk for contracting or transmitting an infection, including inpatients who are acutely ill and those with communicable diseases such as hepatitis B, human immunodeficiency virus (HIV, the virus that causes acquired immune deficiency syndrome or AIDS), tuberculosis, and cytomegalovirus. All of these individuals are in high-risk populations, usually because of their repressed immune systems, complicated medical conditions, and poverty.

In addition, speech-language pathologists have created new roles within shock trauma centers, high-risk neonatal programs, and AIDS programs, and have become responsible for swallowing management programs where the focus may be on working with critically ill patients. Audiologists, too, have created special hearing health programs for high-risk populations. Relatively recent federal legislation (i.e., PL 94-142, Section 504 of the Rehabilitation Act, and PL 99-457) and various state laws focus on the right of disabled individuals to a free, appropriate public education in the least restrictive environment (ASHA, 1991). This means that children with compromised health resistance may be attending public schools and may be in need of communication services. Thus, speech-language pathologists and audiologists in educational settings need to be as vigilant as colleagues in health care institutions of risk-management procedures.

The increase in the prevalence of diseases also necessitates such awareness. Although AIDS may be the best-known infectious disease, in actuality, other diseases are more prevalent, such as herpes simplex and hepatitis B. Contact with individuals with certain infectious diseases such as cytomegalovirus may have health implications for professional women who work during pregnancy.

The nature of our hands-on contact with clients during speech mechanism examinations, respiratory and laryngeal assessments, inspection of the outer ear, hearing aid fittings, swallowing assessments and treatments, and care of clients with laryngectomy and tracheotomy also increases the risk for infection transmission. Any procedure that brings you in direct contact with body fluids necessitates precautions.

Lest we forget, speech-language pathologists and audiologists themselves may be sources of infections that can be transmitted to clients. The state of low resistance to illness of many of our clients already mentioned makes them more susceptible to the infections we might transmit to them. For example, what may appear to be a "common cold" to you may result in bronchitis or pneumonia for frail elderly residents of a nursing facility. These illnesses, in turn, may result in increased nursing care, additional medications, relocation to an acute care hospital, prolonged illness, or death. You may also have a more serious communicable disease that requires the use of precautions to protect your clients.

McMillan and Willette (1988) remind us of the ethical responsibility we have to protect our patients from all health and safety dangers. The most basic ethical responsibility you have regarding spread of infection is to reduce the probability of its occurrence to its lowest possible level in your interactions with clients. When a patient suffers an infection, "progress is slowed, revenue may be decreased due to absence, and the risk of malpractice accusation may increase" (p.37).

Nosocomial infections are infections inadvertently contracted in a health care facility. Health care workers today are highly aware of the fact that hospitals and other facilities are unhealthy environments, in that the risk for exposure to a staphylococcal virus or other infectious agents is much higher in a health care facility than it is at home. Nosocomial infections affect approximately 1 in 10 hospitalized patients, with an estimated annual cost of $6.7 billion per year in the United States (Graves, 2004). This is an increase of more than $2.2 billion from 1992 data provided by the Centers for Disease Control and Prevention (CDC) (1992). Dixon (1987) added that indirect costs such as loss of income are incalculable, though likely high. Various hospital and rehabilitation program accrediting bodies, such as the Joint Commission on Accreditation of Healthcare Organizations, require that facilities have ongoing, comprehensive infection control procedures in place, as part of their Patient Safety Program to maintain their accreditation. Finally, in an era of cost containment, the importance of surveillance of nosocomial infections is critical in providing quality, cost-efficient care. The CDC (1992) estimates that preventing just 6 percent of nosocomial infections would offset the cost for infection control programs in hospitals.

According to the ASHA Code of Ethics, any certified professional must not discriminate in the delivery of professional services on the basis of disability. Thus, certified professionals are required to provide services to high-risk individuals, including those with HIV. ASHA's Legislative Council passed the following resolution in 1988 (ASHA, 1989):

RESOLVED, That it is the position of the American-Speech-Language-Hearing Association that persons with HIV disease (including individuals with AIDS, ARC, and individuals who are seropositive) and those who are regarded by others as having the disease, should be entitled to civil rights protections under Section 504 of the Rehabilitation Act of 1973, as amended (LC-29-88).

INFECTION AND ITS PATHWAY

Infections are caused by microorganisms that are found on your skin, in the air and water, and/or in plants, animals, soil, and people. Some of these are *normal flora,* and others are *pathogens.* Both kinds can cause infections, particularly in people who are at high risk (Engender Health, 2005). Although infections may be acquired in any setting, those acquired *after admission* to a health care institution such as a hospital, nursing facility, psychiatric setting, or outpatient program, are called *nosocomial infections.*

The transmission of an infection follows a predictable pathway. There must be a source of infection, a means of transmission, and a susceptible host. This is referred to as the *chain of infection* (Castle & Ajemian, 1987). The source of infection may be a person, for example, the client or clinician, or it can be an inanimate object such as equipment that has been contaminated by an infected person. Thus, clinicians and clients may infect each other, or one client can infect a second client through indirect contamination of inanimate objects such as toys, a microphone, or speculum (McMillan & Willette, 1988). Clients can also infect themselves (autoinfection). There are many ways an infection can be transmitted, including (1) touching another person, particularly with your hands during assessment, intervention, or daily care; (2) touching one infected client and then using the same hand to touch the oral area of another client; (3) touching an inanimate object that has been contaminated; (4) coughing or sneezing (airborne transmission); (5) ingestion of contaminated food or water; and (6) contact or a bite from an animal or insect such as mosquitoes or fleas.

The final link in the chain of infection is the availability of a susceptible host. It is known that individuals become more vulnerable to contracting an infection when they have reduced immunological defense systems because of their illness(es) and/or malnourishment. Therapies received, such as radiation therapy and insertion of medical equipment (e.g., catheters or intravenous tubes), may also increase their susceptibility. Infants, the elderly, and those with chronic debilitating diseases are more susceptible to infection by the very nature of their frailty.

EXAMPLES OF COMMUNICABLE DISEASES

Examples of infections are so numerous that a complete discussion of all agents is beyond the scope of this chapter. Here, we consider seven common chronic communicable diseases: staphylococcal infections, hepatitis B, HIV/AIDS, cytomegalovirus, herpes, tuberculosis, scabies, and influenza.

Staphylococcal Infections

Staphylococcal infections, often called "staph," comprise a group of infections that are common in hospitals and other medical settings. Staph infections range from simple and localized skin infections such as pimples and boils to serious wounds, urinary, and bloodstream infections, and pneumonia (CDC, 2005c). Newborns, nursing mothers, and patients who have compromised immune systems are at high risk for contracting staph infections (Merck Manual, 2005). Staph infections that become resistant to antibiotics are called *methicillin-resistant staphylococcus aureus* (MERSA). While MERSA is more common in hospitals, 12 percent of the cases involve people in community settings (CDC, 2005c).

Hepatitis B Virus (HBV)

According to statistics compiled for 2003, hepatitis B virus (HBV) is a common, potentially life-threatening infection. It affects about 73,000 persons in the United States per year (CDC, 2005f). About 5,000 people die from the disease each year (CDC, 2005f). Further, the prevalence of hepatitis B is estimated to be at least 1 million persons in the United States, with costs estimated to be at least $700 million per year. HBV incubation is 120 days on average, and the onset of acute disease is insidious. HBV is transmitted via blood, during sexual activity, and

perinatally (CDC, 1999c). Symptoms include loss of appetite or anorexia, malaise, nausea, vomiting, abdominal pain, joint pain, dark urine, clay-colored bowel movements, and jaundice (Occupational Safety and Health Administration, 1992). Such symptoms, which occur in about 70 percent of patients with HBV, usually occur 9–12 weeks after exposure to the hepatitis B virus (CDC, 2005g). Individuals at high risk for harboring or contracting hepatitis B include sexually active individuals, intravenous drug users, patients of hemodialysis units, hemophiliacs, residents of some institutions for the mentally or developmentally disabled and prisons, infants born to infected mothers, and immigrants from areas of high endemicity, including east Asia, Africa, most Pacific Islands, parts of the Middle East, and the Amazon basin (OSHA, 1992; Centers for Disease Control and Prevention, 1999c). Health care workers who come in contact with blood or patient secretions containing blood are potentially among the high-risk groups for contracting HBV. It should be remembered that the risk of contracting hepatitis B is much greater than that for HIV. A preventative vaccine is available for HBV; its immunological effect remains intact for about 15 years (CDC, 2005f, 2005g).

HIV/AIDS

HIV is generally well known by the public. AIDS is the fifth leading cause of death in the United States among people ages 25 to 44 (National Center for Health Statistics, 1999). HIV precedes AIDS, and the disease may be nonsymptomatic for 10 years before AIDS diagnosis. HIV is found in blood, semen, saliva, tears, nervous system tissue, breast milk, and female genital tract secretions, though not all have been found to transmit infection to others. HIV attacks the immune system and increases susceptibility to life-threatening illnesses.

The CDC (2005a) estimates that in 2003 nearly 1.2 million persons were living with HIV/AIDS in the United States. About one quarter of those were unaware of their infection. The majority of these are individuals between 25 and 44 years of age, and the states with the highest cumulative number of cases include New York, California, Florida, and Texas. The most common causes of transmission are male-to male sexual contact and injection drug use (CDC, 2005a). By 2003, more than 524,000 persons diagnosed with AIDS had died (CDC, 2005d). To date, there is no cure for AIDS, although there is active research to develop drug treatments and prevention vaccines. Those at highest risk for contracting HIV include sexually active individuals, intravenous drug users, unborn children of an infected mother, and persons who received blood transfusions or clotting products between 1977 and 1985 (WebMD, 2006a). Transmission is through direct sexual contact and the bloodstream, not casual contact. HIV turns on a mechanism whereby the immune system self-destructs. Once turned on, the destruction continues even if the virus itself is killed.

The many symptoms of HIV/AIDS are listed in Table 21–1. Of particular interest to speech-language pathologists and audiologists are changes in speech and language, impaired cognitive functioning, and hearing loss. Communication difficulties include voice disorders related to Kaposi sarcomas in the larynx, motor speech disorders, language disorders, and general withdrawal from socialization. In addition, should the patient be intubated, an assistive communication device may be necessary (Flower & Sooy, 1987). Conductive and sensorineural hearing impairments are also common and may necessitate the use of a hearing aid or other assistive listening device (Flower, 1991). For a more in-depth discussion of HIV/AIDS and communication disorders, see Flower, 1991.

Cytomegalovirus (CMV)

Cytomegalovirus is a common infection affecting between 50 percent and 85 percent of adults in the United States by age 40 (CDC, 2002) but is most widespread in less developed areas of the world. At high risk are unborn babies of mothers infected with CMV during pregnancy, those who work with children, and those with compromised immune systems such as transplant recipients and those with HIV (ASHA, 1991; CDC, 2002). CMV is a member of the herpes virus group (cold sores, chicken pox, shingles, and mononucleosis) and the Epstein-Barr

TABLE 21–1 Symptoms of HIV/AIDS

Common Symptoms	Additional Symptoms
Prolonged, Unexplained Fatigue	Speech and Language Difficulties
Prolonged Fever	Hearing loss
Chills	Cognitive/Memory Impairment
Swollen Glands/Lymph Nodes	Visual Impairments
Joint Swelling and Bone Pain	Generalized Itching
Mouth Lesions	Chest Pain
Sore Throat	Muscle Pain
Shortness of Breath	Genital Sores
Constipation and/or Diarrhea	Numbness and Tingling
Tumor (Kaposi Sarcoma)	Cold Intolerance
Skin Rashes	
Seizures	
Weight Loss	
Malaise	
Headache	

virus, which causes infectious mononucleosis (CDC, 2002; Crawford & Studebaker, 1990). Transmission is primarily through contact with body fluids such as urine, genital secretions, and eye and nose secretions. CMV is the primary cause of congenital viral infection loss in the United States and creates a variety of problems with hearing, vision, mental abilities, and motor coordination (CDC, 2002). Once infected, the virus remains alive but dormant for life, and recurrence is rare unless the individual's immune system is compromised. There is no current treatment for CMV.

Cytomegalovirus is of concern for women of child-bearing age if they contract the disease during pregnancy (ASHA, 1991). The affected individual may appear asymptomatic or have a protracted mononucleosis-like illness. Any employed woman who is pregnant and who works with young children should be educated concerning CMV and its transmission. Women of child-bearing age may wish to be tested to determine susceptibility to CMV infection. In general, frequent hand washing and appropriate disposal of diapers helps to minimize the spread of infection.

Herpes Simplex Virus (HSV)

Herpes simplex virus (HSV) may take two forms: Type 1 (herpes labialis) usually manifests itself by infections of the lips, mouth, and face. Frequent signs include cold sores or fever blisters in the oral facial region. Most people have been infected with Type 1 virus by the age of 20. Type 1 is precipitated by overexposure to sunlight, fever, stress, and certain foods and drugs (WebMD, 2006b). Type 2 is usually associated with genital infection. Both forms of the infection may be recurrent. The virus is contagious during the blister and wet ulcer stages and can be transmitted through saliva, urine, genital secretions, or contact with broken skin or mucous membranes. Individuals with herpes labialis should refrain from working with infants, burn patients, or immunocompromised patients (Valenti, 1992). Type 2 genital herpes can be spread during vaginal delivery or sexual activity. Infected individuals should seek medical help if herpes symptoms do not resolve within a week or if there are frequent reoccurrences.

Tuberculosis (TB)

Tuberculosis (TB) is a contagious bacterial infection primarily of the lungs and is caused by mycobacterium tuberculosis (CDC, 2005i). In the mid-1980s, a resurgence of TB became evident in the United States after 30 years of decline. The resurgence is attributed to the increase in antibiotic-resistant strains of the disease, the HIV epidemic, an increase in the number of homeless individuals, an increase in immigration from Asian countries, physician nonadherence in prescribing the recommended drug regimen, and few resources for prevention and care. Although TB can affect anyone of any age, it more often is seen in older people who have been exposed to tuberculosis and immuno-compromised individuals. Fortunately, in the United States, the estimated rate of TB cases has seen a steady drop from during the late 1990s and early years of the 21st century (National Center for Health Statistics, 2004).

Populations most at risk for incurring tuberculosis are those living with the consequences of poverty, such as poor nutrition, poor ventilation, crowding, and poor hygiene. Other individuals with weakened immune systems and who are at high risk include those with substance abuse, diabetes, silicosis, cancer of the head or neck, leukemia, and those on specialized treatments for rheumatoid arthritis or Crohn's disease (CDC, 2005i). Of particular concern is that the tuberculosis rate of nursing facility patients is four times higher than that of age-matched community residents (WebMD, 2006d; Boscia, 1986).

According to the CDC (2005i), TB bacteria can attack any part of the body, including the kidney, spine, brain, and lungs. People in the latent stage of the disease do not usually become sick; in the active stage, TB is spread via airborne droplets from sneezes or coughs. Once in the lungs, the bacteria travel to other parts of the body. The primary symptoms of pulmonary tuberculosis are coughing, which spreads the mycobacterium tuberculosis through the air; fatigue; night sweats; chills; coughing up blood; low-grade fever; and weight loss (CDC, 2005i). Should you work in a hospital or nursing home, an annual tuberculosis screening may be mandatory. This may include one or more of the following tests: chest X-ray, sputum cultures, and the tuberculin skin test (WebMD, 2006c). Individuals with latent TB infection will have a positive skin test but a normal chest x-ray and sputum test. Those with active TB can spread the disease to others; they will have a positive skin test and an abnormal chest X-ray or positive sputum test (CDC, 2005i). Treatment for the infection includes a program of medications. Compliance with the medication program is essential because noncompliance leading to treatment failure may result in drug resistance, relapse, increasing disability, and death (Hellman & Gram, 1993). Symptoms often improve within 2 to 3 weeks, although the prescribed medication program must be followed for a lengthy period of time.

Scabies

Scabies is an infectious skin rash caused by infestation with the mite Sarcoptes scabiei. Transmission is through prolonged skin-to-skin contact with an infected individual and may be spread by sharing clothing, towels, and bedding. A quick handshake is unlikely to spread the infestation. Scabies spreads quickly in crowded settings such as hospitals, nursing homes, and child care centers. Again, those with compromised immune systems and the elderly are at risk. Symptoms include pimplelike irritations; burrows or rash on the skin, especially between the fingers and in skin folds throughout the body; intense itching, especially at night; and sores caused by scratching (CDCs, 2005e). It may take 4 to 6 weeks for symptoms to appear for those who have never been infected and only a few days for those with previous infestation. Control measures include mass cleaning of patient bedding, clothing, and food trays, and skin application of a pesticide, usually lindane, for all employees or others who have come in contact with the infected individual (Sherertz & Hampton, 1987). Universal precautions include adequate hand washing, gloving, and gowning, which are essential when working with an infected client (Polder, Tablan, & Williams, 1992).

Influenza Viruses

Influenza, or the "flu," is a highly contagious infection of the respiratory tract. It usually occurs from late fall to early spring. Flu affects all age groups, and its severity can range from mild to severe illness. Each year 20,000 Americans, most of them elderly, die from influenza or secondary complications. Symptoms include some combination of fever, chills, muscle aches and pain, sweating, dry cough, nasal congestion, runny nose, diarrhea, sore throat, headache, malaise, and fatigue (CDC, 2004). Flu spreads in the respiratory droplets of an infected individual who may or not show active flu symptoms. It is especially important to prevent transmission of type A and type B influenza viruses to high-risk groups such as the elderly and patients of all ages with chronic cardiac, pulmonary, renal, or metabolic diseases. Outbreaks of influenza in acute care and chronic care hospitals as well as nursing homes can have serious health care and morbidity implications. Prevention includes yearly vaccine immunization and measures to limit the spread of the disease, including universal precautions such as frequent hand washing, covering your mouth and nose with a tissue when you cough or sneeze, appropriate disposal of tissues, restrictive admission to a facility, separation of infected patients, and prohibition of individuals with respiratory symptoms from visiting high-risk patients (CDC, 2004; Fedson, 1987). Should you contract influenza, it is critical that you check with your employer's infection control personnel for guidelines regarding client contact. Some physicians may prescribe antiviral medications, and all will recommend rest and plenty of liquids.

A new form of influenza, called *avian influenza* or *bird flu*, is a specific type of Influenza A that is spread by infected birds and has seen an increase since 1997. Although rare, the CDC (2005h) recommends that anyone traveling to Asian countries where there are known outbreaks of bird flu avoid poultry farms, contact with animals in farm markets, and surfaces that may be contaminated by poultry or other animals. Research is currently underway on a vaccine for some subtypes of the bird flu.

PROGRAM FOR INFECTION PREVENTION

Most settings in which you practice as a speech-language pathologist or audiologist will have an infection prevention program in place. The general purpose of such programs is to minimize the potential of infection transmission to clients and staff members. Although plans differ according to settings, certain commonalities exist across infection prevention programs. Staff need to (a) be aware of potential risks associated with their settings and professional procedures; (b) know their institutional and departmental infection prevention management plans for minimizing infection spread; (c) know how to implement the infection prevention management plan; (d) know how to modify the plan to meet individual situations; and (e) know when and to whom to report incidents. Common barriers to implementing prevention programs include staff underestimating the risks involved; lack of knowledge of appropriate infection prevention practices and their role in implementing this program; and inadequate supplies, equipment, and space in low-resource settings (Engender Health, 2005).

Should you work in a health care institution such as a hospital or nursing home, there will be a multidisciplinary Infection Control Committee (ICC) responsible for reducing the occurrence of infections through the establishment and monitoring of general policies and procedures for infection control. These rules usually emanate from standards established by federal and state governments and agencies, professional organizations, and accreditation agencies such as JCAHO. The ICC is charged with approving programs of prevention and investigating, reporting, and monitoring infections (Castle & Ajemian, 1987). In addition to complying with

general infection prevention procedures established for the entire institution, individual departments such as Speech-Language Pathology or Audiology will be required to state in writing specific policies and procedures for assuring infection prevention during their contact with clients. See Chapter 19 on Policies and Procedures.

Settings other than hospitals should also have infection prevention programs. For example, home health care programs, educational settings, private practices, and community speech, language, or hearing clinics should each have and implement a systematic written program for ensuring to the highest extent possible the prevention of infection transmission between staff and clients or among clients. Committees similar to the ICC implement and monitor the infection prevention program and provide orientation and continuing education on this topic for all staff.

Preemployment Screening and Follow-Up

A preemployment medical evaluation is one of the requirements of employment in most organizations and certainly in all health care institutions. The purpose of this examination is to identify any individual who may serve as a source of an infectious agent and, therefore, compromise clients, staff, or families with whom they would come in contact. The most important aspects of the screening focus on identification of rubella, hepatitis B, and tuberculosis (Castle & Ajemian, 1987). The preemployment evaluation usually includes a communicable disease history, a history of immunization, and a physical examination. Most organizations also have established policies for immunizations, yearly medical reevaluations, protocols for documentation of employees exposed to communicable diseases, and guidelines for a return to work for these individuals. Information regarding such protocols can be found in your employee handbook or from your institution's infection prevention committee.

Prior to employment and periodically, you will likely need to show evidence of a negative response to the Mantoux skin test for tuberculosis. You may know this test by the acronym PPD for the type of tuberculin used in the test. Two to 3 days after the injection, your arm will be examined and the reaction area measured. In some health care settings, you may be required to take the two-step Mantoux test, which involves testing of the opposite arm 1 to 3 weeks later. In both cases, if there is a positive response, you must check with your primary care physician for a chest X-ray. Keep a copy of all reports in your records and provide one for your employer.

Orientation and Training in Infection Prevention

One of the first tasks you will be required to complete upon employment in most institutions is to participate in a general orientation. Part of this orientation will be devoted to understanding infection prevention needs and protocols along with other protocols aimed at ensuring a healthy and safe work environment. During this orientation, you will become familiar with the management or hygiene plan designed for your department, its rationale, and specific ways to implement the plan into daily practice. In-service education programs to update an existing hygiene plan will also occur as needs arise.

Hygiene Plan

The hygiene plan designed for your department will focus on creating an environment with every reasonable effort made to limit exposure to infectious agents. Potential infectious agents include all body fluids; blood, semen, drainage from scrapes and cuts, feces, urine, vomitus, respiratory secretions, and saliva, along with anything that has come in contact with body fluids (e.g., bandages, prostheses, and instruments). In general, hygiene plans will have as their cornerstone the adoption of *universal precautions*. The underlying premise of *universal precautions* is that one adopts practices that minimize and, if possible, eliminate the risk of transmitting any infection, whether potential or actual. Thus, every clinician, including trainees, working with every client in every setting must assume a preventive

approach to reducing infection transmission. A universal approach to clients ensures that all are treated equally, without discrimination, and with confidentiality regarding their medical status.

Hygiene Plan Techniques

The hygiene plan techniques presented here focus on what you can do to help prevent the transmission of an infectious disease. The first technique discussed, hand washing, is considered the most basic approach to infection prevention. Other techniques include barrier techniques such as the use of gloves, masks, gowns, and lab coats. Finally, sterilization and disinfection are discussed as additional priority methods.

Hand Washing There is no substitute for hand washing in the prevention of infection transmission. Although this is a simple and cost-effective means of preventing the spread of infectious agents to noncontaminated areas and personnel, it is estimated that health care workers wash their hands only about half the time they should (Engender Health, 2005). The goal of hand washing is to reduce as much as possible the presence of contaminating organisms on hands that touch clients or objects in the environment that might be contaminated. Simply, you should wash your hands thoroughly with plain or antiseptic soap and running water before and after contact with each client, even when gloves are worn. The use of liquid soaps is preferred over bar soap. A general minimum guideline for hand washing is 10 seconds, or the amount of time it takes to sing one stanza of "Happy Birthday." Wearing gloves does not negate the need for hand washing. Table 21–2 lists guidelines for when to wash hands, and Table 21–3 lists the recommended steps in washing hands. Should water conservation be an issue in your geographical area, adaptations in the continuous flow of water will be needed. If you do not have access to a water source, you can use disposable antiseptic wipes or alcohol-based hand rubs or gels. Any wipes should be disposed of properly. Be sure to use an emollient lotion after the use of alcohol-based rubs to balance their drying effect.

T A B L E 21–2 Guidelines on When to Wash Hands

- Upon arrival at work.

- Immediately, if they are potentially contaminated with blood or body fluids.

- Between patients.

- After removing gloves.

- Before and after handling inpatient care devices.

- Before preparing or serving food.

- Before and after performing any personal body function.

- When hands are obviously soiled, such as after sneezing, blowing one's nose, or using the bathroom.

- After changing diapers.

- Before leaving your work setting.

- For isolation patients, before removing gown and mask and after removing gown and mask.

SOURCE: American Speech-Language-Hearing Association. (1989). AIDS/HIV: Report: Implications for speech-language pathologists and audiologists. *ASHA, 29,* 33–37. Reprinted with permission.

T A B L E 21–3 Hand Washing Steps

- Remove all jewelry, except for plain wedding bands.

- Obtain paper towel from dispenser.

- Slightly lean forward over sink and avoid touching sink.

- Turn on water to comfortably warm level.

- Wet hands and forearms.

- Apply liquid antiseptic soap.

- Vigorously wash hands, wrists, and forearms, weaving fingers and thumbs together for 30–60 seconds.

- Thoroughly rinse forearms, wrists, and hands.

- Dry hands, then wrist and forearm using a paper towel.

- Avoid rubbing hands too hard to create chapping.

- Use clean paper towel to turn off the faucet and turn the doorknobs if foot or electronic controls are not available.

- Dispose of all paper towels in an appropriate container.

- Use emollient to decrease the risk of skin cracking.

SOURCES: American Speech-Language-Hearing Association. (1989). AIDS/HIV: Report: Implications for speech-language pathologists and audiologists. *ASHA, 29,* 33–37; Palmer, M. (1984). *Infection control: A policy and procedure manual.* Philadephia: W.B. Saunders. Reprinted with permission.

The two most common hand-drying techniques recommended are the use of disposable paper towels and hand dryers. Towels should be disposed of properly and not reused.

Barrier Techniques: Gloves, Masks, Gowns, Shoe Covers, and Lab Coats Gloves, masks, gowns, and lab coats, otherwise known as *personal protective equipment (PPE),* are used to prevent the possibility of transmitting airborne or spattered infectious agents such as droplets of blood or other body fluids onto your skin or clothes. Gloves provide a barrier, though not an impermeable one, to microorganisms that may be transmitted between client and clinician. Wearing gloves becomes particularly important during an oral-facial examination, during middle ear testing, when handling or fabricating ear molds and other prostheses, during swallowing assessments and therapies, and during assessments of respiratory and laryngeal functioning. Gloves should be worn during each of these tasks. Speech-language pathologists and audiologists are most likely to use single use (disposable), nonsterile gloves. Palmer (1984) suggests that the method for putting on disposable, nonsterile gloves should be as consistent as the methods for sterile gloves. If nonsterile gloves are used, hands should be washed before and after gloving. All gloves should be changed before each new client contact. Finally, gloves should be discarded in a properly marked container after each use or when torn during contact with a client.

An acceptable method for putting on nonsterile gloves when no gown is used is recommended by Palmer (1984). Remember not to touch any surface with a contaminated glove that you will later touch without gloves, such as, doorknobs, telephones, and pens. Failure to take this precaution may result in harmful exposure to disease to you and your coworkers and clients. Palmer (1984) provides the following guidelines for gloving.

- Wash and dry hands first.
- Grasp the inside of the right glove with left hand.
- Insert the right hand into glove and pull glove on.
- Place the left hand into the left glove and pull glove on.
- Remove gloves by pulling the contaminated outer side in onto itself.
- Discard gloves in appropriate place.
- Wash and dry hands after gloves are removed.

Remember that masks should only be worn once, donned prior to gown or gloves, and discarded when they become moist. Palmer (1984) suggests

the strings must be tied securely for a snug fit. "If you wear glasses, the mask should fit snugly over your nose and under the edge of your glasses to prevent fogging" (p. 57). Your hands should be washed before and after removing the mask. Isolation gowns must be worn when working with an infected patient or when a patient is in protective isolation. In donning a gown, touch only the inside of the gown. Shoe covers also may be required in isolation areas. All of these protective clothing items should be disposed of in proper containers. Finally, if washable lab coats are used, they should be changed daily or as needed throughout a day, if contaminated. Otherwise, you should use disposable gowns and, after use, dispose of them properly. The Occupational Safety and Health Administration (1992) mandates that any clothing worn as personal protective equipment should be laundered, maintained, or disposed of by the employer and not sent home with the employee for cleaning.

Decontamination: Cleaning, Disinfection, and Sterilization There are three levels of decontamination in infection control. The lowest level of decontamination includes alcohol wipes, mild detergent soap, or agents such as hydrogen peroxide. This type of decontamination is not sufficient for cleaning instruments or contaminated services in a clinical setting (Golper, 1998). Contaminated surfaces need at least moderate decontamination, requiring disinfecting agents. Disinfection and sterilization typically begin with cleaning the surface to remove any obvious foreign material from objects through washing. This step normally precedes both disinfection and sterilization (Rutala, 1987).

Sterilization is considered to be the highest level of decontamination. Sterilization entails a complete destruction of microorganisms and their spores through physical or chemical processes (Rutala, 1987). Sterilization is necessary for any surgical instrument or device or any object that will be used from one patient to another and potentially carries body fluids. Sterlization can be done by use of a steam autoclave, dry heat oven, chemical vapor sterilization, or immersion in a chemical agent (such as Cidex) for

10 hours. Items such as impedance probe tips, oto-scopic specula, and other heat-sensitive instruments must be cleansed of debris prior to being sterilized in a chemical agent, while solid metal items, such as laryngeal mirrors can be sterilized by the first methods (McMillan & Willette, 1988).

Disinfection is a lower level of decontamination than sterilization but will sufficiently destroy most organisms on clinical surfaces. Disinfection involves cleaning objects and the surfaces of materials and furniture touched by a client and staff. Materials include all therapy materials, toys, games, and other items used in assessment or therapy. All surfaces of table tops, chairs, and chair arms should be disinfected after each use. All equipment or materials used during an evaluation that are not inserted in the oral cavity should be disinfected after each use. Metal surfaces should be cleaned by using a registered germicide, and nonmetal surfaces can be disinfected with a solution of household bleach at a 1:10 dilution with water. The items should be sprayed, vigorously washed, lightly misted again, and left moist (McMillan & Willette, 1988). Any used paper towels should be disposed of in proper containers. It is important to point out that the use of any cleaning, disinfection, or sterilization of materials or equipment should adhere to the manufacturers' instructions. Additionally, you should note that cleaning agents or other chemical products can pose a hazard to employee health through skin or aerosol exposure; thus, organizations are required to tell all employees what chemicals are present in their environment. Your facility will have a Material Safety Data Sheets (MSDS) notebook containing a chemical fact sheet on all chemicals in your work area (everything from "White Out" to disinfecting agents), and you will be asked to verify that you have reviewed the MSDS notebook in your area and are aware of the appropriate steps to take should you have a reaction to these agents.

Toys Toys are such a common part of our interaction with pediatric clients that special mention should be made about their place in infection prevention. Whenever possible, use toys that have washable surfaces, especially when working with children in diapers. If possible, each group of children should have their own toys. Avoid furry or fabric dolls and stuffed animals. All toys, game boards and pieces, materials, and furniture should be washed and disinfected after each assessment or therapy session. Toys that have been mouthed by a child should be isolated immediately from other children and then properly washed and disinfected before continued use with other children. See Chapter 16 on early intervention for suggestions on toys.

Regulated Waste Containers

Your setting will have specific guidelines for what is considered "regulated waste" in that agency. OSHA (1992) defines regulated waste as liquid or semiliquid blood or other potentially infectious material (OPIM), items contaminated with blood or OPIM, contaminated sharp objects (sharps), and pathological and microbiological wastes containing blood or OPIM. Individual containers for such regulated waste must be closable, suitable to contain the type of materials enclosed, to prevent leakage, and labeled with the biohazard symbol or color coded (usually red) to warn employees of the potential hazards within. Local and state laws govern where and how regulated wastes will be disposed. You should check with your department's policy and procedure manual section on infection prevention as to appropriate disposal methods for items you use.

ISSUES OF SPECIAL CONCERN

There are three special issues you should be aware of regarding infection control. First, the settings in which we work pose particular infection prevention challenges. The second issue addresses the special needs of female speech-language pathologists or audiologists who work during childbearing years. These professionals should be aware of the relationship of infection prevention and pregnancy. The final issue addressed is how to report a possible infection exposure incident.

Educational Settings

A practical issue that arises in an educational setting such as a public school is how to apply universal precautions. Keep in mind that there are more students attending schools with compromised health than ever before. Hand washing between students may not be easily available or possible because of the location of a therapy room or inability to leave a child or children unsupervised in a room while you go to another room for washing. When possible, the speech-language pathologist or audiologist in this setting should seek a room with or very near hand-washing facilities. A possible alternative to hand washing is to cleanse hands with disposable antiseptic wipes. Hand washing with soap and water should be done as soon as possible thereafter. Professionals in education should be acutely aware of the need to disinfect tables, chairs, and clinical materials between use and appropriate disposal of gloves, tongue blades, or any other potentially infected clinical materials. It is also important that any cleaning materials be kept out of the reach of children at all times.

Long-Term Care Facilities

Although less attention has been paid to nosocomial infections in long-term care facilities (LTCF) compared with acute care hospitals, the 1.6 million resident population in this setting is considered a high-risk group. The increased risk for nosocomial infections among this population is related to living in close quarters, participation in numerous group activities, malnutrition and dehydration, underlying systemic diseases, use of indwelling devices such as catheters, immobility, fecal incontinence, impaired cognitive skills, decreased ability to maintain personal hygiene, and frequent use of multiple medications, including sedatives and tranquilizers (Garibaldi & Nurse, 1992; Gross & Levine, 1987). Ambulatory residents who may be incontinent or coughing also serve as a possible means for spreading infections (Infections in Long-Term Care, 1999). Risk also increases because of decreased staffing and staff who may be unaware of infection prevention procedures. According to the CDC (2005b), at least 250,000 nursing home residents have infections, two out of three receive at least one course of antibiotics annually, and 27,000 have antibiotic-resistant infections. In a study of more than 500 nursing home residents, the most common types included infected decubitus ulcers, conjunctivitis, urinary tract infections, gastroenteritis, and respiratory infections such as influenza, tuberculosis, and pneumonia. It should be noted that the mortality rate for pneumonia among LTCF residents is significantly higher than that of community-based elders.

The high prevalence of nosocomial infections among LTCF residents may be due to the low turnover rate of residents, the high ratio of patients to staff, lack of compensation to staff for sick leave, inadequate immunization requirements, and frequent turnover of nonprofessional employees. Infections that occur at epidemic rates in LTCFs include respiratory tract infections, gastroenteritis, and urinary tract infections (Garibaldi & Nurse, 1992; Infections in Long-Term Care, 1999). Thus, if you work in this setting, consider the higher possibility of transmitting an infection to or contracting one from the population of the institution.

Day Care Centers

Children attending day care centers or nursery programs are at increased risk for contracting and transmitting a variety of diseases (Sherertz & Hampton, 1987). The reasons why infections may spread so easily in this setting are similar to those discussed for nursing home settings. Professionals who work in these settings or whose own children attend them should be aware of the increased potential for contracting and transmitting infections. Of particular concern in day care centers is the issue of proper diapering techniques. The Fountain Valley School District, Fountain Valley, California, provides the following guidelines for diapering and suggests that similar guidelines be used with children who use potty chairs. Be sure to wear gloves during this procedure and dispose of them and the diaper in accordance with your setting's guidelines.

- The professional puts on disposable gloves.
- The child lays on a disposable towel.
- The soiled diaper touches only your hands.
- The diaper is disposed in a plastic bag to be taken home or to an appropriate receptacle.
- There is proper cleansing of the child's bottom.
- There is proper disposal of the wash cloth or towelette.
- The child's hands are washed.
- The diapering area and equipment are cleaned and disinfected.
- The caregiver's gloves are disposed of properly.
- The caregiver's hands are washed thoroughly.

A second concern in day care centers is how to identify a child who is too ill to remain at the center or in need of immediate medical attention. An in-depth discussion of this topic is beyond the scope of this chapter. The reader is referred to an excellent resource, *What You Can Do to Stop Disease in the Child Day Care Center* (CDC, 1984).

SUMMARY

An important aspect of risk management in any work setting is to prevent the transmission of infectious disease. It is your responsibility to understand the risks involved and know and implement universal precautions. The source of an infection can be people, objects, or surfaces (toys, doorknobs, keyboards, phones). Infections are spread through direct contact with the body fluids of another person, through cross-contamination involving the clinician as the means of transmission, from one client to another, through airborne transmission of agents, or through indirect contact with contaminated surfaces of objects. The best precaution to prevent infection transmission is to adhere to

Staff Who Are Pregnant

Staff members who are pregnant may be concerned about contracting an infection that may affect their unborn child. Infections that have the greatest potential for affecting a fetus include those due to rubella, enterovirus, hepatitis B, syphilis, toxoplasma, cytomegalovirus, and varicella. Women who are pregnant should discuss their potential risk for contracting infections in their workplace with their personal physician and the infection prevention personnel in their facilities.

Reporting Exposure Incidents

According to OSHA (1992), you should immediately report any situation in which you have been exposed to a potentially infectious agent. Early reporting will help you receive the medical care you may need, help prevent the spread of the infection to others, and assist your employer in assessing the situation surrounding the exposure incident in an effort to prevent further occurrences. Your employer must provide you with a free medical evaluation and treatment if the exposure occurred during your employment. Again, should you be exposed to a potentially infectious agent, check with your departmental policy and procedure manual for specific guidelines for how and to whom to report the incident.

universal precautions with all clients, regardless of known or unknown pathology. Universal precautions include routine vigorous hand washing before and after client contact; appropriate use and disposal of gloves, masks, and gowns; application of barrier techniques, and proper disinfection/sterilization of clinical tools and materials. The ASHA Code of Ethics requires its speech-language pathologists or audiologists members provide appropriate services to individuals with known infectious disease. Confidentiality regarding protected health information must always be maintained. Remember that infection prevention is a necessary component of quality service delivery.

CRITICAL THINKING

1. Consider your present employment or training setting. What routine precautions do you take to prevent the transmission of infections? How did you learn about these precautions?

2. Why is hand washing one of the best ways to prevent transmission of infections? Practice proper hand-washing techniques.

3. Suppose you worked with a colleague who had a severe cold and cold sores around the lip area. You notice that the coworker does not observe any special precautions to prevent the transmission of her infections to pediatric clients. What would you do?

4. You work in a hospital at which you frequently get referrals to assess patients with AIDS. What ethical and legal issues should you consider in working with these patients?

5. What are some populations and settings that are high risk for infection transmission? Why is the risk higher with these populations?

6. Suppose one of your clients who has a cold coughs and sneezes repeatedly during a session in your presence. What should you do?

7. What infection precautions should you take if you work in early intervention and provide services in children's homes? How would you explain the rationale for your procedures to the family?

REFERENCES

Adam.coy. WebMD. (1999).

American Speech-Language-Hearing Association. (1989). AIDS/HIV: Report: Implications for speech-language pathologists and audiologists. *Asha, 29,* 33–37.

American Speech-Language-Hearing Association. (1991). Chronic communicable diseases and risk management in the schools. *Language, Speech, and Hearing Services in Schools, 22,* 345–352.

Boscia, J. (1986). Epidemiology of bacteriuria in an elderly ambulatory population. *American Journal of Medicine, 80,* 208–212.

Castle, M., & Ajemian, E. (1987). *Hospital infection control: Principles and practice.* New York: John Wiley and Sons.

Centers for Disease Control and Prevention. (1984). *What you can do to stop disease in child day care centers.* Washington, DC: Author

Centers for Disease Control and Prevention. (1992). Public health focus: Surveillance, prevention and control of nosocomial infections. *Morbidity and Mortality Weekly Report, 41,* 783–787.

Centers for Disease Control and Prevention. (1999a). *AIDS/HIV.* Available at http://www.cdc.gov/nchs/fastats/aids-hiv

Centers for Disease Control and Prevention and Prevention. (1999b). *HIV/AIDS Surveillance Report 1999, 11*(1), 1–44.

Centers for Disease Control and Prevention. (1999c). Viral hepatitis B-fact sheet. Available at http://www.cdc.gov/ncidod/diseases/hepatitis/b/fact/htm

Centers for Disease Control and Prevention. (2002). Cytomegalovirus (CMV) infection. Available at http://www.cdc.gov/cmv/

Centers for Disease Control and Prevention. (2004). Key facts about the flu: How to prevent the flu and what to do if you get sick. Washington, DC: Department of Health and Human Services.

Centers for Disease Control and Prevention. (2005a). Basic statistics HIV/AIDs. Available at http://www.cdc.gov/hiv/stats.htm

Centers for Disease Control and Prevention. (2005b). Burden of infections among U.S. nursing home residents. Available at http://www.cdc.gov/drugresistance/healthcare/ltc.htm

Centers for Disease Control and Prevention. (2005c). CA-MRSA Information for the public. Available at http://www.cdc.gov/ncidod/hip/Aresist/ca_mrsa_public.htm

Centers for Disease Control and Prevention. (2005d). Estimated numbers of deaths of persons with AIDS, by year of death and selected characteristics. Available at www.cdc.gov/hiv/stats/2003SurveillanceReport/table7.htm

Centers for Disease Control and Prevention. (2005e). Fact sheet scabies. Available at http://www.cdc.gov/ncidod/dpd/parasites/scabies/factsht_scabies.htm

Centers for Disease Control and Prevention. (2005f). Hepatitis B fact sheet. Available at http://www.cdc.gov/hepatitis

Centers for Disease Control and Prevention. (2005g). Hepatitis B frequently asked questions. Available at http://www.cdc.gov/ncidod/diseases/hepatitis.b/faqb.htm

Centers for Disease Control and Prevention. (2005h). Information about avian influenza (bird flu) and avian influenza A (H5N1) virus. Washington, DC: Department of Health and Human Services.

Centers for Disease Control and Prevention. (2005i). Questions and answers about TB 2005. Available at http://www.cdc.gov/nchstp/tb/faqs/qa_introduction.htm

Crawford, M., & Studebaker, G. (1990). Cytomegalovirus: A disease of hearing. *The Hearing Journal, 43,* 25–30.

Dixon, R. (1987). Costs of nosocomial infections and benefits of infection control programs. In R. Wenzel (Ed.), *Prevention and control of nosocomial infections* (pp. 19–25). Baltimore, MD: Williams and Wilkins.

Engender Health. (2005). Importance of good infection prevention practices. Available at http://www.engenderhealth.org/ip/disease/dt2html

Fedson, D. (1987). Immunizations for health care workers and patients in hospitals. In R. Wenzel (Ed.), *Prevention and control of nosocomial infections* (pp. 116–174). Baltimore, MD: Williams and Wilkins.

Flower, W. (1991). Communication problems in patients with AIDS. In J. Mukand (Ed.), *Rehabilitation for patients with HIV disease.* New York: McGraw-Hill.

Flower, W., & Sooy, C. (1987). AIDS: An introduction for speech-language pathologists and audiologists. *Asha, 27,* 25–30.

Fuchs, P. (1979). *Epidemiology of hospital associated infections.* Chicago: American Society of Clinical Pathologists.

Garibaldi, R. L., & Nurse, B. (1992). Infections in nursing homes. In J. Bennett & P. Brachmann (Eds.), *Hospital infections* (pp. 491–532). Boston: Little, Brown.

Golper, L. A.C. (1998). *Sourcebook for medical speech pathology* (2nd ed.). San Diego, CA: Singular Publishing Group.

Graves, J. (2004). Economics and preventing hospital-acquired infection. Emerging Infectious Diseases, v.10, 561–566. Available at http://www.cdc.gov/eid

Gross, P., & Levine, J. (1987). Infections in the elderly. In R. Wenzel (Ed.), *Prevention and control of nosocomial infections.* Baltimore, MD: Williams and Wilkins.

Hellman, S., & Gram, M. (1993). The resurgence of tuberculosis. *American Association of Occupational Health Nurses Journal, 41,* 66–71.

Infections in Long-Term Care. (1999). Available at http://www.nih.gov/ninr/vol3/Infection.html

McMillan, M., & Willette, S. (1988). Aseptic technique: A procedure for preventing disease transmission in the practice environment. *Asha, 31,* 35–37.

Merck. (2005). Staphylococcal infections. The Merck Manual. Available at http://www.merck.com/

National Center for Health Statistics. (1999). *National vital statistics reports* (v. 27). Hyattsville, MD: Author

National Center for Health Statistics. (2004). *National vital statistics reports* (v. 52) Hyattsville, MD: Author.

National Institute of Allergy and Infectious Diseases. (1999). HIV/AIDs statistics. Available at http://www.niad.niah.gov/factsheets/aisstat.htm

Occupational Safety and Health Administration Fact Sheet. (1992). Washington, DC: Author.

Palmer, M. (1984). *Infection control: A policy and procedure manual.* Philadephia: W.B. Saunders.

Polder, J., Tablan, O., & Williams, W. (1992). Personnel health services. In J. Bennett & P. Brachman (Eds.), *Hospital infections.* Boston: Little, Brown.

Rutala, W. (1987). Disinfection, sterilization, and waste disposal. In R. Wenzel (Ed.), *Prevention and control of nosocomial infections* (pp. 257–282). Baltimore, MD: Williams and Wilkins.

Sherertz, R., & Hampton, A. (1987). Infection control aspects of hospital employee health. In R. Wenzel (Ed.), *Prevention and control of nosocomial infections* (pp. 116–174). Baltimore, MD: Williams and Wilkins.

U. S. Government Manual. (1992/1993). Washington, DC: Office of the Federal Register National Archives and Records Administrations.

Valenti, P. (1992). Selected viruses of nosocomial importance. In J. Bennett & P. Brachman (Eds.), *Hospital infections* (pp. 789–822). Boston: Little, Brown.

WebMD. (2006a) HIV, AIDS; and Older People. Available at www.webmd.com.

WebMD. (2006b) Skin Conditions: Herpes Simplex Viruses. Available at www.webmd.com.

WebMD. (2006c) Tuberculosis Exam Tests. Available at www.webmd.com.

WebMD. (2006d) Tuberculosis What increases your Risk. Available at www.webmd.com.

RESOURCES

Centers for Disease Control and Prevention (CDC)
1600 Clifton Road
Atlanta, GA, 30333
Phone: 404-629-3291.
Web site: http:// www.cdc.gov

Established in 1973, the Centers for Disease Control and Prevention is a federal agency within the United States Public Health Service. The CDC is responsible for national programs aimed at prevention and control of communicable and airborne diseases and other preventable conditions. The agency is composed of nine major divisions that consult with related state and local health programs; develop programs for chronic disease prevention, environmental health, and occupational safety and health; and focus on research, education, information, and epidemiological data collection and analysis. The agency also provides international consultation on these topics.

The CDC can issue recommendations but is not a standard-setting body (U.S. Government Manual, 1992/1993).

Occupational Safety and Health Administration:
U.S. Labor Department
200 Constitution Avenue,
N.W. Washington, DC 20210
Web site: http:// www.osha.gov/

Part of the United States Labor Department, the Occupational Safety and Health Administration (OSHA) develops policies, disseminates information, and enforces occupational safety and health standards. This agency also determines compliance with occupational safety and health standards through inspections and determines and enforces penalties for noncompliance (U.S. Government Manual, 1992/1993).

22

Child Abuse and Elder Mistreatment

ROSEMARY LUBINSKI, EDD

SCOPE OF CHAPTER

Some time during your employment as an audiologist or speech-language pathologist, you may suspect that a child or elder client is a victim of abuse or neglect. Depending on the state in which you are employed, you will have either a professional and/or a mandated obligation to report incidences of suspected abuse. This chapter presents broad definitions and characteristics of various types of child abuse, possible causes for such mistreatment, scope of the problem, and suggestions for what to do when indicators may be present. Similarly, various types of elder abuse and neglect are discussed. This chapter is intended to supplement and not replace individual state definitions, procedures, or requirements for course work on these topics.

CHILD ABUSE AND NEGLECT

Clinicians must be able to identify the signs and symptoms of child abuse and neglect. In addition, you need to be aware of the potential causes and factors that put a child at risk for these forms of maltreatment. Finally, you need to know who may act as an abuser and how common child abuse and neglect are in our society.

Child Abuse

Broadly defined, child abuse occurs when a child under 18 years of age is physically or mentally harmed by a parent or other person legally responsible for his or her care. This may involve physical injury by other than accidental means, sexual offense against the child, or allowing the child to engage in such acts. Physical abuse involves the use of force, such as striking, beating, pushing, shoving, shaking, slapping, kicking, pinching, or burning that result in injury, pain, or impairment. The abuse may or may not be executed with an object. The unjustifiable use of drugs and physical restraints may also be considered physical abuse.

Child abuse may also include other forms of neglect such as malnutrition, dehydration, psychological mistreatment, and failure to treat mental or physical ills that may impair growth and development. Emotional abuse, also called *mental cruelty*, *emotional neglect*, or *emotional maltreatment*, occurs when there is some type of nonphysical actions toward a child that result in psychological stress and may lead to physical or psychological illness. This may be caused by threatening a child verbally or nonverbally, terrorizing, isolating or placing the child in a closed confinement, withholding nurturance and affection, and knowingly permitting the child's maladaptive behavior. Table 22–1 describes potential types and indicators of child abuse and neglect.

Maltreatment and Neglect

Maltreatment occurs when a child under 18 years of age is neglected or has serious physical injury inflicted on him or her by other than accidental means. The parent or other person legally responsible for care has not provided a minimum degree of care and the child's physical, mental, emotional, or educational well-being has been or is in danger of being impaired. Neglect is considered an act of omission. For example, the responsible adult has not provided the child with adequate nutrition, clothing, shelter, protection from safety hazards, personal hygiene, or education although financially able to do so or offered means to do so. Neglect also occurs when the responsible adult has not provided the child with proper supervision or guardianship. This may occur when this individual inflicts or allows harm to be inflicted, places the child at risk of harm, uses excessive corporal punishment, or uses substances that impair self-control.

A child who has been abandoned by his or her parents or other legally responsible person is also considered neglected. Emotional neglect occurs when there is a "state of substantially diminished psychological or intellectual functioning in relation to, but not limited to such factors as failure to thrive, control of aggression or self-destructive impulses, ability to think and reason, or acting out and misbehavior" (Center for Development of Human Services at Buffalo State College, nd, p. 17). Such neglect may cause children to be permanently damaged or may be responsible for more deaths per year than abuse.

Causes and Risks

There are numerous, interrelated possible causes of and risk factors for child abuse and neglect. Table 22–2 lists four major categories that include parent/caretaker characteristics, parent-child relationship characteristics, child characteristics, and environmental factors. It should be noted that these are *potential* risk factors, and the presence of any one is not an absolute predictor of child abuse or neglect. Further, it is likely these factors are not mutually exclusive and do not all arise within the parent/caregiver. Finally, causes and risk factors must be considered within a framework of a cultural background of child-rearing practices, and economic and political values.

Several of these factors bear more discussion. First, 40 percent of physical abuse of children is caused by persons who themselves were abused as

T A B L E 22–1 Types and Potential Indicators of Child Abuse and Neglect

Possible Signs of Physical Abuse

- Unexplained bruises or welts in different places, clusters, in various stages of healings, and/or in shape of instrument used
- Unexplained burns
- Unexplained lacerations or abrasions
- Unexplained skeletal injuries, for example, bites, fracture, bald spots, detached retina
- Inappropriate clothing for weather to conceal injuries
- Extremes in behavior—aggressive to withdrawn
- Easily frightened or fearful—for example, of parents, adults, physical contact, going home, or when other children cry
- Self-destructive
- Hurts others
- Poor social relationships—craves attention, poor relationships with peers, manipulates adults
- Reports fear of parents, injuries, unbelievable reasons for injuries
- Poor academic performance
- Short attention span
- Language delays
- Runaway
- Truancy and or delinquency

Possible Signs of Sexual Abuse

- Difficulty walking
- Abnormalities in genital/anal areas—itching, pain, swelling, bruises, frequent infections, discharge, poor sphincter control
- Venereal disease
- Pregnancy
- Report of abuse
- Drop in academic performance

- Poor peer relationships
- Unwillingness to change, for example, gym clothing
- Unusually sophisticated sexual knowledge and behavior
- Depressed, apathetic
- Suicidal
- Sexually aggressive
- Regression to earlier developmental stages

Possible Signs of Emotional Maltreatment

- Failure to thrive in infancy
- Poor appearance
- Infantile or regressive behavior
- Developmental lags
- Extremes in behavior
- Poor self-concept
- Depressed, apathetic
- Suicidal

Possible Signs of Neglect

- Hunger and malnutrition, begs for or steals food
- Poor hygiene, lice, body odor
- Inappropriate clothing for weather and context
- Unattended physical problems or medical needs
- Lack of supervision especially in dangerous activities or contexts
- Constant fatigue
- Developmental lags
- Extremes in behavior
- Depressed, apathetic
- Seeks attention or affection
- Truancy or delinquency

children (Check, 1989). These adults were inadequately parented during their own childhood and have carried over this negative child-rearing style to their own interactions with children. Second, younger parents, particularly teenagers, appear more at risk for child abuse. Teenagers may be emotionally immature for the responsibilities of parenting and have limited parenting, coping, and homemaking skills. Third, substance abuse contributes to inappropriate parenting styles. Fourth, parents under stress because of unmet internal needs, lack of support, employment, financial or familial crises, and their own health and emotional problems are more vulnerable to child abuse and neglect. Fifth, children who have challenging needs may be more susceptible to abuse and neglect. For example,

T A B L E 22–2 Possible Causes of and Risks for Child Abuse and Neglect

Parent/Caretaker Characteristics

- Personal history of abuse
- History of family violence
- Single parenthood or absence of parent
- Social isolation and lack of emotional support
- Parental/caregiver immaturity or lack of parenting knowledge
- Marital problems of parents
- Physical or mental health problems
- Life crises such as financial problems, unemployment or underemployment, death of spouse
- Substance abuse
- Adolescent parents
- Lack of knowledge in areas of housekeeping, nutrition, and medical care
- Expectation that child act like an adult (e.g., leaves young child alone or to care for other younger children)
- Has low frustration tolerance and poor judgment; cannot delay gratification
- Lack of motivation to learn productive child-raising practices
- Does not believe there is a problem, is unconcerned, or refuses to cooperate

Child Characteristics

- Infant
- Child with special needs (e.g., mental retardation, health problems, sensory impairments, learning difficulties)

- Twins or multiple births
- Premature baby
- Baby born during time of family trauma
- Baby or young child that cries excessively (colicky), has feeding difficulties, resists being held
- Stepchild
- Child of unplanned or unwanted pregnancy
- Adolescence, teenager's striving for independence, teenager's dependency on teenage culture

Parent-Child Relationship Characteristics

- Parent's unrealistic expectations for development, achievement, or responsibility
- Lack of nurturing child-rearing skills
- Use of violence as an accepted means of personal interaction
- Inadequate bonding between parent and child
- Delay or failure to seek needed health care
- Perception that child is evil or different

Environmental Factors

- Lack of social support
- Homelessness
- Poor or inadequate housing
- Large family in crowded housing
- Poverty
- Withdrawal of governmental social, housing, and economic support

children with severe communication problems or those who have continuing, burdensome physical and psychological needs may stress and frustrate parents/caregivers beyond their limits, particularly when there is limited support, financial concerns, education, and respite. Sixth, very young children are at the highest risk for abuse and death from abuse. According to the National Center on Child Abuse and Neglect, children less than 1 year old were more likely to be neglected than at any other time of their lives (United States Department of Health and Human Services, 1994). The demands of infant care

may tax parents or caregivers, particularly those with limited parenting skills, support, or patience.

Munchausen by Proxy

Munchausen Syndrome is a disorder in which an individual deliberately creates factitious physical and/or mental health symptoms to gain attention and sympathy, particularly from medical personnel. When this pattern of exaggeration, fabrication, and inducement is applied to the symptoms of others (usually children), it is called Munchausen by Proxy (MBP).

It is considered a recognized type of maltreatment that may involve physical, sexual, or emotional abuse, neglect, or a combination (Lasher, 2004). MBP perpetrators are usually mothers who appear to be good caretakers, may have extensive health care knowledge and experience, and are convincing in their concern. Some may change health care providers frequently to avoid suspicion and subject their child to unneeded medical tests and procedures. Some may inflict injury to magnify the symptomatology. Most will deny the maltreatment even when confronted with evidence.

Possible indicators of MBP include some combination of the following: frequent emergency room admissions, recurrent episodes of the same complaint, treatment that does not produce expected results, a pattern of the problem arising in the perpetrator's presence and disappearing in his or her absence, and recurrences when the child goes home after treatment. The parent exhibits characteristics commensurate with the pattern described (Lasher, 2004). Confirmation of this diagnosis is difficult but necessary because of the potential for serious harm to a child. SLPs and audiologists who work in medical settings should be alert to this category of child abuse.

Who Is an Abuser?

Child abuse spans all ethnic, social, economic, and racial lines. Abusers may be parents, guardians, relatives, or friends. Eighty percent of abusers are parents, and women (58%) comprise the majority of abusers (National Clearinghouse on Child Abuse, 2005). A typical profile of an abuser is a young adult in his or her mid 20s, with limited education, living at or below the poverty level, and depressed. Nearly all child abusers were inadequately parented in their own childhood, and most were abused as children (Andrews University, 1999; National Clearinghouse on Child Abuse, 2005). It should be noted that child-child abuse also occurs, such as adolescent-child sexual abuse, sibling incest, and cousin-cousin incest.

Extent of the Problem

According to the National Clearinghouse on Child Abuse and Neglect (2005), at least 900,000 children

were abused or neglected in 2003. This was a slight drop in rate from 13.4 children per 1,000 in 1990 to 12.4 per 1,000 in 2003. Neglect accounted for 60 percent of the cases', 19 percent were cases of physical abuse, 10 percent sexual abuse, and 5 percent emotional abuse. Children aged birth to 3 had the highest rates of victimaization (16.4/1,000 children of the same age). High rates were also noted for girls than boys, Pacific Islanders (21.4/1,000), American Indians or Alaska Natives(21.3/1,000), and African-American children (20.4/1,000). In 2003, at least 2.9 million referrals were made about the welfare of 5.5 million children to Child Protective Services agencies in the United States, and 1.9 million of these were accepted for investigation. More than 1,500 children died from abuse in 2003, and again most of these were younger than 4 years old. Only about 8 percent of all confirmed cases of child abuse occur in day care, foster care, or other institutional settings (National Committee to Prevent Child Abuse, 1997).

Financial Costs of Child Abuse

The physical and emotional costs of child abuse are incalculable. The financial costs, are extremely high, totaling more than $94 billion. Direct costs are estimated to be at least $24 billion and include costs for hospitalization, chronic health problems, mental health services, child welfare, law enforcement and judiciary. Indirect costs total another $69 billion from expenses related to special education mental health, juvenile delinquency, lost productivity to society, and adult criminality. These costs, estimated by Prevent Child Abuse America (2001), were gleaned from information provided by the Department of Health and Human Services, the Department of Justice, and the United States Census Bureau.

What to Do If You Suspect Abuse

You cannot ignore signs of abuse. First, you must know if you are a mandated reporter of abuse in your state. You must also know what constitutes abuse in your state, what reasonable cause is, and what to do when you suspect abuse. Your confidentiality will be protected if you have made the report in good faith. If you work in a larger organization, policies and procedures will be in place to guide you about the steps to take when reporting abuse. You are advised to involve your supervisor of your suspicions.

Who Is a Mandated Reporter of Abuse? Each state has specific persons who are mandated or required by law to report suspected child abuse or neglect. For example, according to New York State Law Chapter 544, Identification and Reporting of Child Abuse and Maltreatment—Explaining Reporting Requirements—Study Requirements for Licensing (1989), speech-language pathologists and audiologists are not specifically named in this category. They may, however, be considered under some other mandated personnel category such as a school official, a day care center worker, or a member of hospital personnel engaged in the admission, examination, care, or treatment or patients. It is best to review your school, hospital, or agency's policy and procedure manual for precise guidelines in your facility, locality, and state. Even if you are not a mandated reporter, you have an ethical responsibility to document in writing possible signs of abuse or neglect and report these to your supervisor immediately.

What Is Reasonable Cause? If you suspect a child has *possibly* incurred abuse or neglect, you have reasonable cause to report a possible problem. Reasonable cause is based on personally observed physical and behavioral evidence and/or report from the child, and your own professional training and experience. According to the Center for Development of Human Services at Buffalo State College (nd), "the reporter should only be *able to entertain the possibility that it could have been neglect or nonaccidental* in order to possess the necessary reasonable cause."

When and to Whom to Report Suspected child abuse or neglect should be reported immediately by telephone, at any time of day, 7 days a week. Depending on the state, a written report may be required within a specified time limit. For example,

New York State requires that a written report be filed within 48 hours of the oral report. Where to report cases of child abuse depends on whether you are a mandated reporter. For example, in New York State, mandated reporters and concerned members of the general public call different numbers of the New York State Child Abuse Hotline. Each state will have similar Child Abuse Hotlines listed in the local telephone book. In addition, national phone numbers are listed in the Resource section at the end of this chapter. Again, your agency, hospital, or school will have specific guidelines for policies and procedures regarding reporting of possible child abuse.

Immunity and Confidentiality You have immunity from any civil or criminal liability if you or your agency have reported a suspected case of child abuse or neglect in *good faith*. Your name will be kept confidential unless you provide written permission for its release.

Consequences for Failing to Report If you are a mandated reporter and willfully fail to report a case of suspected child abuse or maltreatment, you may be guilty of a misdemeanor and have a civil liability for damages caused by such failure. Remember that failure to report your suspicion may result in continued and more severe harm to a child.

ELDER ABUSE, NEGLECT, AND EXPLOITATION

Elders are among the most vulnerable in our society. Their ability to protect themselves may be hampered by cognitive and communication problems. As with child abuse, you need to be aware of the signs and symptoms of elder abuse and what to do should you suspect such maltreatment. Remember that elder abuse or neglect can take place in the home or in formal care settings.

Elder Abuse

Elder abuse is a general term that describes actions by a person(s) in trust who causes harm to an elder (Bourget, 1999). Such mistreatment may be because the person either does something or fails to do something that harms the elder. Elder abuse may occur in the home, in institutional settings, or may be self-imposed (Administration on Aging, 1998). The seven most common forms of elder abuse include physical abuse, sexual abuse, emotional or psychological abuse, neglect, abandonment, financial or material exploitation, and self-neglect. Signs of elder abuse may characterize more than one or more types of maltreatment. Table 22–3 provides a summary of the seven major types of elder abuse and potential signs or symptoms of each type.

Elder Neglect

Elder neglect is defined as "an act of omission, of not doing something, of withholding goods or services" (Quinn & Tomita, 1986, p. 34). When neglect is due to ignorance or stress on the part of the caregiver, it is considered passive neglect. It becomes active when the caregiver deliberately neglects the elder. Sometimes considered less serious than abuse, neglect can result in serious harm to elders as can abuse.

Specific Types of Elder Abuse

Many types of elder abuse are similar to that of child abuse, including physical abuse involving injury, pain, or impairment and sexual abuse whereby individuals receive inappropriate and unwanted sexual activities imposed on them. Several other types of abuse that are particular to elders or have different characteristics are described in the following sections.

Emotional or Psychological Abuse Elders who experience undue emotional pain or distress are said to be emotionally abused. A common type of emotional abuse is administered verbally through verbal attacks, insults, threats, intimidation, humiliation, or harassment or by giving the elder the "silent

treatment." Other forms of emotional abuse include infantilization of the elder and isolation from persons and activities of choice.

Neglect Neglect involves deliberately ignoring the needs of elders. Neglect may take the form of financial neglect, by failing to attend to financial obligations, and physical neglect, when the elder receives inadequate food, water, clothing, shelter, personal hygiene, medicine, comfort, or personal safety (Administration on Aging, 1998). Neglect can be intentional (active), characterized by a conscious effort to inflict harm, or unintentional (passive), which is associated with laziness or lack of knowledge (Cicirelli, 1986).

Abandonment Abandonment is the deliberate desertion of an elder by a person who has responsibility for that elder. Abandoned elders are left alone frequently and for extended time periods in their home or other setting by caregivers. This is particularly dangerous for those elders who cannot provide for their own daily needs such as food, personal care, and medications. In addition, the loss of socialization opportunities may have a deleterious effect on the elder and contribute to cognitive and emotional decline.

Financial or Material Exploitation This type of abuse occurs when an elder's funds, property, or material assets are illegally or improperly used, usually without authorization or permission. Examples of financial or material exploitation include fraudulent check cashing; forgery of signature; misuse or theft of property or other possessions; coercion into signing a document (e.g., a will); or the improper use of conservatorship, guardianship, or power of attorney (Administration on Aging, 1998).

Self-Neglect Self-neglect occurs when elders harm themselves. For example, elders may improperly or inadequately care for their own health, safety, clothing, nutrition, hygiene, or shelter. This category excludes mentally competent elders who consciously engage in these behaviors.

T A B L E 22–3 Types and Potential Indicators of Elder Abuse, Neglect, and Exploitation

Possible Signs of Physical Abuse

- Cuts, wounds, punctures, choke marks
- Unexplained fractures, broken bones, skull fractures
- Bruises, welts, discolorations
- Detached retina, hematoma, pressure sores
- Untreated or improperly cared-for injuries
- Poor skin hygiene or condition
- Dehydration without illness-based cause
- Malnourishment without illness-based cause
- Loss of weight
- Cigarette or rope burns
- Soiled clothing or bed
- Broken eyeglasses, hearing aids, other assistive devices
- Signs of being restrained
- Sudden change in elder behavior
- Elder report of physical abuse
- Death or murder

Possible Signs of Sexual Abuse

- Bruises around breasts or genital area
- Unexplained sexually transmitted diseases
- Unexplained vaginal or anal bleeding
- Torn, stained, or bloody underclothing
- Elder report of sexual abuse

Possible Signs of Psychological/Emotional Abuse

- Hesitancy to express feelings in public
- Ambivalence, deference to others, passivity, cowering
- Lack of eye contact
- Clinging, trembling
- Depression
- Confusion or disorientation
- Fear
- Withdrawal
- Denial
- Helplessness, hopelessness
- Severe anxiety
- Anger

- Confabulations
- Elder report of verbal or emotional mistreatment
- Extreme withdrawal
- Elder becomes noncommunicative, especially in presence of caregiver
- Attempted suicide

Possible Signs of Financial or Material Exploitation

- Improper signatures on financial documents or unusual activity in bank accounts
- Financial statements do not come to elder's home without explanation
- Power of attorney given or changed without explanation
- Change(s) in will or other documents without explanation
- Financial mismanagement of funds, including unpaid bills
- Elder states that he or she has been signing papers without understanding their content
- Missing personal items
- Heightened concern by elder regarding financial management
- Lack of amenities, including appropriate clothing, entertainment, and so on that elder could afford
- Promises of care by caregiver or family
- Provision of unnecessary services or purchase of items
- Unauthorized withdrawal of funds using an ATM or credit card
- Elder receives eviction notice from house he or she owned
- Elder report of financial or property mismanagement

Possible Signs of Abandonment

- Desertion of an elder at a hospital, nursing home, or other institution
- Desertion of an elder at a public location
- Report by elder of being abandoned

Possible Signs of Neglect

- Dirty environment
- Fecal or urine smell

T A B L E 22–3 *(Continued)*

- Environmental safety hazards
- Rashes, sores, lice, or other infestation
- Untreated medical condition
- Malnourishment or dehydration
- Inappropriate or inadequate clothing and grooming

Possible Signs of Self-Neglect

- Inability to handle activities of daily living, including personal care and meal preparation
- Suicide attempts

- Inadequate financial management
- Dirty, unsafe living environment
- Homelessness
- Refusing medical or personal care
- Willful isolation
- Alcohol or other drug abuse
- Slovenly appearance
- Malnourishment or dehydration
- Not keeping medical or other important personal appointments.

Who Is Abused?

According to the National Center on Elder Abuse (1999), the majority of elder abuse victims are female (67.3 percent). The median age of elders abused by others was 77.9 years and 77.4 years for elders who neglected themselves. Two-thirds of the victims of domestic abuse were white, 18.7 percent were African American, and 10 percent were Hispanic.

Who Is at Risk?

Any elder is at risk for abuse, although those who have mental or physical disabilities are at the greatest risk. Both men and women are equally at risk of abuse (Bourget, 1999). Elders are at risk when their caregivers over- or underestimate their abilities and thus have unreasonable expectations for performance. Elders are also at risk if there is a history of domestic abuse in their family or in that of a professional caregiver. The likelihood of abuse increases when caregivers have difficulty with temper control; physical, mental, or substance abuse problems; and immature personalities. Elders themselves may increase their risk for abuse if they verbally insult or psychologically taunt their caregivers, especially with threats of withholding inheritances (Quinn & Tomita, 1986). Other factors that place elders at risk include dependency and isolation, family conflict, poverty

or financial stress (American Gerontological Society, 2005).

Who Is an Abuser?

Anyone may abuse elders. Abuse transcends all racial, economic, educational, and socioeconomic strata (Quinn & Tomita, 1986). The National Center on Elder Abuse (1999) reports that in 1996 there was no difference in the percent of male versus female abusers. They also found that adult children are the most frequent abusers of the elderly (36.7 percent); spouses ranked second (12.6 percent), and other family members third (10.8 percent). It should be noted that other studies have identified spouses as the most frequent abusers. Formal caregivers who have poor working conditions, low salary, and limited education are at higher risk for becoming an abuser.

Extent of the Problem

A recent national study of elder abuse in domestic settings (Administration on Aging, 1998) estimated that at least 500,000 older persons were abused and/or neglected or experienced self-neglect in 1996. These data are considered gross underestimations of the true number of cases. It is predicted that for every reported incident of elder abuse, there are five that go unreported. This study found that nearly half of all reports of elder abuse were substantiated after investigations. Another 40 percent were unsubstantiated, meaning that either there was no abuse or the criteria for abuse or neglect were not sufficiently met, although abuse or neglect may have occurred. The most common types of elder maltreatment were in decreasing order of frequency: neglect (49 percent), emotional/psychological abuse (35 percent), financial/material exploitation (30 percent), physical abuse (27 percent), abandonment (4 percent), sexual abuse (3 percent), and other (1.4 percent). These frequency data are not mutually exclusive, as more than one type of abuse may be reported for an incident.

Why Does Elder Abuse Occur?

Elder abuse and neglect are generally attributed to these factors:

- Physical and mental impairment of the elder
- Caregiver stress
- Violence as a problem-solving strategy
- Individual problems of the abuser
- Society's negative portrayal of elderly
- Greed (Quinn & Tomita, 1986)

It is likely these hypothesized causes work in tandem rather than individually. Meeting the needs of frail, physically and/or mentally challenged elders is a time- and effort-consuming task, especially for caregivers with limited personal resources and reduced or immature psychological stamina. In some cases, a "triggering crisis" may instigate an incident of abuse. In other cases, long-term, unrelieved stress and physical fatigue may result in an explosion of violence. Some families may have routinely used abuse as a problem-solving strategy. Some elders may purposely antagonize their caregivers, whereas others with reduced intellectual abilities may not understand or appreciate the care received. Finally, society stigmatizes the disabled and their caregivers. Limited financial or social incentives are available for caregivers who may sacrifice career and social lives for their elder family member. Some caregivers may deliberately hasten the progression of decline because it will result in a greater or earlier financial inheritance. Reinharz

(1986) commented that elder abuse is not a modern problem and represents "twin cultural themes of honor and contempt" toward the elderly.

Certain caregiving contexts appear to trigger abuse, and many of these are related to the stress involved. For example, feeding, incontinence, interrupted sleep, and incessant vocalizations are all extremely stressful for caregivers, especially when they occur repeatedly and without respite. These situations become even more problematic if the caregiver is an alcohol or drug abuser or has a history of being abused or abusive.

Elders may be afraid to report abuse because of their fear of what will happen to them if their caregiver is removed. Many elders greatly fear they will be forced to leave their home and relocate to an institutional setting where there will be less independence, loss of control, and loss of familiar surroundings and property. Thus, many elders refrain from mentioning incidents of abuse because they perceive the alternative of institutionalization to be worse than the abuse they receive in their home.

Elder Abuse in Long-Term Care Facilities

Working with elders in long-term care facilities can be a challenging job, particularly when residents have high physical and psychological needs, salary and societal regard are low, and training is minimal. Pillemer and Moore (1990) state that possible risk factors for staff abuse of elders in long-term care settings include patient aggression and provocation, staff burnout, staff age, and conflict regarding daily routines. More than 75 percent of staff had observed psychological abuse, 41 percent admitted to committing such abuse, about 33 percent had observed physical abuse, and 10 percent had committed physical abuse. Physical abuse is the most commonly reported abuse against elders in nursing homes, followed by sexual abuse, neglect, and monetary abuse. Male nurses aides committed two-thirds of the reported cases of abuse. Prevention undoubtedly lies in higher qualifications for staff, more staff training, and enforcement of mandatory abuse reporting (Quinn& Tomita, 1997).

WHAT TO DO?

Whether audiologists and speech-language pathologists are mandated to report child or elder abuse is determined by each state. If you suspect elder abuse, it is best to document in writing the indicators and discuss the policy and procedure of your setting for reporting these potential signs of elder abuse.

In most states, the Adult Protective Services agency (APS) is the major site responsible for both investigation of reported cases of elder abuse and for providing help to victims and their families.

This agency is often contained within the county level department of social services. Other organizations that have primary roles in investigation and follow-up of elder abuse referrals include the Area Agency on Aging, county Departments of Social Services, the local law enforcement agency, the medical examiner/coroner's office, hospitals, the state long-term care ombudsman's office, mental health agencies, and facility licensing or certification organizations. See the Resources section for more specific information.

SUMMARY

Audiologists and speech-language pathologists need to be vigilant for signs that abuse has occurred against clients for whom they provide assessment or intervention services in home, community, or institutional settings. Young children and elders with communication problems and other disorders are particularly vulnerable to abuse because of their high-intensity needs. Abuse may take a variety of forms, including physical, psychological, sexual, financial, or neglect. Abuse and/or neglect can occur in any age, ethnic, or economic group; in urban, suburban, or rural settings; and in any type of setting by paid caregivers, family members, or others. Speech-language pathologists and audiologists need to know their individual state regulations regarding mandated reporting of child or elder abuse and should know their agency's particular guidelines for reporting suspected cases of child abuse. Identification of abuse against those with whom we work may help prevent further abuse and provide the abuser with the help he or she needs to refrain from this type of dangerous and humiliating behavior.

CRITICAL THINKING

1. What are possible indicators of abuse among children and elders?

2. What steps would you take if you suspected child or elder abuse?

3. How would you consider cultural differences in child-raising practices in deciding if a child had possibly been abused?

4. What might be the effects if you do not report a suspected case of child or elder abuse?

5. Should speech-language pathologists and audiologists be legally described as "mandated" reporters of child abuse in every state? Why or why not?

6. When visiting a home for an early intervention evaluation, you noticed that the children in the home were dirty, dressed inappropriately for the heating conditions in the home, and frequently scratched themselves. The physical environment of the home was also filthy. The mother, however, was an excellent informant and greatly interested in the speech and language development of her children. The mother and children appeared to have a warm relationship. What would you do?

7. Create scenarios that might be indicative of child or elder abuse. Consider what you should do in each situation.

REFERENCES

Administration on Aging. (1998). *The national elder abuse incidence study; Final report Sept 1998*. Available at http://www.aoa.dhhs.gov/

American Gerontological Society. (2005) Elder mistreatment. Available at http://www.healthinaging.org/

Andrews University. (1999). Child abuse. Available at http://www.andrews.edu/

Bourget, B. (1999). Elder abuse. Available at http://www.cyberbeach.net/

Center for Development of Human Services at Buffalo State College. (nd). *Identification and report of child abuse and maltreatment: A course for mandated reporters*. Buffalo, NY: Author.

Check, W. (1989). *Child abuse*. New York: Chelsea House Publishers.

Cicirelli, V. (1986) The helping relationship and family neglect in later life. In K. Pillemer & R. Wolf (Eds.), *Elder abuse conflict in the family* (pp. 49–66). Dover, MA: Auburn House Publishing.

Lasher, L. (2004). MBP overview and definitions. Available at http://www.mbexpert.com/definition.html

National Clearinghouse on Child Abuse. (2004). Child abuse and neglect fatalities, statistics and interventions. Available at http://nccanch.acf.hhs.gov

National Clearinghouse on Child Abuse. (2005). Definitions of child abuse and neglect. Available at http://nccanch.acf.hhs.gov

National Committee to Prevent Child Abuse. (1997). Available at http://www.childabuse.org/

National Council on Elder Abuse. (1999). *The basics. Elder abuse information series #3*. Available at http://www.gwjapan.com/NCEA/

New York State Law Chapter 544, Identification and Reporting of Child Abuse and Maltreatment—Explaining Reporting Requirements—Study Requirements for Licensing. (1989).

Pillemer, K., & Moore, D. (1990). Highlights from a study of abuse of patients in nursing homes. *Journal of Elder Abuse and Neglect, 2,* 5–29.

Prevent Child Abuse. (2001). Total estimated cost of child abuse and neglect in the United States. Available at www.preventchildabuse.org

Quinn, M. J., & Tomita, S. (1986). *Elder abuse and neglect*. New York: Springer Publishing.

Quinn, M. J., & Tomita, S. (1997). *Elder abuse and neglect* (2nd ed.). New York: Springer Publishing.

Reinharz, S. (1986). Loving and hating one's elders: Twin themes in legend and literature. In K. Pillemer & R. Wolf (Eds.), *Elder abuse conflict in the family* (pp. 25–48). Dover, MA: Auburn House Publishing.

U.S. Department of Health and Human Services, National Center of Child Abuse and Neglect. (1994). *Child maltreatment 1992: Reports from the states to the national center on child abuse and neglect*. Washington, DC: U.S. Government Printing Office.

RESOURCES

Note that the web addresses and phone numbers of these resources are fluid and should be checked for currency at time of use.

Administration on Aging
    U.S. Department of Health and Human Services
    330 Independence Avenue, SW
    Washington, DC 20201
    Phone: 202-619-0724
    Web Site: http://www.aoa.gov

Adult Protective Service (APS)
    Call directory assistance and request the number for the department of social services or aging services in your county.

American Academy of Pediatrics
    Check this Web site for a listing of medical diagnostic child abuse programs developed by the American Academy of Pediatrics:
    http://www.aap.org/
    sections/scan/medicaldiagnostic/
    medicaldiagnostic.htm

Area Agency on Aging
Look in the government section of your telephone directory under the terms "aging" or "elderly services." This agency can provide the phone number for the local long-term care ombudsman in your area.

Child Help USA Hotline
Phone: 800-422-4453 (24 hrs)
Web site: http://www.childhelp.org

Eldercare Locator
For those who want to identify aging services in specific communities, call this Administration on Aging agency.
Phone: 800-677-1116

Medicaid Fraud Control Units (MFCU):
Every State Attorney General's Office has an MFCU to prosecute Medicaid provider fraud and patient abuse in long-term care or home health care settings.

Mental Health Net
Provides information and referral numbers for numerous national hotlines. Web site: http://mentalhelp.net/

National Center for Missing and Exploited Children
Helps families and professionals
Phone: 800-843-5678

National Committee to Prevent Child Abuse
Web site: http://www.childabuse.org

National Domestic Violence Hotline
Helps children, parents, friends, and offenders of family violence
Phone: 800-799-7233

National Respite Locator Service
Helps parents, caregivers, and professionals caring for children with disabilities, terminal illnesses, or those at risk of abuse
Phone: 800-677-1116

Youth Crisis Hotline
Helps individuals reporting child abuse of children 12–18.
Phone: 800-448-4663

23

Service Delivery for Culturally and Linguistically Diverse Populations

HORTENCIA KAYSER, PHD

SCOPE OF CHAPTER

During the past 30 years, speech-language pathologists and audiologists have become increasingly aware of the needs of culturally and linguistically diverse populations. Professionals are faced daily with the challenges of providing appropriate assessment and treatment to populations that historically have received little attention. This chapter provides an overview of issues you will confront as a speech-language pathologist or audiologist in working with diverse populations.

The chapter begins with a demographic profile of culturally and linguistically diverse individuals in the United States. You will then be introduced to factors that define and affect professional and clinical practice such as ASHA's positions statements concerning individuals who are culturally and linguistically diverse (CLD), and specific issues affecting assessment and treatment of communication disorders in these populations.

DEMOGRAPHICS
AND DEFINITIONS

Culturally and linguistically diverse populations historically include Native, Hispanic, African, and Asian Americans. ASHA (2005) has expanded the definition to encompass issues related to age, experience, ability, gender, race, ethnicity, language, religion, politics, sexual orientation, and socioeconomic status. For this section demographics will focus on those populations that have been highlighted by the United States Census Bureau.

The Hispanic population has become the largest ethnic group in the United States (United States Census Bureau, 2000). Asian American and African American populations are increasing rapidly, and all of the immigrant populations that have entered the United States in the last 10 years are becoming an important factor in the nation's sociocultural, economic, and educational planning. The United States Census Bureau (2000) reported that of the 281.4 million people residing in the United States, approximately 87 million identified themselves as members of a racial or ethnic minority. Of that population 13.4 percent are Hispanic, 12.8 percent are African American, 4.2 percent are Asian Pacific Islander, and 1.5 percent are American Indian/Alaskan Natives (see Figure 23–1).

Approximately 11.7 percent or 31 million U.S. residents are foreign born. Forty-seven million (18.4 percent) between the ages of 5 and 17 speak a language other than English at home. The 5.5 million English language learners (ELLs), also referred to as *Limited English Proficient* (LEP) students, in U.S. public schools speak more than 276 languages. Eighty percent of ELL students speak Spanish as their first language. This demographic profile is considered to be conservative and documents those immigrants who participated in the census. It does not include the possibly large number of immigrants who were not counted or have an illegal resident status.

School caseloads also reflect the growing diversity among students (see Figure 23–2). In 2001, of the 5.9 million school-aged children (ages 6–21) served under the Individuals with Disabilities Education Act (IDEA), approximately 1.1 million had a speech or language impairment, and 74,000 had a hearing impairment. Of these 1.1 million students who received services for speech or language impairment, 20.5 percent were African American, 14.6 percent were Hispanic, 1.9 percent were Asian/Pacific Islander, and 1.3 percent were American Indian/Alaskan Native students. Note that although Hispanics and African Americans make up 13.4 percent and 12.8 percent of the national population, respectively, these two groups are overrepresented in special services. Assessment of these school populations is a difficult process and is reflected in the numbers of children in special education.

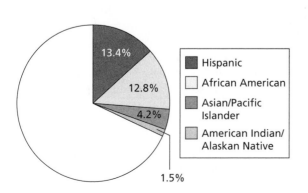

FIGURE 23–1 Growing Diversity in Population (2000)

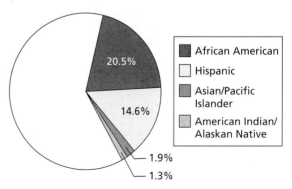

FIGURE 23–2 Growing Diversity in Caseloads (2001)

The United States Census Bureau predicts significant growth in CLD populations over the next 25 years. By 2030, 60 percent of the United States population is projected to be white, non-Hispanic, and 40 percent will be members of other diverse racial and ethnic groups. ELLs will account for approximately 40 percent of the entire school-aged population in the United States (United States Census Bureau, 2003).

ASHA estimates that 10 percent of the United States population has a communication disorder (Battle, 2002). This same figure may be used to estimate the prevalence of communication disorders among culturally and linguistically diverse populations, translating to a possible figure of 8.7 million Americans. This estimate may be conservative considering that many CLD groups have health and social problems particular to their race or ethnicity. For example, hypertension and sickle cell anemia are common among African Americans and affect growth in children's hearing, and increase the risk of stroke. Diabetes is prevalent among Hispanics and is a factor in higher incidences of hypertension and stroke. The high incidence of otitis media among Native Americans affects hearing sensitivity and language delays. The estimate that 10 percent of the population have a communication disorder may be conservative, and greater numbers of culturally and linguistically diverse children may have communication disorders identified or unidentified because of language barriers. As an example, children with communication disorders may not be served because of a lack of personnel who speak a child's language, or professionals may not consider a child to have a communication disorder because a school district policy dictates that children have to speak English before they are assessed or treated for a communication disorder. Thus, a child may not receive appropriate speech, language, or hearing services.

The United States Department of Health and Human Services (1985) reported that economically disadvantaged populations are more likely to be predisposed to disorders caused by environmental,

teratogenic (causing developmental malformations), nutritional, and traumatic factors than other groups. These and other variables such as child abuse in low-income families, single parent families, homelessness, teenage pregnancies, and educational achievement may increase the number of individuals from culturally and linguistically diverse populations with communication disorders. The *National Healthcare Disparities Report* (United States Department of Health and Human Services, 2004) stated that the circumstances for racial and ethnic minorities have not changed, and these individuals often experience worse access to care and lower quality of preventive, primary, and specialty care. The United States Census Bureau reported that racial and ethnic minorities are more likely than non-Hispanic whites to be poor or near poor. In 2002, 24 percent of African Americans, 22 percent of Hispanics, 10 percent of Asians, and 16.6 percent of the foreign-born populations were classified as poor. Poverty and a lack of medical insurance combine to affect millions of individuals who may have diseases and injuries that affect communication disorders and thus are untreated.

Minority Speech-Language Pathologists and Audiologists

In 2004, approximately 8,400 of ASHA's 118,437 members (7.1 percent) identified themselves as belonging to a racial minority or multiracial. One percent or 1,200 speech-language pathologists and audiologists have identified themselves as bilingual. ASHA does not provide a mechanism to determine the language proficiency of these professionals and depends upon self-identification through the Office of Multicultural Affairs. Recruiting and retaining bicultural and bilingual students, educators, clinicians, and scientists has become an important priority for ASHA (2004).

Recruitment of bilingual personnel begins in the elementary schools, through participation of audiologists and speech-language pathologists in recruitment fairs, parent programs, health fairs, and other community events that will expose children to our professions. High school recruitment fairs are excellent avenues for young adults to hear about these professions. Universities can also promote recruitment programs that target bilingual students during recruitment trips, career fairs, and university events that inform students of our professions. Retention of students from CLD groups will mean commitment to these students from the administration through scholarships, tuition waivers, graduate assistantships, graduate fellowships, and a financial aid package to help students meet the challenges of a postsecondary education. Student academic assistance in the form of academic services such as writing centers, tutoring sessions, and support groups from other CLD students all support students to achieve and succeed in colleges and university programs in Communication Sciences and Disorders. The need for professionals who are culturally proficient and bilingual is of utmost importance for the profession to provide effective services for an increasingly diverse nation.

Although there is an insufficient number of culturally and linguistically diverse professionals to provide the services needed for CLD populations, ASHA has been proactive in educating its largely mainstream membership. Technical reports and position statements that affect the practice with diverse groups are summarized chronologically. Each of these papers was developed to guide speech-language pathologists and audiologists and also protect CLD populations and professionals.

ASHA POSITION STATEMENTS

Six position statements and one technical report have made a major impact on service delivery to culturally and linguistically diverse populations with communication disorders. These statements embody decades of discussion among speech-language pathologists, audiologists, and university researchers concerning best practices and the ethical responsibility of clinicians and researchers. As the decades have passed, the

issues have become clearer and the commitment to resolve these concerns has become greater among CLD professionals and the association. The following is a summary of each of these important Position Statements.

Social Dialects

The purpose of the *Position Paper on Social Dialects* (ASHA, 1983a) was to clarify the association's view of social dialects. The policy document makes it clear that dialectal variation of English is not a communication disorder. According to the position, all social dialects are adequate, functional, and effective varieties of English. Thus, children and adults are not to be admitted to treatment programs or identified as disordered solely on the basis of their dialect. However, individuals who speak a nonstandard English dialect may elect to have speech and language services to develop Standard English. If a speech-language pathologist provides this service, the practitioner must work to preserve the integrity of the client's dialect. The speech-language pathologist must also have the clinical competency to provide this service by knowing the linguistic characteristics of the client's native dialect.

This paper is important because many children in the public schools may be identified as speech and language disordered because of their use of African American English (AAE) or Spanish Influenced English, or other social dialects that are viewed as nonstandard use of English. Individuals with these speech and language characteristics are not communicatively disordered. Recognition of these dialects becomes important in the scope of practice of speech-language pathologists and audiologists.

Clinical Management of Communicatively Handicapped Minority Language Populations

The purpose of the clinical management position statement (ASHA, 1985) recommended those clinical competencies necessary to assess and treat communication disorders in culturally and linguistically diverse populations and to describe alternative strategies when these competencies are not met. Five competency areas were identified for bilingual speech-language pathologists and audiologists: (1) language proficiency (native or near-native fluency in both the minority language and the English language), (2) normative processes (ability to describe the process of normal speech and language acquisition for both bilingual and monolingual individuals, and how those processes are manifested in oral and written language), (3) assessment (the ability to administer and interpret formal and informal assessment procedures to distinguish between communication difference and communication disorders), (4) intervention (the ability to apply intervention strategies for treatment of communicative disorders in the native language), and (5) cultural sensitivity (the ability to recognize cultural factors that affect the delivery of speech-language pathology and audiology services to non English language speaking communities).

The position paper acknowledged that there may be difficulty in acquiring bilingual speech-language pathologists and audiologists; therefore, five alternative strategies for acquiring bilingual personnel were included: (1) establish contacts (e.g., find consultants who can provide the service); (2) establish cooperatives (e.g., a group of agencies or school districts could share one bilingual speech-language-pathologist or audiologist); (3) establish networks (e.g., ties could be developed between agencies and university programs that might have bilingual graduate students, and these students can then be recruited by the agencies); (4) establish clinical fellowship and graduate practicum sites (e.g., bilingual graduates could be used to assist personnel in school and other facilities); (5) establish interdisciplinary teams (e.g., a team approach could be developed among the monolingual speech-language-pathologist or audiologist and bilingual professionals such as teachers, psychologists, and nurses who are knowledgeable of nonbiased assessment procedures and development of the client's language).

The final recommendation in the position paper listed those individuals who may serve as interpreters or translators. Interpreters can be recruited from language banks, bilingual professional staff, family members, or friends of the client. Note that use of the family or friend is the last resort because interpreters must have training and knowledge of the clinical procedures. Family members may not interpret accurately because of cultural roles, protection of the family member, or not understanding the professionals' statements (Kayser, 1998).

This position statement was of particular importance because it served as the basis in curriculum development for many minority emphasis graduate programs in speech-language pathology and audiology. The majority of the competencies for clinicians who serve CLD clients are stated clearly, but the language proficiency competency for speech-language pathologists and audiologists was not well defined. Since the acceptance of this paper by the ASHA's Executive Board and Legislative Council, research and best practices with English language learners has advanced our understanding in assessment and treatment practices with diverse populations. The Clinical Management Paper is in the process of revision with current evidence-based practice.

Bilingual Speech-Language Pathologists and Audiologists

The primary purpose of this ASHA position paper was to define the term *bilingual,* to protect the public from clinicians who claim to have bilingual abilities, and to serve as a model for clinicians who aspire to become bilingual (ASHA, 1989). The definition states that speech-language pathologists or audiologists who identify themselves as bilingual must be able to speak their primary language and speak (or sign) at least one other language with native or near-native proficiency in semantics, phonology, morphology/syntax, and pragmatics during clinical management. Many bilingual professionals have attempted to meet the intent of this definition and, through continuing education, have met the academic competencies as outlined in the 1985 Clinical Management position statement (ASHA, 1985).

Language proficiency in the second language can be evaluated through testing services in university language programs or by state education agencies that certify teachers. Regardless of the method chosen by clinicians to document their academic competencies and language proficiency, they are bound by the ASHA Code of Ethics to provide quality services to all clients (ASHA, 1994).

The Speech-Language Pathologist and English as a Second Language

The growing number of children in schools from culturally and linguistically diverse populations has increased the likelihood of professionals serving as instructors of English as a Second Language (ESL). School districts may not have ESL instructors and thus view the speech-language pathologist as the alternative language service provider for a child who does not speak English. The position statement on provision of ESL instruction by speech-language pathologists in school settings (ASHA, 1998) states that ESL instructors require specialized academic preparation in areas such as second language acquisition, comparative linguistics, and ESL pedagogy. Speech-language pathologists may not have had the academic preparation in their graduate studies program. Speech-language pathologists must therefore examine their education and experience relative to their state's credentialing for ESL teachers. The clinician who does not have this specialized background should not provide direct instruction in ESL, but should collaborate with ESL instructors in providing preassessment, assessment, and intervention with children who are English language learners.

This is an important statement because it defines for school speech-language pathologists ASHA's position on our scope of practice, how we can enhance service delivery systems, how to appropriately identify and serve students from culturally and linguistically diverse groups, and how important it is to comply with the ASHA Code of Ethics (ASHA, 1994), state and federal mandates, and school district policy.

Students and Professionals Who Speak English with Accents and Nonstandard Dialects: Issues and Recommendations

This paper was a combined position statement and technical report (ASHA, 1997). The technical report was developed to describe the inequities and discrimination reported to the National Office concerning employment practices, clinical training, and selection of CLD graduate students into graduate programs in Communication Sciences and Disorders. The technical paper provided guidelines and suggestions for clinical and graduate faculty to improve circumstances for graduate students with accents or dialects viewed as nonstandard English. ASHA's position is that students and professionals in communication sciences and disorders who speak with accents and/or dialects can effectively provide speech, language, and audiology services to persons with communication disorders as long as they have the expected knowledge. There is no research that reports that individuals who speak with accents are less likely to perform well in clinical situations than a Standard English speaker. Additionally, ASHA members must not discriminate against persons who speak with an accent and/or dialect in educational programs, employment, or service delivery. This paper was a critical turning point in the fair treatment of professionals and graduate students in communication sciences and disorders. The recruitment and retention of CLD students in speech-language pathology and audiology is an important outcome of this paper.

Knowledge and Skills Needed by Speech-Language Pathologists and Audiologists to Provide Culturally and Linguistically Appropriate Services

This competency paper was written to encourage clinicians to continue lifelong learning to develop those knowledge and skills required to provide culturally and linguistically appropriate services. It specifies the knowledge and skills needed to provide culturally and linguistically appropriate services (ASHA, 2004). It also serves as a guide to identify those weaknesses and strengths in our knowledge in serving CLD populations. The seven areas addressed in this paper expanded our scope of practice in the following areas: (1) cultural competence, (2) language competencies of the clinician, (3) language, (4) articulation and phonology, (5) resonance/voice/fluency, (6) swallowing, and (7) hearing/balance. Each section identifies specific areas of knowledge and skills necessary to appropriately serve culturally and linguistically diverse populations. Professionals who work in different clinical settings may view the whole document as daunting, but its purpose is to identify those sections that are of critical importance for an individual's clinical practice and to develop those specific knowledge and skills.

Cultural Competence

The ASHA Board of Ethics (2005) provided a definition of cultural competence with the purpose of promoting sensitivity and increasing awareness to cultural diversity. The board used specific sections of the Code of Ethics and related these to cultural diversity. For example, Principle of Ethics I, Rule C speaks directly to the issue of clinical and research activities by prohibiting discrimination in the delivery of services or the conduct of research and scholarly activities on the basis of race, ethnicity, gender, age, religion, national origin, sexual orientation, or disability. Rules A and B direct members to provide services competently and to use every resource, including referral when appropriate. Referral is necessary when cultural or linguistic differences negatively influence outcomes. Principle of Ethics II, Rule C states that members shall continue professional development throughout their careers. This means that clinicians should develop the knowledge and skills required to provide culturally and linguistically appropriate services. Principle of Ethics I, Rule E, prohibits delegation of tasks that are beyond the competence of the assistant or interpreter without adequate supervision from a certified clinician. This is particularly important when the clinician does not speak the language that the assistant is using in treatment. The final principle, Ethics IV, Rule H, provides guidance in our interactions with colleagues and students, prohibiting discrimination against these individuals for any reason. Discrimination against individuals for any reason ultimately dishonors the professions.

The position statements have provided guidance and proactive commitment to diversity within the fields of speech-language pathology and audiology. As the association has grown through the past three decades, the professions have become aware of the ethical responsibility to cultural competence and appropriate services to culturally and linguistic diverse populations. See Chapter 4 on ethics for further discussion.

CLINICAL ISSUES AFFECTING CULTURALLY AND LINGUISTICALLY DIVERSE POPULATIONS

Four major clinical issues confront speech-language pathologists and audiologists when providing services to CLD populations. The first is an understanding of bilingualism and second language acquisition and its impact on the assessment and treatment process. The second issue relates to the assessment of children and adults from diverse cultures and languages. The third relates to the culture and language(s) during treatment, and the fourth issue affects both assessment and treatment, working with an interpreter and/or paraprofessional. All of these issues will be briefly discussed.

Bilingualism and Second Language Acquisition

Baetens-Beardsmore (1986) has stated that the term *bilingualism* has different meanings for different individuals. For some, it may be equal abilities in two languages. Bilingualism has been defined with varying degrees of strictness, depending on how proficient or competent a speaker must be to be considered bilingual. Valdes and Figueroa (1995) defined bilingualism as knowledge of "more than one" language. Their framework for bilingualism is described as a continuum of proficiencies. Children may be fluent in Spanish, L1, but have limited proficiency in English, L2. There are children who are fluent in English but may have limited fluency in Spanish. Between these points there is individual variation in the proficiency for each language. Baetens-Beardsmore (1986) suggested that this continuum is a result of societal and individual variables. Children are exposed to societal variables that affect their bilingualism such as urban or rural habitation, distance from the native tongue country, frequency of visits to the homeland, numbers of speakers of the language in the community, length of residence in the United States, native literacy in the community, native language education, and church or community centers that serve as a gathering place for use of the native language. Individual variables that influence bilingualism include ethnic identity, emotional attachment to the native language, emphasis on family ties, language attrition (loss), motivation to use the home language, attitude toward the mainstream community, and need for use of the native language and English. Societal and individual variables affect the individual differences in children's bilingualism and proficiency in the two languages.

Recently, internationally adopted children have become an important population for service delivery. In the last 30 years, more than 265,000 children have been internationally adopted. The majority have come from Asia and European countries (Adoption Institute, 2004). The speech and language reports on these children have had mixed results. For example, Glennon and Masters (2002) reported few delays in language development 21 to 36 months post-adoption for children from Eastern Europe and China. Yet, Glennon (2002) reported that children adopted from Eastern Europe are at risk of developing language and learning problems if scaled scores were below 75 on the *Communication and Symbolic Behavior Scales-Developmental Profile* (Wetherby & Prizant, 2002) and/or if the child had significant delays in symbolic play.

Research continues at more than 60 agencies across the country. The majority of these centers focus on the health, growth, and well-being of these children and are located in medical centers. Centers for speech and language development are still in development across the country. The majority of these children come from different environmental backgrounds that either have supported or not supported these children's growth and development, including speech and language. Hearing health and sensitivity may not have been addressed while the children were in orphanages. Losing their first language will likely be inevitable unless the adopting parents insist on supporting the language through involvement in a native language community or educational programming.

How children progress in their development of English while they lose their native language is still unknown. It is likely that the majority of these children, if adopted before the age of 1 year and placed in rich language environments and homes, will learn English and become academically successful in American schools. Older children may have more difficulty. Research is needed for clinicians to appropriately respond to the needs of internationally adopted children and their families. See Chapter 11 on Special Populations for more discussion of this group.

Assessment

Professionals are concerned with the correct identification of speech, language, and hearing disorders in individuals who are second language learners or who are culturally and linguistically different. The profession recognizes that many speech-language pathologists and audiologists lack the knowledge to serve these CLD populations (Roseberry-McKibben, 2005), and yet we are bound by the ASHA Code of Ethics to do all that we can to serve them (ASHA, 2005).

The first step toward appropriate services is to recognize that test instruments are to serve us in identifying the strengths and weaknesses of these clients' English capabilities, which includes their perception of English sounds. The test instruments alone do not tell us whether a CLD client has a speech, language, or hearing disorder. As clinicians, we must use resources beyond the test instrument to help identify communicatively impaired individuals who are from CLD backgrounds.

Test instruments are important for accurate and objective assessment of individuals with communication disorders in monolingual English-speaking populations. They help determine the client's communication abilities by comparing the performance to a "typically developing" population. Norms are usually developed from a population that is primarily middle class, English speaking, and of European background. Some test instruments include a small percentage of CLD populations but once the means are calculated, this only serves to lower the norms and not appropriately assess the CLD groups.

When clinicians assess individuals who do not fit this norm, accurate assessment becomes problematic for a number of reasons. First, it is inappropriate to use English tests with a population that is different from the test instrument norm group. If the test instrument is translated, this compromises test validity and reliability. In addition, cultural and linguistic differences may affect the interactions between the client and clinician and thus the results of the testing.

Using tests that are insensitive to the diversity of the population results in invalid data. Culture must play a dominant role in the development of any diagnostic or behavioral test. Clients may perform differently when tested because of their cultural background (Kayser, 1998). Because of a client's linguistic differences, results in levels of communicative competence may vary from those of the mainstream population. Test instruments typically reflect the culture of the test developer and present speech and language stimuli thought to be familiar to all individuals. A CLD client may not, however, have had the same cultural and language

experiences as the majority population. Because many cultures and languages are served in the schools, tests developed for these populations have not been possible.

The use of nonstandard or modified procedures in the assessment of linguistically diverse clients (Erickson & Iglesias, 1986; Kayser, 1989a, b, 1995) is a common practice among clinicians. The clinician initially administers a test using standardized procedures. The clinician readministers the test by altering the procedures to allow more response time or allow for dialectal variations in the client's responses. Other modified procedures include rewording instructions, providing more examples, having the child explain the "error" response, administering items beyond the test ceiling, and allowing other similar test responses. The purpose of these modified procedures is to obtain as much information about a client's strengths and weakness in communication and not rely on the final test score and how the client compares to a mainstream English-speaking population.

Another suggestion is to adapt a test instrument so that it becomes culturally appropriate for the target population (Kayser, 1995a). The test instrument is adapted so that the content and/or tasks become culturally familiar to the client. For example, the vocabulary may be adapted to words used in the community. The task used to elicit a response may be unfamiliar or unnatural to the individual; therefore, a change is made so that the area of speech and language tested can be assessed using a more culturally acceptable task. Once tests are adapted, the original test no longer exists. The norms are now invalid and inappropriate for comparisons. The danger of adapting a standardized test is loss of standardization, thus reducing validity and reliability. The clinician must then describe the performance of the individual and compare this performance to known developmental norms for a particular population.

An alternative approach to testing is using systematic observations of the target individual, ethnographic interviewing of the family concerning the client's use of language and communicative competence, published questionnaires for parents and teachers, reviewing supporting documents from other agencies, and dynamic assessment.

Dynamic assessment includes a test-teach-retest protocol for observing and evaluating the learning process of a child or adult from a CLD background (Gutierrez-Clellen, Pena, & Quinn, 1995; Pena & Gillam, 2000; Pena, Iglesias, & Lidz, 2001). The clinician begins by assessing children's abilities in areas such as vocabulary or narratives. The teach session, also called *mediation,* requires the clinician to attempt to teach the child something about what is expected in the assessment phase. The retest phase is repeated to assess the outcomes of the learning process. Dynamic assessment allows the clinician to make inferences about the child's learning potential and what strengths the child has in learning. Significant research supports dynamic assessment in distinguishing children who are language impaired from children with typical language skills. How this system can be used reliably is a variable researchers must address.

Testing does not give speech-language pathologists and audiologists all of the answers to our questions about clients from CLD backgrounds. Clinicians will have to explore new methods of assessment to determine language difference from disorders in these populations.

Treatment

Culturally diverse communities may have their own traditional ways of caring for individuals with disabilities. When families hold beliefs that are different from the mainstream, they may be unlikely to seek out educational, medical, or other health care services (Saenz & Huer, 2003). Hwa-Froelich and Westby (2003) described a conflict relating to our educational system and families' perceptions. Children were typically referred to special education programs by mainstream staff who viewed special services as a right of children living in a literate, highly technological society that values independent functioning. Many of the children came from nonliterate, nontechnological backgrounds where the children were socialized to be dependent on their families and communities for all of their needs. Thus,

children were displaced, were denied services, or received services that were not valued or wanted by the family because of misunderstandings and lack of cultural knowledge (Hwa-Froelich & Westby, 2003).

Intervention requires that a client's communication needs are met through an understanding of what the family needs and values and what constitutes appropriate intervention services. When clinicians plan therapy for CLD clients, there should be three considerations: (1) the clinician and client's cultural backgrounds and how these might influence the clinical process; (2) the individual's bilingualism and need for the first language, and (3) the content of therapy that is culturally sensitive and would facilitate learning.

Clinician versus Child's Culture Taylor (1986) describes the interactions between the clinician and client as a social event. Each person comes into this social event, called *therapy,* with his or her own perceptions, values, mores, attitudes, customs, conversational rules, grammatical rules, and culture. When the clinician and client have different cultural and linguistic backgrounds, miscommunication and misunderstanding of treatment goals and objectives may result. Scudder and Holmskog (1989) studied the repair strategies of Spanish-speaking children between the ages of 6 and 11 years. They interacted with Anglo and Hispanic adults. The results indicated that the children used different revision strategies depending upon whether the adult was Hispanic or Anglo. Children would change the form of the utterance but not the semantic content with the Anglo listener and also added information to the original response. With the Hispanic listener, the children repeated all or part of the original utterance. Scudder and Holmskog (1989) state that the children viewed the nonnative listener as needing more clarification than the native Spanish listener. Kayser (1995b) reported the interactions of three Anglo and three Hispanic clinicians as each screened 20 typically developing Hispanic children. Group A was tested in English and group B was tested in Spanish. The verbal and nonverbal behaviors of the Anglo and Hispanic clinicians were strikingly different. The Anglo clinicians kept a social distance of 48–60 inches from the children, while the Hispanic clinicians kept within a range of 18–48 inches. Hispanic clinicians touched the children to control their behavior while the Anglo clinicians did not touch the children. The Hispanic clinicians used facial gesture to communicate affirmation, confusion, agreement, and disagreement with the child. It was observed that eye gaze was also used to control the children's behavior. The Anglo clinicians were observed only to smile.

The verbal communication styles between the children and clinicians were also different. The Anglo clinicians used verbal reinforcements, questions, permission statements, statements of need, hints, explanations concerning a task, and if–then statements, such as "if you show me the car, then we can play with the toys" to coax children. The Hispanic clinicians were directive with the children, such as "di" (say), "ensename" (show me), and "haz esto" (do this). During clarifications, Hispanic clinicians repeated the utterances, while Anglo clinicians rephrased the utterances. Hispanic clinicians also had verbal behaviors not observed among the Anglo clinicians. They complimented the children's beauty, appearance, clothes, names, and names of family members. This was observed throughout the sessions. These interactions may have influenced the testing results, because 80 percent of the children tested by the Anglo clinicians failed the screening. Only 10 percent of the Hispanic children tested by Hispanic clinicians failed the screening.

Clinicians come into the clinical setting with their own set of norms for interactions that are based upon their cultural expectations. Children and adults from culturally and linguistically diverse groups also have their own set of norms for interactions that are based upon their cultural expectations. Speech-language pathologists and audiologists must recognize that the interactions during testing and treatment may affect the outcomes of treatment.

Language of Instruction   English has been the language of choice for intervention for the majority of minority clients in many agencies, whether or not the client speaks English. Choice may not exist, however, if intervention in the home language is possible. There is research to support the use of the native language in therapy. Perrozi (1985), Perrozi and Chavez-Sanchez (1992), and Kiernan and Swisher (1990) began the investigation of language of instruction with Spanish-English speaking and Native American children. Their work with single subject designs supported native language instruction. They concluded that it may be instrumental in helping CLD children with language impairments to develop skills in both the native and the majority language. Both research groups suggested that a bilingual curriculum is better than teaching only in English. Gutierrez-Clellen (1999) reviewed the literature concerning language choice in intervention with bilingual children and presented evidence from bilingual education in Canada and the United States that concluded that instruction in the native language is beneficial to learning the English language. Gutierrez-Clellen (1999) and Kohnert, Yim, Nett, Kan, and Duran (in press) recommend the use of the native language for instruction because of an additive effect that occurs for those children who maintain the use of the native language while learning English. Additive bilingualism occurs in children, and the results are higher performance in academic achievement as well as higher proficiency in two languages than if children were instructed only in English.

Treatment Content   Cultural sensitivity has been the theme among advocates for culturally and linguistically diverse individuals with communication disorders (Kayser, 1993; Saville-Troike, 1986). This cultural sensitivity may then affect the content of the therapy. Kayser (1993) states that background research about a culture may be necessary to plan appropriate culturally sensitive therapy. Preparation may include observations of the community and discussion with bilingual professionals and families to understand those aspects of culture that may be unfamiliar, offensive, and inappropriate within the therapy session. Becoming knowledgeable about a different culture will require interactions with families and communities. Understanding a different culture will also produce sensitivity to what is necessary, appropriate, and not offensive to the client who is receiving speech, language, or hearing services.

Recognizing the values and community activities also will provide clinicians with a wealth of content and materials for speech and language treatment as well as aural stimuli for the audiologist. An example is illustrated when a clinician told me that she had just read about an Easter custom among Mexican American families. Children and adults cracked colorful dried eggshells filled with confetti over each other's heads. These eggshells are called *cascarones*. She had worked with Hispanic children for 20 years and never had heard of this custom. She introduced the topic in therapy with groups of Hispanic children on her caseload and was surprised that the children could explain, describe, and sequence the making of these cascarones (Kayser, 1995b).

Lynch and Hanson (2004) recommends four effective ways to begin to gather information about other cultures: (1) learning through books, the arts, and technology; (2) talking and working with individuals from the culture who can act as cultural guides and mediators; (3) participating in the daily life of another culture; and (4) learning the language of another culture. Working with clients from other cultures will take an investment of time, effort, reading, and recognizing when to ask more questions to fully understand what else you need to know.

Paraprofessionals and Interpreters

Using a nonprofessional as an interpreter may appear to be an adequate solution to an immediate need, but the process of interpretation can be problematic. Interpreting for another individual is a learned skill and not an ability that comes naturally. Langdon (1988) reports that interpreters may omit, add information, use the wrong word, or transpose information. Interpreters must be trained carefully before they are used for client-family conferences, assessment, and treatment.

Paraprofessionals and interpreters provide two separate clinical roles that require different training. The *paraprofessional,* as defined by ASHA (1983b, 1993), is any person who, after receiving on-the-job or academic training, provides clinical services that are prescribed and directed by a certified speech-language pathologist or audiologist. An *interpreter* is one who conveys information from one language to the other in the oral modality; a *translator* conveys information in the written modality (Langdon, 1992). Both paraprofessional and interpreter should have a minimum of a high school diploma with communication skills that are adequate for the tasks assigned by the clinician. Interpreters should have oral and written abilities in English and the minority language. All bilingual persons are not capable of acquiring these skills. Professional interpreting requires training and advanced linguistic skills in two languages (Kayser, 1995a, 1998). Langdon (1992) suggests that the role of the interpreter requires an ability to stay emotionally uninvolved with the discussions. The interpreter must maintain confidentiality and neutrality, accept the clinician's authority, and be able to work with other professional staff (Kayser, 1995a, 1998). When a family member or friend becomes the interpreter, information relayed to the family may be omitted or misunderstood (Kayser, 1995a, 1998). Interpreters are increasingly part of the practice of speech-language pathologists and audiologists. Training for both the professional and the interpreter will produce valid and reliable interactions with the client who does not speak English.

The paraprofessional/interpreter's role may include screening of speech, language, and/or hearing, treatment activities that do not require clinical decision making, chart recording, clinical record maintenance, preparation of clinical materials, and testing of hearing aids. The paraprofessional and/or interpreter should not be responsible for interpreting data, determining caseloads, transmitting clinical information to other professionals, preparing reports, referring clients to other professionals, or using a title other than assigned by the professional (ASHA, 1993). See Chapter 10 on the topic of paraprofessionals.

AUDIOLOGY AND MULTICULTURAL POPULATIONS

Audiologists may believe that pantomime is a sufficient skill when testing children and adults who do not speak English. Unfortunately, language barriers and cultural differences do influence the audiometric evaluation of non-English speaking populations (Hodgson & Montgomery, 1994). Clients who do not understand English can have a frustrating experience when they are uncertain about what is expected of them for a response and what exactly the audiologist will be administering during the evaluation. It becomes especially frustrating for both the clinician and client when questions arise during the protocols. Hodgson and Montgomery (1994) recommend answering three questions during an evaluation (1) How great is the loss of hearing sensitivity? (2) What type of hearing loss is present? (3) How good is word recognition ability as a function of clarity of hearing? The first two questions can be answered with little to no ability of the audiologist to speak the client's language. The third question must be answered with the use of speech. Perception of another language with the confounding variable of hearing loss makes the evaluation less likely to be valid. Testing with words that are familiar makes the evaluation much more reliable and valid.

The audiologist should also consider culture. Culturally and linguistically diverse groups have different prevalence of hearing disorders and ear infections. Native Americans have persistent ear infections, presumed to be caused from an anatomical difference in the angle of the Eustachian tube. Many cultures have specific beliefs about the appropriate interactions of opposite genders, such as the audiologist touching the patient's head or ears. Sensitivity to these possibilities is important. The reporting of the test results becomes problematic when there is no interpreter who can relay the information to an individual who does not understand English. Sensitive information such as a progressive hearing loss or the effects of sickle cell on a hearing mechanism, should be provided with cultural sensitivity (Scott, 2002). The use of interpreters who understand audiometric terminology becomes extremely important to the audiologist in explaining the procedures and results with sensitivity to the client's cultural background.

SUMMARY

This chapter introduced those issues that confront speech-language pathologists and audiologists working with culturally and linguistically diverse populations with communication disorders. ASHA position statements were briefly described concerning culturally and linguistically diverse populations. Each of these issues has an impact on the quality of service provided to multicultural populations. Issues discussed included demographics, communication disorders in culturally and linguistically diverse populations, testing, treatment, and paraprofessionals/ interpreters. ASHA has been a leader among professional associations in providing its membership with information concerning culturally and linguistically diverse people and continues to provide information to the public and its members.

CRITICAL THINKING

1. The ASHA position statements concerning culturally and linguistically diverse populations have made a tremendous impact on the clinical practice in our fields of speech-language pathology and audiology. Describe how you feel about these position statements and how you might approach cultural competency in service provision to CLD populations.

2. Standardized testing is only one part of the diagnostic evaluation of CLD populations. How would you describe the inadequacies of tests to another professional? To the client? To parents? What nonstandardized assessment procedures are useful for CLD populations? How would you report these results in your documentation?

3. Providing treatment to children and adults who speak another language different from yours is a challenge to most professionals. How would you approach this challenge and who would you ask to assist you? What difficulties might you have in using family or professional interpreters?

4. Everyone has a culture. How do you think your own cultural background affects your provision of clinical services?

5. What are some ways you could increase your understanding of another culture that is near you at home, work, or school? Suppose you take a clinical position that serves a CLD population. How would you upgrade your knowledge base and skills to work effectively?

6. What ethical issues might you face in working with individuals from different cultural and linguistic backgrounds? Review the ASHA or AAA Code of Ethics for issues that affect service to CLD populations.

7. How can we attract more individuals from diverse backgrounds into speech-language pathology and audiology?

REFERENCES

Adoption Institute. (2004) Available at http://www. adoptioninstitute.org/

American Speech-Language-Hearing Association. (1983a). Position paper: Social dialects and implications of the position on social dialects. *Asha, 25,* 23–27.

American Speech-Language-Hearing Association. (1983b). *Guidelines for the employment and utilization of supportive personnel.* Rockville, MD: Author.

American Speech-Language-Hearing Association. (1985). Clinical management of communicatively handicapped minority language populations. *Asha, 27,* 29–32.

American Speech-Language-Hearing Association. (1989). Bilingual speech-language pathologists and audiologists. *Asha, 31,* 93.

American Speech-Language-Hearing Association. (1993). *Position statement and guidelines for the education/training, use, and supervision of support personnel in speech, language pathology and audiology.* Rockville, MD: Author.

American Speech-Language-Hearing Association. (1994). Code of ethics. *Asha, 36* (Suppl. 13), 1–2.

American Speech-Language-Hearing Association Joint Subcommittee of the Executive Board on English Language Proficiency. (1997). Students and professionals who speak English with accents and non-standard dialects: Issues and recommendations. *Asha, 40* (Suppl. 18).

American Speech-Language-Hearing Association. (1998). Provision of English as-a-second-language instruction by speech-language pathologists in school settings. *Asha, 40* (Suppl. 18).

American Speech-Language-Hearing Association. (2004). ASHA counts for 2004: Highlights and trends. Table 4: Summary counts of ethnicity and race and cCCs. http://www.asha.org/

American Speech-Language-Hearing Association. (2004). Knowledge and skills needed by speech-language pathologists and audiologists to provide culturally and linguistically appropriate services. *ASHA* (Suppl. 24).

American Speech-Language-Hearing Association. (2005). Cultural competence. *ASHA* (Suppl. 25).

Baetens-Beardsmore, H. (1986). *Bilingualism: Basic principles.* San Diego, CA: College Hill Press.

Battle, D. (Ed.) (2002). *Communication disorders in multicultural populations* (2nd ed.). Boston: Butterworth-Heinemann.

Erickson, J., & Iglesias, A. (1986). Assessment of communication disorders in non-English proficient children. In O. Taylor (Ed.), *Nature of communication disorders in culturally and linguistically diverse populations* (pp. 181–218). San Diego, CA: College-Hill Press.

Glennon, S. (2002). Language development and delay in internationally adopted infants and toddlers: A review. *American Journal of Speech-Language Pathology, 11*(4), 333–339.

Glennon, S., & Masters, M. G. (2002). Typical and atypical language development in infants and toddlers adopted from Eastern Europe. *American Journal of Speech-Language Pathology, 11*(4), 417–433.

Gutierrez-Clellen, V. F., Pena, E., & Quinn, R. (1995). Accommodating cultural differences in narrative style: A multicultural perspective. *Topics in Language Disorders, 15,* 54–67.

Hodgson, W. R., & Montgomery, P. (1994). Hearing impairment and bilingual children: Considerations in assessment and intervention. *Seminars in Speech and Language, Vol. 15, 2,* 174–182.

Hwa-Froelich, D., & Westby, C. (2003). Frameworks of education: perspectives of southeast Asian parents and Head Start staff. *Language, Speech, and Hearing Services in Schools, 34,* 299–319.

Individuals with Disabilities Education Improvement Act of 2004. (PL 108-446).

Kayser, H. (1989). Speech and language assessment of Spanish-English speaking children. *Language, Speech, and Hearing Services in Schools, 30,* 226–244.

Kayser, H. (1993). Hispanic cultures. In D. Battle (Ed.), *Communication disorders in multicultural populations* (pp. 114–157). Boston: Andover Medical Publishers.

Kayser, H. (1995a). *Bilingual speech-language pathology: An Hispanic focus.* San Diego, CA: Singular Publishing Group.

Kayser, H. (1995b). Intervention with children from linguistically and culturally diverse backgrounds. In M. E. Fey, J. Windsor, & S. F. Warren (Eds.). *Language Intervention: Preschool through the elementary years* (pp. 315–332). Baltimore, MD: Paul H. Brookes.

Kayser, H. (1998). Hispanic cultures and language. In D. Battle (Ed.), *Communication disorders in multicultural populations* (2nd ed., pp.157–196). Boston: Butterworth-Heinemann.

Kiernan, B., & Swisher, L. (1990). The initial learning of novel English words: Two single-subject experiments with minority-language children. *Journal of Speech and Hearing Research, 33,* 707–716.

Kohnert, K., Yim, D., Nett, K., Kan, P. F., & Duran, L. (In Press). Intervention with linguistically diverse preschool children: A focus on developing home language(s). *Speech, Language Hearing Services in Schools.*

Langdon, H. (1988). Working with an interpreter/translator in the school setting. Dimensions of appropriate assessment for minority handicapped students: Recommended practices. Presented at the State Conference for School Superintendents, Tucson, AZ.

Langdon, H. (1992). Speech and language assessment of LEP/bilingual Hispanic students. In H. Langdon & L. R. L. Cheng (Eds.), *Hispanic children and adults with communication disorders* (pp. 201–271). Gaithersburg, MD: Aspen Publishers.

Lynch, E. W., & Hanson, M. J. (2004). *Developing cross-cultural competence* (3rd ed.). Baltimore, MD: Paul H. Brooks.

No Child Left Behind Act. Available at http://www.nclb.gov.

Pena, E. D., & Gillam, R. B. (2000). Dynamic assessment of children referred for speech and language evaluations. In C. Lidz & J. Elliott (Eds.), *Dynamic assessment: Prevailing models and applications* (Vol. 6, pp. 543–575). Oxford, England: Elsevier Science.

Pena, E., Iglesias, A., & Lidz, C. (2001). Reducing test bias through dynamic assessment of children's word learning ability. *American Journal of Speech-Language Pathology, 10,* 138–154.

Perozzi, J. A. (1985). A pilot study of language facilitation for bilingual, language handicapped children: Theoretical and intervention implications. *Journal of Speech and Hearing Disorders, 50,* 403–406.

Perozzi, J. A., & Chavez-Sanchez, M. L. (1992, October). The effect of instruction in L1 on receptive acquisition of L2 for bilingual children with language delay. *Language, Speech, and Hearing Services in Schools, 23,* 348–352.

Roseberry-McKibbin, C. (2002). *Multicultural students with special language needs.* Oceanside, CA: Academic Communication Associates.

Saenz, T. I., & Huer, M. B. (2003). Testing strategies involving least biased language assessment of bilingual children. *Communication Disorders Quarterly, 24*(4), 184–193.

Saville-Troike, M. (1986). Anthropological considerations in the study of communication. In O. Taylor (Ed.), *Nature of communication disorders in culturally and linguistically diverse populations* (pp. 1–19). San Diego, CA: College-Hill Press.

Scott, D. M. (2002). Multicultural aspects of hearing disorders and audiology. In D. E. Battle (Ed.), *Communication disorders in multicultural populations* (3rd ed.) Boston: Butterworth-Heinemann.

Scudder, R., & Holmskog, S. (1989). *Spanish-speaking children's repairs during conversation with an Anglo adult.* Unpublished manuscript.

Taylor, O. (1986). Historical perspectives and conceptual framework. In O. Taylor (Ed.), *Nature of communication disorders in culturally and linguistically diverse populations* (pp. 1–19). San Diego, CA: College-Hill Press.

U.S. Census Bureau. (2002). *Census 2000 Special Reports, Series CENSR-4, Demographic Trends in the 20th century.* Available at http://www.census.gov/prod/2002pubs/censr-4.pdf

U.S. Census Bureau. (2002). *Annual demographic supplement to the March 2002 current population survey.* Washington, DC: Author.

U.S. Department of Health and Human Services. (1985). *Report of the secretary's task force on black and minority health* (Vol. 1, Executive Summary, Publication 491-313/44706). Washington, DC: Government Printing Office.

U.S. Department of Health and Human Services. (2004). *National healthcare disparities report. Priority populations: Racial and ethnic minorities* (pp. 87–100). Washington, DC: Author.

Valdes, G., & Figueroa, R. (1995). *Bilingualism and testing: A special case of bias.* Norwood, NJ: Ablex Publishing.

Wetherby, A. M., & Prizant, B. M. (2002). *Communication and symbolic behavior scales—Developmental profile.* Baltimore, MD: Brookes Publishing.

RESOURCES

American Speech-Language-Hearing Association Link to Multicultural Tools http://www.asha.org/

Battle, D. (Ed.). (2002). *Communication disorders in multicultural populations* (2nd ed.). Boston: Butterworth-Heinemann.

Bialystok, E. (2001). *Bilingualism in development: Language, literacy, & cognition.* Cambridge, England: University of Cambridge.

Genesee, F., Paradis, J., & Crago, M. B. (2004). *Dual language development & disorders: A handbook on bilingualism & second language learning.* Baltimore, MD: Brookes Publishing.

Goldstein, B. A. (2004). *Bilingual language development & disorders in Spanish-English speakers.* Baltimore, MD: Brookes Publishing.

Stone, J. H. (2005). *Culture and disability.* Thousand Oaks, CA: Sage.

24

Supervision and the Supervisory Process

ELIZABETH S. MCCREA, PHD
LEE ANN C. GOLPER, PHD

SCOPE OF CHAPTER

The supervisory process is an important contributor to the education, training and career development of personnel in the professions. This chapter will first discuss supervision in speech-language pathology from a historical perspective. Subsequently, a model of supervision in clinical education will be presented that has the flexibility to support the development of speech-language pathologists and audiologists at all stages of professional development and in varied service delivery settings. In the course of presenting the model, implementing strategies and tools will also be suggested and issues of supervisor competency and accountability will also be discussed. Finally, we will examine supervision in the work place to promote staff development and job satisfaction.

HISTORICAL OVERVIEW

The supervisory process and supervisors have been a part of the preparation and training of members of the professions of speech-language pathology and audiology almost since their beginning. For a summary of the very early years in the development of the process, Anderson (1988), Farmer and Farmer (1989), and Ulrich (1985) offer accounts of the evolution of supervision.

During the decade of the 1960s, the first conferences concerning aspects of the supervisory process (Anderson & Milisen, 1965; Kleffner, 1964; Miner, 1967; Villareal, 1964) were held. Reports and articles were published at the conclusion of these conferences, and a monograph by Darley (1967) and an article on supervision (Halfond, 1964) also contributed to the early literature in supervision.

The interest in supervision quickened during the 1970s. Conferences continued (Anderson, 1970; Turton, 1973), and the ASHA Committee on Supervision was established in 1975. The Council of College and University Supervisors of Practicum was founded in 1970 and soon expanded its membership in 1974 as it became the Council of University Supervisors in Speech-Language Pathology and Audiology (CUSPSPA) and began publishing its own quarterly newsletter, *SUPERvision*. For the first time, books on supervision in the field were published (Oratio, 1977; Rassi, 1978; Schubert, 1978). In addition, training programs in Communication Sciences and Disorders began offering course work to prepare individuals for their work as supervisors.

The 1980s saw several important events that continued to develop interest in supervision. The Council of Graduate Programs in Communication Sciences and Disorders (now the Council of Academic Programs in Communication Sciences and Disorders) held a conference devoted entirely to student supervision. CUSPSPA held two national conferences, one in 1987 and the second in 1989. Proceedings from each of these conferences were published and continued to build the literature base in supervision. ASHA certification

and accreditation bodies began to recognize the need for quality supervision through enhanced requirements for educational and service programs (ASHA, 1983). Most importantly, the ASHA Legislative Council adopted a position statement that outlined 13 tasks and 81 associated competencies describing appropriate supervision. Four major books were published (Anderson, 1988; Casey, Smith, & Ulrich, 1988; Crago & Pickering, 1987; Farmer & Farmer, 1989).

CUSPSPA continued its leadership in supervision during the 1990s by sponsoring three national conferences, each of which published proceedings (Bruce, 1994; Dowling 1992b; Wagner, 1996). Two books (Dowling, 1992a; Rassi & McElroy, 1992) combined theory and practice in supervision. ASHA accreditation and certification bodies continued their emphasis on the importance of quality clinical education, and therefore supervision, as they developed new standards for program accreditation and certification of personnel. New standards require documentation of knowledge and skill and stipulate both formative and summative assessment of students' courses of study (ASHA, 2000).

ASHA also recognized the importance of supervision in the development of other levels of personnel within the professions. In 1993 the Clinical Certification Board recognized the importance of quality supervision during the clinical fellowship (CF) experience and revised the ASHA Membership and Certification Handbook in speech-language pathology to document the nature of supervision during the CF (ASHA 1997). Appropriate supervision was also seen as an important component in the utilization of support personnel; a position statement was adopted in 1995 (ASHA, 1995) and a set of guidelines in 1996. Both of these specify supervisory activities necessary in the appropriate training and use of speech-language pathology assistants (ASHA, 1996). As a result of organizational restructuring within ASHA, CUSPSPA was sunsetted; however, Special Interest Division 11, Administration and Supervision, took its place and currently has a membership of more than 700 (Newman, 2005). This Division publishes three newsletters (*Perspectives*) each year for its members.

In the first half of this decade, Division 11 sponsored three national conferences on administration and supervision in 2001, 2002, and 2003. In addition two primary books were published that continued the merging of theory and practice in supervision (Dowling, 2001; McCrea & Brasseur, 2003). Importantly, the Council of Academic Programs in Communication Sciences and Disorders began to include clinic directors in university training programs in their annual conferences. These meetings regularly offer presentations relative to best practices in clinical education and provide supervisors the opportunity for face-to-face networking regarding issues important to the development of personnel in the professions.

DEFINITIONS

It was not until late in the decade of the 1970s that a concrete notion of what supervision was and what supervisors did in clinical education was developed. The ASHA Committee on Supervision (1978) began to differentiate the clinical process from the supervisory process. It defined *supervision* as the "interaction that takes place between the supervisor and clinician and may be related to the behavior of the clinician or the client or to the program in which the supervisor and clinician are employed" (ASHA, 1978, p. 479). The committee went further to distinguish two primary categories of tasks that supervisors often complete. *Clinical teaching* was defined as the "interaction between supervisor/supervisee in any setting which furthers the development of clinical skills of students or practicing clinicians as related to changes in client behavior" (ASHA, 1978, p. 479). *Program management* was defined as "those activities that relate to the administration or coordination of programs, for example, scheduling, budgeting, program planning, employing, or dismissing personnel" (p. 479). Clearly, these two kinds of activity are different, yet at the same time are related and overlaid on each other. Clinical teaching may receive greater emphasis in educational programs, but it is also a primary means through which continuing growth and development of clinicians is implemented after they enter the workforce. Program management, on the other hand, may be the predominant responsibility of the supervisor in service delivery settings.

A decade later, Anderson (1988) proposed a definition of supervision that has guided much of the study and development of the supervisory process within the professions in the last 25 years. She defined supervision as:

> A process that consists of a variety of patterns of behavior, the appropriateness of which depends upon the needs, competencies, expectations, and philosophies of the supervisor and the supervisee and the specifics of the situation (task, client, setting, and other variables). The goals of the supervisory process are the professional growth and development of the supervisee and the supervisor, which it is assumed will result in optimal service to clients. (p. 12)

This was the first time that a definition of supervision which identified the variables inherent in the process was published in the professional literature. Just as important, it offered a perspective on the process that is applicable across all levels of supervisees (i.e., from preprofessional to professional).

CONTINUUM MODEL OF THE SUPERVISORY PROCESS

Anderson's definition of supervision recognizes that supervision is a dynamic process for the professional development of both the supervisor and supervisee. It is based on the assumption that professionals will be involved in some supervisory or consultative experience beginning during their training and continuing for the duration of their careers and that the expectations and needs of those involved in the process change over this period. The continuum mandates a change in the amount and type of involvement of both the supervisor and supervisee. Further, the supervisor's major responsibility is to assist the supervisee in achieving competent independence so that their relationship becomes one of peer consultation rather than dependency. This concept of supervision negates the earlier belief that supervision should be directive, controlling, and evaluative. In this older

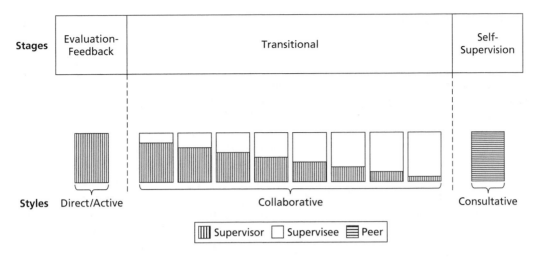

FIGURE 24–1 Anderson's Continuum of Supervision

SOURCE: Adapted from *The Supervisory Process in Speech-Language Pathology and Audiology (p.62)* by J.L. Anderson, 1988, Boston: College-Hill Press/Little Brown and Company. Reprinted with permission.

model, supervisees were expected to be passive participants in the process, responding to supervisor comments, requests, and direction. The continuum model of supervision, however, parallels supervisory practices described by Blumberg (1980), Cogan (1973), Goldhammer (1969), Goldhammer, Anderson, and Krajewski (1980), and Costa and Garmston (1985) and the clinical education process described by McAllister (2000). Importantly, this dynamic continuum model of supervision is consistent with the current standards for accreditation of academic training programs in communication sciences and disorders (ASHA, 2000). These standards necessitate supervisory practices that are appropriate to the supervisee's level of knowledge, experience, and emerging competence. The goal of contemporary supervision is to develop speech-language pathologists and audiologists who can think critically, make decisions, and solve problems in changing educational and medical contexts with a variety of patient/client types and disorders.

Stages of the Continuum

Given the variables listed earlier (i.e., needs, expectations, philosophy, and competency of both supervisor and supervisee as well as the specifics of the

setting) in Anderson's definition (1988), it is clear that there probably is not one way to supervise. In fact, the model is based on the belief that supervision exists on a continuum and uses different strategies and styles appropriate at different points in time and determined by the variables in the definition (task, client, organizational structure, etc.). See Figure 24–1. The continuum requires a change over time in the amount and type of involvement of both supervisor and supervisee in the process. For example, as the degree of dominance of the supervisor decreases, the responsibility and participation of the supervisee increases. Most importantly, none of the stages of the continuum are time bound; individual supervisees may be found at any point on the continuum throughout their career, depending upon personal and professional situational variables. The three stages are (1) evaluation-feedback, (2) transitional, and (3) self-supervision.

Evaluation-Feedback Stage In the initial stage the supervisor plays a traditional, leading, information giving, and directive role in the supervisory relationship. Supervisees tend to be at an entry level with minimal knowledge and skill in working with a particular type of client or disorder. They may also be those students who are struggling to meet expectations and have not demonstrated the ability to think, implement, and self-evaluate. They are unable to demonstrate independent professional competence that is necessary for professional practice. Whatever the reason for placement in the evaluation-feedback stage, the goal for both supervisor and supervisee is to work together in a productive way to move quickly from this point.

Transitional Stage   In this stage, the supervisor and supervisee gradually become more collaborative in their interaction. As supervisees demonstrate more consistent and higher levels of knowledge and skill in the clinical context, their relationship with their supervisors become more peer-like and the focus becomes one of joint problem solving. In this stage, supervisees participate in varying degrees in decision making. They are learning to analyze their clinical behavior and to plan future strategies on the basis of that analysis. For example, they can problem solve before and after a clinical experience, and this ability in turn makes them better able to make modifications during their clinical sessions, as opposed to waiting to discuss changes with their supervisors between clinical sessions. Supervisees may move back and forth within this stage depending upon many variables—the tasks, their experience level, and the setting in which the training takes place. If supervisees lose ground on the continuum for whatever reason, the important factor in this movement is that they can "recover" their position in the transitional stage because of their previous experience within the clinical process and their growing understanding of themselves as clinicians.

Self-Supervision Stage   Self-supervision is the ultimate goal of clinical teaching and the stage in which supervisees have the ability to accurately analyze their clinical behavior and its outcomes and to change it based on these analyses. They are no longer dependent upon supervisors for observation, analysis, and feedback about their work. It is also the stage in which supervisees become responsible for their own professional growth. But, as rapidly as research and regulation change the dynamics in the professions, it is the stage in which

supervisees also continue to desire peer interaction and consultation.

Supervisors need to be aware of the continuum as they plan for each supervisee. Additionally, they need to possess the flexibility that will enable them to adjust their behaviors as they move back and forth along the continuum and between supervisees. The task of identifying the placement of a supervisor/supervisee dyad on the continuum is one of the most fundamental and important decisions within the supervisory process because it determines how supervisor and supervisee will work together.

Striving to reach the self-supervision stage is important in speech-language pathology and audiology because many professionals work alone or without supervision or consultation from persons trained in their own profession. When working in such situations, the responsibility for professional growth lies with the individual. This increases the need for educational programs to produce self-analytical supervisees and for practicing professionals to have way(s) of continuing their professional growth. The continuum model of supervision presented here and its attendant phases and styles of behavior offer a process for accomplishing this goal (McCrea & Brasseur, 2003).

Styles of Supervisor Behavior

The appropriate style for each stage of the continuum—direct-active, collaborative, or consultative—is determined by the skill level of the supervisee and the nature of the task as it relates to client needs.

Direct-Active Style   The direct-active style of supervisory interaction is most appropriate for the evaluation-feedback stage of the continuum. It embodies the behavior described in the early descriptive studies in supervision: telling, suggesting, and evaluating. In this style the supervisor is controlling and directive while the supervisee is respondent, if not passive, and in a subordinate position. The direct-active style can be appropriate for supervisees early in their development when they have difficulty analyzing the client's behavior and their own; however, the decision to use it should be made carefully. Several questions should be answered to help determine if this style is indeed appropriate:

- By whose judgment is the supervisee determined to be inexperienced or unskilled?

- On what basis has the judgment been made that the supervisee is in the evaluation-feedback stage?

- Has the judgment been based on objective data?

- Or, is the judgment the result of subjective appraisal by the supervisor?

- Is this the supervisor's style with all supervisees? (McCrea & Brasseur, 2003)

A certain amount of directing, suggesting, and modeling by supervisors is certainly appropriate at times, especially in light of possible answers to these questions. Protracted use of this style, however, may also be a deterrent to the independence and growth of the supervisee.

Collaborative Style The collaborative style is the appropriate style for moving away from the evaluation-feedback stage/direct-active style of supervision. The supervisor's role becomes increasingly less direct but certainly not inactive. Both supervisor and supervisee assume responsibility and provide input in varying degrees at different times about both the clinical and supervisory process. Objectives for client, supervisee, and supervisory interaction are jointly established. The supervisor provides feedback but also encourages input from the supervisee, accepts the supervisee's ideas, problem solves with the supervisee, analyzes clinical behavior, and encourages self-analysis and further planning by the supervisee. All of these actions recognize and respect the supervisee as a developing professional. The supervisee, in turn, accepts increasing responsibility for participation in the clinical and supervisory process, provides input, accepts suggestions, questions the supervisor, requests rationale and justification for supervisor statements, and engages in self-analysis and problem solving. Again, these activities encourage greater independence. Supervision is

seen as a joint process in which the supervisor and supervisee share responsibilities and interact as professionals to meet common objectives (McCrea & Brasseur, 2003).

Consultative Style As supervisees assume greater responsibility, they move logically toward the self-supervision stage. Self-supervision requires a continuing search for professional growth through self-analysis of professional behavior and work. The supervisee at this stage will be able to self-identify strengths and weaknesses, make appropriate behavioral modifications, and seek assistance though further knowledge when necessary. As with other stages, self-supervision is not time bound, and therefore, the consultative style may be used at appropriate times in the educational program, the off-campus/externship or CF experience, or the employment setting. A supervisor using the Consultative Style will be mainly listening, supporting, problem solving, and when appropriate, giving direct suggestions. This supervisory style is closely aligned with the concept of mentoring in which collaboration and support without direct evaluation are hallmarks (McCrea & Brasseur, 2003).

PHASES OF SUPERVISION

While the continuum of supervision provides a conceptual model of the supervisory process, what is also needed is a strategy that will facilitate the development of supervisees across the continuum. Anderson (1988) postulated five phases of the supervisory process, which are cyclical and, over time, permit the increasing independence of supervisees in problem solving and thinking critically. (1) understanding, (2) planning, (3) observation and data collection, (4) analysis, and (5) integration.

Understanding Phase

This phase prepares both supervisors and supervisees for meaningful participation in the supervisory process and encourages them to communicate about the supervisory process throughout their entire period of interaction. The purpose of this preparation is the development of mutual understanding of the various components of the supervisory process so that supervisory interactions are enriched. Thus, participants are better able to use the process to strengthen clinical performance and promote professional growth. This mutual understanding will come from basic knowledge about the supervisory process. Both participants should discuss their expectations and needs. In fact, this sharing of goals and objectives, defining needs and expectations, and clarification of the differences and similarities in perception of roles may well be one of most important components of the entire supervisory interaction, probably forming the pattern for the entire relationship (McCrea & Brasseur, 2003). The Resource section identifies several tools to begin the dialogue during the understanding phase and to continue to use throughout the supervisory relationship.

Planning Phase

Behavior change for clients and professional growth for supervisees and supervisors comes as the result of fourfold planning: for the client, for the clinician, for the supervisee, and for the supervisor (Anderson, 1988; McCrea & Brasseur, 2003). It is insufficient to plan only for the clinical improvement of the client. The supervisory process deserves equal attention so that the supervisee and supervisor also learn and develop from their interaction. Both supervisor and supervisee must plan and set goals for the supervisory context and must determine how they will document their own progress in this relationship. From the data collection of their own work together, they will be able to plan for their own evolution in the supervisory process.

Basic to the success of the planning phase is determining the ability level of the supervisee and matching that with an appropriate supervisory style (McCrea & Brasseur, 2003). This determination is important to supervision in any setting but takes on added importance in light of the new ASHA standards for accreditation and ultimately for certification (ASHA, 2000). These standards state that

the amount of supervision of clinical practicum "must be appropriate to the student's level of knowledge, experience, and competence" (p. 7). Several issues are important in making this determination:

- The supervisee's ability to solve problems
- The degree of dependency/independency of supervisees as clinicians and as supervisees
- The ability of supervisees to self-observe and analyze their behavior
- The supervisors' flexibility in adapting their style to supervisee levels of development (McCrea & Brasseur, 2003)

Tools to facilitate this assessment are identified in the Resource section.

Observation and Data Collection Phase

This phase of the supervisory process requires the collection of objective data so that events can be reconstructed accurately enough for analysis (Goldhammer, Anderson, & Krajewski, 1980). It is also the phase of supervision that moves it from a subjective to an objective process. Anderson (1988) stated that "observation without data collection is a waste of time" (p. 123). It is crucial to collect observational facts without coloring them with personal perception or commentary.

Specific observation/data collection activities will be, in great measure, tied to the goals and objectives developed during the planning phase. It is important for the observer to have a purpose for the observation activity. For instance, is it to collect baseline data? Monitor quality assurance services? Measure progress toward therapy goals? Or is it to identify patterns of supervisee behavior that facilitate or impede the clinical process? Whatever the purpose for observation, the resulting data should be organized in such a way that will enable the observer to relate the behavior of the supervisee to the consequences of that behavior for the client (McCrea & Brasseur, 2003). Suggestions for tools to facilitate the observation/data collection phase can be found in the Resource section.

Analysis Phase

The purpose of the analysis phase is to make sense of the data that have been collected. At this time, behaviors of the supervisee are related to the behaviors of the client and when those of the supervisor are related to those of the supervisee. This is the point that the continuum model and process of supervision differs most from traditional supervision described in the early literature. Developing analytical skills may well be the most important contributor to producing thoughtful, analytical professionals (McCrea & Brasseur, 2003).

If supervisees are to become clinically competent and independently functioning professionals, they must develop expertise in self-analysis. It is important for them to become cognizant of their behavior and the effect of that behavior on their clients if they are to modify or strengthen those behaviors. The analysis process enables clinicians to extract from a mass of behaviors a design from which they can begin to see what is happening, to draw inferences, to construct hypotheses about what was effective and what was not, to test those hypotheses, and then to plan for the future on the basis of their findings. Analysis, particularly when it is conducted jointly between supervisee and supervisor, contributes in a major way to meeting expectations of supervisees for fair and rational feedback and evaluation. Thus, their evaluation emanates from objective data, and they become involved in analyzing and evaluating their own behavior (McCrea & Brasseur, 2003).

Cogan (1973) identified several objectives for the analysis phase:

- Determining if objectives from the planning stage were met
- Identifying salient patterns in the teacher's (supervisee's) behavior
- Identifying unanticipated learning by the student (client)
- Identifying critical incidents in the interaction (behavior that significantly affects the learning or relationship between teacher and student)

- Organizing the data to determine what was learned
- Determining if what was planned was carried out
- Developing a database for the rest of the supervision program

Whatever the focus of analysis, this phase of the continuum process should increasingly become the responsibility of supervisees. As they accept this responsibility, they become similarly responsible for their own behavior and professional growth.

Integration Phase

This final stage involves purposeful feedback and communication between supervisor and supervisee and employs data and analyses to understand the behavior of the client, the supervisee, and/or the supervisor. Typically, this communication takes place in regularly scheduled conferences between supervisees and supervisors. Supervisor behavior is important to the implementation of this phase and to the development of collaborative and ultimately consultative styles of supervision that permit increasingly more active, responsible, independent supervisees.

The content of supervisory conferences should be determined by individual needs, placement on the continuum, supervisory objectives, and other factors important to both supervisee and supervisor. The provision of feedback, whether oral or written, is an important part of conference dialogue. Kurpius and Christie (1978) suggest the following criteria in regard to providing feedback:

- It should be descriptive and objective rather than evaluative.
- It should be specific rather than general.
- It should be appropriate for the recipient.
- It should be about something on which the recipient can act.
- It should be well timed with regard to events.
- It should be checked with regard to its clarity.
- The recipient should want/expect the feedback.

The integration phase is the culmination of all the effort and time that has thus far gone into the supervisory process. The process, however, does not end here. Once a specific set of outcomes has been achieved, the process and phases repeat themselves with new focus, new planning, and new dynamics. Goals that have been previously achieved now must be revisited and refined, hopefully with greater insight and independence on the part of the supervisee.

CONSIDERATIONS ACROSS DIFFERENT LEVELS OF SUPERVISEES

The continuum model of supervision is flexible enough to accommodate all levels of supervisees throughout their training. The key decision that needs to be made, however, is the placement of the supervisee on the continuum and what this decision means for both the amount of supervision and the supervisor's style. In addition to the information referenced earlier in the chapter, the following supervisee-specific information will help a supervisor individualize his or her work with a supervisee:

- Experience with similar clients/disorders
- Academic preparation for disorder management
- Supervisee's perception of his or her own strengths/needs in terms of the client
- Anxieties about management of the client/disorder
- Types of previous supervisory experiences
- Perception of self in terms of general clinical dependence/independence
- Prior responsibility for data collection and analysis of client behavior and his or her own clinical behavior

Whalen (2001) also suggests 10 generic abilities that are also important to supervisees' ability to generalize from one context to another and to successfully apply their knowledge and skill with clients and their families in practice settings:

- Commitment to learning
- Interpersonal skills
- Communication skills
- Effective use of time and resources
- Use of constructive feedback
- Problem solving
- Professionalism
- Responsibility
- Critical thinking
- Stress management

Some perspective on these domains of behavior would also be helpful to fully understand supervisees' appropriate placement on the continuum.

Even with this specific information to consider, some general statements can be made about continuum placement based on supervisee prior clinical experience and course work. Typically, beginning students, whether at the undergraduate or graduate level, will be placed in the evaluation-feedback stage of the continuum and appreciate supervisors who use a direct-active style of supervision (i.e., teaching, structuring, directing, evaluating). A unique adaptation of the direct-active style and a downward extension of this stage/style is the apprenticeship model; an example of this approach to supervision was described by Gillam & Pena (1995) and Gillam (1999). In the initial stages of this training approach, supervisees are assigned to supervisors who function as master clinicians and who model and interpret clinical behavior for supervisees during an initial period of highly structured, specific observation. Gradually, supervisors encourage supervisee participation at a comfortable, yet challenging, level and provide a bridge for generalizing skills and knowledge from familiar to novel situations. The contemporary ASHA standards (ASHA, 2000) that require competent and independent demonstration of clinical skill by supervisees require that supervisors move away from this direct modeling of behavior and help students become active clinical problem solvers. This requires the active engagement of supervisees in planning and decision making about clients and their treatment programs and necessitates a supervisory approach that will facilitate the ability of supervisees to monitor and modify their own behavior. The transitional and self-supervision stages of the continuum provide a means to meet this challenge.

CRITICAL THINKING AND THE SUPERVISORY PROCESS

Simply put, critical thinking is the complexity of one's thought and is itself thought to be developmental in nature (Moses & Shapiro, 1996). The most simplistic level of thought is binary in nature: something is right or wrong, black or white. This is followed by early logical decision making in which solutions are determined based on one's experience or opinion. Later, logical decision making permits solutions to be determined based on the nature of the supporting arguments for or against a course of action. The last and highest level of critical thinking is the awareness that truth is conditional and that an appropriate solution in one situation might not be appropriate in another.

The ASHA standards (ASHA, 2000) require the education and training of students "who can think critically." The continuum model of supervision makes maximal use of objective data and self-analyses by both the supervisor and supervisee and emphasizes an analytical approach to understanding and creating change in behavior. The process of supervision that implements the model is compatible with the developmental aspects of critical thinking:

- Dichotic thinking—Evaluation-Feedback Stage
- Early and late logical decision making—Transitional Stage
- Awareness that truth is relative—Self-Supervision Stage (Moses & Shapiro, 1996)

Levels of critical thinking are increasingly evidenced across the continuum of supervision by supervisees' abilities to analyze their own behavior and its consequences and to propose appropriate modifications with greater independence.

Mature critical thinking skills are clearly important in training programs, but they are also important to organizational effectiveness in professional settings (Dowling, 2001). Here again, the continuum model of the supervisory process has the potential to contribute to the development of critical thinkers who will serve not only their clients but their employers in positive ways.

EXPECTATIONS OF STUDENTS ABOUT SUPERVISION

There are few data in the literature of the professions about the expectations of supervisees with regard to the supervisory process. Dowling (2001) indicated that supervisees want to be actively involved in conferences, particularly as they gain experience and do not expect to assume a passive role in which they are told what to do. They want and expect feedback and guidance from their supervisor. Most importantly, they want the opportunity to contribute their thoughts and have their ideas respected, incorporated, and responded to in a thoughtful manner. They want to be valued as emerging professionals. The continuum model of supervision and its associated stages, styles of interaction, and process phases offer a way of meeting student expectations about the supervisory process and their participation in it.

SUPERVISION IN SERVICE DELIVERY SETTINGS

The environments in which speech-language pathologists and audiologists work are increasingly varied, and individuals who work in these settings are experiencing significant change and reconfiguration. Changes are often associated with decreases in the financial resources necessary to maintain an appropriate array of services for those with communication disorders. This in turn has prompted managers of service delivery systems in the professions to find ways to extend appropriate and effective service to patients and clients in cost-effective ways.

UTILIZATION AND SUPERVISION OF SPEECH-LANGUAGE PATHOLOGY ASSISTANTS

The use of speech-language pathology assistants (SLPAs) who are supervised by certified speech-language pathologists is one way to "increase the frequency of service to clients while maintaining service quality and controlling cost" (ASHA, 2001). In 1996 ASHA approved guidelines for the training, credentialing, use, and supervision of assistants. This document detailed a scope of responsibility and defined the parameters of work for both assistants and the speech-language pathologists who supervise them. These guidelines make it clear that while assistants can complete a variety of tasks, including direct service to clients, they must work under the direction of a certified and, if appropriate, licensed speech-language pathologist who retains all legal and ethical responsibility for the client. In addition to ASHA guidelines, individual states may regulate the utilization and supervision of assistants. When ASHA and state regulations governing the supervision of assistants are not consistent, the speech-language pathologist should follow the more conservative set of requirements (McCrea & Brasseur, 2003). Chapter 10 discusses paraprofessionals in more detail.

Supervision Standards of SLPAs

The profession of speech-language pathology adopted minimum standards for supervision of speech-language pathology assistants that involve both indirect and direct supervisory activities (ASHA, 2001). *Indirect* supervision involves demonstration, record review, and review and evaluation of taped sessions. *Direct* supervision is defined as on-site, in-view observation and guidance by the speech-language pathologist while the assistant performs the assigned activity. In addition to the nature of the supervisory activity, the guidelines also specify the minimum amount of supervision that must be documented when SLPAs are part of the service delivery system. During the first 90 days, 30 percent of all assistant activity must be supervised:

- No less than 20 percent direct supervision should be provided during client contact.
- Indirect supervision may make up the remaining 10 percent.
- Each client assigned to the assistant must have direct contact with the supervising speech-language pathologist at least once every 2 weeks.
- The supervising speech-language pathologist must review data on clients seen by the assistant each week.

After the first 90 days of employment, as appropriate, the amount of supervision may be adjusted, dependent upon the assistant's competency and need; however, a minimum of 20 percent supervision must be maintained throughout the period of employment, 10 percent of which is direct.

Amount of Supervision for SLPAs

One of the most significant concerns surrounding the use of assistants, particularly when they contribute to the service delivery mission of a facility, is the determination of how much supervision is necessary for each client interaction carried out by the SLPA. In addition to variables associated directly with the assistant (e.g., training, experience), Hagler and MacFarlane (1997) suggest that issues of degree of client contact, the complexity of client contact, and the degree of interpersonal interaction required by that contact are also important in this decision. Generally, the more complex the activity and the more intensively a client is seen, the greater the need for greater levels of supervision, even levels of supervision that exceed the minimum levels required by the ASHA guidelines.

Phases of SLPA Supervision

In addition to administrative and regulatory considerations in the utilization of speech-language pathology assistants, supervising speech-language pathologists must also think about the content of their supervision. McCrea and Brasseur (2003) suggest that a modified continuum perspective is a viable methodology for the supervisory process with assistants. If growth is to occur on the part of assistants within their scope of responsibilities and their assigned tasks, then there must be a shift between the supervisor and the assistant with regard to responsibility for the substantive content of the process and conferences. The supervision of the assistant should not just focus on the evaluation of the assistant by the supervisor. It should develop opportunities for joint problem solving in an effort to enhance the assistant's knowledge and skill within his or her scope of responsibility.

The phases of supervision (i.e., understanding, planning, observation, analysis, and integration) provide a concrete framework for building a supervisory program that will support the assistant's ongoing development. The discussion of these phases earlier in the chapter continues to be cogent with regard to supervision of assistants. In addition, ASHA (1999) and Mullins and McCready (2002) have developed activities and forms consistent with the continuum model to use in the supervision of speech-language pathology assistants.

SUPERVISION IN THE WORK PLACE

Clinical service delivery in audiology and speech-language pathology is a human enterprise. We are people providing services to better the lives of other people. The people who provide clinical services,

the organization's employees, are its greatest asset (Golper & Brown, 2005); thus, the primary purpose for supervision in clinical service delivery settings is *personnel management.*

In a clinical service delivery setting, the supervisee is a paid employee, not a student; nonetheless, the same supervisory skills apply in either context. In the work setting, just as in the clinical training program, the supervisor plans, observes, analyzes and responds to the behavior of the supervisee. In the work setting, however, the supervisor is less concerned with the supervisee's acquisition of new knowledge or developing basic clinical skills and independent decision making and more concerned with ensuring the supervisee is qualified and capably managing all of his/her job performance expectations. In clinical service delivery, supervision is the responsibility of those individuals who hold positions with a designated supervisor title—department or division *directors, managers,* program *coordinators, team leaders,* and the like. Supervisors may be responsible for supervising only one or two people, or whole departments. Depending upon the structure of the program, supervisors may also be held accountable for overseeing a budget for their program area. In clinical service settings, supervisors typically have four interrelated areas of responsibilities:

1. Provision of quality services that meet client expectations
2. Compliance with standards
3. Oversight of program budgets
4. Management of human resources

Management of human resources includes an array of activities such as: providing staff orientations and conducting performance appraisals; rewarding and recognizing employees for exemplary performance; approving vacation and other leave requests; setting staff development goals; approving purchases; and recommending salary increases. Supervisors are also required to take corrective actions when employees are not meeting expectations. Knowing how to motivate others and how to provide effective counseling or training for performance improvements, and take disciplinary actions as needed, are essential qualities for effective supervision of employees.

An important aspect of the management of human resources is staffing. Supervisors must ensure that the programs are *adequately staffed* (have enough people to meet the workloads) and *competently staffed* (have the right skill mix within the staff for the types and complexities of cases seen). Supervisors also must ensure that the clinical staff has the materials, equipment, and resources to do their jobs and that the services they provide meet quality standards; satisfy clients and their families; comply with accrediting and payer regulations; and adhere to budgetary expectations. Supervisors ensure that the productivity expectation for each staff member is achievable and will adequately contribute to the organization's performance expectations. Productivity expectations are a part of any employee's job responsibility regardless of where they work (e.g., schools, clinics, hospitals), and those expectations need to be clearly explained at the time of hire. Productivity may be defined as a *caseload*, or the number of clients assigned to an individual clinician, or some targeted metric, such as a certain number of visits per day, or a certain amount of billed time per day.

Supervision of Clinical Fellows and Audiology Externs

Supervisors in clinical work settings view the clinical fellowship (CF) for speech-language pathologists (SLPs) and the externship year at the end of the Doctor of Audiology (AuDs) curriculum, essentially as *trainee level* staff positions. When clinical fellows (CFs) and AuD externs are hired into these entry level staff positions, they are expected to meet essentially all of the incumbent obligations and responsibilities of any other employee and perform as an independent member of the staff. The exceptions include any activity that would require oversight and supervision by certified and/or licensed personnel. Because trainees have not yet completed all requirements for certification and/or licensure and are required to be supervised by more senior

clinicians, the trainees' supervisors serve as preceptors and mentors. Preceptors or mentoring supervisors typically plan out an individualized program of development building based upon the trainee's résumé (courses, clinical rotations, and experiences acquired during graduate training) and fleshing out areas identified as needing more extensive clinical exposure or further knowledge and skill development. CFs and AuD externs are expected to function fairly independently but in accordance with the regulations that apply within a given state, setting, and facility. For example, hospital programs may require all documentation be reviewed and cosigned by the supervising licensed clinician prior to filing in the client's medical record.

Credential Verifications

Once an applicant has been identified as a potentially good candidate for a clinical position, the following information in the application typically will be verified by the supervisor or hiring manager at the time of, or shortly following the interview:

- Academic credentials
- Previous employment or clinical affiliations
- References

Additionally, many facilities require that a background check be completed before a formal offer can be made to a potential employee. The supervisor may make additional verifications of credentials and experience during the initial orientation phase. The new employee will be asked to provide evidence of degrees, licensure, and any special certifications or training claimed in the application, such as cardiopulmonary resuscitation (CPR) training or evidence of having completed a continuing education workshop cited in the résumé. A copy of a transcript from graduate school is often requested to verify the new employee has had the required course work needed to perform his/her job. Transcripts and course work verifications may be waived if the applicant is a graduate of an accredited graduate program (i.e., accredited by the Council on Academic Accreditation, for example). In addition to verifying information new employees listed on their application, supervisors may ask them to verify that they have the specific competencies they will need to perform their specific job. This verification can include a skills assessment by the supervisor or a peer clinician or a self-assessment and rating of specific competencies related to the problems and populations they will encounter on the job. For example, new employees may be asked to rate their competency or familiarity with various standardized tests or procedures. If new employees lack some of the competencies required of a given position, they may be assigned a mentor to assist them with developing those competencies within a designated time frame, usually by the end of the employment probationary period.

Orientations and Probationary Periods, and Performance Appraisals

Supervisors are required to ensure that each employee they supervise knows what his or her particular job expectations are and, at least annually, to evaluate performance related to those job expectations. To ensure new employees know all of the elements of their job, supervisors in clinical programs are required to provide a comprehensive orientation during the first few days/weeks on the job. This orientation covers everything from the organization's vision statement to how to use the copy machine. This initial staff orientation requires that employees review and confirm that they understand the expectations and policies and procedures that will apply to their work. During the orientation period any training that is mandatory for all employees within the facility or program will also be completed (e.g., safety training, universal precautions, CPR, confidentiality). At a minimum, orientations include the following broad areas of review: (a) organizational overview (mission, vision, and goals of the organization); (b) office functions and logistics (e.g., phone procedures, computer access); (c) personnel policies (e.g., leave policies, mandatory training, dress code, salary, and benefits); and (d) clinical activities (e.g., productivity expectations, activities required to do the job, scheduling clients, documentation practices).

Most of the larger clinical service programs will require a probationary period, typically 3 to 6 months, for new employees. Probationary employees become regular employees after the initial performance appraisal has been conducted by the supervisor and when employees have demonstrated they can perform all job expectations. The time frame for the probationary period may vary depending upon the nature of the position; clerical staff usually have a briefer probationary period than professional staff. At the end of the probationary period and at the time of the probationary performance evaluation, a decision to either discontinue or continue the probationary period is made. Personnel policies vary somewhat between organizations, but usually probationary employees who clearly are not performing up to job expectations can be terminated by their supervisor *at will*. The typical due process rights do not apply until the employee is no longer in a probationary status.

Performance Appraisals

During the probationary performance appraisal and at the time of annual performance appraisal, supervisors must determine if the employee has met all of his or her key responsibilities and has demonstrated mastery of the competencies required for the job. Performance appraisals typically require the supervisor to review and rate each performance component, or key responsibility, across some kind of scale, such as "0 = does not meet performance expectations, 1 = meets performance expectations, 2 = exceeds performance expectations." The annual performance appraisal is intended to be a time when the supervisor and employee can reflect on the past year, review the goals that were achieved, and set goals for the next year. It is a time for constructive feedback and an opportunity to reward and recognize outstanding performance. Golper and Brown (2005) list the purposes of the supervisor's performance appraisal as follows:

- Express recognition and appreciation for contributions made by the employee during the past year.

- Discuss the employee's performance, including strengths and weaknesses.

- Address the quality and quantity of the employee's work.

- Assess and foster the employee's potential for further advancement and development.

- Build and strengthen the supervisor/employee mentoring relationship.

- Examine how goals and objectives were met during the previous year.

- Plan goals and objectives for the coming year. (p. 109)

360 Degree Assessments

Increasingly, organizations are using multiple sources of input in performance appraisals, or what is termed *360 degree assessments*. Research has demonstrated that performance evaluations based solely on a supervisor's ratings are less reliable and valid than those based on a variety of sources (U.S. Office of Personnel Management, 1997). There may be aspects of an individual's key responsibilities that would necessarily be better evaluated by a peer than a supervisor. Figure 24–2 illustrates the variety of sources of input that would comprise a 360 degree assessment.

Evaluating the Supervisor

Issues related to supervisor accountability are discussed in detail later in this chapter. When considering a 360 degree approach to performance assessments in the work setting, it should also be noted that multiple sources of input may be used in clinical work settings to evaluate the performance of supervisors as well as supervisees. In a 360 degree context, the performance appraisal of the supervisor would include: input from the support and clinical staff who directly report to the supervisor; input from peers within the program; input from external customers, such as supervisors in other departments; and an assessment by the administrator to whom the supervisor directly reports. Research indicates supervisors become more effective managers when they receive feedback from their supervisees as a part of their performance evaluation (United States Office of Personnel Management, 1997).

Professional Development

Another important concern for a supervisor in a clinical work setting is encouraging professional growth and career development among the staff. Large organizations may have an established career ladder. As the name implies, career *ladders* are a stepwise recognition of achievements in professional development spanning the entry level, trainee position through senior level, master clinician. Career ladders encourage employees to take on additional responsibilities within the program (lead a committee or team), acquire new skills, master an area of specialization, and represent the organization within the professional community through educational presentations or volunteer service in professional organizations. Career ladders allow employees to advance without having to seek promotion to a supervisor position. Advancement within an organization is a way to recognize the individual's achievement with a new title (e.g., Audiologist II) and usually includes a bonus or salary increase.

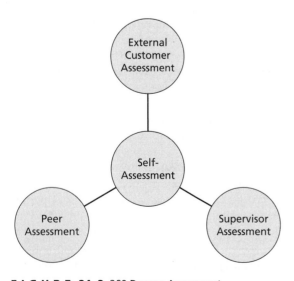

F I G U R E 24–2 360 Degree Assessment

SUPERVISOR COMPETENCIES

The ASHA (1985) position statement on clinical supervision specified 13 tasks supervisors in speech-language pathology and audiology should be able to do:

■ Establish and maintain an effective working relationship with the supervisee.

■ Assist the supervisee in developing clinical goals and objectives.

■ Assist the supervisee in developing and refining assessment skills.

■ Assist the supervisee in developing and refining clinical management skills.

■ Demonstrate for and participate with the supervisee in the clinical process.

■ Assist the supervisee in observing and analyzing assessment and treatment sessions.

■ Assist the supervisee in developing and maintaining clinical and supervisory records.

■ Interact with the supervisee in planning, executing, and analyzing supervisory conferences.

■ Assist the supervisee in evaluation of clinical performance.

■ Assist the supervisee in developing skills of verbal reporting, writing, and editing.

■ Share information regarding ethical, legal, regulatory, and reimbursement aspects of professional practice.

■ Model and facilitate professional conduct.

■ Demonstrate research skills in the clinical or supervisory process.

Each task then is broken down into 81 competencies distributed across these 13 tasks; however, since the time of the position statement and in light of the revision of standards for training program accreditation and certification of personnel (ASHA, 2000), an additional task (and associated competencies) should be added to this list:

■ Interact with the supervisee in the formative assessment process, which would include determining the dependence/independence of supervisees as well as the appropriate amount of supervision based on this determination.

These tasks and competencies only reflect the "technical" aspects of supervisory knowledge and skill. In addition, it is important for supervisors to think about the way they accomplish these tasks/competences—that is, how they mediate the technical aspects of their role through their own behavior. These may be termed *process* competencies and include skills such as:

■ Active listening

■ Self-analysis of their behavior in their role as supervisor

■ Demonstration of cultural competency

■ Demonstration of interpersonal immediacy through nonverbal and verbal relational communication strategies as well as nondefensive communication strategies

All of these tasks, whether in the technical or process domain, underscore the complexity as well as the subtlety of the supervisory process. They are also reflective of the fact that supervision both in a clinical training setting and in the work place is a distinct area of professional practice and requires specific knowledge and skill to implement it appropriately. Strong clinical skills, the Certificate of Clinical Competence, or having been a supervisee oneself at one time do not directly translate into the ability to supervise successfully and comfortably (McCrea & Brasseur, 2003).

Specific preparation of those who function as supervisors is highly recommended (McCrea & Brasseur, 2003). Despite the professions' reliance on "appropriate" supervision to ensure quality of training and of service delivery, currently there is a paucity of formal coursework or continuing education (CE) to fulfill this need for preparation. ASHA continues to present CE sessions at its annual convention and teleconferences on the supervisory process. Special Interest Division 11–Administration and Supervision publishes *Perspectives* three times a year for which CE credit may be earned. State associations should similarly be proactive for their members in providing CE opportunities in the supervisory process. Likewise, training programs should provide support to those members of the profession who provide supervisory support to students in their on- and off-campus practica. Finally, two comprehensive books on the supervisory process remain in print to support members who function as supervisors for any portion of their professional responsibility (Dowling, 2001; McCrea & Brasseur, 2003); both works discuss conceptual models for supervision and suggest strategies and tools implementing them with supervisees.

INDIVIDUAL SUPERVISOR ACCOUNTABILITY

Little is known about what educational programs or service delivery settings expect or require from faculty or staff supervisors in regard to the clinical education aspects of their positions. If supervisors are evaluated, it is more likely than not an administrative evaluation or one that focuses on subjective impressions of global aspects of supervisor behavior. It is not an evaluation that will necessarily provide insight into the efficiency and effectiveness of an individual supervisor's practice (McCrea & Brasseur, 2003) even when organizations may use a 360° feedback process for evaluation of leaders, managers, and supervisors, described earlier.

Evaluations from supervisees in and of themselves, although they do have some relevance, cannot be assumed to provide sufficient data for evaluation of supervisors. Supervisees may not have sufficient understanding of the supervisory process to know what to expect or evaluate. As the historical data indicated, supervisees seldom question or challenge their supervisor, even though they may disagree or complain in private. Further, unless complete anonymity is assured, the likelihood of honest and complete feedback is doubtful (McCrea & Brasseur, 2003).

Since there are no validated guidelines for the outcomes achieved by supervisors and none appear to be on the horizon, supervisors must look to other, more informal resources to gain an understanding of the results of their behavior and work. A great deal has been said in this chapter about the importance of planning, observing, and analyzing supervisee behavior. Data on clinician behavior as it relates to what has been planned, implemented, and discussed might provide one measure of supervisor effectiveness. Supervisors who might measure their own effectiveness in this way could design any number of data collection techniques to help answer relevant questions.

Supervisors might also use the task and competency list from the ASHA Position Statement on Clinical Supervision (ASHA, 1985). Casey (1985) developed a *Supervisory Skills Self-Assessment* using this list. In this procedure, supervisors ask and answer two questions about each competency:

- How important is this competency for effectiveness in my program?

- How satisfied am I with my ability to perform this skill?

They then record their actual or perceived and ideal score. The greater the gap between the actual and ideal score, the higher the priority for development of the competency within the supervisor's behavioral repertoire.

For example, a supervisor may score him or herself high on the importance of the competency "Ability to interact with supervisee in a manner that facilitates the supervisee's self-exploration and problem solving" but low on the way it is performed. This lack of satisfaction may be related to that fact that the supervisor recognizes that a supervisee cannot identify areas of need and consequently does not actively participate in conference problem-solving discussions. In addition, the supervisor may determine that the supervisee has a difficult time collecting and analyzing client performance data that also contribute to his or her inability to participate meaningfully in planning conferences. In response to these observations, the supervisor may develop an action plan to modify his or her approach with the supervisee with a goal of more active student participation. In this way, a supervisor can set an objective and determine whether it was accomplished on the basis of the outcomes achieved by the supervisee. Ultimately, the supervisor should determine if the supervisee's change in behavior results in client improvement.

Self-study within the supervisory process is the first step to accountability in the clinical training aspect of the supervisory process. It should be seen as an opportunity for supervisors to develop their own quality assurance mechanisms rather than having inappropriate accountability systems imposed on them. Studying the manner in which one might implement and/or enhance the dynamics of the supervisory process in one's own practice is also the foundation upon which a program of lifelong learning can be built (McCrea & Brasseur, 2003).

SUMMARY

Supervision is a distinct area of professional responsibility and practice with specific tasks and competencies (ASHA, 1985). It is a key aspect of staff development and accountability in the work place. It is also an area of practice that is important to achieving the outcomes specified in the new ASHA standards for accreditation and certification. This chapter presented a model of supervision that is flexible enough to accommodate all levels of supervisee: preprofessional, support personnel, and professional staff. Supervision remains an integral component to the education of clinical practitioners and to the quality of service provided in professional settings. It requires in-depth study. Clinical mastery is not necessarily equivalent to supervision mastery. Preparation for and continued study of the supervisory process by supervisors is critical to preparing the next generation of clinicians. Supervisors of assistants and professionals also need to find ways to document their effectiveness in providing state-of-the-art effective clinical services.

CRITICAL THINKING

1. From your perspective, compare the challenges of supervising preprofessional and professional supervisees.

2. Which of the five phases of the supervisory process, in your estimation, is the most important? Why?

3. Are analysis and evaluation of behavior related? If so, how, and if not, why not?

4. Why is it important to remove subjectivity from supervisory feedback?

5. Consult the ASHA Position Statement on Clinical Supervision (available on the ASHA Web site). Complete an audit of your own supervisory behavior across the tasks and competencies. Which of them is the greatest challenge to you in your work setting? Design an intervention plan for yourself to enhance your behavior.

6. What skills are needed by supervisors of assistants and professionals? How do these differ from that needed for supervision of students in training?

7. What skills and competencies do you look for in your supervisors? If they do not meet these expectations, what can you do to improve your supervision experience?

8. What unique skills would you need to develop to become a supervisor in a service-delivery setting?

REFERENCES

American Speech-Language Hearing Association. (1978). Committee on Supervision in Speech-Language Pathology. Current status of supervision in speech-language pathology and audiology. *ASHA, 20,* 478–486.

American Speech-Language Hearing Association. (1983). *ASHA membership and certification handbook.* Rockville, MD: Author.

American Speech-Language Hearing Association. (1985). Committee on Supervision in Speech-Language Pathology and Audiology: Clinical supervision in speech-language pathology and audiology. *ASHA, 27,* 57–60.

American Speech-Language Hearing Association. (1995). *Practical tools for supervising speech-language pathology assistants.* Rockville, MD: Author.

American Speech-Language Hearing Association. (1996). Guidelines for training, credentialing, use and supervision of speech-language pathology assistants. *ASHA, 38*(16), 21–24.

American Speech-Language Hearing Association. (1997). *ASHA membership and certification handbook.* Rockville, MD: Author.

American Speech-Language Hearing Association. (1999). *Practical tools and forms for supervising speech-language pathology assistants.* Rockville, MD: Author.

American Speech-Language Hearing Association. (2000). *Background information and standards for implementation for the certificate of clinical competence in speech-language pathology.* Rockville, MD: ASHA, Council on Professional Standards in Speech-Language Pathology and Audiology.

American Speech-Language Hearing Association. (2001). *Knowledge and skills for supervisors of speech-language pathology assistants.* Rockville, MD: Author.

Anderson, J. (Ed.). (1970). *Proceedings of Conference on Supervision of Speech and Hearing Programs in the Schools.* Bloomington: Indiana University.

Anderson, J. (1988). *The supervisory process in speech-language pathology and audiology.* Boston: College-Hill.

Anderson, J., & Milisen, R. (1965). *Report on pilot project in student teaching in speech and hearing.* Bloomington: Indiana University.

Blumberg, A. (1980). *Supervisors and teachers: A private cold war* (2nd ed.). Berkeley, CA: McCutchan Publishing.

Bruce, M. (Ed.). (1994). *Proceedings of the 1994 International and Interdisciplinary Conference on Clinical Supervision: Toward the 21st Century.* Council of Supervisors in Speech-Language Pathology and Audiology, Cape Cod, MA.

Casey, P., Smith, K., & Ulrich, S. (1988). *Self-supervision: A career tool for audiologists and speech-language pathologists* (Clinical Series No. 10). Rockville, MD: National Student Speech-Language-Hearing Association.

Cogan, M. (1973). *Clinical supervision.* Boston: Houghton Mifflin.

Costa, A., & Garmston, R. (1985). *The art of cognitive coaching; Supervision for intelligent teaching.* Sacramento, CA: The Institute for Intelligent Behavior.

Crago, M., & Pickering, M. (Eds.). (1987). *Supervision in human communication disorders: Perspectives on a process.* San Diego, CA: Little Brown-College Hill Press.

Dowling, S. (1992a). *Implementing the supervisory process: Theory and practice.* Englewood Cliffs, NJ: Prentice Hall.

Dowling, S. (Ed.). (1992b). *Proceedings of the 1992 National Conference on Supervision-Total Quality Supervision: Effecting Optimal Performance.* Council of Supervisors in Speech-Language Pathology and Audiology, Nashville, TN.

Dowling, S. (2001). *Supervision: Strategies for successful outcomes and productivity.* Boston: Allyn and Bacon.

Farmer, S., & Farmer, J. (1989). *Supervision in communication disorders.* Columbus, OH: Merrill.

Gillam, R. (1999). ISSUE III: Models of clinical instruction. Adopting an integrated apprenticeship model in a university clinic. In P. Murphy (Ed.), *Proceedings of the Annual Conference in Graduate Education* (pp. 97–99). Minneapolis, MN: Council of Academic Programs in Speech-Language Pathology and Audiology.

Gillam, R., & Pena, E. (1995). Clinical education: A social constructivist perspective. In R. Gillam (Ed.), *The supervisor's forum, 2,* 24–29. The Council of Supervisors in Speech-Language Pathology and Audiology.

Goldhammer, R. (1969). *Clinical supervision.* New York: Holt, Rinehart, and Winston.

Goldhammer, R., Anderson, R., & Krajewski, R. (1980). *Clinical supervision* (2nd ed.). New York: Holt, Rinehart, and Winston.

Golper, L., & Brown, J. (Eds.). (2005). *Business matters: A guide for speech-language pathologists.* Rockville: MD. American Speech-Language-Hearing Association.

Hagler, P., & MacFarlane, L. (1997). *Collaborative service delivery by assistants and professionals* (Rev. ed.). Edmonton, Alberta, Canada: Alberta Rehabilitation Coordinating Council.

Halfond, M. (1964). Clinical supervision-stepchild in training. *ASHA, 6,* 441–444.

Irwin, R. (1976). Verbal behavior of supervisors and speech clinicians during micro-counseling. *Central States Speech Journal, 26,* 45–51.

Irwin, R. (1981). Training speech-language pathologists through microtherapy. *Journal of Communication Disorders, 14,* 93–103.

Kleffner, F. (Ed.). (1964). *Seminar on guidelines for the internship year.* Washington, DC: American Speech and Hearing Association.

Kurpius, D., & Christie, S. (1978). A systematic and collaborative approach to problem solving. In D. Kurpius (Ed.), *Learning: Making learning environments more effective.* Muncie, IN: Accelerated Development.

McAllister, L. (2000). Where are we going in clinical education: A review of current status and some theoretical and philosophical guideposts for new directions. *Proceedings of the Council of Academic Programs in Communication Sciences and Disorders 2000 Conference,* Minneapolis, MN.

McCrea, E., & Brasseur, J. (2003). *The supervisory process in speech-language pathology and audiology.* Boston: Allyn and Bacon.

Miner, A. (1967). A symposium: Improving supervision of clinical practicum. *ASHA, 9,* 471–482.

Moses, M., & Shapiro, D. (1996). A developmental conceptualization of clinical problem solving. *Journal of Communication Disorders, 29,* 199–221.

Mullins, J., & McCready, V. (2002). *The SLP assistant supervisor's companion.* East Moline, IL: Linguisystems.

Oratio, A. (1977). *Supervision in speech-language pathology: A handbook for supervisors and clinicians.* Baltimore, MD: University Park Press.

Rassi, J. (1978). *Supervision in audiology.* Baltimore, MD: University Park Press.

Rassi, J., & McElroy, M. (Eds.). (1992). *The education of audiologists and speech language pathologists.* Timonium, MD: York Press.

Schubert, G. (1978). *Introduction to clinical supervision.* St. Louis, MO: W.H. Green.

Turton, L. (Ed.). (1973). *Proceedings of a workshop on supervision in speech pathology.* Ann Arbor, MI: University of Michigan, Institute for the Study of Mental Retardation and Related Disabilities.

Ulrich, S. (1985). Continuing education model of training. In K. Smith (Moderator), *Preparation and training models for the supervisory process.* Short course presented at the annual convention of the American Speech-Language-Hearing Association, Washington, DC.

U.S. Department of Personnel Management. (1997). *360 degree assessment: An overview.* Available at http://www.opm.gov/perform/wppdf/360asess.pdf

Villareal, J. (Ed.). (1964) *Seminar on guidelines for supervision of clinical practicum.* Washington, DC: American Speech and Hearing Association.

Wagner, B. (Ed.). (1996). *Proceedings of the 1996 Conference on Clinical Supervision—Partnerships in Supervision: Innovative and Effective Practices.* Council of Supervisors in Speech-Language Pathology and Audiology, Cincinnati, OH.

Whalen, T. (2001). *Incorporating professional behavior expectations into performance appraisals.* Paper presented at ASHA Special Interest Division 11 Leadership Conference: Power Tools for Leadership and Supervision, Chicago.

RESOURCES

Tools to Facilitate the Understanding Phase
    Larson's Supervisory Expectations Rating Scale

Larson's Supervisory Needs Expectations Rating Scale
    Larson, L. (1982). Perceived supervisory needs and expectations of experienced vs. in-experienced student clinicians. (Doctoral dissertation, Indiana University, 1981). *Dissertation Abstracts International, 42,* 4758B. (University Microfilms No. 82-11, 183).

Tihen's Expectations Scale
    Tihen, L. (1984). Expectations of student speech/language clinicians during clinical. (Doctoral dissertation, Indiana University, 1983). *Dissertation*

Abstracts International, 44, 3048B. (University Microfilms No. 84-01, 620).

Clinical Supervisory Survey of Perceived Effectiveness of Various Supervision Strategies

Broyles, S., McNiece, E., Ishee, J., Ross, S., & Lance, D. (1999). *Influence of selected factors on the perceived effectiveness of various supervision strategies.* Poster session presented at the annual convention of the American Speech-Language-Hearing Association, San Francisco, CA.

Powell's Attitude Toward Clinical Supervision Scale

Powell, T. (1987). A rating scale for measurement of attitudes toward clinical supervision. *SUPERvision, 11,* 31–34.

Supervisory Conference Rating Scale

Brasseur, J., & Anderson, J. (1983). Observed differences between direct, indirect, and direct/indirect videotaped supervisory conferences. *Journal of Speech and Hearing Research, 26,* 349–355.

Tools to Facilitate the Planning Phase

The Wisconsin Procedure for Appraisal of Clinical Competence (W-PACC)

Shriberg, L., Filley, F., Hayes, D., Kwiatkowski, D., Schatz, J., Simmons, K. & Smith, M. (1974). *The Wisconsin procedure for appraisal of clinical competence (W-PACC).* Madison, WI: Department of Communicative Disorders, University of Wisconsin-Madison.

Bartlett's Action Plan

Bartlett, S. (2003). In E. McCrea & J. Brasseur (Eds.), *The supervisory process in speech-language pathology and audiology* (pp. 154–156). Boston: Allyn and Bacon.

Appraisal Instruments Unique to Individual Training and/or Service Delivery Programs

Tools to Facilitate the Observation/Data Collection Process

Individually constructed observation/data collection tools:

1. Tallies of behaviors identified in goals/ objectives
2. Full verbatim transcripts of clinical interaction
3. Selected verbatim transcripts of targeted verbal behavior

Structured Observation/Data Collection Tools

Kansas Inventory of Self-Supervision

Mawdsley, B. (2003). In E. McCrea & J. Brasseur (Eds.), *The supervisory process in speech-language pathology and audiology* (pp.177–183). Boston: Allyn and Bacon.

Boone-Prescott Content and Sequence Analysis System

Boone, D., & Prescott, T. (1972). Content and sequence analysis of speech and hearing therapy. *ASHA, 14,* 58–62.

Analysis of Behavior of Clinicians (ABC) System

Schubert, G., Miner, A., & Till, J. (2003). In E. McCrea & J. Brasseur (Eds.), *The supervisory process in speech-language pathology and audiology* (pp. 187–189). Boston: Allyn and Bacon.

25

Technology as a Professional Issue

JOHN M. TORRENS, PHD

SCOPE OF CHAPTER

This chapter provides an overview of technology and how it can be used in the practice of speech-language pathology and audiology as well as research in communication science and disorders. This chapter cannot provide an up-to-date accounting of technology and applications available to clinicians as this information would be outdated immediately. However, the reader will gain an understanding of computing basics, the importance of computer technology in professional life, various forms of technology, recommended competencies, the future of technology in clinical practice, and ethical issues in the use of technology. Technology is commonly defined as the science of the application of knowledge to practical purposes, or *applied science*.

TECHNOLOGY TIME LINE

As current technology builds on past technology, there is an exponential increase in the speed with which practical applications for a variety of situations become available. Consider that there was a span of nearly 5,000 years between the abacus, widely considered the first mechanical counting device, and the first personal computer. Next consider the fact there was a span of only 50 years between the first personal computer and the widespread use of personal digital assistants. Every new application of science creates the possibility for many more applications.

The abacus may not come to mind as an example of technology. It is, however, an example of a technological solution to a problem faced by society at the time, which was the need for a faster, more accurate way to perform calculations. Eons ago, the abacus was a cutting-edge device which in today's terminology might be referred to as *high tech*. In the 21st century, the abacus is more appropriately viewed as low tech because advances in technology have produced faster and more effective calculating machines. High tech and low tech are relative terms. A product that was once considered high tech, such as the abacus, is now viewed as obsolete. Similarly, products that are considered high tech today because they represent the most recent advances in applied science may be viewed as low-tech products in 10 years.

COMPUTING BASICS

Most people relate technology to computers. Indeed, the vast majority of today's technological innovations are computer-based. Fifty years ago, complex tasks such as surgery or designing a building were done without computers. Similarly, clinicians were evaluating clients, writing reports, and providing therapy all without computers. Early examples of speech-language and audiology tools include amplifying sound by cupping one's hand around the ear, funnel-like devices to improve auditory acuity, and analog tape recorders for the capture of voice and speech sounds. Given the ubiquity of computers and their relevance to everyday professional life, it is important to understand the basic components of a computer system: the processor, input, output, storage, and software.

- **Processor:** Sometimes referred to as the *central processing unit,* or CPU, this is essentially the brains of the computer, where the control unit and logic units are housed.
- **Input Device:** As the name suggests, this component feeds data into the computer. Examples include a mouse, keyboard, or microphone.
- **Output Device:** This component takes information from a computer and produces a way for us to interface with data. Examples include a printer, monitor, or speaker.
- **Storage:** This component maintains data for retrieval. Primary storage such as random access memory, or RAM, stores data temporarily, while secondary storage devices, such as magnetic tape, disks, CDs, or universal serial bus (USB) key chains store data permanently.
- **Software:** Software is a series of coded instructions that can be read by a computer. We interact with our computers through software, which serve different practical functions. For example, word processing programs allow us to write reports, and spreadsheets allow us to collect and analyze outcomes data.

Machine Language

Despite all the complex functions a computer can perform, every action can be boiled down to a series of 1s and 0s, or a string of binary digits. This binary system correlates to the computer's internal state. That is, an electronic state of "on" is represented by a 1 and "off" is represented by a 0. The various combinations of 1s and 0s produce the letters, shapes, colors, sounds, and images on our computer.

Machines communicate with one another through 1s and 0s using encoding systems. The most prevalent encoding system is the American Standard Code for Information Interchange (ASCII). This system uses seven-bit encoding to distinguish alphanumeric characters.

Similarly, the most extraordinary sounds and images can be broken down into a series, however long, of 1s and 0s. Sound was once represented by wave forms, or analog signals. Voice transmission via telephones and recordings of music were primarily analog. The problem with analog is that it does not work well with computers, which speak in a binary machine language. Another problem is that analog does not duplicate well, as illustrated by difficulties in copying a VHS tape. With each duplication of the tape comes a decrease in quality. Digital sounds, or sound represented by 1s and 0s, can be handled by computers and can be copied with absolute perfection. As a result, there has been a movement of music and telephone companies toward digital sound.

The practice of speech-language pathology and audiology as well as research in communication sciences and disorders has benefited from this change. For example, digital copies of voice and speech samples can be reproduced and segmented without any reduction in quality, and digital hearing aids can be programmed with a higher level of accuracy and efficiency.

The Network

Computers by themselves seem hardly useful today without connection to some type of network. It is not always practical to hold every bit of information you need on one PC or even on an external memory device. Consequently, access to a network gives the user the advantage of storing and retrieving large amounts of information from a number of computers and locations. The Internet is a common network that connects individual computers to an incomprehensible amount of information. Smaller networks, like those in corporate, academic, or even home settings (local area networks) can also add convenience and safety. Some advantages of networking include the ability to centrally manage critical functions such as virus and spam protection, backup, firewalls, and parental controls. A local area network can also allow multiple users to access and interact with the same program, application, or file in real time. Local networks also provide a degree of mobility for users in that they do not always need to work from the same machine or location. Computers can be connected to a network by network cables or wirelessly.

No discussion of networks would be complete without mention of bandwidth. The volume of information that can be moved through a network is determined by the bandwidth available. The network cable is much like a pipe, and wider pipes allow more water to flow through them. Likewise, broader bandwidth allows for information, represented as 0s and 1s, to flow through the network cable. Anyone with a dial-up connection who has ever tried to download music can attest to the difference broader bandwidth makes regarding transmission speed.

Transmission speed is generally expressed in terms of bits per second, or bytes per second. Remember that a bit is a single binary digit, and a byte is a series of bits arranged to represent a character.

Kilobyte (KB):	1,000 bytes per second
Kilobit (Kb):	1,000 bits per second
Megabyte (MB)	1,000,000 bytes per second
Megabit (Mb)	1,000,000 bits per second
Gigabyte (GB)	1,000,000,000 bytes per second
Terabyte (TB)	1,000,000,000,000 bytes per second

Broader bandwidth permits greater speed of transmission and results in larger amounts of data transferred more quickly. Broader bandwidth, however, is associated with higher cost and reduced availability in some areas.

The speed with which information is transmitted from one point to another depends largely on the type of wire and/or cable being used. This is commonly referred to as a *transmission medium*:

- **Dial-up:** This is also referred to as a *plain old telephone system* or POTS connection, or *land lines.* Information is transmitted through telephone lines at speeds of up to 56Kb per second.

- **Integrated Services Digital Network (ISDN):** This type of broadband connection, including T1 and T4 connections, are run through telephone lines at speeds ranging from 64 Kb per second (abbreviated as 64 Kbps) to 128 Kbps depending on the specifications and configuration of the equipment.

- **Satellite:** Information is transmitted through air and space via satellite at uplink speeds of 50–128 Kbps (average speed: 50 Kbps) and Downlink speeds of 400–500 Kbps, with bursts of 1.5 Mb.

- **Cable:** Information is transmitted through coaxial copper cable at uplink speeds of up to 10 Mbps and downlink speeds up to 27 Mbps.

- **DSL (Digital Subscriber Lines):** Information is transmitted through telephone lines at speeds of 1.544 to 6.1 Mbps downstream and 16 Kbps to 1.5 Mbps upstream.

The World Wide Web One of the most popular features of the Internet is the World Wide Web (WWW), commonly referred to as the Web. The Web is a network of information repositories called Web sites that can be accessed by users by way of hypertext transfer protocol (HTTP) and universal resource locator (URL) links.

Web sites can range from basic sources of information, much like an online brochure, or they can provide powerful functionality. For example, many people now have the option to manage their bank accounts, trade stocks, review and submit their children's homework, and shop online. Likewise, clients use the Web to gather information about communication sciences and disorders and to research diagnostic and treatment options. With the ubiquity of Web functionality in other areas of life, speech-language pathologists and audiologists are also offering more than information on their Web sites. For example, practitioners can provide their clients with access to scheduling, progress notes, reports, and other resources. They can also use the Web to provide services. This is described in the section on telepractice.

As in any other computer or network environment, protection of private health information or educational records is required. If speech-language pathologists or audiologists intend to store and transmit clinical information by way of a professional Web site, it is advisable to engage the services of a professional or a firm to ensure the protection of records. Those interested in using a Web site as electronic brochures can often develop and maintain these sites on their own after completing some basic course work or training. If a clinician decides to self-publish a professional Web site, there are several basic considerations:

- **Intellectual property rights:** It is easy to cut and paste information from one Web site to another. However, this can often result in plagiarism. As in any type of publication, one should reference the source of information and seek permission to reprint information if used in its entirety.

- **Static vs. dynamic sites:** Visitors to Web sites expect that the information is up to date and useful. It is important to verify the currency and accuracy of information on a professional Web site and to ensure that links to other sites remain active.

- **User-friendliness:** A professional Web site is clear and simple to navigate. Graphics should be used judiciously since some visitors may not have the bandwidth necessary for large images or sound files to load quickly.

IMPORTANCE OF TECHNOLOGY TO PRACTICE

The use of modern technology is an important aspect of professional practice for audiologists, speech-language pathologists, and communication scientists. It is more important, however, that our use of technology be wise and judicious. Employment of technology simply for the sake of it may or may not have a positive effect on clinical services or research findings. Furthermore, the types of technology employed by one user may not necessarily be the best options for another. To be effective as clinicians and scientists, we must choose tools that will help us attain an improved level of quality, accuracy, and productivity. It is equally important that clinicians be able to identify and evaluate technological tools for clients' use. Technological applications can be used for improving workflow as well as clinical outcomes.

Imagine managing a caseload of 40 clients or conducting clinical trials without the use of modern technology. The limitations would quickly become apparent in today's academic, educational, medical, and private practice arenas. This is not to say that clinicians in past eras were not accurate, productive, or providing the highest quality services possible at that time. Rather, modern clinicians have professional and ethical responsibilities to use appropriate technology that will benefit our clients.

The use of modern technology itself will not guarantee that clinical services will be of high quality. It is the expertise and discretion in the application of this technology that will yield benefits. For example, the use of videofluoroscopy is of limited value unless the clinician is competent in performing and interpreting the exam. Similarly, the use of a spreadsheet to track data will be of little use to scientists who do not know how to use one. However, if these same individuals would learn how to use a spreadsheet, they would open up a wide range of possibilities for improving their services. For example, if they could set up, enter, sort, and analyze data in a table, they would have access to a quantity of information. Clinicians could tabulate progress and provide outcome-based data for clients, third party payers, and the clinical community. Clinicians could thus become involved in active data collection and research.

There are regular improvements in technology involving clinical applications. One of the most striking areas where this is evident is augmentative and alternative communication (AAC). Even a simple picture board, arguably the most low-tech AAC application, benefits from the use of software that helps find, size, print, store, and change pictures, icons, or words being used. On the high-tech end of the spectrum, there have been marked improvements in the outdated "robot voices" of speaking devices, often allowing for customization and selection of different voices based on the client's preference. In general the cost, applicability, flexibility, and usefulness of many high-tech devices have shown great improvements recently. For clinicians working with AAC, this requires constant learning and exploration to keep up with the changes and improvement.

Beyond the ability to improve accuracy in data collection and quality of data analysis, one of the clear advantages in using technology is increased productivity. By doing routine tasks in a more efficient and effective way, more clients can be served without a concomitant decrease in quality of service. This benefits clients who are in need of services and frees the clinician to do other tasks that, in turn, increase the available billable time for the facility. From the use of word processing software to write, edit, and store clinical reports to the quality of a new digital microphone, there are many ways to improve the quality, accuracy, and productivity of our clinical work through the wise use of modern technology. Similarly, modern scientists can collect and analyze much more data in less time than could their cohorts 50 years ago, which increases the speed with which findings can be shared with the professional community. Manuscript editing and peer review of scholarly work have also increased in efficiency and effectiveness as a result of the productivity gains from software and the connectivity provided by networks.

ETHICS AND TECHNOLOGY

Within ASHA's Code of Ethics are statements that explicitly address the use of technology and statements that imply applicability to the use of technology. For example, Principle II, Rule F states "Individuals shall ensure that all equipment used in the provision of services or to conduct research and scholarly activities is in proper working order and is properly calibrated" (ASHA, 2003, p. 2). This clearly addresses the use of instrumentation and other clinical equipment. Other rules imply an ethical responsibility when it comes to technology. Take for example the concept of competence, which is addressed later in this chapter and mentioned in Principle 1, Rule A, which states "Individuals shall provide all services competently" (p. 1). This rule has a wide range of implications and includes competent use of technology in the provision of clinical services. Principle 1, Rule B is even less explicit, yet has technological implications: "Individuals shall use every resource, including referral when appropriate, to ensure that high-quality service is provided" (p. 1). One possible interpretation of this rule of ethics is that clinicians have an ethical responsibility to use technology as a resource, when appropriate, to ensure high-quality services.

Ethical responsibilities weave through every part of clinical practice and research, including the use of technology. Rather than trying to think of specific principles and rules that relate specifically to the use of technology, it is more useful to understand the Code of Ethics as a whole and apply the spirit and intent to all parts of clinical practice. Some areas of practice are more susceptible to ethics violations due to the use of technology, as described elsewhere in the chapter. For example, the use of electronic documentation requires heightened awareness of the technology being used in order to meet the privacy and confidentiality requirements of the Health Insurance Portability and Accountability Act of 1996 (HIPAA) (Centers for Medicare and Medicaid Services, 1996). Similarly, the growing use of telepractice (i.e., the use of technology to deliver professional services at a distance) presents novel clinical and research situations that require careful consideration regarding ethics issues. Read Chapter 4 on Professional Ethics for a more in-depth discussion.

OFFICE SOFTWARE

One area of clinical practice that benefits greatly from the use of technology is documentation. Often the bane of busy clinicians, documentation is the written record of what we do; it provides the client, agency, and third party payers with accountability for our services. Technology makes this task easier and more efficient. Clinicians in all settings are expected to produce and submit reports in a timely and effective manner to obtain services for clients and to receive payment. In settings where bills are generated and sent to payers electronically, nearly immediately following a clinical service, the electronic documentation of the procedures charged may be required to be attached. Timely access to electronic records by the billing office can effectively eliminate denials and can streamline collections.

The most widely used application for documentation is a word processor, which is a common component of office tools. The ability to write, edit, store, and retrieve documentation electronically has marked advantages over pen-and-paper-based documentation. Treatment notes, evaluation reports, professional correspondence, and other documents are all efficiently handled by word processing applications. Some programs offer a variety of tools such as mail merge, track changes, spell check, thesaurus, and the ability to link with other applications in a suite (e.g., spreadsheets).

Databases and spreadsheets are also useful tools for managing client data such as demographics, contact and insurance information, goals, and outcomes. Presentation software is useful in preparing client, teacher, and caregiver education materials that augment direct clinical service. In addition, these applications help clinicians prepare exciting professional presentations. All of these basic tools offered in an office suite can be useful to clinicians who take the time to familiarize themselves with them.

In addition, there is a growing number of clinical documentation applications, most of which can automate some part of the evaluation or treatment documentation process. In many cases these programs can be linked to other office management applications, and some even have them built in. For example, there are programs that allow a clinician to create the format of a report in advance and then enter important data into fields through a graphical user interface (GUI). One benefit of this type of program is that data for a specific field (e.g., client's first name) need to be manually entered only once. The program then populates all other similarly labeled fields with what was originally entered.

In more advanced applications, the data are entered into the initial intake form (e.g., name, address, identification number, primary care physician) and populated in other forms that are ready to print. For example, if a receptionist enters demographic information for a client into an intake form, the software will automatically populate the same fields (e.g., name, address, phone number) on other forms that need to be printed, such as a consent form, parent interview form, or physician cover letter.

Despite its advantages, electronic documentation does have drawbacks. One such concern is the potential for breaches of confidentiality and privacy. Regardless of the type of device used (laptop, personal computer, personal digital assistant) and the environment in which it is used (e.g., stand-alone, networked), there is the possibility that private information can be viewed by individuals not involved in the care of the client. In the worst case, the information can be used for criminal activities such as identity theft. Professional responsibility to clients has always required that clinicians take reasonable and appropriate measures to protect client information, and this responsibility is now given the weight of law.

Two laws, the Health Insurance Portability and Accountability Act of 1996 (HIPAA), and the Family Educational Rights and Privacy Act (FERPA) (U.S. Department of Education, 1974) have critical documentation implications. Depending on a clinician's work setting, at least one of these laws will apply. While HIPAA was designed to make the sharing of health information easier, there are high standards for privacy and confidentiality. Violations of these standards can result in heavy fines and even jail time. It is incumbent upon all providers in health and educational settings to treat client information with a high degree of confidentiality.

Good practices that protect privacy include locking your PC when you leave your desk and providing password protection on client files in addition to the password on your PC. In a network environment, client file access should be strictly limited to those with responsibility for client care. Care should also be taken in printing or faxing documents so that client information is not inadvertently accessed by individuals not involved in the care of the client. For example, printed information should be immediately retrieved from a copier to eliminate the possibility of unauthorized viewing or duplication of the information.

CONSIDERATIONS FOR USING ELECTRONIC DOCUMENTATION

While there is much to be gained from using an electronic records system, some serious issues also must be considered. When using electronic documentation tools, consider the following:

- **Usefulness:** What will be gained from using electronic documentation tools? Will there be tangible improvements in quality, efficiency, cost effectiveness, accuracy, legibility, and/or productivity? Are the gains in these areas worth the cost in time and money to implement?

- **Authentication:** A provider's signature generally needs to appear after a report or note. This can present a challenge if all documentation is electronic, or paperless. Do the recipients of these reports have security systems in place to accept and verify electronic signatures?

- **Modifications:** If a change is made in the original record, how will it be documented? The convention for paper notes is to strike a line through the corrected text and initial it. How will the reader recognize altered text in electronic documentation?

- **Access:** In a paper filing system there is typically a sign-out procedure. How will this work in electronic records? Will the system log who has viewed what files and for how long? Is this information easy to retrieve for accountability purposes? How will access rights be granted? Is there a security mechanism in the system that will allow all providers who need access to have it? How will it know when access is no longer needed?

- **Privacy:** How will client information be protected from unauthorized use in an electronic records environment? The use of passwords, security rights, encryption software, and even security hardware such as biometrics (e.g., retina scan, fingerprints) should all be considered.

- **Storage:** How will electronic records be stored and archived? What is the requirement for record retention in your setting? Will paper files be kept for a certain period of time or destroyed after a digital copy is made? Will the records be backed up and replicated for safety purposes?

Therapy Tools (Noninstrumental)

There is a myriad of tools available for the treatment of speech, language, and hearing problems. Adaptive and assistive technology is one example of how clients and clinicians can benefit from technological advancements. Sound quality, weight, cost, interoperability with other software, user interfaces, and portability continue to improve as a result of improved technology. Even the use of low-tech options such as picture boards has been made easier by programs that store, change, sort, and print pictures that can be used for a number of clients. Clearly, such programs have advantages over cutting with scissors, pasting with glue, and photocopying.

The use of software for the treatment of language disorders can also be useful. Adults with aphasia and adolescents with learning disabilities have a range of applications that can help them improve their conditions. While the availability of such programs can be beneficial in therapy as well as independent practice for a client, clinicians must be aware of their professional responsibility to their clients. Not all programs or applications will be applicable to all clients. Furthermore, not all programs may live up to their claims. Clinicians must assess the skill levels of their clients and match them to the range of products available. It is important to avoid the trap of using the one-size-fits-all mentality and not assume that a tool that works for one client will work for all. When choosing a high-tech or low-tech option, be it for evaluations or treatment, candidacy criteria must be considered.

Some considerations for choosing a technological treatment tool:

- Is the vendor reputable?
- Do you know anyone else using this product?
- Is there evidence to support its efficacy?
- Can you compare this tool to other similar products?
- Is it dependent on a skill that your client does not have (e.g., mobility in upper extremities, visual tracking, or manual dexterity)?
- Can it be used to address a range of goals, or is it specific to a few?
- Is it functional and relevant to the client's daily life?
- Will the vendor let you test it out on your client and return it if it is not a fit?
- Will the client's family be able to use it?
- Is it of interest to the client?
- Does the vendor provide a warranty or support service?

Instrumentation

Technological advancements have resulted in more tools that can be used in the evaluation and treatment of clients. Using instrumentation enables scientists and clinicians to quantify perceptual measures with objective instrumental measures. For example, a physician can perceive that a patient has a broken bone after a clinical exam and years of experience, and this clinical impression can be quantified through instrumentation, in this case an X-ray.

Some tools used by other health professionals are important to audiologists, speech-language pathologists, and communication scientists. For example, magnetic resonance imaging (MRI) is used by radiologists and can be useful for speech-language pathologists who work with stroke patients. Speech-language pathologists do not conduct the MRI study, but the resulting information can be critical to client care.

In addition to clinical applications, instrumentation also plays a key role in research in communication sciences and disorders. Though they are not necessarily used on a daily basis by practicing clinicians, several devices are helpful in contributing to the knowledge base in the professions. Some examples of instrumentation used by speech-language pathologists, audiologists, and communication scientists in research include the following:

- **Electroglottograph (EGG):** This noninvasive device is used to analyze the vibratory characteristics of the vocal folds.

- **Laryngoscope:** This camera allows for direct viewing of the larynx and vocal folds.

- **Manometer:** This instrument measures air pressure, airflow, air volume, and movements of the respiratory muscles by way of a subject blowing through a tube.

- **Pneumotachograph:** This measures similar variables as a manometer, but differs in that it measures oral and nasal airflow separately through a mask worn on the subject's face.

- **Sound level meter:** This device measures environmental sounds and displays the sound in decibel levels.

- **Sound spectrograph:** This instrument processes complex sound, such as speech, and displays it as a spectrogram or waveforms that can be manipulated, analyzed, and stored.

- **Spirometer:** This measures subglottal airway variables such as tidal volume and vital capacity and displays it graphically.

- **Stroboscope:** This emits light at regular intervals to enable the user to view vocal fold movement.

- **Videokymography (VKG):** This relatively new technique uses a device that captures the high-speed motion of the vocal folds and records it for later display.

Clinicians use more common forms of instrumentation as well. While they may not be directly involved in research, the use of instrumentation by practicing clinicians allows for the collection, analysis, and storage of data that can be used to establish levels of evidence, efficacy, and outcomes. One important example of multidisciplinary instrumentation in the medical setting is videofluoroscopy. This is an X-ray study of a swallow on videotape, which speech-language pathologists use to evaluate the physiology of a swallow. Similarly, fiber optic endoscopy, which is a way to study a swallow using a video camera on the end of a flexible scope, can also improve client care by adding another dimension to a comprehensive evaluation by providing a real-life image of the anatomy. Electromyography (EMG) is a type of instrumentation used in the treatment of swallowing disorders. Electrodes are placed on the skin near muscles that are being treated or studied, and muscle activity is displayed for clinical analysis and storage.

Other instruments are helpful in evaluating and treating speech and resonance disorders. For example, the Visi-Pitch IV by KayPENTAX® is a device that provides speech biofeedback as well as measurements of speech and voice behavior. These types of devices can be used to evaluate, treat, and conduct research on a variety of conditions such as voice disorders, motor speech disorders, fluency, foreign accent and second language articulation, and hearing impaired speech. Additional instrumentation such as a nasometer or palatometer is also useful for evaluating, treating and researching resonance disorders resulting from cleft palate, motor speech disorders, functional nasality problems or a palatal prosthesis.

In audiology, the use of instrumentation is more prevalent due to the nature of the profession. Audiologists often are required to provide specific biometric measurements in their diagnoses and therefore must rely on instrumentation. For example, an audiometer measures auditory thresholds in a way that a clinical perceptual exam cannot. Similarly, a tympanometer provides information about middle ear compliance that cannot be measured perceptually. Other instruments, such as an otoscope or video otoscope, provide audiologists with a visual display of the ear canal and tympanic membrane. The benefit of a video otoscope is that the image can be displayed on a monitor for collaboration, teaching, or research purposes whereas an otoscope merely provides the user with a view of the structures.

More recent advances include instrumentation that allows an audiologist to measure the sounds made by the cochlea, to assess otoacoustic emissions (OAE) through Vivography™, or to test the neural integrity of the auditory system for hearing or balance through auditory brainstem response (ABR). Audiologists who evaluate or study balance disorders also use videonystagmography (VNG) and electronystagmography (ENG), in which electrodes are placed on the face of clients or subjects, and they follow lights on a bar and have cool and warm air introduced to their ears. Computers analyze the responses for an audiologist's interpretation. For treatment of hearing disorders, digital programmable hearing aids and the continued development of cochlear implant technology represent significant advancements in the care of clients.

TECHNOLOGICAL COMPETENCIES OF CLINICIANS

As with clinical applications, clinicians are expected to possess certain technological competencies prior to using a tool or application. As discussed earlier, to the extent that technological incompetence would be harmful to a client, clinicians have an ethical responsibility to become proficient in the use of a tool, device, or application prior to using it with clients. This is obvious in the case of instrumentation due to the direct applicability to client care. The use of technology for activities indirectly related to client care and research are also important. The good news is that the current and future generations of clinicians are growing up with a pervasive exposure to technology.

- **Basic keyboarding:** Speech-language pathologists and audiologists should be able to enter information into a computer or similar device with reasonable proficiency. Be familiar with shortcut keys and the operation of a mouse.

- **Computer navigation and file management:** Clinicians should know how a computer stores and organizes files as well as how to customize files. Understanding basic menu conventions and how to access online help features is also useful.

- **Security:** As mentioned earlier, there are many ways to protect access to computers and files. Following the password protection guidelines at your facility is important. Generally passwords should be no less than 6 characters and include numbers, letters, and characters. This makes it much harder for someone to decipher a password using "brute force" software (i.e., a program that attempts random strings of characters with exceptional speed until the password is broken). Avoiding the use of familiar names and important dates is fundamental.

- **Research:** Practicing clinicians today must know where to go to find information. For example, you should understand the basic conventions of a Boolean search on popular search engines and know how to use facility resources, such as accessing scientific information through an online library or other service.

- **Awareness:** It is important for clinicians to know that there is likely a technological solution for just about any data management problem and to understand how to evaluate these solutions for acceptability to the intended application.

- **Critical thinking:** Clinicians should also be able to compare products, devices, and solutions to others in the marketplace, understand the features of each, and be able to explain the advantages and disadvantages of each to a client and his or her family.

- **Troubleshooting:** Clinicians must know how to use online help and refer to troubleshooting documentation in the event a device or program is not working as intended, and how to contact the manufacturer or distributor when needed.

THE FUTURE OF CLINICAL PRACTICE

It is reasonable to assert that the practices of speech-language pathology and audiology will continue to evolve based on the continuity of scientific contributions to the professions, the increase of evidence-based practice, medical and educational advancements, and prevention programs. It is also reasonable to stress that technology will be at the center of this evolution. In much the same way that humanity in general has benefited from technological advances and their everyday applications, communication sciences and disorders will benefit from advancements in technology.

The continuity of research using new technology in research methodology will surely lead to a greater understanding of communication disorders. The new findings will in turn lead to innovative approaches to evaluation and treatment. The new approaches will then lead to the invention of new tools for speech-language pathologists and audiologists. The role of science and research in our professions is vital, and the prospects for future advancements are exciting.

As we continue to develop more evidence regarding evaluation and treatment techniques in communication sciences and disorders, we will be able to harness unprecedented efficiencies in our clinical work. For example, we will be able to abandon traditional techniques for which there is low-level evidence in favor of techniques for which there is high-level evidence. In turn, this will improve outcomes, decrease costs, and allow us to focus our time and energy on new problems for which we are uniquely equipped.

As in other fields, medicine and education will continue to develop new insights and breakthroughs. Applying the lessons learned from these broad disciplines will inevitably help us understand how to better serve our own clients. Some of these breakthroughs may be in the area of prevention, resulting in a whole new landscape for our professional practice. For example, imagine a school clinician's caseload in a world where autism is preventable or a pharmacological innovation that resulted in a profound decrease in damage to the brain's language centers after a stroke. Better yet, imagine the impact if the medical community discovers a mechanism by which the brain can repair itself and restore damaged pathways. Clearly, the outlook for the future of the professions is inextricably linked to technology and technological advances.

TELEPRACTICE

No discussion of technology in clinical practice would be complete without mention of telepractice, which is defined as "the application of telecommunications technology to deliver professional services at a distance by linking clinician to client, or clinician to clinician for assessment, intervention, and/or consultation" (ASHA, 2005a, 2005b, 2005c, 2005d). As with all technological applications in clinical practice, it is important to understand the benefits and the disadvantages of telepractice. In addition to a position statement on telepractice in speech-language pathology (ASHA, 2005b) and audiology (ASHA, 2005a), ASHA has also published a technical report for audiologists (ASHA, 2005c) and speech-language pathologists (ASHA, 2005d) using telepractice.

A growing body of literature supports the use of telepractice in the delivery of professional services. This is especially true when distance, geography, or mobility limit access to care. A number of articles describe the use of telepractice to evaluate and treat a variety of disorders, such as fluency (Kully, 2002), voice (Mashima, 2003), dysphagia (Perlman & Witthawaskul, 2002), brain injury (Brennan, Georgeadis, Baron & Barker (2005), and other adult neurological disorders (Duffy, Werven, & Aronson, 1997).

In the audiology literature, a growing number of services are available, including video-otoscopy (Burgess et al., 1999; Heneghan, Sclafani, Stern & Ginsburg, 1999; Sullivan, 1997), counseling and audiologic rehabilitation services (Office of the Advancement of Telemedicine, 2004), Internet-based hearing assessment (Givens & Elangovan, 2003), and auditory brainstem response (ABR) and newborn hearing screening (Krumm, Ribera, & Schmiedge, 2005).

It is useful to think of telepractice as simply another tool in a clinician's repertoire that is subject to the same standards as any other service delivery model or procedure. This includes ensuring provider competence, assuring that equipment and transmission modes are of sufficient quality and reliability, obtaining informed consent, examining effectiveness, and tracking outcomes. The use of telepractice does not excuse providers from any legal or ethical responsibilities they would have in any other clinical encounter.

There are two basic types of telepractice. *Asynchronous* techniques, commonly referred to as store-and-forward, involve capturing data at a remote site and forwarding it to a clinician for review. Examples of this include a voice sample that is sent as a sound file to a voice specialist for perceptual analysis or an audiogram that is sent electronically to an audiologist. *Synchronous* techniques, commonly known as interactive techniques, involve the interaction of client and clinician in real time and can include interactive video or audio. Examples of synchronous techniques include use of the public Internet or closed circuit TV to treat voice patients and videophones to provide treatment to stroke patients.

Despite the promises and the growing support in research and practice, there are several significant barriers to the use of telepractice:

- **State licensing:** Since licensing laws exist to protect the consumer, clinicians need to be licensed in the patient's state if services are to be delivered via telepractice where the patient and clinician are in different states.

- **Professional liability/malpractice:** Coverage from the majority of professional liability plans ends at state lines. In addition to licensure, malpractice coverage needs to include coverage in the home state where the client is located when receiving services.

- **Reimbursement:** While this is slowly improving, there is no generally recognized reimbursement mechanism for services delivered via telepractice. Some state Medicaid programs and third party insurance carriers will provide reimbursement, but most telepractice programs are grant-funded or supported by private pay clients.

- **Candidacy:** As with any other clinical tool or protocol, some patients who will not benefit from telepractice. Candidacy criteria include aspects of their condition (e.g., mobility or visual acuity), support system (e.g., family members or aids that can assist in telepractice sessions), and familiarity and comfort with technology.

- **Confidentiality:** Any time information is captured, stored, or transmitted electronically, there is the potential for a security breach. While there are ways to secure protected health information, the perception of insecurity is an obstacle for reimbursement as well as patient acceptance.

- **Ethics:** As with any other tool, clinicians providing service at a distance via telepractice need to be qualified and competent in the delivery of clinical services rendered as well as the delivery of the service in this manner. Providing clinical services via telepractice requires knowledge and skills that are different from providing face-to-face services. ASHA has produced technical papers on this subject.

DISTANCE LEARNING

Technology is also making distance learning more available for speech-language pathologists and audiologists. Professional associations and private companies offer an array of continuing education programs that bring educational opportunities right into the workplace or to clinicians' homes via telephone and video conferences and computer-based programming. Numbers of graduate distance education programs have emerged in recent years to provide opportunity for working audiologists to upgrade to the AuD. Thus, technology is an asset to practicing clinicians who want continuing education and opportunities to connect with other clinicians and resources across the country and world. Clinicians can easily access a variety of current educational programs at usually less financial cost and with more convenience.

SUMMARY

This chapter provided an overview of technology, which is commonly defined as the science of the application of knowledge to practical purposes and how it can be used in research and clinical practice. Readers were exposed to computing basics, the importance of computer technology in professional life, various forms of technology, including instrumentation, recommended competencies, the future of technology in clinical practice, technology and education, and ethical issues in the use of technology. The future of our professions is inextricably related to current and future advances in technology.

CRITICAL THINKING

1. Is there a case to be made that the human body is essentially a highly complex binary machine? Consider that in human genetics, the four components of a DNA strand are adenine, thymine, guanine, and cytosine. Furthermore, consider the fact that the only possible pairings are Adenine-Thymine (A-T), and Guanine-Cytosine (G-C). How is this analogous to binary machine language? What parts or functions of the human body are analogous to input, output, memory, and software? Of these, which ones are directly related to communication?

2. What are the benefits of technology in today's clinical practice? What are some of the current demands, barriers, obstacles, or issues in service delivery that can be mitigated by the use of technology?

3. What parallels can you draw between the overall advances in humanity compared to the communication sciences as a result of technology?

4. How has your life changed as a result of technology? How do you think your professional life will change over the course of your career as a result of technology? What will you do to keep up with the rapid changes in technology in your profession?

5. The manufacturer of a new assistive technology device is promoting its new product by offering free Continuing Education workshops to speech-language pathologists (SLPs). At the workshop they learn all about the device, observe it in action with an actual user, and get hands-on experience with the device. The manufacturer also provides examples of insurance and Medicaid documentation that will facilitate reimbursement. It is clearly a quality product, and the company has been gathering evidence of its usefulness beyond expert opinion. In fact, they have conducted a few comparison studies between their product and that of a competitor, whose product you have

been recommending to your clients. The company announces it will provide an all-expenses paid trip to a tropical island for SLPs who get 20 devices approved by an insurance company or Medicaid. What are some of the ethical issues in this scenario, and what is your responsibility to your clients?

6. How can audiologists keep abreast of changes in hearing aid technology without feeling tied to the manufacturers? What other ethical issues do audiologists face with regard to technology?

7. Think about the clinical settings in which you have worked. What types of technology did

you use? What measures were taken to ensure that the technology was current, in good working order, and calibrated? Whose responsibility was this, and how was it documented?

8. What precaution does your clinical environment take to protect the confidentiality of clients? How can office technology help or hinder confidentiality?

9. How do you plan to use technology to maintain your professional currency? What are the advantages and disadvantages of using technology as an educational tool?

REFERENCES

American Speech-Language-Hearing Association. (2003). Code of ethics (revised). *ASHA Supplement, 23,* 13–15.

American Speech-Language-Hearing Association. (2005a). Audiologists providing clinical services via telepractice: Position statement. *ASHA Supplement 25,* in press.

American Speech-Language-Hearing Association. (2005b). Speech-language pathologists providing clinical services via telepractice: Position statement. *ASHA Supplement 25,* in press.

American Speech-Language-Hearing Association. (2005c). Audiologists providing clinical services via telepractice: Technical report. *ASHA Supplement 25,* in press.

American Speech-Language-Hearing Association. (2005d). Speech-language pathologists providing clinical services via telepractice: Technical report. *ASHA Supplement 25,* in press.

Brennan, D. M., Georgeadis, A. C., Baron, C. R., & Barker, L. M. (2004). The effect of videoconference-based telerehab on story retelling performance by brain injured subjects and its implications for remote speech-language therapy. *Telemedicine and e-Health, 10*(2), 147–154.

Burgess, L., Holtel, M., Syms, M., Birkmire-Peters, D., Peters, L., & Mashima, P. (1999). Overview of telemedicine applications for otolaryngology. *Laryngoscope, 109*(9), 1433–1437.

Centers for Medicare and Medicaid Services. (1996) Health Insurance Portability and Accountability Act of 1996 (HIPAA). Available at http://www.cms.hhs.gov/hipaa/

Duffy, J. R., Werven, G. W., & Aronson, A. E. (1997). Telemedicine and the diagnosis of speech and language disorders. *Mayo Clinic Procedings, 72,* 1116–1122.

Givens, G. D., Blanarovich, A., Murphy, T., Simmons, S., Blach, D., & Elangovan, S. (2003). Internet-based tele-audiometry system for the assessment of hearing: A pilot study. *Telemedicine Journal and e-Health, 9,* 375–378.

Givens, G. D. & Elangovan, S. (2003). Internet application to tele-audiology—"Nothin' but Net." *American Journal of Audiology, 12,* 59–65.

Heneghan, C., Sclafani, A., Stern, J., & Ginsburg, J. (1999). Telemedicine applications in otolaryngology. *IEEE Engineering in Medicine & Biology Society, 18* (4), 53–62.

Krumm, M., Ribera, J., & Schmiedge, J. (2005). Using a telehealth medium for objective hearing testing: implications for supporting rural universal newborn hearing screening programs (UNHS). *Seminars in Hearing, 26,* 3–12.

Kully, D. (2000). Telehealth in speech-language pathology: Applications to the treatment of stuttering. *Journal of Telemedicine and Telecare, 6*(2) 39–41.

Mashima, P., Birkmire-Peters, D., Syms, M., Holtel, M., Burgess, L. & Peters, L. (2003). Telehealth: Voice therapy using telecommunications technology. *American Journal of Speech-Language Pathology, 12,* 432–439.

Office for the Advancement of Telemedicine. (2004). Dramatic consultations using Telemedicine: Northern California Telemedicine Network (NCTN) Santa Rosa Memorial Hospital (SRMH) Santa Rosa, CA. [On-line]. Available at http://telehealth.hrsa.gov/grants/success.htm#aud.

Perlman, A.L. & Witthawaskul, W. (2002). Real-time remote telefluoroscopic assessment of patients with dysphagia. *Dysphagia, 17*(2), 162–167.

Sullivan, R. (1997). Video-otoscopy in audiologic practice. *Journal of American Academy of Audiology, 8,* 447–467.

U.S. Department of Education. (1974). The Family Educational Rights and Privacy Act (FERPA), 20 U.S.C. § 1232g; 34 CFR Part 99. Available at: http://www.ed.gov/policy/gen/guid/fpco/ferpa/index.html

RESOURCES

Berman, A. & Orlikoff, R. (1997). Instrumentation in voice assessment and treatment: what's the use? *AJSLP, 6*(4), 9–16. Available at: http://www.asha.org/

Golper, L. C. & Brown, J. E. (Eds.). (2005). *Business matters: A guide for speech-language pathologists.* Rockville, MD: American Speech-Language-Hearing Association.

Kuster, Judith Maginis. Net connections for communication disorders and sciences. Available at: http://www.mnsu.edu/comdis/Kuster2/welcome/html.

Lubinski, R. & Higginbotham, D. (1997). *Communication technologies for the elderly: vision, hearing, and speech.* San Diego, CA: Singular Publishing Group.

McGuire, R. (1995). Computer-based instrumentation: clinical applications. *Language, Speech, and Hearing Services in Schools, 26*(4), 223–231.

26

Stress, Conflict, and Coping in the Workplace

ROSEMARY LUBINSKI, EDD

SCOPE OF CHAPTER

Although most professionals experience some fatigue and frustration related to professional life, some professionals will experience such depleting stress from one or a variety of sources that they may be a candidate for burnout. In both of the cases described in the following scenarios, these professionals' lives are in jeopardy because of a variety of internal and external factors. In some cases, individuals may try to remediate the problem. Others opt to leave the profession or change jobs, but most just carry on despite feelings of chronic stress and burden. As the best treatment for burnout is prevention, this chapter is presented to introduce students and professionals to this potential problem, provide strategies for self-identification, and suggest prevention and management through positive coping.

Maslach (1982) says, "The risk of burnout is less likely to become reality if you get a head start on it" (p. 131). Academic and clinical training programs, as well as professional agencies and organizations, have a responsibility to concentrate on knowledge and skills but also on how to become and remain a "totally healthy" professional. Additional beneficiaries of this humanistic approach are clients, coworkers, and families.

Rick   ❋ ❋ ❋

Rick is a 41-year-old audiologist who recently completed the requirements for an AuD at an university about 75 miles from his home. His position as an audiologist at a large medical center did not require this advanced degree, nor was it required for licensure in his state. Rick felt that the degree was to his advantage, although he knew it would consume his personal time and would involve financial expense. None of the other five audiologists in his program intended to do this and teased him about his motivation to "run the hospital" some day. Rick's wife was also skeptical but supportive about the added costs and the time it would take away from his job and family. Rick and his wife had adopted a preschooler with special needs 2 years previously. Rick worked full time while going to school for 18 months and traveled to classes two nights a week.

During his 2nd year, he was in a serious accident that totaled his car and resulted in minor injuries to his passenger. Rick then decided to take a 3-month leave of absence so that he could finish his program, deal with his father's death, and provide support to his mother. When Rick returned to his job, he found that one of his colleagues had been promoted to Program Director and that his office had been moved. There was no public recognition of his having received the advanced degree and no salary increase. He overheard a colleague say, "Did he think we'd roll out the red carpet for him when he got a doctorate?" In the next several months following his return to work, Rick lost 15 pounds and resumed smoking. Feeling demoralized and depressed, Rick considered leaving audiology.

Susan   ❋ ❋ ❋

After working full time as a speech-language pathologist in a medical setting for 10 years, Susan felt that a part-time position in home care would offer her more flexibility considering her recent divorce and need for after-school child care for her preteen twin daughters. Upon joining a home care company, Susan was placed on a team headed by nurse and included occupational and physical therapists, a social worker, and several personal care aides. Susan looked forward to this type of work since it paralleled the adult population of her former job. She knew that she needed to adapt to the new computer-based reporting system of the agency and the demands made by travel and scheduling to home sites.

On the day when the team met to discuss Mr. JB, a patient with aphasia whose care was shared by all of the team, Susan was surprised that the nurse did not ask her to give suggestions for communicating with the patient and shocked when she was told it would be sufficient to put suggestions in the patient's file. Susan was equally amazed when she overheard the nurse say to one of the team members that there "really isn't anything you can do for speech patients. I rarely encourage doctors to refer for it. They get

much more out of PT and OT." During a home care visit to a patient with global aphasia, the nurse told the patient that he was improving "far beyond" expectations in all areas but speech and that area did not have a good prognosis. Susan felt that the nurse's comments did not reflect the gains the patient had made thus far and were detrimental to the patient's motivation. During other team meetings, Susan noted that the nurse consistently omitted reference to or humorously referred to speech "therapy" while praising other rehabilitation programs. With their hectic schedules, Susan had little opportunity to get to know the other team members. She believed, however, that they were generally unaware of the negativity toward speech-language pathology. When Susan talked to the nurse about her perceptions, she was told that she was "just too sensitive. . . . Your divorce, you know, puts a lot of stress on you. Of course we all know speech can be valuable for some patients. What's important is for you to concentrate on is getting your reports in on time." Susan could not envision working on this team for months or years and seriously contemplated leaving the home care position.

Speech-language pathologists and audiologists also need to be aware of signs and symptoms of stress in their clients and families. Prolonged and unrelieved stress may diminish clients' motivation for and efforts in therapy, carryover to functional contexts, and ability to problem-solve strategies for effective communication. Similarly, family members' stress may have a detrimental effect on our assessment and intervention. The topic of client and family stress and burden is far too extensive for this chapter, but a section of the chapter is devoted to helping communication disorders specialists appreciate the importance of stress and burden as a related professional issue. Read the previous two case studies as a preface to the topic of stress, burden, and coping.

DEFINITIONS AND SYMPTOMS

The first step in dealing effectively with stress, burnout, and conflict is to know their characteristics. Remediation strategies follow logically from this identification.

Stress

Although there are many definitions of stress, one definition that appears sufficiently comprehensive and applicable to professionals in communicative disorders is that by Monet and Lazarus (1977). They state that stress "consists of any event in which environmental demands, internal demands, or both tax or exceed the adaptive resources of an individual, social system, or tissue system" (p. 3). Thus, stress may emanate from some combination of professional and/or personal events of our environment, our individual capacity to cope with stressors and their effects, our perception of the situation, and our biologic capacity to respond to stress.

Each of us is able to cope with life's demands. For any number of reasons, however, one's internal and external coping resources may be so strained at certain times that adaptation is ineffective to meet the problem. In the case of acute stress, the individual is thrown off-balance for a short period of time before stability returns. For example, when preparing for a final examination, students may focus only on studying for that test for a week, while their other academic and personal pursuits, or health, suffer. After the test, students resume their regular daily routine. In contrast, chronic stress occurs when a person is challenged over a long period of time by mild to severe stressors. Persistent stress tends to result in a snowball or pileup effect. Individuals may not even be completely conscious of the nature or severity of the stressors affecting them or of the numerous serious effects. They may be aware, however, that their ability to cope effectively is diminished.

Chronic stress, in particular, takes an insidious and vicious physical and psychological toll on an individual. Physical effects of stress can range from mild to extreme. Such effects include fatigue, insomnia, headaches, gastrointestinal disorders, dermatological disorders, susceptibility to infection, hypertension, and heart disease (Farmer, Monahan, & Hekeler, 1984). Psychologically, the person may feel some degree of anxiety or depression. How the person perceives and eventually copes with chronic stress may in itself cause further problems. For example, skipping meals may lead to unnecessary weight loss, and self-medicating through the use of drugs, alcohol, or overeating may lead to a dependency or health issues. Social withdrawal may lead to feelings of even greater despair. Consider the varieties of stress both Rick and Susan felt in the earlier case studies. Stress can be brought on by a single catastrophic life event (e.g. death, moving to a new location, divorce) or by a series of events that in combination overwhelm the individual's capacity to cope.

Burden

The effect on family members of caring for individuals of all ages who have significant and prolonged physical or psychological impairments is called *burden*. Burden consists of the physical, psychological or emotional, social, and financial problems that family members caring for such persons can experience (George & Gwyther, 1986). Burden is a multidimensional and complex phenomenon and can be considered objectively by measuring the degree of disruption in health status, social life, and finances. Burden can also be considered from a subjective viewpoint by including the caregiver's perception of psychological or emotional impact. Burden can result in deterioration of a caregiver's physical and mental health and ability to carry out activities of daily living. Most important, burden appears to be related to the amount of caregiver social support and the caregiver's subjective perceptions of caregiving (Novak & Guest, 1989). Again, both Susan and Rick had a certain amount of burden associated with their own family situations.

Burnout

A special effect of chronic stress is burnout. Maslach (1982) defines burnout as a "syndrome of emotional exhaustion, depersonalization, and reduced personal accomplishment that can occur among individuals who do 'people work' of some type" (p. 3). Burnout is a cumulative process rather than an event (Farber, 1983); it is the result of a sustained burden in a caregiving relationship. Burnout is rooted in the relationship between caregiver and care receiver. Many clients with communication disorders and their families may have such a multitude of serious and complicated problems. Trying to meet the needs of another person can tax anyone's internal and external resources, even if meeting those needs is an expected part of our job. In some clinical situations, the caseloads may be so high that there is not enough time to provide the counseling and support that appear so needed to enhance traditional therapy. In yet other clinical situations, clients may get little assistance from family or significant others and depend even more on the speech-language pathologist or audiologist for support. Some clients are unmotivated and noncompliant, and clients and families may show little or no obvious appreciation for professional skill and support.

Burnout can emanate from many other sources as well. Table 26–1 lists sources of burnout adapted from research by Macinick and Macinick (1990), Maslach (1982), Scheller (1990), and Tschudin (1990). Unreasonable demands of the professional position, incompetency on the part of coworkers

and supervisors, lack of training to perform the job expectations, and stringent policies and procedures governing the agency collectively or individually contribute to burnout. In some clinical positions, there will be a lack of autonomy and opportunity for self-actualization. Job insecurity and low pay, combined with increased financial pressures, may also be critical. A perception of discrimination based on age, race, sexual preference, ethnic group, or gender can also lead to stress. Inadequate supervision, unclear criteria for job expectations or performance evaluations, and evaluations that focus only on the negative ("what you could do better") are all detrimental to happiness at work. Finally, negative relationships with coworkers or a supervisor create a hostile situation where burnout is likely to occur.

The clinician's own personality characteristics may be a source of burnout. Maslach (1982) uses such adjectives as *submissive, anxious, fearful, passive, impatient, insecure,* and *intolerant* to describe the personality profile of someone at risk for burnout. In light of the foregoing discussion, consider factors that contributed to a feeling of burnout for Rick and Susan. Maslach cautions, however, that *all* individuals, given the right (or wrong) degree of stressful circumstances, are candidates for burnout. Burnout may occur with the strongest of personalities when stresses are prolonged, intense, or unresolved. In both Rick's and Susan's cases, numerous familial pressures added to the pressures inherent within their professional situations.

The issue of competing demands from job and family deserves special attention because the profession of speech-language pathology, in particular, is dominated by women. It should be remembered, however, that many professional men share in caregiving and homemaking duties and thus also experience difficulties in balancing competing demands of professional and family life. In a study of caregiving needs of our professions, Shewan and Blake (1991) found that while the median number of dependents for affiliates of ASHA was only one, caregiving duties consumed 20 hours per week. Full-time speech-language pathologists spent more time on caregiving duties than did audiologists; women spent more time on caregiving duties than did men.

T A B L E 26–1 Sources of Burnout

Client Factors

- Overly demanding clients and/or families
- Complicated, serious problems of clients and/or families
- Lack of client/family responsiveness
- Lack of client /family appreciation

Professional Situation Factors

- Size of caseload
- Too many responsibilities
- Lack of autonomy
- Little opportunity for self-actualization
- Low pay; few salary increases
- Job insecurity
- Little opportunity for continuing education
- Tedium
- Excessive paperwork and inadequate time to complete it
- Inadequate working conditions and/or resources
- Discrimination: sexism, ageism, racism
- Inadequate supervision
- Unclear criteria for professional evaluation

- Evaluation based on negative factors only
- Coworker competition or incompetence
- Lack of coworker support
- Bullying behavior by coworkers
- Interdisciplinary conflict or competition
- Unprofessional attitudes on part of supervisor or coworkers
- Lack of positive reinforcement from supervisor
- Rigid or unrealistic institutional policies

Personal Factors

- Unrealistic expectations; perfectionism; need for control and to "do it all"
- Inability to say "no"
- Inability to delegate work to others
- Lack of confidence
- Need for approval from others
- Hostility
- Impatience
- Personal and/or family health problems
- Family pressures
- Competing demands of job and family

Bonnar (1991) states that caregiving is not valued in our society and is perceived as "invisible work." Caregiving involves other than housework duties and tends to be considered within the female domain of responsibilities. The recipients of caregiving are children and the elderly. The U.S. Department of Labor (1990) reports that 65 percent of women who had children less than 18 years of age were employed. Scharlach and Boyd (1989) found that 23 percent of employees had some caregiving duties for elderly parents. Stone and Short (1989) reported that close to 1 million working women were faced with caregiving responsibilities for both children and adults. These statistics are likely to have implications for benefits from individual employers as well as for

federal policy and legislation affecting maternity, parental, or family leave (McGovern & Matter, 1992).

Another source of burnout that deserves special mention is the presence of coworkers who exhibit bullying behavior. Known as "toxic coworkers" (Cavaiola & Lavender, 2000), these individuals tend to be convincing, charming, and manipulative persons who have excellent verbal ability but a decided need to criticize and humiliate others. Their goals include attaining their personal self-interests and self-esteem by degrading others, usually those they perceive as a threat. It is estimated that one in six workers is bullied each year, most targets are women, and more than half of the bullies are women (Mezger, 2004). This is interesting since

T A B L E 26–2 Examples of Bullying Behavior by a Coworker

- Convincing liar; Jekyll and Hyde personality
- Verbally agile—nonspecific and evasive
- Sense of superiority
- Needs to control and attain power
- Compulsive need to criticize, intimidate, dominate, and humiliate
- Manipulative
- Acts out of self-interest and self-preservation
- Distorts or fabricates allegations for control
- Creates arbitrary rules and unreasonable demands
- Makes a fuss over trivia while ignoring important things
- Uses gossip, rumor, and innuendo to discredit and isolate target
- Excludes and "ices out"
- Tries to erode the confidence of the target
- Has a short selective memory regarding what they said or did
- Does not value others or their achievements
- Cannot distinguish between aggression and assertive behavior
- Poor listening skills
- Tends to rely on written communication such as e-mail rather than face-to-face contact
- May take credit for other's work
- Threatens job loss

SOURCE: Adapted from The Serial Bully, 2005, available at http://bullyonline.org/workbully.serial.htm; and R. Mezger, "Battling the Workplace Bully," *Cleveland Plain Dealer*, July 25, 2004.

women are supposed to be nurturing and protective of each other. Note that toxic coworkers are often in superior positions but may also be peers (Downs, 2005). Table 26–2 lists other signs of bullying that a coworker may exhibit.

The insidious nature of these individuals may take a serious toll including depression, post-traumatic stress disorder, other physical and psychological stresses, absenteeism, lost productivity, and financial loss to the targets and their employers. Some targets of bullying experience panic attacks and have difficulty concentrating and making decisions. Unfortunately, it is more common that the targets often feel so stressed that they leave their positions while the bully remains in a position of power. Some employers, however, do take action against employees who can be proven to have committed psychological harassment. An excellent resource for information on workplace bullies is *The Bully at Work: What You Can Do to Stop the Hurt and Reclaim Your Dignity on the Job*, by Namie and Namie (2003).

Several themes emerge from this discussion of sources of burnout. The sources of burnout are idiosyncratic, diverse, and multiple. The stressors can range from mild to catastrophic. Given the combination of circumstances, anyone in a helping profession such as speech-language pathology or audiology is a candidate for burnout. Critical to prevention of burnout is awareness and self-perception of stressors and knowing how to access your internal and external resources for coping successfully with them.

Stages of Burnout

Cherniss (1980) postulates there are three stages to the process of burnout in the helping professions. Stage 1 is an imbalance between the demands and resources to deal with job stress. There are too few personal or institutional resources to equalize increasing demands. This leads to Stage 2, when the individual reacts to this strain with feelings of anxiety, tension, fatigue, and exhaustion. Finally, in Stage 3, defensive coping emerges, characterized by emotional detachment, withdrawal, cynicism, and rigidity. A vicious and insidious cycle emerges: The greater the demands placed on the professional, the greater the demand for and depletion of the individual's energy and resources for coping.

Effects of Burnout

The effects of burnout are as numerous and complex as are the causes. Table 26–3 divides the effects of burnout into four major categories: professional

T A B L E 26–3 Signs and Effects of Burnout

Professional Effects

- Detachment/depersonalization
- Sense of inadequacy
- Irritation with clients
- Diminished listening skills
- Decreased work output
- Deteriorating work performance
- Leave work earlier than usual/increased absenteeism
- Negative impact on finances of individual or agency

Psychological Effects

- Sadness
- Anger
- Frustration
- Loss of satisfaction or accomplishment
- Overly self-critical
- Cynical and negative
- Tension
- Anxiety
- Depression
- Forgetfulness
- Feeling of helplessness
- Suspiciousness
- More risk taking

- Paranoia
- Suicide

Physiological Effects

- Feeling of exhaustion and chronic fatigue
- Reduced autoimmune response
- Increased susceptibility to illness and infection
- Rapid heart rate
- Hormonal abnormalities
- Shortness of breath
- Poor eating habits
- Addiction to controlled substances or alcohol
- Frequent headaches
- Insomnia
- Gastrointestinal disorders
- Dermatological disorders (e.g., hives, eczema, acne)
- Back and neck disorders
- Hypertension
- Heart attack
- Stroke

Effects on Significant Others

- Marital conflict
- Family discord
- Loss of intimacy
- Estrangement from others

effects, psychological effects, physiological effects, and effects on significant others. According to Maslach (1982), one of the most obvious signs of burnout is a sense of *emotional exhaustion* in which the professional feels frustrated, physically exhausted, and emotionally depleted. The individual feels hopeless and as though there is "no more to give." The natural strategy to cope with such emotional exhaustion is to try to distance oneself from work. The professional perceives that with self-withdrawal from the source(s) of the problem, particularly the persons involved, stability will be recovered.

Unfortunately, this response leads to *depersonalization* in which the professional resents and denigrates clients, coworkers, or others who are perceived to be the root of the problem. Maslach adds that such a negative perception eventually leads to a sense of *personal inadequacy*. In this state, one feels a deep sense of failure and inability to accomplish one's goals. All of these feelings blend and lead to poor quality and quantity of work performance as well as depression. Consequently, some individuals may change careers or job positions, reduce work load, and/or seek counseling.

The psychological effects are also apparent and range from feelings of sadness, anger, and frustration to depression, suspicion, and paranoia. Conflicting feelings abound. Feelings such as being annoyed and frustrated lead to detachment; irritation and overload lead to depersonalization; reduced self-esteem leads to depression.

One of the most common physiological effects is a sense of chronic exhaustion. The persistent negative responses of emotional depletion, depersonalization, and sense of inadequacy combined with pervasive deleterious psychological effects may lead to serious health problems. These health problems can take any individual or combination of forms, such as headaches, susceptibility to infections, insomnia, gastrointestinal disorders, and hypertension. At the most serious end of the continuum, some individuals may suffer a heart attack or stroke. Numerous other obvious health problems may also occur such as poor eating habits, alcohol abuse, smoking, and overuse of or dependency on tranquilizers or other drugs. Some individuals may even resort to suicide.

The effects of stress and burnout are also evident in work productivity and efficiency. According to a 2003 study of the effects of depression on work productivity, Stewart found that the total cost of depression was $44 billion. Workers with depression lost more than 8 hours of work per week whereas those who were not depressed lost only about 1.5 hours of productive time.

The effects of burnout may reach to coworkers and family. For example, a professional who is experiencing burnout may withdraw from coworkers, view them in a suspicious manner, or become dependent on them for completing a job. When burnout is rampant within an agency, a negative climate may pervade the institution, and job satisfaction and morale are likely to be low (Cherniss, 1980). Frequent job turnover is also a result and has economic and quality improvement implications.

Family members are likely to bear some of the brunt of professional burnout. Marital conflict and family discord are well documented by many professionals who feel burned out (e.g., *social work*: Siefert, Jayaratne, & Chess, 1991; *teaching*: Sakharov, & Farber, 1983; *medicine*: Mawardi, 1983; *nursing*: McLaughlin & Erdman, 1992; *day care workers*: Maslach & Pines, 1977). Spouses and children may make such comments as "Dad's grumpy all the time," "I can't seem to do anything right for Mom any more," and "Since you got that job, you've not been the person I married." The professional may be unaware that the angry outbursts at home are a reflection of professional burnout. A professional who is emotionally and physically exhausted from stresses in the workplace cannot magically leave them at the door when family time begins. In addition, the effects of stresses associated with marriage, family life, finances, and other outside issues complicate and magnify professional stresses and their effects. A vicious and insidious cycle of stress and maladaptive coping is likely to occur.

STRESS IN HUMAN SERVICE PROFESSIONS

A logical question you might ask is, "Why is burnout so common among human service professionals?" A helping relationship involves an investment of knowledge and skill blended with facilitating interpersonal qualities to effect change in another individual. Individuals drawn into helping professions such as speech-language pathology and audiology tend to be oriented to people rather than things and to helping those in trouble (Pines, 1983). Other helping professions include, but are not limited to, those related to teaching, psychology, counseling and social work, medicine, and nursing. The fact that so many human service professions work in impersonal institutions further complicates the situation. Farmer and colleagues (1984) identify at least four stressful factors inherent in helping professions: (1) the complexity of our clients and their needs; (2) the difficulty in evaluating "success" in the helping professions; (3) poor perception of helping relationships by others; and (4) the decision-making process inherent in many helping relationship agencies. Maslach (1982) calls burnout the "cost of caring."

The fact that human services are frequently offered through governmental and institutional settings further complicates the situation. Caplan and Jones (1975) list stresses particular to institutional settings, including role ambiguity, role conflict, and role overload. For example, in some institutional settings there are unclear job definitions, discipline boundaries, and criteria for success. Role conflict emerges from inappropriate or unclear demands on the professional or when faced with disparity between individual and institutional ethics and values. Role overload develops from caseloads that are too large or too demanding. The setting by its very nature may be insensitive to the demands on or needs of individual professionals. Farber (1983) cautions that this attitude may increase as economic resources to support human service programs decrease. Recent changes in Medicare and other insurance funding have caused instability in some health care settings and apprehension concerning employment. Such concern can exacerbate feelings of burnout.

BURNOUT IN SPEECH-LANGUAGE PATHOLOGY AND AUDIOLOGY

Several studies have addressed the topic of burnout among speech-language pathologists (Miller & Potter, 1982; Potter, Hellesto, Shute, & Dengerink, 1988; Potter & Rudensey,1984). In Miller and Potter's 1982 study of speech-language pathologists, 43 percent of the respondents considered themselves to have experienced moderately severe burnout. Burnout appeared related to job dissatisfaction, job effectiveness, and lack of management and support services for coping. Interestingly, burnout was not related to setting, years of employment, caseload, client severity level, paperwork demands, or collegial relationships.

In a second study that investigated how speech-language pathologists coped with burnout, Potter and Rudensey (1984) found that 16 percent of their respondents were leaving the profession because of burnout. Effective coping strategies included adapting personal career goals to be more realistic, understanding motivations for being within a helping profession, increasing communication with administrators, and developing a self-change attitude. They also found that there were some effective strategies generated by agencies to reduce burnout among speech-language pathologists. These strategies included systematic solicitation and implementation of employee suggestions, group discussions, flexible scheduling, released time for continuing education, and clear communication about job expectations. Potter and Rudensey concluded that a team approach involving a speech-language pathologist and an administrator could be effective in improving the mental health of clinical staff.

Two studies have specifically addressed burnout among audiologists (Potter et al., 1988). In the first study of 184 clinically certified audiologists, 40 percent of the respondents considered themselves mildly burned out, 30 percent as moderately or severely burned out, and 29 percent as not experiencing burnout. Factors contributing to burnout included feelings of job ineffectiveness and dissatisfaction. In a follow-up survey of audiologists that explored causes and coping strategies related to burnout, the same authors found 15 percent of their respondents were leaving the profession, with another 67 percent having considered this option. The authors concluded that strategies that might reduce burnout among audiologists include (1) having employees participate more in organizational policy setting; (2) reducing caseloads and paperwork; (3) including more uninterrupted flexible break time; (4) matching supervisor's and employee's role expectations; and (5) providing accurate job descriptions. Nemes (2004), in a recent article on burnout in audiology, cautioned audiologists to walk a fine line between deriving too much satisfaction from working with patients and burnout. Burnout is a real possibility for those professionals who work with hearing impaired for many years and make their professional work the total focus of their personal satisfaction.

Self-Identification Strategies

Perhaps in reading this chapter you have said "That's me" or "Could that really happen to me?" At times, most professionals will have negative experiences associated with professional life. What is critical, however, is prolonged, excessive, and destructive experiences and perceptions that lead to professional burnout. Recognition of warning signs and symptoms mentioned in this chapter is the first step in prevention or recovery from burnout. Three inventories by Farmer and colleagues (1984) focus on the sources of stress, the effects of stress, and the behaviors used to cope with stress in human services. Although there are many other well-established stress and burnout inventories available in the literature (e.g., Derogatis, 1977; Vitaliano, Russo, Carr, Maiuro, & Becker, 1985; Pfifferling, 2005) these inventories serve as good starting points for self-evaluation. Each of these inventories requires that you identify and/or rate sources of stress, effects of stress, and strategies you use to cope with perceived difficulties.

A second method of identifying burnout is to talk with trusted coworkers and family about your behaviors and reactions. These individuals may be well aware of changes in your attitude and behavior that may signal potential burnout. It should be noted, however, that many colleagues may be hesitant to comment spontaneously on another's behaviors even when concerned.

REMEDIATION OF STRESS AND BURNOUT

Both professionals and their employment settings have a vital interest in remediating or preventing stress and burnout. Thus, changes that will reduce stress and foster productive coping strategies can emanate from you and/or your setting. There are two basic ways to approach this problem: (1) change yourself and your attitudes or (2) remove the cause(s) of the stress (Tschudin, 1990). Excellent

sources for more in-depth reading on how to cope with burnout include works by Maslach (1982) and Pines, Aronson, and Kafry (1981). Numerous studies on the effects of stress-reducing programs tend to show positive outcomes for the professional and the setting (e.g., Lees & Ellis, 1989). Also see Namie and Namie (2003) to read more about bullying in the workplace.

Changing Yourself and Your Attitudes

Macinick and Macinick (1990) and Maslach (1982) are among many authors who suggest that at least some remediation of burnout stems from changing one's attitudes. Systems rarely change, individuals do. Thus, remediation begins with understanding yourself and understanding, accepting, and working smart even within a flawed system. Thus, professionals who feel burned out need to self-analyze goals, expectations, and value systems governing their professional life. Changing one's attitudes also involves development of problem-solving strategies that maximize inner strengths and accomplishments. Productive problem solving entails problem identification, presentation of alternative solutions and their potential benefits, and consideration of the costs involved in solving the problem.

An initial step in coping with burnout is to assess your strengths. Personal strengths may be ignored by a professional who feels stressed. Farmer and colleagues (1984) suggest you begin by listing what you consider to be your physical, emotional, social, intellectual, spiritual, and other strengths. Such analysis may lead you to affirm your positive qualities, cultivate a more positive self-image, and call up these resources when stressed. You must regain control and sell yourself to yourself. In the case of bullying, remember that the bully has the problem, not you.

If you are feeling burned out professionally, you may need to analyze your own motivations influencing the practice of your job. Tschudin (1990) suggests that many professionals bring "personal luggage" to work such as carryover of childhood expectations to adulthood, guilt, vague resentments, perfectionism, inability to say no, overcaring for others, and lack of confidence. Examine your personal values and live by them. Tschudin states that:

> When you look at the stress produced from within yourself, you begin to see that the responsibility lies with you, and within you. But it takes a lot of personal strength to accept this, cope with it and use it positively. (p. 41)

Some individuals can do this self-analysis and self-change alone, and others need the help of a mentor or counselor. Remember that seeking help is not a sign of weakness but of strength.

Working Smarter A second strategy that professionals may adopt to change themselves is to "work smarter." Professionals who feel burned out do not need to work harder but do need to make a more productive investment in their work life. Working smarter, according to Maslach (1982), involves changing your job to be less stressed and more efficient. This can be achieved by setting realistic goals, doing the same thing differently, improving time management, taking breaks, and taking things less personally.

Setting realistic goals stems from an analysis of what *really* needs to be done, resources for completion, and available time. "Setting realistic goals involves a recognition of your limitations as well as your abilities" (Maslach, 1982, p. 91). The value of changing how things are done is that you will feel more in control of the situation. This strategy begins with analysis of the steps involved in tasks and their eventual elimination or modification. For example, one clinician may want to begin the day at 7 A.M. with completion of paperwork from the previous day, whereas another would rather come in later and do this at the end of the day. Taking a planned break from work is also essential in remediation of burnout. Some professionals need quiet times dispersed between clients; others need to "go out for lunch," and still others divert some of their professional time to less intense or stressful tasks. Finally, and perhaps most difficult, professionals need to perceive difficult situations as objectively as possible.

Working smarter may also involve taking action. For example, you may keep a log of bullying behavior to identify patterns of such actions. Keep a copy of memos, e-mails, or other written or recorded harassment for future reference in a safe place. If harassment is the source of your stress and burnout, check your employer's harassment policy and work with your occupational health office ("How to Deal with Workplace Bullying," 2005). For example, if you choose to approach the bully, discuss your grievance with your grievance officer first and focus on the undesirable behaviors, not the person. At times, a formal written complaint may be necessary.

Nutrition Proper nutrition is key to relieving stress. Alcohol and food abuse may only add to the problems and reduce your physiological reserve. Check with your physician and/or a nutritionist for dietary guidance.

Decompression Activities Taking care of yourself outside the work situation helps relieve burnout. Maslach (1982) states that "the demands of a caring profession necessitate that professionals take good care of their body and spirit" (p. 95). Examples of physical decompression activities include exercise, noncompetitive physical activities, a healthy diet, plenty of rest, yoga, and relaxation techniques.

Exercise, one of the most popular stress reduction techniques, helps to condition the cardiovascular system to withstand stress (e.g., Tatelbaum, 1989). Exercise activities such as walking, jogging, swimming, and other aerobics all result in direct medical, endurance, flexibility, and emotional benefits (Farmer et al., 1984). Relaxation activities include deep breathing, progressive muscle relaxation, autogenic training, biofeedback, yoga, imagery, and meditation (Peddicord, 1991). Many people find listening to music to be a natural "tranquilizer" (Parachin, 1991). Many of these relaxation activities can be done throughout the workday.

Psychological decompression activities include participation in meaningful and enjoyable outside activities. As the song goes, "accentuate the positive." Participation in recreation activities such as hobbies can help counterbalance a day of stress. Taking an occasional day off from work or going on a planned vacation can contribute to well-being. Unfortunately, because of demanding caseloads, financial needs, and competing demands from work and home, some professionals have or make little time available just for themselves. Maslach (1982) states that "frustrations and failures can be put into perspective when balanced by satisfactions and successes" (p. 95). To help others effectively, you consistently need to fortify yourself physically and psychologically.

Continuing Education Participation in continuing education programs offered through the workplace or professional organizations is an excellent strategy for dealing with burnout. Continuing education helps you gain new skills to work more effectively and efficiently, stimulates creative thinking and problem solving, and opens networks with other professionals. In-services offered through your employment setting might focus not only on assessment and intervention issues related to communication disorders but also to time management, conflict resolution, and stress management.

Attendance at regional, state, or national meetings provides an opportunity for many professionals to combine educational enhancement with the opportunity to "get away" from the stresses of both work and family. Generally, there are social activities at these events where you can initiate or renew professional and personal friendships. In order not to be disappointed with the continuing education program offered, you should be sure to review carefully announcements and to determine if the stated objectives match your background and needs at the time. Finally, you may find yourself "recharged" when you are the presenter at a continuing education program. The challenge and intellectual stimulation inherent in the preparation and the positive feedback afterward may help relieve burnout.

Support and Counseling Social support is defined as "information that leads individuals to believe that they are cared for and loved, esteemed, and valued and that they participate in a network of communication and mutual obligation" (Pines, 1983, p.156). Cobb (1976) considers support an "immunization" against stress. A supportive individual is an active listener who provides nonjudgmental emotional backup, assistance, insight, and feedback. The primary vehicles for offering support are open communication, active listening, and accessibility.

In many institutional settings, individual mentors are available to discuss technical and psychological aspects of the job. The clinical fellowship or internship supervisor may assume this role for the first-year professional, with coworkers, formally or informally, possibly adopting this relationship. Pines and colleagues (1981) suggest that even staff meetings can help reduce burnout if they focus on articulation of shared problems and staff development. Similarly, in some settings, particularly large institutional settings such as school districts or hospitals, work-setting support groups may be available. These groups focus on developing staff effectiveness and problem solving through free expression of feelings, offering of suggestions and feedback, and realistic goal setting (Scully, 1983). There may be specific topic agendas such as techniques for stress management, methods of conflict management, development of self-esteem, and assertiveness (Tschudin, 1990).

Support offered by family and friends is also valuable, although "bringing home" stressful topics may exacerbate burnout rather than relieve it. Maslach (1982) states that family and friends tend to offer comfort, appreciation, and positive experiences. Her research has also identified the critical importance of a good marriage or intimate relationship in "counterbalancing" the stresses of a job. Some authors suggest that spirituality may sustain individuals through stressful times. Spirituality goes beyond participation in formal religious organizations and focuses on a person's perception of his or her place in the universe and the creation of a personal value system (Farmer et al., 1984). Prayer and meditation may provide relief and serve as decompression activities.

Humor

In his autobiography, Norman Cousins (1981) called humor a form of internal jogging. It moves your internal organs around, increases your heart rate, and reduces your blood pressure. It also enhances respiration. Laughter is an "igniter of great expectations" (p. 217). Maslach (1982) also states that humor is an important supportive coping technique. "Being able to joke and laugh about a stressful event reduces the tension and anxiety—it also serves to make the situation less serious and less overwhelming" (p. 60). These two quotes serve to remind us that humor is one of the most powerful techniques to reduce stress and to cope with burden. Murphy and Murphy (2000, p. 24) offer seven strategies on how to incorporate humor in our lives:

1. Select humor that complements your life and work.

2. Quantify humor by using it as part of your therapy goals and measure the results.

3. Keep in mind that the very best humor is when you can laugh at yourself.

4. Know where to find good, funny stuff fast.

5. Know and believe what humor can do for you and your patients.

6. Remember: You can't always be in control, but you always have choices.

7. Reward yourself.

Humor can be shared with clients, families, and coworkers through jokes, funny stories, quotes, and anecdotes, through nonverbal communication, through cartoons, posters, bulletin boards, and via the Internet. Professionals should only use humor that is culturally and linguistically appropriate.

Conflict Resolution on the Job

Remember that all of us experience some conflict in the course of our professional lives, but it must be handled carefully so that work can be meaningful and productive. There will be times when the strategies featured here do not help relieve stress and burden, particularly when the stress involves a conflict with a colleague. You will need to identify who is involved in the conflict, what critical issues are involved, what each person's position is regarding the conflict, and what strategies might be used to settle the conflict. Conflict resolution will involve your ability to create a dialogue with the other person. This conversation should stem from your basic sense of respect for this individual. It is best to have your dialogue in a neutral place that is physically and psychologically comfortable for you both. Be prepared to define the issue as something you need to solve together. Fittro (2005) suggests that you describe the behaviors, feelings, consequences, and desired changes you envision by starting sentences with "I" rather than "you." Empathic listening is critical to the process so that you understand the other as a precursor to being understood. The next step is for each person to brainstorm possible solutions followed by a positive evaluation of each one. The goal is to identify solutions or compromises that are acceptable to each person and provide a "win-win" context. Solutions should be tried and evaluated after some period of time.

Should personal conflict resolution not solve the issue, a third party or mediator may be involved. Mediation provides both parties with a safe and neutral environment where they can offer their perspectives and solutions. Mediators create a context where individuals feel they can speak openly. They also facilitate the meeting, clarify issues as needed, and provide possible suggestions. Mediation has been found to be a positive context for solving conflicts, particularly one where individuals perceive that they have had fair and equitable treatment (Roehl and Cook, 1989).

Unfortunately, the best strategies for resolving conflicts do not always work. Some individuals are so entrenched in their own perspectives and unwilling to work toward a solution that a positive resolution is impossible. Their own personalities and communication styles may be barriers to a productive dialogue. Yet others may be unwilling to discuss issues and want to avoid any context where the issues are openly discussed.

Changing Jobs

There may be times in your professional life when despite your concerted efforts to adapt to and cope with stresses, a change in employment may be the best alternative. Maslach (1982) cautions us to consider carefully what a change means and its expected outcome. "Change does not automatically guarantee success and happiness" (p. 107). Change may involve assuming another position within the same organization, such as becoming a supervisor or administrator. Pines et al. (1981) describe this as "quitting upward." It may also mean changing employment settings to work in a comparable position or a new one. Finally, change may mean leaving the professions of speech-language pathology or audiology.

In considering a change, you need to assess if the new position really results in a removal of current stressors. It is possible a position in a new agency entails similar stressors to your present position. Further, a new position may have unique or additional stressors with which you are not prepared to cope. Before you change positions, remember there is a certain degree of stress inherent in changing positions. For example, there may be unfamiliar duties and routines associated with the new position, philosophical differences in service delivery, and "great expectations" for performance. Should you be changing geographical areas, there is the added stress of relocation perhaps to an unfamiliar area that lacks a personal support system.

Notwithstanding these cautions, change can be invigorating and challenging. A new position may be a true antidote for burnout. This may be the perfect opportunity to use coping skills learned in a previous position. It may also be a chance to demonstrate heretofore unrecognized abilities and to fulfill personal career goals. Reflect back on Susan's situation. Should she leave her position because of the bullying behavior of her coworker and supervisor? What other strategies can she use other than leaving the job? Also, is it reasonable for Rick to consider leaving audiology? What options does he have?

PREVENTION OF BURNOUT

Early identification of burnout is the most effective way to cope with burnout. As Maslach (1982) states, the key to prevention is early action. The risk of burnout is less likely to become reality if you are forewarned. Thus, students and professionals alike can benefit from an awareness of the presenting signs of burnout and the development of work and lifestyles that help prevent its emergence.

What are some practical ways to discourage burnout? Knowing the scope of your professional duties helps to define your job in realistic terms. If some of the duties are beyond your abilities, these should be discussed with your supervisor to determine how you might gain needed skills or how the duties might be reassigned. Discussion with your supervisor should also focus on how you will be evaluated in your position so that you have a clear conception of the agency's performance expectations. Unless you have this information, you may assume too many duties, assume duties for which you are unprepared, and work toward goals that are unrealistic or unappreciated.

A second strategy for preventing burnout is to enlist the help of a mentor who can provide objective feedback to you about your performance and with whom you can discuss potential and real problems. This person may be an excellent resource for helping you to work smarter and more effectively within your agency. Maslach (1982) states that colleagues may serve as an "early warning system" to each other when early burnout symptoms appear. A third strategy for preventing burnout is to incorporate the burnout coping strategies into your life from your student days and your earliest professional employment. For example, you should periodically and objectively self-analyze your professional goals and motivations, participate in exercise, recreation, and continuing education programs, and seek support when needed.

NEEDED RESEARCH

The professions of audiology and speech-language pathology have undertaken little specific research in the area of professional burnout (e.g., Miller & Potter, 1982; Potter & Rudensey, 1984). There appears to be little reason to suspect that these professions are more immune to burnout than other helping professions such as social work, nursing, and education. Our professions are undergoing scrutiny and modification of such national issues as changing demographics of our target populations, the focus on increasing costs of health care, education and rehabilitation, demands for definition of efficacy of treatment, and technological advancements within our own professions. The time is ripe for inclusion of the topic of burnout in our training programs to prepare future professionals to function effectively at an emotional and interpersonal level within their work settings. Finally, although burnout affects both genders, being female-dominated professions, we should be particularly sensitive to the competing demands and stress many women experience in balancing work and family life. Much can be gained from an exploration of the stressors and the productive strategies women and men use to meet competing demands. Our professions and the individuals we serve would benefit from closer introspection into such professional issues.

STRESS AND BURNOUT AMONG CAREGIVERS

Families carry the primary responsibility for the care, management of, and rehabilitation of their chronically ill and/or disabled family members of all ages. Froggatt (1990) described care as having a "dual" nature in that it is both labor and love intensive. Unpaid caregiving offered by family members usually in the home is considered informal in contrast with paid services of professionals. Family caregiving may be provided by any member, but it tends to be a female role, often relegated to wives and mothers, adult daughters, or daughters-in-law.

Middle-aged women have been labeled the "sandwich generation" because of their responsibilities to older frail parents and to the needs of children. Smaller and different types of families, changing patterns of marriage and companion relationships, and increased mobility of individual family members suggest that who will provide informal caregiving will change in years to come.

Caregiving has been conceptualized from a number of models, but what appears constant is that caregiving is a multidimensional role depending on the needs of the care recipient and the abilities and motivations of the care provider. Caregiving can involve a wide variety of roles but is most often associated with providing help with instrumental tasks such as providing physical care and direct assistance with activities of daily living. Caregiving is also likely to include other types of tasks, including communicating with medical, rehabilitative, and educational professionals, acting as an advocate for the care recipient, assisting with financial affairs, helping with decision making, and providing social stimulation. Thus, providing care can involve a number and variety of roles for which the care provider can be more or less prepared.

Caregiving by family members can result in positive feelings of fulfillment and self-esteem, especially since the care is usually given to a loved family member. Caregiving can, however, also result in a wide variety and degree of stress for the care provider. For example, stress can emanate from (1) restrictions on the caregiver's personal and professional lifestyle; (2) competing demands with intergenerational obligations and workplace; (3) the physical and cognitive characteristics and demands of the care recipient; (4) financial changes; (5) lack of training to provide care; (6) lack of help or respite; and (7) social isolation. Caregiving becomes stressful when there are drastic lifestyle changes and when the caregiver feels overwhelmed by or trapped in the situation (Wilson, 1989). Caregivers adjust their lives to meet the needs of the care recipient by giving up those things that are most "marginal" or "elastic," such as personal time, socialization and leisure activities, and personal interests (Cantor, 1983). Caregivers who have a closer relationship or bond with the care recipient, such as spouses, parents, and adult children, usually experience greater stress.

Burden is the adverse consequence of accumulated stress in one or more domains of caregivers' lives, including physical, psychological or emotional, social, and financial areas. Burden can be objective in that there are quantitative changes in caregiver time, health status, finances, social roles, and occupation. Burden can also be subjective in that the care provider perceives a range of emotions related to the caregiving situation, including embarrassment, resentment, overload, anxiety, depression, and feelings of exclusion (e.g., Morycz, 1980; Vitaliano, Young, & Russo, 1991).

Speech-language pathologists and audiologists need to be aware of the variety of caregiving roles and the related stress and burden family members may experience. Family members who are overloaded may be unreliable information receivers or givers, opposed to intervention suggestions, or too absorbed in caregiving to concentrate on communication needs. Their own coping difficulties may mitigate their ability to participate fully in assessment or intervention, not because of lack of desire but because of the aggregate of real and perceived caregiving stresses. Thus, speech-language pathologists and audiologists need to be aware of signs of caregiver stress and burden and know how to address these needs through counseling and family support groups. In some cases, referral to mental health professionals is warranted and should be done with consultation with the family physician, the hospital or agency, or the health/educational care team. Unfortunately, limited interaction with caregivers may make such identification more difficult, although the effects of caregiver strain will be no less significant and detrimental to the carryover of audiology or speech-language pathology services.

SUMMARY

At some point in a professional career, audiologists and speech-language pathologists may incur prolonged stress that leads to burnout. Burnout is defined as emotional and physical exhaustion, a feeling of incompetence and depersonalization. Burnout arises from an intermingling of factors, including the nature of our clients' problems, complex work setting factors, and one's own personal makeup. It results in deterioration in work performance, psychological disorders, physiological changes, and changes in relationships with clients, coworkers, and significant others.

Coping with burnout involves changing one's own attitudes about work and success; working smarter; incorporating exercise, recreation, and other decompression techniques into daily life; participating in continuing education; and seeking peer, family, or professional support. The best antidote for burnout is prevention, which involves discussion of burnout etiology and symptoms during preprofessional training. Approaching employment with a self-monitoring attitude will also help prevent burnout.

Finally, speech-language pathologists and audiologists need to be aware of the serious impact of the caregiving process on care providers. Family members may experience significant changes in their physical and emotional health as well as their social and professional lives that diminish our effectiveness in assessment or intervention. Care providing, whether it be informal assistance given by family or friends or professional services, can exact an expensive physical, psychological, or social toll, often to the detriment of the care receiver. Speech-language pathologists and audiologists who consider a holistic approach to working with clients or patients that focuses on balancing theoretical and technical knowledge with psychological support will surely provide quality services to those who can benefit.

CRITICAL THINKING

1. What are some warning signs of burnout?

2. What would you do if one of your colleagues demonstrated signs of burnout?

3. What societal factors do you believe contribute to burnout within human service professions?

4. What are some possible signs of stress and burden that family caregivers may exhibit? How do these influence your professional services?

5. What direct and indirect roles do speech-language pathologists and audiologists have in addressing stress and burden in family caregivers? Why is this often a neglected area in our professional service?

6. What suggestions would you have for both Rick and Susan in the case studies beginning this chapter? What internal and external difficulties add to their stress and create conflicts for them?

REFERENCES

Bonnar, D. (1991). The place of caregiving work in contemporary societies. In J. Hyde & M. Essex (Eds.), *Parental leave and child care*. Philadelphia: Temple University Press.

Cantor, M. (1983). Strain among caregivers: A study of experience in the United States. *The Gerontologist, 23*, 597–604.

Caplan, R., & Jones, K. (1975). Effects of workload, role ambiguity, and type A personality or anxiety, depression, and heart rate. *Journal of Applied Psychology, 60*, 713–719.

Cavaiola, A., & Lavender, N. (2000). *Toxic coworkers: How to deal with dysfunctional people on the job*. Oakland, CA: New Harbinger Publishers.

Cherniss, C. (1980). *Staff burnout job stress in the human services*. Beverly Hills, CA: Sage Publications.

Cobb, S. (1976). Social support as a moderator of life stress. *Psychosomatic Medicine, 38*, 300–314.

Cousins, N. (1981). *Human options*. New York: W. W. Norton.

Derogatis, L. (1977). *SCL-90 administration, scoring and procedures manual*. Privately published.

Downs, M. (2005). *Putting a workplace bully back in line*. Available at http://my.webmd.com/

Farber, B. (1983). Dysfunctional aspects of the psychotherapeutic role. In B. Larker (Ed.), *Stress and burnout in the human services professions* (pp. 97–115). New York: Pegasus.

Farmer, R., Monahan, L., & Hekeler, R. (1984). *Stress management for human services*. Beverly Hills, CA: Sage Publications.

Fittro, J. (2005). *Resolving conflict constructively and respectfully*. Available at http://ohioline.osu.edu

Froggatt, A. (1990). *Family work with elderly people*. New York: Macmillan.

George, L., & Gwyther, L. (1986). Caregiver well-being: A multi-dimensional examination of family caregivers of demented adults. *Gerontologist, 26*, 248–252.

How to deal with work place bullying: advice, guidance and help with adult bullying. (2005). Available at http://www.bullyonline.org/

Lees, S., & Ellis, N. (1989). The design of a stress-management program for nursing personnel. *Journal of Advanced Nursing, 15*, 946–961.

Macinick, C., & Macinick, J. (1990). Strategies for burnout prevention in the mental health setting. *International Nursing Review, 37*, 247–250.

Maslach, C. (1982). *Burnout: The cost of caring*. Englewood Cliffs, NJ: Prentice Hall.

Maslach, C., & Pines, A. (1977). The 'burnout' syndrome in day care settings. *Child Care Quarterly, 6*, 100–113.

Mawardi, B. (1983). Aspects of the impaired physician. In B. Farber (Ed.), *Stress and burnout in the human service professions* (pp. 119–128). New York: Pergamon Press.

McGovern, P., & Matter, D. (1992). Work and family coping demands affecting worker well being. *American Association of Occupational Health Nurses Journal, 40,* 24–35.

McLaughlin, A., & Erdman, J. (1992). Rehabilitation staff stress as it relates to patient acuity and diagnosis. *Brain Injury, 6,* 59–64.

Mezger, R. (2004). Battling the workplace bully. *Cleveland Plan Dealer,* July 25, 2004.

Miller, M., & Potter, R. (1982). Professional burnout among speech-language pathologists. *ASHA, 24,* 177–180.

Monet, A., & Lazarus R. (Eds.). (1977). *Stress and coping.* New York: Columbia University Press.

Morycz, R. (1980). An exploration of senile dementia and family burden. *Clinical Social Work Journal, 8,* 16–27.

Murphy, J., & Murphy, A. (2000). Seven strategies for reducing stress. *Advance, 10,* 24.

Namie, G., & Namie, R. (2003). *The bully at work: What you can do to stop the hurt and reclaim your dignity on the job.* Naperville, IL: Sourcebooks.

Nemes, J. (2004). Professional burnout: how to stop it from happening to you. *The Hearing Journal.* Available at http://www.highbeam.com/

Novak, M., & Guest, C. (1989). Application of a multidimensional caregiver burden inventory. *The Gerontologist, 29,* 798–803.

Parachin, V. (1991). Pressure-proof your life: Creative ways to reduce stress. *Today's Nurse, 13,* 9–11.

Peddicord, K. (1991). Strategies for promoting stress reduction and relaxation. *Nursing Clinics of North America, 26,* 867–874.

Pfifferling, J. (2005). *Burnout risk appraisal.* Available at http://www.cpwb.org/

Pines, A. (1983). On burnout and the buffering effects of social support. In B. Farber (Ed.), *Stress and burnout in the human service professions* (pp. 155–174). New York: Pergamon Press.

Pines, A., Aronson, E., & Kafry, D. (1981). *Burnout.* New York: The Free Press.

Potter, R., Hellesto, P., Shute, B., & Dengerink, J. (1988). Burnout among audiologists: Its incidence and causes. *The Hearing Journal, 41,* 18–25.

Potter, R., & Rudensey, K. (1984). Coping with burnout. *Asha, 26,* 35–37.

Roehl, J., & Cook, R. (1989). Mediation in interpersonal disputes: Effectiveness and limitations. In K. Kressel, D. Pruitt, & Associates (Eds.), *Mediation research* (pp. 31–52). San Francisco: Jossey-Bass.

Sakharov, M., & Farber, B. (1983). A critical study of burnout in teachers. In B. Farber (Ed.), *Stress and burnout in the human service professions.* New York: Pergamon Press.

Scharlach, A., & Boyd, S. (1989). Caregiving and employment: Results of an employee survey. *The Gerontological Society of America, 29,* 382–387.

Scheller, M. (1990). *Building partnerships in hospital care.* Palo Alto, CA: Bull Publishing.

Scully, R. (1983). The work setting support group: A means of preventing burnout. In B. Farber (Ed.), *Stress and burnout in the human service professions.* New York: Pergamon Press.

Shewan, C., & Blake, A. (1991). Caregiving: A common role for ASHA members. *Asha, 35,* 35.

Siefert, K., Jayaratne, S., & Chess, W. (1991). Job satisfaction, burnout, and turnover in health care social workers. *Health and Social Work, 16,* 193–202.

Stewart, W. (2003). Cost of lost productive time among U.S. workers with depression. *JAMA, 289,* 3135–3144.

Stone, R., & Short P. (1990). The competing demands of employment and informal caregiving to disabled elderly. *Medical Care, 28,* 513–526.

Tatelbaum, J. (1989). *You don't have to suffer: A handbook for moving beyond life's crises.* New York: Harper and Row.

The Serial Bully. (2005). Available at: http://www.bullyonline.org/

Tschudin, V. (1990). Support yourself. *Nursing Times, 86,* 40–42.

U.S. Department of Labor, Women's Bureau. (1990, September). *20 facts on women workers.* Fact sheet No. 90–92. Washington, DC: Author.

Vitaliano, P., Russo, J., Carr, J., Maiuro, R., & Becker, J. (1985). The ways of coping checklist: Revision and psychometric properties. *Multivariate Behavioral Research, 20,* 3–26.

Vitaliano, P., Young, H., & Russo, J. (1991). Burden: A review of measures used among caregivers of individuals with dementia. *The Gerontologist, 31,* 67–75.

Wilson, H. (1989). Family caregiving for a relative with Alzheimer's dementia: Coping with negative choices. *Nursing Research, 38,* 94–98.

Evidence-Based Practice

27

The Future of Science

RAY D. KENT, PHD

SCOPE OF CHAPTER

Research is intrinsically futuristic, always directed to the next experiment, the next theoretical advance, the next challenge to the standard view. Research is a frontier phenomenon, and its practitioners work on a horizon of possibilities. To dare any specific forecast into what research may bring is uncertain at best, foolish or irrelevant at worst. The challenge is also great because communication sciences and disorders constitute a field of broad and expanding horizons. Manifold opportunities for future developments can be imagined, and a single chapter can do little justice to such large scientific capital. But because research is a human enterprise that rests on intellectual and economic resources, one can make some general projections, taking into account the historic pattern and the present-day foundation for future development.

This chapter takes a general view of research on human communication and its disorders. The purpose is not so much to predict particular scientific accomplishments as it is to assay the socioeconomic trends and various influences that will govern funding for research and the parameters of its application. The expenditure for research on communication sciences and disorders is quite small compared to that for the major diseases such as cancer or heart disease, but all areas of research, whether large or small, are subject to the major forces of social policy. To put it in other words, "Science policy implements a social contract" (Pielke & Byerly, 1998, p. 42). The future of science will be defined by the social contract through which society provides the resources for science and, in turn, reaps the benefits of scientific achievements.

SCIENCE AND THE SOCIAL CONTRACT

The social policy that provides economic support for science in the United States appears to be at the threshold of, if not within, a period of fundamental change. Because this change has multiple ramifications, it is important to gain some understanding of it. Until quite recently, the social policy that undergirded research support was the Bush contract, named after Vannevar Bush, who in 1945 published a document of extraordinary influence. As noted by Pielke and Byerly (1998), the Bush contract is based on three fundamental assumptions. First, it assumes that scientific advances are essential to meet national needs. Few people would argue with this contention, and the expectation that science will benefit society is critical to the public support of science. Second, the way in which science meets national needs can be described through a simple linear/reservoir model. In this model, science creates a reservoir of knowledge that is tapped by society. Third, science is practiced in relative autonomy, isolated from the direct influence of society. This isolation ensures a freedom of scientific inquiry. In this model, society provides the resources for, but does not govern, the scientific enterprise. Ideally, science would grow continuously, and as it does, the reservoir of knowledge would expand and society would benefit from this vast pool of information. However, science can become highly expensive, and some commentators believe that exponential growth is unlikely (Nalimov, 1981; Price, 1963). Inevitably, then, science must compete for resources with other social institutions, such as those addressing needs in defense, health, education, national disasters, and other social services. Even if there were general agreement that the reservoir of knowledge should be as large as possible, it may be economically prohibitive to support vigorous programs of research in all specialties at all times. The conduct of science can also be affected by ethical issues, as in the case of reproduction science, the harvesting of fetal tissues for stem cell research, and genetic engineering.

Accordingly, the social contract may change in favor of a model in which economic and moral priorities are established for the support of science. These priorities would determine the allocation of funds for various areas of research. Some sense of the difficulties involved can be gained from an examination of the factors that determine funding for research by the National Institutes of Health. It has been proposed that the funding for different areas and disorders can be gauged by the burden of disease (Gross, Anderson, & Rowe, 1999) or by the amount and effectiveness of lobbying (Gottlieb, 1999). (See Curran, Effinger, Pantel, & Curran, 1983, for further discussion of priorities and policy.)

There is indeed a growing conviction that the level and breadth of research funding enabled by the Bush contract may not be sustainable under current and projected resources. As the social contract that defines science policy undergoes change, there are broad implications for research. Science has come to a point that might be called "the end of growth," a period in which "the frontiers of knowledge still seem endless, but the financial and human resources needed to extend those frontiers now seem to be increasingly limited" (Sigma Xi, 1987, p. 32). The "end of growth" is not necessarily abrupt; indeed, warnings of a budgetary limitation for science have sounded for some time, even while federal appropriations for science have continued to increase. The expectation of change is evident in recent discussions that relate to definitions of what science should be (Notturno, in press) and whether science is at a socioeconomic crossroads (Charlton, in press). It should not be assumed that science is immune to social, political, and economic forces; to the contrary, science is affected by each of these factors and the science of the future will be molded by exogenous influences. The dependency of science on its sociopolitical environment is captured in the following quotation, "Historians and economists have recognized that while scientific innovation has occurred in many settings, it has prospered most when talent, supportive institutions, mobility, free communications, and financing are available in significant measure" (Moses, Dorsey, Matheson, & Their, 2005).

Current and future scientists probably will have to consider very carefully how their work might be supported by the available resources. But this is not the only reason for a change in the social contract. It is also clear that many problems will not be solved solely by scientific methods. As Pielke and Byerly (1998) observed, "Infectious diseases develop resistance to antibiotics" and "Proliferation of wastes and weapons mars the nuclear option" (p. 44). Scientific accomplishments surely can produce benefits, but they also can incur side effects or long-term consequences that are not entirely desirable. Furthermore, some advances may bring about ethical dilemmas, as has been widely discussed with respect to modern genetics and various developments in molecular biology. The implication is that science today is not a completely autonomous enterprise but rather one that seeks solutions within a broader framework of personal and social benefits and risks. In certain circumstances, governments impose restrictions on the ways in which research can be done, especially when humans or human tissues are involved.

A demand for immediate applicability of all research could greatly impair the health of the research enterprise. Frequently, research on fundamental scientific problems yields enormous benefits, not all of which were even imagined at the time of the initial discovery. Funding agencies must take care that research into fundamental questions is not harmed by a drastic reallocation of funds to research that addresses applied problems of high priority. The value of a given research project cannot always be determined from a narrow set of immediate priorities. Consider the instructions (see Appendix 27-1 at the end of the chapter) that the National Institutes of Health provide to the reviewers of research grant applications. The fundamental dimensions by which an application is judged are the significance of the research, the approach to be used, the innovation of the proposed research, the capabilities of the investigator, and the appropriateness of the environment. These five yardsticks are the evaluation tools used by the world's largest funding agency for research on human health.

The Committee on Science of the United States House of Representatives took a major step in defining the new federal science policy with its report, "Unlocking Our Future: Toward a New National Science Policy" (September, 1998; excerpts of the report appear in *Science Communication, 20,* 328–336). Some basic issues are summarized here. An important point is that the report affirms the importance of federal funding for fundamental scientific, or basic, research. It also endorses a program of research grants to individual investigators that offset indirect costs and are evaluated by a peer-reviewed selection process. The report recommends that funding be provided for creative, groundbreaking research that might be considered too risky in a conservative review process. Mention also is made of the Governmental Results and Performance Act, which mandates a review of outcomes of federally supported programs, including research. The report recommends that funding agencies evaluate outcomes by using a research portfolio rather than evaluating outcomes for individual research grants.

An obligation that falls to scientists is to inform the public and policy makers about what kinds of scientific advances are likely and at what cost. For example, Feigin (2005) considers how research may affect the prospects for child health. The National Institutes of Health accomplish a similar goal with the preparation of strategic research plans that typically summarize major research accomplishments and identify particular opportunities for new discoveries and their clinical application.

THE CLINICAL IMPERATIVE: DOING GOOD AT AN ACCEPTABLE COST

Research in clinical fields, including speech-language pathology and audiology, confronts another major issue, the general problem of demonstrating desired outcome at an affordable cost. This issue enfolds a range of topics known by such names as *clinical outcome, efficacy, effectiveness,* and *efficiency.* Clinical outcome is the effect of a treatment or intervention. Considerable emphasis is now placed on *functional outcomes*, which are effects that pertain to the basic dimensions of human life, such as activities of daily living. Efficacy is the comparison of two or more treatments when performed by competent specialists under ideal conditions. Research on efficacy tells us which of two procedures is better or more successful. Effectiveness is the outcome of intervention when it is conducted under conditions available in the community. Efficiency is the relationship between the benefit of an intervention and the cost of its delivery. An intervention may be judged as efficacious and effective, but could be so expensive as to be prohibitive to implement on a large scale. For a more extensive discussion of issues in clinical outcome, see Frattali (1988).

The problems are complex, but in the simplest sense, the question to be answered is: Do the clinical treatments provided by specialists provide functional benefits at a cost that society is willing to pay? The word *functional* implies that the benefits can be measured for activities that are part of daily living (e.g., basic self-care), educational achievement, or occupational placement and performance. It is not sufficient to demonstrate that a client or patient improves to some degree on a test developed for a specific kind of performance. For example, even if a child receiving treatment for a language disorder can be shown to produce a greater variety of linguistic structures in a clinical setting, this improvement may not necessarily translate to functional changes in the child's school performance or interaction with peers. The willingness of society to pay for clinical services depends partly on the perceived consequences of the illness or disability and the perceived benefits of a particular kind of clinical intervention.

Evidence-based practice is the logical result of demands for scientific documentation of clinical practice. The importance of evidence-based practice in communication sciences and disorders is readily seen in the efforts of the American Speech-Language-Hearing Association to publish technical reports (ASHA, 2004), form a central committee to coordinate activities related to evidence-based practice (Advisory Committee on Evidence-Based Practice), and devote resources to a national center (National Center for Evidence-Based Practice). These are fundamental steps that pave the road on which clinicians and clients will surely travel. See Chapter 28 for a thorough discussion of evidence-based practice.

DISSEMINATION: THE FIRST FRUITS OF RESEARCH

The discovery of new information in any scientific domain is exciting and satisfying to the scientists involved, but unless the knowledge is disseminated, it could well be of little or no real value to the general public. Research is not only discovery but also the accurate and effective dissemination of the new knowledge to other researchers, to clinical practitioners, and to the public. Dissemination of research information is already changing quickly because of (1) new technologies such as the World Wide Web; (2) an increasingly active role of the media in presenting new results to the public; and (3) the urgent demands by insurers and others for certain kinds of data (e.g., data on the value of clinical interventions). Dissemination is not a simple pipeline between the scientific laboratory and the consumer of research. Rather, dissemination presents its own complex decisions about quality control, reliability, efficiency, and access. The ethical burden on authors of scientific articles is considerable, as considered in the excellent papers by Benos and colleagues (2005) and Claxton (2005a, 2005b).

The editor-in-chief of *The New England Journal of Medicine* commented that "The capacity to convert information of all kinds (print, audio, video) into a digitized form and to send digitized data out over an expanding number of networks has the potential of completely revolutionizing our definition of a journal" (Kassirer, 1993, p. 178). Although many obstacles remain in the legal and economic domains, it is relatively simple to replace (or partner) print journals with electronic versions made available over the World Wide Web. Today, subscribers to some journals have the choice of a traditional hard copy, a compact disk, or a Web site. A positive result of the new technology is that recently acquired knowledge can be accessed quickly by anyone with the technological resources. This includes the lay public. Clinical specialists frequently discover that patients and clients (or their caregivers) have searched the World Wide Web for information on diseases or disabilities. Consequently, consumers may be considerably better informed today than was the case even a decade or so earlier. But the ease of access to information can be offset by some disadvantages, not the least of which is questionable quality control over some of the information.

The media play an important role in announcing new scientific knowledge to the public. Many major discoveries attract the attention of the broadcast and print media almost as soon as they are released to the scientific community. Coverage by the media can be crucial to science because it demonstrates to the public the fast pace of discovery and the potential benefits to society. But at times, the advantages of such public dissemination are offset by inattention to limitations of the research or the need for corroboration of the findings. On occasion, clinical practitioners may feel caught between consumer demands for services (which may be fueled by powerful statements in the public media) and the need for scientific investigation into a type of intervention. The public may fail to understand that acceptance of a new intervention is not necessarily straightforward. Frequently, scientific studies may yield conflicting, or not entirely consistent, results. Some of the ways in which this problem is addressed are meta-analyses and consensus conferences, considered later in this chapter.

Dissemination enables the next step in the research-to-practice sequence, the application of evidence to clinical practice. The ultimate goal of clinical research is to improve clinical assessment and intervention. The vitality of research in a clinical discipline can be gauged by the responsiveness of clinical practice to new discoveries. Obviously, research by itself will not accomplish this goal. It is imperative that the results of research be disseminated to clinicians who have the discernment to use these results to modify clinical practice as indicated. This is not a simple process. It demands a breed of

practitioner who is committed to a vigorous kind of professional education. This education can be summarized as follows:

> Eventually, self-directed lifelong learning and the teaching of evidence-based medicine may take hold, so that practitioners learn during their training how to learn for the rest of their professional lives, becoming adept at keeping up with new evidence and applying it to the betterment of their patients' health. (Haynes, 1993, p. 220)

The new evidence can come in several forms, but it is well to recognize that certain types of evidence have a higher degree of acceptability than others.

Clinical Trials

The randomized controlled clinical trial is the definitive assessment of clinical intervention (Brook, 1993; Greenberg, 1993). Clinical trials are particularly important in medicine to evaluate interventions such as drugs or surgery, but trials can be applied to behavioral interventions as well. Clinical trials in communicative disorders are relatively few but the number is growing. For a general discussion of clinical trials in communication disorders, see Baum, Logemann, and Lilienfeld (1998). As important as clinical trials (and the nearly inevitable meta-analyses) are and will be, enthusiasm for their application should be balanced by recognition of several limitations. Some of these, discussed by Brook (1993) and Cohen, Stavri, and Hersh (2004), are as follows. First, it is likely that many clinical decisions by practitioners of all kinds will have to be made without convincing data, even if a robust program of clinical trials were initiated—and communicative disorders are far from having a robust program. The research enterprise simply is not large enough to provide evidence for every decision that must be made by the practicing clinician. Second, the procedures used in clinical trials may be sufficiently different from those actually used clinically that the results of the clinical trials may not be totally relevant to the clinical situation. The disparity is not always easily recognized and may require conscientious attention. Third, there is a need for methods that combine knowledge *and* expert judgment. Brook's comments pertain to medicine, but they should apply equally well, if not more so, to a discipline such as communicative disorders in which scant data from clinical trials are available.

Placebos

Placebos are commonly used in medical research as a control condition. A placebo is a treatment for which no particular benefit is expected aside from the benefit that may follow any procedure the patient believes could be effective. Sugar pills are one form of placebo used in evaluating the benefit of a drug that is administered in a similar kind of pill. Interestingly, the placebo, which is ostensibly without any expected health benefit, can be beneficial in one third or more of a given study group (Turner, Deyo, Loeser, Von Korff, & Fordyce, 1994). The benefit of the placebo is sufficiently strong that it has come to be called "the placebo effect." This effect is not limited to clinical trials involving drugs. It can occur in virtually any kind of treatment, including behavioral interventions.

Like active treatments, the placebo can have time-effect curves, peak effects, cumulative effects, and carryover effects. One lesson of the placebo effect is that the human response to intervention is not as simple as might be the case in studies with animals or computer models.

Reviews and Meta-Analyses

The path to accepted scientific knowledge is not always straightforward. In many areas of research, published papers are not entirely congruent in their conclusions and sometimes are even contradictory. For this reason, reviews and meta-analyses, also called *overviews* have become an important source of information. These terms are not used consistently by all authors.

For the purposes of this chapter, a *review* is a survey of an area of scientific study or clinical practice. Properly done, a review considers information from all (or nearly all) published articles pertaining to a given subject. A review may be a survey prepared by

a recognized authority in the field, or it can be a synthesis resulting from a systematic review prepared by individuals trained for this purpose. As important as these synthesizing activities may be, it is sobering to read the conclusion of one article: "These results also cast doubt on the wisdom of relying on experts to be solely responsible for preparation of review articles. Our data suggest that experts, on average, write reviews of inferior quality" (Oxman & Guyatt, 1993, p. 129). Guidelines for readers of reviews can be found in Oxman and Guyatt (1988).

A *meta-analysis* is a consolidation of data from different publications or from different ongoing clinical trials (Robey, 1998; Robey & Dalebout, 1998). The morpheme *meta* in this context means comprehensive or transcending, and a central purpose of a meta-analysis is to go beyond any individual publication or research study. A meta-analysis uses mathematical methods to derive a synthesis of independent research results. Unlike a primary research study, in which the units of observation are typically individual subjects, the meta-analysis uses as its units the outcomes of tests of null hypotheses as reported in a number of primary studies. Meta-analysis is particularly important for clinical outcome studies because it is "the preferred method for determining the preponderance of evidence in clinical-outcome research relating to questions of treatment efficacy and treatment effectiveness" (Robey & Dalebout, 1998, p. 1227). The undertaking is not without difficulties. It is well for anyone who attempts to prepare such a synthesis to consider the pitfalls, as described by Oxman and Guyatt (1993) and Matt and Cook (1994).

Consensus Conferences

A consensus conference is a group judgment process for the synthesis and evaluation of scientific data. Unlike a meta-analysis, which can be conducted by one individual who has access to a collection of independent primary studies, the consensus conference brings together a group of acknowledged experts who typically have dissimilar opinions on some or all aspects of the problem. Especially for controversial issues with potentially great impact on public health, the consensus conference can be highly effective. The consensus conferences sponsored by the National Institutes of Health (NIH) have become an international model (Ferguson, 1993). These conferences conform to three basic standards:

1. The conference is a public meeting.
2. The scientific topic is suitable for NIH, and the conference embraces a variety of viewpoints on the topic.
3. An unbiased panel weighs the evidence.

Whether supported by NIH or not, conferences can be the clearing ground for issues on which conflicting or uncertain conclusions have been drawn.

TRANSLATIONAL RESEARCH

Translational research is the application of emerging scientific knowledge to therapeutic advances. Translational research may take at least two forms, one being the translation of animal research or "bench" research to research on humans and another the translation of basic (preclinical) research on humans to research on humans with disease or disorder. A "translation gap" results from disproportionate efforts in basic research and clinical applications. Several factors contribute to this gap, including industry's preference for late-stage clinical trials, a static distribution of NIH support for basic and applied research, and the inclination of venture investors to seek companies that have products that are close to market (Moses et al., 2005). The degree of concern that NIH has for this problem is reflected in the recent plans for the "NIH Roadmap," which features initiatives to encourage clinical and translational research (Zerhouni, 2005).

TECHNOLOGY

Technology and science are not the same thing, although some in the lay public may confuse them. Science, as an enterprise that produces new ideas, typically uses technology and often produces new technologies, but technologic proficiency alone does not define a science or a scientist. And yet technologic sophistication often is perceived to be an important credential of the scientist, and technologic apparatus may be taken to define the scientific workplace. Technology extends the faculties and senses of the scientist, making possible a degree of accuracy and sensitivity that can be quite remarkable. Unquestionably, technology will have profound effects on research in all disciplines. Technology also may facilitate the transfer of knowledge from the laboratory to the clinic. For example, computer-generated analyses perfected in the laboratory may be transported to the clinic to increase the power and accuracy of clinical observations. Of course, technological transfer demands resources. Clinical personnel must be trained in the use of the technology, and the necessary instruments must be acquired and maintained.

As Nalimov (1981, p. 153) observed, "science creates the ecological situation favorable for itself." That is, science promotes education in the sciences, communication of scientific information, technological and engineering resources, and even the demand for more science. It is difficult to separate science from its resources, especially as the resources, including technology, enable the growth of science and the social impact of its discoveries. Science is not an encapsulated human activity, but rather an activity that tends to affect the way we conceptualize the world and the way we work in the world.

INTERDISCIPLINARY RESEARCH

Both the complexity of many research problems and the powerful benefits of hybrid expertise favor the continued development of interdisciplinary research. Teams of investigators and technicians are often required in areas such as neuroimaging, prosthetics (mechanical and electrical), genetic studies, surgical monitoring, nanotechnology, and many others. Collaborations and consortia will be the rule rather than the exception in certain kinds of research, and disciplinary specialists need to learn the skills of interdisciplinary and multidisciplinary communication and project management.

It is almost bromidic to say that the field of communication sciences and disorders draws from many different disciplines. But mere proclamation does not guarantee the desired result. The most sophisticated kind of interdisciplinary or multidisciplinary research requires an aggressive crossing of borders and an enlightened understanding of what each discipline has to offer. The future of science will require scientific personnel to seek interdisciplinary and multidisciplinary projects. Multidisciplinary centers are being formed in several areas and are particularly suited to fields of study in which there are ample data but difficult problems. Ideally, the multidisciplinary center integrates scientists with different specialties to work on a complex problem.

One of the most important divides to be bridged in interdisciplinary or multidisciplinary initiatives is that between behavioral and natural sciences. Poor behavioral choices by individuals can induce, maintain, or exacerbate health problems. Just one behavioral issue—compliance with a clinical specialist's recommendations—is critical to the success of intervention. Behavioral and natural science can be mutually informative, but bringing them together in the desired symbiotic relationship is not as easy as one might hope. Glass and McAtee (2005) recommended three innovations to promote the integration of behavior and natural sciences. The first is an elaboration of the "stream of causation" metaphor along the two axes of time and levels of nested systems of social and biological organization. The second is an inquiry into the proposition that "upstream" features of social context are themselves causes of disease. The third is the concept of a risk regulator to advance the investigation of behavior and health in populations.

THE CHALLENGE
OF POPULATION DIVERSITY

If personal characteristics such as age, gender, and ethnicity had no effect on a behavior of interest or on a particular clinical treatment, then research could be done on virtually any group of subjects and the results could be generalized to an entire population. However, it is frequently the case that these and other personal variables can individually, or in their combination, influence behavioral patterns and the degree to which a clinical treatment is effective. In fact, it is often unwise to assume that personal characteristics are not important in evaluating outcome for a particular procedure. Males and females do not always experience the same consequences of a disease process, and they do not necessarily derive the same benefit from a clinical treatment (Christen, 1991; Glucksmann, 1981; Pool, 1994).

Speech and voice are inherently sexually dimorphic, and even language processes such as syntax and pragmatics may reflect the gender of the communicator. The same statement could be made concerning age, ethnicity, and several other variables. This perspective leads to an ambitious program of research in which major demographic features are taken into account. Some steps have been taken, as exemplified in the construction of databases structured according to gender, age, and other features. It is essential that this direction of research be continued.

INTERNATIONAL PERSPECTIVES

Many scientific advances have a value that is not limited by cultural or national boundaries, and a major scientific advance can have the potential for worldwide benefit. Discovery of a new vaccine, a potent antibiotic, a new source of fuel, or an efficient means of waste management can affect people in every continent and every nation for generations to come. Research in communication sciences and disorders also can bring benefits to the international community, but these benefits are not always as straightforward as in other sciences.

Particularly when a discovery is in some way specific to a given dialect or language, the application to other speech communities or languages cannot be immediately assumed. Nonetheless, it is clear from cross-language studies that important commonalities can exist. But aside from the question of the immediate application of scientific discoveries, there is a fundamental issue concerning international cooperation. The issue is the education of scientists and the development of research facilities on the international stage. The United States is one of the world's leaders in research on communicative disorders, and it is not surprising that students from many other nations have come to the United States to study in the disciplines of speech-language pathology and audiology. Academic programs therefore have the potential for international influence. Thinking about communication and its disorders should become increasingly international in its character, even as the new communication technologies (e.g., machine translation) begin to erase linguistic barriers in their careers.

PROMOTING RESEARCH AND RESEARCH TRAINING WITHIN THE PROFESSION

The lifeblood of science in any discipline is the preparation and retention of investigators. Unlike many, if not most, specialties, communicative disorders and sciences has faced, and continues to face, a shortage of trained research personnel. This problem has been recognized for many years and has been addressed by initiatives within ASHA and the Council of Academic Programs in Communication Sciences and Disorders (CAPCSD). In 1997, ASHA and CAPSCD formed a joint committee, the Working Group on Recruitment, Retention, and Academic Preparation of Researchers and Teacher-Scholars. This working group made a number of recommendations, some of which were realized in

the development of an ASHA-focused initiative in 2004 and 2005. This initiative, called the *Doctoral (Ph.D.) Shortage,* identified three issues:

Issue 1: There is a critical shortage and continuing attrition of PhD level faculty in higher education that will affect preparation of professionals as well as the conduct of research in communication sciences and disorders.

Issue 2: Tradition has limited the role of research instruction in all levels of the curriculum resulting in a lack of coordinated academic culture and scientific/research personnel preparation experiences in the discipline that promote careers as teachers/researchers in higher education.

Issue 3: There is no coordinated data collection and dissemination system related to doctoral programs that allows for the exchange of information on research training experiences, funding levels, scholarship activities, and those who enter academia upon completing the PhD degree.

The challenge of preparing future generations of researchers is formidable, but the attention given to this problem is the first step toward a solution. At least two points are clear; (1) newly graduated PhD students should find excellent professional opportunities in the field, and; (2) educational programs must increase their generation of PhD students. With respect to the second point, the need is not only for more PhD graduates, but for PhD graduates who are prepared to work in a research and scholarly environment that is increasingly multidisciplinary and international.

SUMMARY

Communicative disorders and sciences is but one small slice of a gigantic research enterprise. To some degree, the progress of research in any one discipline is affected by the overall vigor of science in its broadest scope. For example, the budgets for major federal funding agencies determine the number of

research grants that will be funded in a given fiscal period. Directly or indirectly, budgets can also determine the amount and kind of preparation of new scientists. Different priorities for funding can enrich one area while impoverishing others. It is likely that there will be intense competition among scientific disciplines for financial support of research. Especially because there appears to be a major change in the social contract that underlies science policy, those who are concerned about the state of the science in the discipline should be prepared to take an active role in encouraging scientists and in providing the resources needed for a healthy research environment.

CRITICAL THINKING

1. What is the Bush contract? Why is this contract important to understanding the public policy behind scientific research?

2. What is a placebo, and why is it used in research on clinical treatments? Define a placebo condition that might be used in a treatment study for a communicative disorder (select any disorder and treatment), or find a published article that uses a placebo condition.

3. Discuss the relationship between science and technology. How do they differ? How do they benefit one another?

Think of some examples of the interaction between science and technology from communication sciences and disorders. In these examples, delineate science from technology.

4. What is the role of meta-analyses and consensus conferences in research? Why are these vehicles necessary or desirable to the application of scientific information?

5. What experiences in your undergraduate or graduate education encouraged/discouraged you to participate in research? How and why should a practicing clinician participate in research?

REFERENCES

American Speech-Language-Hearing Association. (1994). *Handbook of research education in communication sciences and disorders.* Rockville, MD: Author.

American Speech-Language-Hearing Association (2004). *Evidence-based practice in communication disorders: An introduction.* Available at http://www.asha.org/

Anonymous. (1999). Excerpts from unlocking our future: Toward a new national science policy. *Science Communication, 20,* 328–336.

Baum, H. M., Logemann, J., & Lilienfeld, D. (1998). Clinical trials and their application to communication sciences and disorders. *Journal of Medical Speech-Language Pathology,* 55–64.

Benos, D. J., Fabres, J., Farmer, J., Guterrez, J. P., Hennessy, K., Kosek, D., Lee, J. H., Olteanu, D., Russell, T., Shakh, F., & Wang, K. (2005). Ethics and scientific publication. *Advances in Physiology Education, 29,* 59–74.

Bossuyt, P. M., Reitsma, J. G., Bruns, D. E., Gatsonis, C. A., Glasziou, P. P., Irwig, L. M., Moher, D., Rennie, D., de Vet, H. C., & Lijer, J. G. (2003). Standards for Reporting of Diagnostic Accuracy. The STARD statement for reporting studies of diagnostic accuracy: Explanation and elaboration. *Annals of Internal Medicine, 138,* W1–W12.

Brook, R. H. (1993). Using scientific information to improve quality of health care. In K. S. Warren & F. Mosteller (Eds.), Doing more good than harm: The evaluation of health care interventions. *Annals of the New York Academy of Sciences* (Vol. 703, pp. 74–84). New York: New York Academy of Sciences.

Bush, V. (1945; reprinted 1960). *Science: The endless frontier.* Report to the President on a program for postwar scientific research. Washington, DC: U.S. Government Printing Office.

Charlton, B. G. (in press). Boom or bubble? Is medical research thriving or about to crash? *Medical Hypotheses.*

Charlton, B. G. (2006). Boom or bubble? Is medical research thriving or about to crash? *Medical Hypotheses, 66,* 1–2.

Christen, Y. (1991). *Sex differences: Modern biology and the unisex fallacy* (N. Davidson, Trans.). New Brunswick, NJ: Transaction Publishers.

Claxton, L. D. (2005a). Scientific authorship. Part 1. A window into scientific fraud? *Mutation Research, 589,* 17–30.

Claxton, L. D. (2005b). Scientific authorship. Part 2. History, recurring issues, practices, and guidelines. *Mutation Research, 589,* 31–45.

Cohen, A. M., Stavri, P. Z., & Hersh, W. R. (2004). A categorization and analysis of the criticisms of evidence-based medicine. *International Journal of Medical Informatics, 73,* 35–43.

Committee on Publication Ethics (COPE). (1999). Guidelines on good publication practice. Available at http://www.publicationethics.org.uk/

Curran, A. S., Effinger, A. W., Pantel, E. S., & Curran, J. P. (1983). Public health: Priorities and policy-setting in the real world. In F. S. Sterret (Ed.), Science and public policy III. *Annals of the New York Academy of Sciences* (Vol. 403). New York: New York Academy of Sciences.

Feigin, R. A. (2005). Prospects for the future of child health through research. *Journal of the American Medical Association, 294,* 1373–1379.

Ferguson, J. H. (1993). NIH consensus conferences: Dissemination and impact. In K. S. Warren & F. Mosteller (Eds.), Doing more good than harm: The evaluation of health care interventions. *Annals of the New York Academy of Sciences* (Vol. 703, pp. 180–198). New York: New York Academy of Sciences.

Frattali, C. M. (1998). Outcomes measurement: Definitions, dimensions, and perspectives. In C. M. Frattali (Ed.), *Measuring outcomes in speech-language pathology* (pp. 1–27). New York: Thieme.

Glass, T. A., & McAtee, M. J. (in press). Behavioral science at the crossroads in public health: Extending horizons, envisioning the future. *Social Sciences and Medicine.*

Glass, T. A., & McAtee, M. J. (2006). Behavioral science at the crossroads in public health: Extending horizons, envisioning the future. *Social Sciences and Medicine, 62,* 1650–1671.

Glucksmann, A. (1981). *Sexual dimorphism in human and mammalian biology and pathology.* London: Academic Press.

Gottlieb, S. (1999). U.S. research funding depends on lobbying, not need. *British Medical Journal, 318,* 1715.

Graduate Council of the University of Arizona. (nd). *Mentoring: The faculty graduate student relationship.* Tucson: The University of Arizona.

Greenberg, H. (1993). On the proper use of clinical trials. In K. S. Warren & F. Mosteller (Eds.), Doing more good than harm: The evaluation of health care interventions. *Annals of the New York Academy of Sciences* (Vol. 703, pp. 41–43). New York: New York Academy of Sciences.

Gross, C. P., Anderson, G. F., & Rowe, N. R. (1999). The relation between funding by the National Institute of Health and the burden of disease. *New England Journal of Medicine, 340,* 1881–1887.

Haynes, R. B. (1993). Some problems in applying evidence in clinical practice. In K. S. Warren & F. Mosteller (Eds.), Doing more good than harm: The evaluation of health care interventions. *Annals of the New York Academy of Sciences* (Vol. 703, pp. 210–225). New York: New York Academy of Sciences.

Kassirer, J. P. (1993). Dissemination of medical information: A journal's role. In K. S. Warren & F. Mosteller (Eds.), Doing more good than harm: The evaluation of health care interventions. *Annals of the New York Academy of Sciences* (Vol. 703, pp. 173–179). New York: New York Academy of Sciences.

Matt, G. E., & Cook T. D. (1994). Threats to the validity of research synthesis. In H. Cooper & L. V. Hedges (Eds.), *The handbook of research synthesis* (pp. 503–520). New York: Russell Sage Foundation.

Minghetti, N. J., Cooper, J. A., Goldstein, H., Olswang, L. B., & Warren, S. F. (1993). *Research mentorship and raining in communication sciences and disorders: Proceedings of a national conference.* Rockville, MD: American Speech-Language-Hearing Foundation.

Minifie, F. D. (1996, October). The future of the discipline. *Newsletter of the Special Interest Division on Speech Science and Orofacial Disorders, 6,* 1–4.

Moses, H., Dorsety, E. R., Matheson, D. H. M., & Their, S. O. (2005). Financial anatomy of biomedical research. *Journal of the American Medical Association, 294,* 1333–1342.

Nalimov, V. V. (1981). *Faces of science.* Philadelphia: ISI Press.

Notturno, M. (in press). Rethinking science as an area of concern [Editorial]. *Medical Hypotheses.*

Notturno, M. (2006). Rethinking science as an area of concern [Editorial]. *Medical Hypotheses, 66,* 217–219.

Oxman, A. D., & Guyatt, G. H. (1988). Guidelines for reading literature reviews. *Canadian Medical Association Journal, 138,* 697–703.

Oxman, A. D., & Guyatt, G. H. (1993). The science of reviewing research. In K. S. Warren & F. Mosteller (Eds.), Doing more good than harm: The evaluation of health care interventions. *Annals of the New York Academy of Sciences* (Vol. 703, pp. 125–133). New York: New York Academy of Sciences.

Pielke, R. A., Jr., & Byerly, R., Jr. (1998, February). Beyond basic and applied. *Physics Today,* 42–46.

Pool, R. (1994). *Eve's rib: The biological roots of sex differences.* New York: Crown Publishers.

Price, D. J. D. (1963). *Little science, big science.* New York: Columbia University Press.

Robey, R. R. (1998). A meta-analysis of clinical outcomes in the treatment of aphasia. *Journal of Speech, Language, and Hearing Research, 40,* 172–187.

Robey, R. R., & Dalebout, S. D. (1998). A tutorial on conducting meta-analyses of clinical outcomes research. *Journal of Speech, Language, and Hearing Research, 40,* 1227–1241.

Sigma Xi. (1987). *A new agenda for science.* New Haven, CT: Author.

Turner, J. A., Deyo, R. A., Loeser, J. D., Von Korff, M., & Fordyce, W. E. (1994). The importance of placebo effects in pain treatment and research. *Journal of the American Medical Association, 271,* 1609–1614.

Zerhouni, E. A. (2005). U.S. biomedical research: basic, translational, and clinical sciences. *Journal of the American Medical Association, 294,* 1352–1358.

APPENDIX 27–1

Guidelines for Written Review

SOURCE: THE FOLLOWING INFORMATION IS FROM THE NATIONAL INSTITUTES OF HEALTH GUIDE
(VOL. 26, NO. 22, JUNE 27, 1997).

The goals of NIH-supported research are to advance our understanding of biological systems, improve the control of disease, and enhance health. In your written review, you should comment on the following aspects of the application in order to judge the likelihood that the proposed research will have a substantial impact on the pursuit of these goals.

(1) **Significance.** Does this study address an important problem? If the aims of the application are achieved, how will scientific knowledge be advanced? What will be the effect of these studies on the concepts or methods that drive this field?

(2) **Approach.** Are the conceptual framework, design, methods, and analyses adequately developed, well integrated, and appropriate to the aims of the project? Does the applicant acknowledge potential problem areas and consider alternative tactics?

(3) **Innovation.** Does the project employ novel concepts, approaches, or methods? Are the aims original and innovative? Does the project challenge existing paradigms or develop new methodologies or technologies?

(4) **Investigator.** Is the investigator appropriately trained and well suited to carry out this work? Is the work proposed appropriate to the experience level of the principal investigator and other researchers (if any)?

(5) **Environment.** Does the scientific environment in which the work will be done contribute to the probability of success? Do the proposed experiments take advantage of unique features of the scientific environment or employ useful collaborative arrangements? Is there evidence of institutional support?

28

Applying Evidence to Clinical Practice

LEE ANN C. GOLPER, PHD
KAREN E. BROWN, PHD

SCOPE OF CHAPTER

Audiologists and speech-language pathologists are increasingly being asked to justify their procedures and practices by evidence-based methods. Looking to research evidence and using decision tools that are a part of evidence-based practices can help answer basic clinical questions: Is my diagnosis correct? Is this test needed? What is the expected outcome, or prognosis, with and without treatment? Is this particular intervention likely to improve my client's condition? Could this intervention cause harm? What is the cost-benefit of an assessment or treatment protocol?

Evidence-based practice is based on the premise that the answers to these questions lie with "the integration of the best research evidence with clinical expertise and patient values" (Sackett, Straus, Richardson, & Haynes, 2000, p. 1). These authors define *best research evidence* as coming from clinically relevant research examining the precision and accuracy of diagnostic tests and the efficacy of treatment and its application to everyday practices. That evidence is to be considered in the context of the clinician's own expertise and the client's expressed wishes and values.

In this chapter we will consider some of the terminology, concepts, practices, and methodologies that are a part of evidence-based practices. We will look at how we can examine research and draw recommendations from systematic reviews (SRs); how research is ranked, or classified; how the predictive validity of assessment methods and diagnostic tests might be evaluated; and what these analyses mean to clinical practice. The goal of this chapter is to convince the reader that all clinicians have the tools at hand to evaluate the strength of the evidence available to guide their clinical decisions.

RANKING RESEARCH AND RECOMMENDATIONS

When we talk about the "best" evidence, we are referring to applying specific criteria to determine the credibility of a research study or a group of studies under review. It is important that our diagnostic and treatment decisions be guided by the least biased sources. Systematic reviews and rankings of the evidence are key features of evidence-based practices. There are several different general approaches to ranking evidence. Some provide fine-tuned distinctions and criteria within levels (e.g., the Oxford Centre for Evidence-Based Medicine Levels of Evidence, n.d.), while others might group different types of studies into a single category if they appear to have equivalent risks for bias. Rating systems for the strength of the recommendations are typically graded in some manner. For example, Grade A recommendations are supported by one or more randomized controlled trials; Grade B recommendations are supported by one or more well-designed retrospective, prospective, or outcome study(ies); Grade C recommendations are supported by case series reports of outcome studies without a control or comparison group; and Grade D recommendations are supported by expert opinion without explicit appraisal (Centre for Evidence-Based Medicine, 1999). Other reviewers apply descriptive systems with recommendations designated as based on experimental (highest ranked), observational, or authoritative (lowest ranked) evidence (Beukelman, 2001).

Evidence-ranking systems are applied in systematic reviews; examples include the approach used by the Quality Standards Subcommittee of the American Academy of Neurology (Miller et al., 1999):

- Class I. Evidence provided by one or more well-designed, randomized controlled trial(s) (RCTs).

- Class II. Evidence provided by one or more well-designed, observational clinical study(ies) with concurrent controls (such as single case controlled or cohort-controlled studies).

- Class III. Evidence provided by expert opinion, case series, case reports, and studies with historical controls.

The ASHA Research and Scientific Affairs Committee (RSAC) (2004) presented an adaptation of a rating scale used in the Scottish Intercollegiate Guideline Network (SIGN), provided in Table 28–1.

Such rankings of evidence and classifications of recommendations allow for a systematic assessment of the strength of the evidence in support of a given approach to treatment or a specific procedure—the higher the ranking, the more credible the evidence.

T A B L E 28–1 Levels of Evidence for Studies of Efficacy

Level	Description
Evidence is ranked according to quality and credibility from highest/most credible to lowest/least credible.	
Ia	Well-designed meta-analysis of > 1 RCT
Ib	Well-designed randomized control study
IIa	Well-designed controlled study without randomization
IIb	Well-designed quasi-experimental study
III	Well-designed nonexperimental studies (i.e., correlational and case studies)
IV	Expert committee report, consensus conference, clinical experience or respected authorities

SOURCE: ASHA Research and Scientific Affairs Committee, 2004. Adapted from the Scottish Intercollegiate Guideline Network. Available at http://www.sign.ac.uk

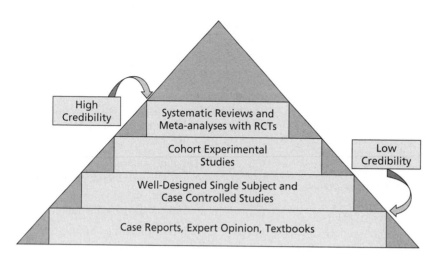

F I G U R E 28–1 Ranking Sources of Evidence

Within these ratings, *meta-analyses* (discussed in detail later in this chapter) that include at least one RCT and/or a systematic review (SR) that includes at least one RCT are viewed as highly credible, while committee recommendations, expert opinions, or other sources not explicitly supported by research (such as in textbooks) are the least credible. That does not imply that less-credible sources are bogus, only that the evidence available has not been tested with the level of scrutiny of higher-ranked evidence. When considering the evidence, one goes to the "best available," most highly ranked, evidence. When Level I or II evidence is not available to answer a clinical question, we move to the next level of evidence for guidance, appreciating that uncertainty increases as a function of an increased potential for bias (Figure 28–1).

Research and Scientific Affairs Committee (RSAC) Report

When considering evidence rankings and evidence reviews, the ASHA RSAC report (ASHA, 2004) identified five themes:

1. **Independent confirmation and converging evidence:** Systematic reviews of evidence are encouraged and supported by a number of organizations. The purpose behind these reviews is to look for converging evidence from multiple, credible studies. At times these systemic reviews reveal conflicting findings in the literature; thus, the reviewers may be more persuaded by the higher-ranked evidence or may advise caution in interpreting the evidence.

2. **Experimental control:** Systematic reviews include a close examination of the controls imposed and design of the study. The RSAC report points out that evidence from quasi-experimental studies ranks lower than controlled studies, only because controls and random assignment ought to reduce experimenter bias.

3. **Avoidance of subjectivity and bias:** Any steps taken to reduce subjectivity and bias will increase a study's credibility. For example, the extent to which both the participant and the experimenter are "blinded" to the therapy would enhance the credibility of the results. The extent to which the outcome measurements are taken by someone other than the investigator would also presumably reduce bias. The investigators should explain what happened to any participants who did not complete the study as there should be an "intention to treat" all participants.

4. **Effect size and confidence intervals:** Another prominent theme in EBP is the expectation that studies specify the magnitude of differences and provide data to indicate that there was sufficient statistical power to detect a clinically important effect in the sample (e.g., the *effect size* should be reported). Several standardized metrics are now routinely applied to calculate effect size (Robey, 2004; Wilkinson & APA Task Force on Statistical Inference, 1999). Investigators should also report the *Confidence Interval* (CI) that is associated with a given effect. Statistical significance does not provide evidence of the strength of an observed association (Riegelman, 2000). The underlying assumption in any statistical sampling is that there is potential for a sampling error—that is, that the findings occurred by chance rather than by design. The CI is the range within which the investigator predicts "with confidence" that a given value is the true value for the trait being studied. The CI is the estimated difference range or variation around the "true" value. A narrow CI provides stronger evidence than a wide CI. For this reason, studies with more subjects are likely to be ranked higher than studies with smaller samples. In EBP it is common for reviewers to look for a CI of 95 percent (Riegelman, 2000).

5. **Relevance and feasibility:** Finally, the RSAC report suggests EBP looks for the applicability, relevance, and feasibility of the research. Can this treatment or test be applied to the real world?

Meta-analysis

Meta-analysis is a statistical method for combining data from two or more published studies in a somewhat similar to conducting multisite studies (Riegelman, 2000). Meta-analysis is usually intended to examine the effect of a given procedure or area of treatment by applying statistical methods to combine the results from a group of studies examining the same or similar questions and hypotheses. Meta-analyses can only be performed when the data in the reference studies have been presented in sufficient detail. Meta-analysis presents a number of limitations and confounding variables.

For example, there may be bias or methodologic flaws in the reference studies; also, since positive findings are more likely to be published than negative findings, the problem of a selection bias is always a consideration with meta-analyses. The analysis itself is not unlike the type of analysis required in any clinical investigation: estimating effect size, testing the statistical significance, adjusting for confounding variables, and looking for homogeneities (Riegelman, 2000; Sackett et al., 2000). Robey's (1998) meta-analysis of the efficacy of aphasia treatment provides an excellent step-by-step illustration of its application to clinical questions.

Conducting Systematic Reviews

Several organizations and groups support and conduct ongoing systematic reviews of research evidence across many professional enterprises, including law, medicine, rehabilitation, and education, and information in this area is expanding rapidly. There has been a high degree of interest in evidence reviews in audiology and speech-language pathology to support clinical decisions. For example, in 1997 the Academy of Neurologic Communication Disorders and Sciences (ANCDS) identified the need for a systematic analysis of the research evidence related to neurogenic communication disorders and has an ongoing project aimed at a systematic review across neurogenic communication disorders and treatment procedures (Golper et al., 2001).

Reviews such as these require considerable time and effort to complete. The introduction to the ANCDS project provides a model for conducting systematic searches and reviews, which includes: forming the review committee, defining the questions, identifying the references, establishing criteria for classifying and ranking the evidence, conducting the searches, preparing the evidence table(s), identifying the strength of the recommendations for procedures or therapies based on the best evidence, and publishing evidence-based practice guidelines in clinical articles (Yorkston et al., 2001). ASHA has a 3-year Focused Initiative aimed at educating its members about EBP and emphasizing EBP in research to improve the availability of systematic reviews and research-guided clinical practices. Access to current information related to EBP is available on the ASHA Web site, including links to articles about evidence-based guidelines (ASHA, 2004). Kuster (n.d.) also has prepared and shared an "efficacy" Web site to help students and clinicians access information related to treatment studies in speech-language pathology and audiology. Her review references cross the gamut of outcomes research, including general child language disorders, literacy, autism, augmentative and alternative communication, aphasia, dysphagia, motor speech disorders, traumatic brain injury, phonological disorders, stuttering, and voice disorders.

Along with sites providing specific access to research evidence in audiology and speech-language pathology, the Agency for Healthcare Research and Quality (AHRQ) (n.d.), Cochran Collaboration (2005), and the Scottish Intercollegiate Guideline Network (n.d.) are excellent resources. The National Guideline Clearinghouse (n.d.) provides direct links to reviews to health services research and summary statements (as well as research in other areas such as law and education). The AHRQ also provides funding opportunities (n.d.) for EBP projects.

CONDUCTING PHASED RESEARCH

As Kent states in Chapter 27 of this text, one of the of the problems with conducting systematic reviews of research evidence is that the pool of published research literature in any given area does not necessarily accumulate in a logical, systematic way, and widespread application of a given therapy can proceed before the efficacy has been examined. An exciting finding may be reported on the evening news immediately after the preliminary results are presented at a professional meeting or released by the public relations service in the investigator's university. Often these are premature findings that

have not undergone controlled investigation. These headline-making claims will be followed by a caveat from the principal investigator who, if interviewed, might say something like, "Although the findings are encouraging, further research is required to verify and understand the clinical significance."

Robey and Schultz (1998) help us to frame and conceptualize a logical plan for experimentation, one that progresses from discovery to real-world application. These concepts and terminology were proposed nearly 30 years ago by the Office of Technology Assessment (OTA, 1978). We will include this model in our discussion of EBP for two purposes: (1) when conducting systematic reviews of research evidence, it may be useful to consider where a given investigation fits within the ideal schema for systematic investigation, from discovery to application; and (2) readers will encounter the terms *outcomes, efficacy,* and *effectiveness* used interchangeably in the research literature, when in fact these terms refer to different types and phases of investigation.

Outcomes, Efficacy, and Effectiveness

An *outcome* merely designates an observed consequence, usually an observation made at one point in time compared to an observation made later. An outcome does not index efficacy or effectiveness (Wertz & Irwin, 2001). Clinicians are constantly engaged in collecting "outcomes." If an individual clinician conducts outcome ratings and submits the data in the prescribed manner, outcome data can be pooled, as with the National Outcomes Measurement System (NOMS), an ASHA-sponsored program. This project requires systematic collection of pre- and post-treatment data, including the use of functional rating scale measures, to evaluate treatment outcomes across communication disorders by a number of variables (e.g., service delivery setting, diagnosis type, number of visits). In individual cases, the clinician's own clinical data are key factors in treatment decisions and provide the justification for the need for therapy. As empirical evidence, however, clinician-gathered treatment data would be viewed as potentially biased and would probably not be considered equivalent to even the weakest evidence, "consensus opinion."

Outcome data are sometimes gathered to make comparisons between facilities, such as morbidity and mortality data comparisons between hospitals. Or outcome data may be examined within a payer type (e.g., Medicare) for benchmarking or fiscal adjustment purposes, or to look to see if particular provider professionals or facilities have better or worse outcomes than their peers. Since data are required to be submitted electronically to third party payers, comparisons of outcomes can be made from large data pools within these organizations.

Collecting and comparing outcome data are problematic. Cornett (1998) points out that outcome measures in health service delivery are not statistically meaningful, not comparable across institutions, and not adjusted for severity or risk. Outcome measures may have no direct link to a provider action, may be difficult to collect due to technological restraints, are expensive to collect, and are easily manipulated. Nonetheless, treatment outcome information is increasingly important in service delivery, and the clinician's own data may be the best available and only evidence upon which to justify treatment recommendations. Individual outcome data can also be used to examine if assessment methods, particularly screening assessments, are under- or overselecting individuals with certain conditions, by applying EBP methods for making calculations of sensitivity, specificity, and likelihood ratios, which we will discuss later. To better appreciate the universe of outcome measurement as applied to our discipline, the reader is directed to Frattali (1998); however, the important caution to make here is that an outcome, whether it is derived from observing an individual client or a pool of thousands of clients, does not tell us much about either the efficacy or effectiveness of a given procedure. Let's consider why the Office of Technology Assessment (1978) and Robey and Schultz (1998) advise care in the use of the terms *efficacy* and *effectiveness:*

Efficacy: The probability of benefit to individuals in a defined population from a procedure applied for a given disorder in *ideal* conditions (OTA, 1978).

Effectiveness: The probability of benefit of a given procedure in the general population of individuals with a given disorder under *average* conditions (Robey & Schultz, 1998).

Ideally, effectiveness studies would be conducted after efficacy has been demonstrated. Unfortunately, the distinctions between outcomes, efficacy, and effectiveness are not always appreciated nor consistently applied in the literature; consequently, claims regarding efficacy are made from studies that lack the required controls, particularly in early literature looking at the efficacy of various treatments in single subject experiments or small group studies. As Robey and Schultz (1998) observe,

> . . . efficacy is a property of a treatment delivered to a population and inference to a population requires a group experiment . . . and, as single-subject experiments do not provide inference to a population . . . they do not and cannot index efficacy. (p. 805)

Looking at the Robey and Schultz (1998) model for progressive phases of research helps us to appreciate the qualitative differences among studies and also helps to underscore a point made by Dollaghan (2004). In her discussion of the myths and realities of evidence-based practices, she reminds us:

> The EBP orientation disavows the longstanding belief that all basic science findings are relevant to clinical practice. The goals, designs, and methods of studies aimed at providing strong answers to questions about clinical practice are in some respects quite different from those of studies aimed at understanding basic mechanisms of disease. In the EBP framework, evidence from studies of basic mechanisms plays a similar role to evidence derived from personal

experience or the opinions of authorities; all of those sources can provide fruitful "leads," but these must be followed up in subsequent studies explicitly designed to address questions about clinical practice. (p. 4)

Phase I: Discovery In this phase of research, hypotheses are initially developed and refined. A new treatment is introduced and tested with a small number of cases, typically patients who have not been adequately treated by other methods. A hypothesis based on a theory, or perhaps an incidental observation, is tested on a small sample without a control group, to see if the treatment might be fruitful. In this phase of research, the experimenter is asking, "Is this therapy *active*? Does this help?"

Let's look at Botox therapy for an illustrative example: Dolly, Black, Williams, and Melling (1984) published a report in *Nature* on the effect of botulinum neurotoxin on motor nerve terminals, producing paralysis without loss of sensation. Shortly afterward, clinical applications of this therapy with various dystonias were explored by researchers and botulinum toxin (Botox) was found to have therapeutic effects for segmental dystonias of the face and neck. It seemed reasonable, therefore, to predict that Botox might have a therapeutic benefit in treating a focal dystonia of the laryngeal musculature in patients with spasmodic dysphonia (SD). Once the drug was approved for clinical investigations in the late 1980s, patients were recruited to determine if a small injection of Botox into the vocal folds could effectively reduce SD without inordinate risk to the patient. Pre- and post-treatment outcome measures were taken and case reports were published (Miller, Woodson, & Jankovic, 1987; Friedman, Brybauskas, Toriumi, & Applebaum, 1987). At that point randomized controlled trials had not been conducted (efficacy studies), nor had there been any subsequent or large-scale examination of the application in real clinical practice (effectiveness studies). Clinicians did not know yet what the efficacy or effectiveness of Botox for SD was. We knew only that Botox therapy was "active." That is, it could be demonstrated to be a treatment that resulted in a desired outcome surpassing what might be expected from other therapies, such as behavioral voice therapy and surgery, and the risks and complications were minimal. Studies examining variables to determine ideal candidacy for Botox (e.g., age, gender, duration of the disorder, associated medical problems, smokers versus nonsmokers, abductor versus adductor types of SD, severe versus mild disorders) had not been conducted. Studies of the best injection sites, injection methods, dosages, or the optimal assessment and follow-up protocols did not appear until the mid-1990s (Inagi, Ford, Bless, & Heisey, 1996; Langeveld, Drost, & Baatenburg de Jong, 1998; Meleca, Hogikyan, & Bastian, 1997). If we look at a recently completed systematic review of research in the use of Botox for SD completed by Duffy and colleagues (2003), it would appear that there is currently strong, converging evidence to support the effectiveness of Botox with certain SD candidates, but the development of much of this body of evidence lagged behind the routine use of Botox in clinical practice. This is a pattern commonly seen in many medical, surgical, and behavioral therapies.

In should be noted that since its introduction, Botox has undergone testing in a number of Phase I and Phase II type studies, in addition to clinical trials for several conditions. Currently, a variety of therapeutic uses are being studied in National Institutes of Health Randomized Controlled Trials clinical investigations, with studies ranging from treatment of drooling in amyotrophic lateral sclerosis (ALS) to idiopathic toe walking in children. Information on these types of studies is available online at PubMed, a service sponsored by the National Library of Medicine and the National Institutes of Health (see Resources at the end of this chapter.

Phase II: Refinement of the Methods The investigator continues the experimentation begun in Phase I by refining the methods, establishing the participant selection criteria, determining the variables that need to be controlled, establishing the assessment protocol, and laying out a plan for the conditions required to test the efficacy of the treatment. Phase I and II are preliminary steps needed prior to initiating large group clinical trials.

Phase III: Efficacy Research In this clinical trial phase of research, studies are conducted with rigid experimental controls applied according to the ideal conditions defined in Phase II. In Phase III, the experimenter applies criteria to the subject selection, recruits robust numbers of subjects who are randomly assigned to groups, and both participants and investigators are blinded to the treatment (i.e., neither the participants or investigators is aware of who did or did not receive the treatment under investigation). Treatment versus no treatment designs or a comparison of two treatments design may be also applied, if more appropriate. Robey and Schultz (1998) point out that during this phase, new discoveries may be made and there may be refinement of methods; however, all research activities today must be highly scrutinized and governed by Institutional Review Boards (IRBs). IRB review and approval is required with any change in a research protocol, however tantalizing, to ensure the Health Insurance and Portability and Accountability Act (HIPAA) protections are maintained. All clinical investigators are required to follow strict guidelines enforced by their IRBs regarding the protection of human subjects. These guidelines were delineated in the *Belmont Report* from the National Commission for the Protection of Human Subjects of Biomedical and Behavioral Research (1976). This statement addresses basic ethical principles and guidelines to assist researchers in resolving ethical problems that may arise in the conduct of research with human subjects.

Phase IV: Effectiveness Research In this phase treatment procedures found to be efficacious in Phase III are tested in subpopulations in real-life clinical practice to determine their effectiveness. Effectiveness research tests the therapeutic applications in less ideal, average, and noncontrolled conditions. In this phase variations in participant compliance, clinician training, and amount (dosage),

duration, frequency, and timing of the treatment can be evaluated.

Phase V: Application Research The final step in the analysis involves exploration of the efficiency and relevance of treatment by considering client satisfaction, cost-effectiveness of the treatment, cost utility (quality of life outcome) and cost-benefit.

EVALUATING DIAGNOSTIC AND SCREENING PROCEDURES

Clinicians use a variety of tests to help them make assessment and management decisions for their clients. Testing can be time consuming and expensive, and it is important to conduct the minimum amount of testing necessary to arrive at an accurate diagnosis. Most diagnostic tests that are quick and easy to administer (checklists, screening tests) may not be completely accurate. They are typically used to determine if further evaluation with a more sophisticated instrument is needed. Since additional testing can be costly and difficult to access, clinicians should know how much confidence to have in the results of a preliminary or screening test. In some cases, it may not be possible to conduct further testing or to refer the client for more comprehensive assessment. This makes it all the more important for clinicians to understand the strengths and weaknesses of the tests they administer.

Specificity and Sensitivity

The practice of using the results of one test to determine the need for further evaluation with another test, or a battery of tests, is common in the field of medicine, where there is great concern about the costs of ordering multiple tests of dubious or redundant diagnostic value. For example, a person with a family history of diabetes and positive test results on a blood glucose screening is likely to be referred for a glucose tolerance test and careful evaluation of clinical symptoms to rule in or rule out diabetes

(Pagana & Pagana, 2002). Within the practices of speech-language pathology and audiology are many instances in which the results of a screening test prompt the clinician to pursue further testing. A school-age child's poor performance on a hearing screening may result in a referral to an audiologist for a comprehensive hearing evaluation. A bedside screening for dysphagia that suggests the presence of aspiration may be followed by a modified barium swallow study to confirm or rule out aspiration. A child who performs poorly on an articulation screening may be scheduled for comprehensive speech and language testing to determine if the child will qualify for school-based speech pathology services. In such cases, clinicians must interpret the results of the screening test and decide if the evidence supports the need for further testing to ensure an accurate diagnosis.

Decisions based on test results should take into account the statistical probability that the results are wrong. Clinicians need to know how likely it is that a test will fail to identify an individual with a specific disorder, or, conversely, that the test will incorrectly indicate that an individual has the disorder when, in fact, it is not present. Determining the *sensitivity* and *specificity* of a diagnostic finding is one of the tools available in EBP to evaluate the diagnostic accuracy of a test, what Riegelman (2000) referred to as "testing a test" (p. vii). Using fairly simple 2×2 table calculations, sensitivity measures how well a test identifies individuals who have the target disorder, and specificity measures how well a test identifies individuals who do not have the target disorder. Both provide uniquely important information, and both are reported as the percentage of correct results.

To evaluate the specificity and sensitivity of a particular measure, we need to have an independent "gold standard" test for comparison. A gold standard is a test or some measure that has been found to be consistently close to 100 percent accurate for diagnosing the target condition. This standard is used as the reference for determining the accuracy of screening test results. To calculate sensitivity and specificity, a screening test is given to a group of

Sensitivity = The percentage of true positives: (number of True Positives)/(number of True Positives + number of False Negatives), or the proportion of affected individuals caught by screening

Specificity = The percentage of true negatives: (number of True Negatives)/(number of True Negatives + number of False Positives), or the proportion of unaffected individuals who pass screening

F I G U R E 28–2 Calculating Specificity and Sensitivity

individuals, and the same individuals are given the gold standard, or reference test. The results of the screening test are then compared to the results of the gold standard test. Sensitivity is the percentage of positive screening test results that correctly identify individuals who have the target condition, as verified by the reference test. Specificity is the percentage of negative screening test results that correctly identify individuals who do not have the target condition, as verified by the reference test. Figure 28–2 shows the calculations for specificity and sensitivity.

The results of the screening test and the reference test are entered into a 2×2 contingency table (see Figure 28–3). Test results that are positive for both the screening test and the reference test are referred to as *true positive* results. The number of true positive results is entered into quadrant a on the table. When the screening test result is negative for a disorder that was positively identified by the gold standard test, the screening test result is known as a *false negative* result. The number of false negative results is entered into quadrant c on the table. Test results that are negative for both the screening test and the reference test are known as *true negative* results, and that number is entered into quadrant d. Finally, if the target condition is absent, as confirmed by the gold standard test, but the screening test results are positive, the results are referred to as *false positives*. The number of false positives is entered into quadrant b.

The formula for sensitivity is $a/(a + c)$. A screening test with "high" sensitivity produces a large proportion of true positives. The formula for specificity

		Gold standard test for language delay	
		Language delay: Present	Language delay: Absent
Screening test for language delay	Positive screening test results	80 True Positives a	b 7 False Positives
	Negative screening test results	c 15 False Negatives	d 81 True Negatives
	Totals	a + c 95	b + d 88

Sensitivity = $a/(a+c)$ = 80/95 = .84 (84%)
Specificity = $d/(b+d)$ = 81/88 = .92 (92%)

F I G U R E 28–3 2 × 2 Contingency Table for Calculating Sensitivity and Specificity of a Hypothetical Screening Test for Developmental Language Delay

is $d/(b+d)$. A screening test with "high" specificity produces a large proportion of true negatives.

For example, consider a group of 183 children who are given a screening test to detect developmental language delay. If 95 of the children actually have developmental language delays, and 80 of those children are correctly identified with positive screening test results (true positives), the sensitivity of the test would be 80/(80 + 15), or 84 percent. If the remaining 88 children have typically developing language, and 81 of those children are correctly identified with negative test results (true negatives), the specificity of the test would be 81/(7 + 81), or 92 percent. The 2 × 2 table and calculations for this example are shown above in Figure 28–3.

Describing how well a test performs in terms of its sensitivity alone or specificity alone is problematic. The sensitivity of a test does not provide the necessary information to tell a true positive result from a false positive result. Sensitivity would be 100 percent for a test that simply identified every person who took it as having the target condition.

Obviously, such a test would produce many false positive results. A clinician reviewing the test results would have no way of telling the true positives from the false positives.

Likewise, specificity does not provide information for distinguishing between negative test results that are true negatives and those that are false negatives. A test would achieve 100 percent specificity by identifying every person who took it as being free of the target condition. This test would misidentify (false negative results) all individuals who had the disorder. Such a test would be useless for identifying individuals who had the target condition.

Both sensitivity and specificity must be known to evaluate how well the test discriminates between individuals who do and do not have the disorder. Reports of sensitivity and specificity, when considered in isolation, can be misleading. Sensitivity, in particular, can overrepresent the value of a test. For example, consider a method of a hearing screening test for which the sensitivity is reported to be 95 percent. In evaluating this method, the test correctly identified

		Gold standard test results	
		Disorder Present	Disorder Absent
Screening test results	Positive	95 True Positives a	b 75 False Positives
	Negative	c d 5 False Negatives	25 True Negatives
	Totals	a + c = 100	b + d = 100

Sensitivity = $a/(a+c)$ = 95/100 = .95 (95%)
Specificity = $d/(b+d)$ = 25/100 = .25 (25%)

F I G U R E 28–4 Example of a Hearing Screening Procedure with Excellent Sensitivity and Poor Specificity

95 percent of the test takers who actually had significant hearing loss. Without knowing the specificity of the test, 95 percent sensitivity sounds good. Now consider what happens if the specificity for that test is reported to be only 25 percent. Look at quadrants *a* and *b* in Figure 28–4. Of the 200 individuals who were given the test, 100 of whom actually had notable hearing loss and 100 of whom who had normal hearing, there were 75 false positive screening test results. A total of 170 individuals had positive

screening test results, and almost half (75/170) of those results were wrong. If a clinician administered that test and a client produced a positive test result, the clinician would have little to go on in deciding if the result was a true positive or a false positive.

The same type of example can be used to demonstrate the problems that would arise from using a test that had excellent specificity and poor sensitivity. Figure 28–5 shows what would be found with a screening procedure with 98 percent

		Gold standard test results	
		Disorder Present	Disorder Absent
Screening test results	Positive	30 True Positives a	b 2 False Positives
	Negative	c d 70 False Negatives	98 True Negatives
	Totals	a + c = 100	b + d = 100

Sensitivity = $a/(a+c)$ = 30/100 = .30 (30%)
Specificity = $d/(b+d)$ = 98/100 = .98 (98%)

F I G U R E 28–5 Example of a Hearing Screening Test with Excellent Specificity and Poor Sensitivity

specificity and 30 percent sensitivity. The test correctly ruled out the hearing loss in all but two of the individuals who had normal hearing; however, the 70 false negative results show that this test failed to identify the hearing loss in most of the individuals who had actually had the condition.

The closer both the sensitivity and specificity values are to 100 percent, the more predictive information they provide about the presence or absence of the target disorder. Sackett and colleagues (2000) state that high sensitivity is most useful for ruling out the disorder in individuals with negative test results, and they suggest applying the mnemonic *SnNout* (Sensitivity Negative, rule out) to such findings. They also propose that high specificity is most useful for ruling in the disorder in individuals with positive test results. They suggest that *SpPin* (Specificity Positive, rule in) is an appropriate mnemonic for these findings. This is the converse for how most clinicians typically think about sensitivity and specificity.

To understand how to use SnNout and SpPin, look again at Figure 28–4. The high sensitivity of this test, 95 percent, is of little use because it would not help a clinician distinguish between true positive and false positive test results. But notice that the negative screening test results are primarily true negatives. Since most of the individuals who had the disorder (as verified by the gold standard test) produced true positive screening test results, there were very few false negative results. Although positive screening test results would not be diagnostically meaningful, a clinician could feel confident that an individual with a negative screening test result did not have the disorder. When sensitivity is high and the test result is negative, the condition may be ruled out (SnNout).

Figure 28–5 illustrates how SpPin can be applied. The high specificity of this test (98%) indicates that most individuals who did not have the disorder produced negative screening test results. Of the 100 individuals who were free of the disorder, only two had positive test results. Therefore, a clinician whose client had a positive result on the screening test would feel confident that additional testing or management strategies were appropriate

for that individual. When specificity is high and the test result is positive, the condition may be ruled in (SpPin).

When test makers create a screening test for a specific disorder, they must consider the consequences of erroneous results. Tests with high sensitivity and low specificity err on the side of overidentifying cases of the disorder. This can result in referrals for unneeded additional testing or unneeded treatment. Tests with low sensitivity and high specificity err on the side of missing the condition and in favor of correctly ruling out individuals who are disorder free. This could mean that some individuals who would benefit from further evaluation and treatment are missed. The choice of whether to use a test that tends to overidentify or underidentify cases of the disorder must balance the risks and expense of failing to detect the condition relative to the risks and expense of subjecting the individual to unneeded testing and treatment.

In choosing a test, the clinician must consider the consequences of failing to identify the condition as well as the consequences of misdiagnosing a condition that is not present. Where possible outcomes are serious, the clinician may choose to be overly cautious. A clinician working in an acute care hospital setting may choose a bedside screening test for dysphagia that has high sensitivity, but low specificity, for the presence of aspiration. Referrals for instrumental swallow evaluation, such as a Modified Barium Swallow (MBS) or Fiberoptic Endoscopic Evaluation of Swallowing (FEES), can be expensive and require specialized equipment. Nevertheless, the risks associated, and cost-benefit ratio, with misidentifying an aspirator as a nonaspirator usually outweigh the risks associated with performing an instrumental test on a person who does not aspirate. On the other hand, a school-based clinician may choose an articulation screening test for preschoolers that has greater specificity compared to sensitivity. Missing the chance to provide early intervention for a child with speech deficits is not desirable, but neither is it life threatening. In addition, overidentifying articulation problems at the preschool level can produce serious problems related to caseload levels and availability of funding.

Likelihood Ratios

Sensitivity and specificity are the most basic and the most frequently reported test evaluation statistics, but they have some inherent limitations that are addressed by other statistics. The 2 × 2 contingency table is used to calculate a number of other statistics that are useful for test evaluations, including *likelihood ratios*, *predictive values*, and *posttest probability*. These metrics take into consideration the demonstrated accuracy of the screening instrument and the prevalence of the target condition within a particular population. Sackett and colleagues (2000) refer to the "old-fashioned concepts of sensitivity and specificity and the new-fangled and more powerful ideas around likelihood ratios" (p. 72). They suggest that clinicians become familiar with the more advanced assessment tools. An excellent discussion of the expanded role of sensitivity and specificity to aid in clinical decision making is presented by Riegelman's (2000, 2005) *Studying a Study and Testing a Test*.

Calculating Likelihood Ratios Likelihood ratios (LRs) are easy to calculate if the accompanying manual describing test development reports the sensitivity and specificity (see Figure 28–6). Likelihood ratios for positive tests (LR+) compare the proportion of true positive screening test results to the proportion of false positive screening test results. As discussed previously, one problem with sensitivity is that it does not provide any information about the

relationship between true positive results and false positive results. For the example shown in Figure 28–3, the proportion of true positive results (sensitivity) was 84 percent (80/95), and the proportion of false positive results (1 − specificity) was 8 percent (1 − .92). The formula for the likelihood ratio for positive tests is *sensitivity ÷ (1−specificity)*, or the proportion of true positive results divided by the proportion of false positive results, 84%/8% = 10.5. This means that a positive test result was 10.5 times more likely to have been produced by a person with the condition than a person who was free of the condition. The greater the LR+, the higher the likelihood that a positive test result is a true positive.

Likelihood ratios for negative tests (LR−) compare the proportion of false negative screening test results to the proportion of true negative results. This statistic shows how likely it is that a negative test result is a false negative. In other words, how likely is it that a negative test result is wrong and that the person who produced it actually has the target condition? The lower the LR−, the better. A low LR− means that there is little chance that a negative test result will be produced by a person who has the target condition. For the example shown in Figure 28–3, the proportion of false negative results (1 ÷ sensitivity) was 16% (1 − .84), and the proportion of true negatives was 92% (81/88). The formula for the likelihood ratio for negative tests is (1−*sensitivity*) ÷ *specificity*, or the proportion of false negative results divided by the proportion of true negative results, 16/92 = 0.174. A negative test result was much less likely to have been produced by a person with the target condition than to have been produced by a person without the condition. Since equal likelihood is represented by a LR of 1.0, a LR− of 0.174 indicates that there is little likelihood that a negative test response would be wrong.

How can an understanding of sensitivity, specificity, and likelihood ratios help clinicians make the best use of a screening test? Here is an example. Suppose that a new screening test has been developed for the early detection of autism in children. A clinician administers the screening test to a

---

Likelihood Ratio (LR) for a Positive Test =

$$\frac{\text{Probability of a true positive (sensitivity)}}{\text{Probability of a false positive (100\% − specificity)}}$$

Likelihood Ratio (LR) for a False Test =

$$\frac{\text{Probability of a false negative (100\% − sensitivity)}}{\text{Probability of a true negative (specificity)}}$$

F I G U R E 28–6 Calculating Likelihood Ratios

		Gold standard test for autism	
		Autism Present	Autism Absent
Screening test for early detection of autism	Positive	263 (60%) True Positives a	b 51 (7%) False Positives
	Negative	173 (40%) c False Negatives	d 633 (93%) True Negatives
	Totals	a + c = 436	b + d = 684

N = 436 + 684 = 1120

Sensitivity 263/436 = 60%   false positives = 51/684 = 7%
Specificity 633/684 = 93%   false negatives =173/436 = 40%

LR + = 60/7 = 8.6
LR − = 40/93 = .43

F I G U R E 28–7 Hypothetical Screening Test for Early Detection of Autism

child, and the result is positive. Based on the positive result, should the clinician rule in autism and conclude that the child is a candidate for further evaluation and/or intervention? The literature that accompanies the test states that it was administered to 1,120 children, and the resulting sensitivity was moderate, 60 percent, and specificity was high, 93 percent. The results are shown in Figure 28–7. The clinician sees that the test failed to identify 40 percent of autistic children, but it correctly ruled out autism in almost all children who did not have the condition. The SpPin mnemonic can be applied here to rule in autism because specificity is high.

When discussing the result of the test with the parents, or making a referral for further evaluation, the clinician would like to have a more precise way of describing the child's performance. This is where the likelihood ratio can help. How likely is it that the positive result is correct? The likelihood ratio for a positive test result is 8.6 (60 percent/7 percent). Therefore, the clinician can say that the positive result indicates that the child is about eight and a half times more likely to be autistic than a child whose test result was negative.

What if the same test were administered to a child and the result was negative? The clinician would know that the test is likely to miss 40 percent of children who have the condition. Also, the likelihood ratio for a negative test is an unimpressive 0.43 (40%/93%). Is there enough information to rule out autism? This is where clinical judgment plays a critical role. The screening test alone is not strong enough to engender confidence that a negative test result is accurate. This is a situation in which the long-term effects of failure to identify the condition are usually worse than subjecting a child who is free of the condition to more extensive testing. The clinician's personal assessment of the child, based on medical history, observation, and other measures, must be used to decide if further evaluation is needed.

Positive Predictive Values Positive predictives (PVs) indicate the probability a disorder is present or absent, which has important implications for screening tests. The predictive value for a positive finding, or positive predictive value, refers to the percentage of individuals who actually have a disorder after having a positive test or screen for that condition. Conversely, the predictive value for a negative finding, or negative predictive value, refers to the percentage of individuals who did not have the disorder after a negative test or screen for that condition. Riegleman (2005) points out the importance of considering the effect of pretest probability on a predictive value—that is, the predictive value of a given test or screen will be dramatically different between groups that have different probabilities of having the disease. Some tests may be useful for screening in populations with a high probability of a given disorder (such as screening for memory problems in a population of individuals with traumatic brain injury) but useless in the general, healthy population where the suspicion of having a disorder is low.

SUMMARY

Clinicians are pressured to demonstrate the efficacy and effectiveness of their treatment methods. Access to available systematic reviews across several topics is as easy as typing in a Web site. Dollaghan (2004) described these searches as good "high yield" sources for busy clinicians. Unfortunately, in these reviews, like other areas of health service delivery, audiologists and speech-language pathologists do not yet have a deep pool of Level I or Level II research evidence to guide them in every clinical decision. Thus, clinicians must look to the best available evidence, which frequently will be Phase I or Phase II types of studies, or Level III studies, such as case reports and/or consensus or expert opinions. Those sorts of evidence are not as highly ranked as investigations using random assignment to group or other controls (RCTs), so recommendations to guide clinical decision are made with caution. Randomized controlled trials are referenced as the "gold standard" for evidence; however, such studies are not explicitly designed to answer real world clinical questions in audiology and speech-language pathology, and it is difficult to construct RCTs with a complete "blinding" of patients and clinicians (Dollaghan, 2004). It is the responsibility of the clinician to make informed decisions that take into account the best evidence available coupled with their own clinical experience and the unique treatment conditions and attributes of an individual client.

CRITICAL THINKING

1. Under the current Medicare regulations for skilled nursing facilities and rehabilitation facilities, the costs of off-site diagnostic studies (hearing tests, modified barium swallow evaluations) for clients receiving care in the facilities are borne by the facility. Consequently, the medical director in an inpatient rehabilitation facility has decided to reduce orders for outpatient evaluations, including videofluoroscopic swallow studies that require transportation and costly evaluation in another facility. The medical director has recommended implementing an in-house bedside dysphagia screening program as first-line assessment to guide feeding and swallowing management with dysphagic patients. The medical director has announced a goal of reducing the number of orders for outside radiologic studies by 50 percent and has asked you, the SLP member of the care team, to design a "best practices" protocol for the new bedside dysphagia screening program. How might you use EBP tools and methodologies to help determine the best practices for appropriately diagnosing dysphagia? Are there any studies or evidence-based guidelines currently available related to evaluation or management of dysphagia that might be brought into the discussion? Apply what you know about determining specificity and sensitivity of a screening test to determine best

practices. Is there evidence available in the research literature or in your own clinical records to guide you in assessing the cost-benefit of misdiagnosis of aspiration risk?

2. What does the current evidence tell us about the usefulness of newborn hearing screening?

3. What are some of the issues or difficulties faced when designing a randomized, double-blind controlled study in audiology and speech-language pathology? Can you think of ways to circumvent those difficulties?

4. Based on the evidence at hand, do we know if *not treating* an aphasic person is harmful?

5. How would misidentifying a child as having a mild hearing loss be problematic?

6. Locate a current journal in communication sciences and disorders, and select and review a research article. Describe the following: type of study (single case research design, case report, treatment/no treatment design, comparison of treatments design, other); number of participants; variables controlled (e.g., age, gender, handedness, health status, medications); and random or nonrandom assignment to groups. Where might this study fit in the Robey and Schultz (1998) phases of research? Is this an efficacy or effectiveness study? Was the effect size reported? Can you rank the evidence in the article using the rankings provided in Table 28–1?

REFERENCES

Agency for Healthcare Research and Quality (AHRQ). (n.d.). Available at http://www.ahrq.gov

American Speech-Language-Hearing Association. (2004). *Evidence-based practice in communication disorders: An introduction.* Available at http://www.asha.org/

Beukelman, D. (2001). State of the science report, 2001. *Rehabilitation Research Center in Communication Enhancement.* Durham, NC: Duke University.

Centre for Evidence-Based Medicine. (1999). *Levels of evidence and grades of recommendation.* Available at http://www.cebm.net/levels_of_evidence.asp

Cochrane Collaboration. (2005). *Cochrane data base of systematic reviews.* Available at http://www.cochrane.org

Cornett, B. S. (1998). Outcomes measure in health care settings. In C. Frattali (Ed.), *Measuring outcomes in speech-language pathology* (pp. 453–476). New York: Thieme.

Dollaghan, C. (2004, April 13). Evidence-based practice: Myths and realities. *The ASHA Leader, 12,* 4–5.

Dolly, J. O., Black, J., Williams, R. S., & Melling, J. (1984). Acceptors for botulinum neurotoxin reside on motor nerve terminals and mediate its internalization. *Nature, 307,* 457–460.

Duffy, J. R., Yorkston, K. M., Beukleman, D., Golper, L. A., Miller, R., Spencer, K., Strand, E., & Sullivan,

M. (2003). *Medical interventions for spasmodic dysphonia and some related conditions: A systematic review.* (ANCDs Technical Report No. 2). Available at http://ancds.org/

Frattali, C. M. (Ed.) (1998). *Measuring outcomes in speech-language pathology.* New York: Thieme.

Friedman, M., Grybauskas, V., Toriumi, D. M., & Applebaum, E. L. (1987). Treatment of spastic dysphonia without nerve section. *Ann Otol Rhinol Larygol, 96,* 590–596.

Golper, L., Wertz, R. T., Frattali, C. M., Yorkston, K. M., Myers, P., Katz, R., Beeson, P., Kennedy M. R. T., Bayles, K., & Wambaugh, J., (2001). Evidence-based practice guidelines for the management of communication disorders in neurologically impaired individuals: An introduction. Available at http://www.ancds.org

Inagi, K., Ford, C. N., Bless, D. M., & Heisey, D. (1996) Analysis of features affecting botulinum toxin results in spasmodic dysphonia. *Jour. Voice, 10,* 306–313.

Kuster, J. (n.d.). Efficacy information on the Internet in speech-language pathology and audiology. Available at http://www.mnsu.edu/comdis/efficacy/efficacy.html

Langeveld, T. P. M., Drost, H. A., Battenburg de Jong, R. J. (1998). Unilateral versus bilateral botulinum toxin injections in adductor spasmodic dysphonia. *Ann Otol Rhinol Laryngol, 107, 280.*

Meleca, R. J., Hogikyan, N. D., Bastian, R. W. (1997). A comparison of methods of botulinum toxin injection for abductor spasmodic dysphonia. *Otolaryngology/Head and Neck Surgery, 117,* 487–492.

Miller, R. G., Rosenberg, J. A., Gelinas, D. F., Mitsumoto, H., Newman, D., Sufit, R., Borasio, G. D., Bradley, W. G., Bromberg, M. B., Brooks, B. R., Sasarskis, E. J., Munsat, T. L., & Oppenheimer, E. A. (1999). Practice parameter: The care of the patient with amyotrophic lateral sclerosis (an evidence-based review). *Neurology, 52,* 1311–1325.

Miller, R. H., Woodson, G. E., & Jankovic, J. (1987). Treatment options for spasmodic dysphonia. *Otolaryngology Clinics of North America, 24,* 1227–1237.

National Commission for the Protection of Human Subjects of Biomedical and Behavioral Research. (1979). *The Belmont report.* Available at http://ohsr.nih.gov/guidelines/belmont.html

National Guideline Clearinghouse. (n.d.). Available at http://www.guideline.gov

National Institutes of Health. (n.d.). Available at http://clinicaltrials.gov

Office of Technology Assessment. (1978). *Assessing the efficacy and safety of medical technologies* (OTA-H-75). Washington, DC: U.S. Government Printing Office.

Oxford Centre for Evidence-Based Medicine Levels of Evidence. (n.d.). Available at http://www.cebm. net/toolbox.asp

Pagana, K. D., & Pagana, T. J. (Eds.). (2002). *Mosby's manual of diagnostic and laboratory tests* (2nd ed.). St. Louis: Mosby.

Riegelman, R. K. (2000). *Studying a study and testing a test* (4th ed.) Philadelphia: Lippincott, Williams & Wilkins.

Riegleman, R. K. (2005). *Studying a study and testing a text* (5th ed.). Philadelphia: Lippincott, Williams & Wilkins.

Robey, R. R. (1998). A meta-analysis of clinical outcomes in the treatment of aphasia. *Journal of Speech, Language, and Hearing Research*, 41, 172–187.

Robey, R. R., & Schultz, M. C. (1998). A model of conducting clinical-outcome research: An adaptation of the standard protocol for use in aphasiology (review). *Aphasiology, 12,* 787–810.

Robey, R. R. (2004). Reporting point and interval estimates of effect-size for planned contrasts: fixed within effect analyses of variance. *Journal of Fluency Disorders, 29,* 307–341.

Sackett, D. L., Straus, S. E., Richardson, W. S., & Haynes, R. B. (2000). *Evidence based medicine: How to practice and teach EBM* (2nd ed.). New York: Churchill Livingstone.

Scottish Intercollegiate Guideline Network. (n.d.). Available at http://www.sign.ac.uk

Wertz, R. T., & Irwin, W. (2001). Darley and the efficacy of language rehabilitation in aphasia. *Aphasiology*, *15,* 231–247.

Wilkinson, L., & American Psychological Association Task Force on Statistical Inference. (1999). Statistical methods in psychology journals: Guidelines and explanations. *American Psychologist, 54,* 594–604.

Yorkston, K. M., Spencer, K., Duffy, J., Beukelman, D., Golper. L. A., Miller, R., Strand, E., & Sullivan, M. (2001). Evidence based practice guidelines: An application to the field of speech-language pathology. *Journal of Medical Speech-Language Pathology, 4,* 243–256.

RESOURCES

Academy of Neurologic Communication Disorders and Sciences (n.d.). Available at http://www.ancds.org

National Guideline Clearinghouse
Public resource for evidence-based clinical practice guidelines
Web site: http://www.guidelline.gov

National Library of Medicine
National Institute of Health
PubMed
Web site: http://www.pubmed.gov

Index